Pain Control in Obstetrics

PAIN CONTROL IN OBSTETRICS

Ezzat Abouleish, M.D., M.B., Ch.B., D.A., D.M., M.D. (Anesth.)
Associate Professor of Clinical Anesthesiology
University of Pittsburgh School of Medicine;
Director of Obstetric Anesthesia
Magee-Womens Hospital
Pittsburgh, Pennsylvania

With Seven Contributors

J. B. Lippincott Company
Philadelphia · Toronto

ISBN 0-397-50376-8

Library of Congress Catalog Card Number 77-13971

Printed in the United States of America

1 3 5 6 4 2

Library of Congress Cataloging in Publication Data

Abouleish, Ezzat.
    Pain control in obstetrics.

    Bibliography: p.
    Includes index.
    1. Anesthesia in obstetrics. 2. Analgesia.
I. Title. [DNLM: 1. Anesthesia, Obstetrical.
W0450 A155p]
RG732.A26   617'.9682   77-13971
ISBN 0-397-50376-8

To my wife, Atiya, whose quiet love, proper understanding, and exceptional talents made this work possible

Contributors

Steve N. Caritis, M.D.
Assistant Professor of Obstetrics, Gynecology and Pediatrics
University of Pittsburgh School of Medicine;
Active Staff, Magee-Womens Hospital
Pittsburgh, Pennsylvania

Sofronio B. de la Vega, M.D.
Assistant Professor of Clinical Anesthesiology
University of Pittsburgh School of Medicine;
Staff Anesthesiologist, Magee-Womens Hospital
Pittsburgh, Pennsylvania

Daniel Edelstone, M.D.
Research Fellow, Cardiovascular Research Institute
University of California San Francisco Medical Center
San Francisco, California

Ray McKenzie, M.B., Ch.B. (N.Z.), M.D., F.F.A.R.C.S. (Eng.)
Associate Professor of Clinical Anesthesiology
University of Pittsburgh School of Medicine;
Associate Professor, University of Pittsburgh School of Dentistry;
Director of Anesthesia, Magee-Womens Hospital
Pittsburgh, Pennsylvania

Eberhard Mueller-Heubach, M.D.
Assistant Professor of Obstetrics, Gynecology and Pediatrics
University of Pittsburgh School of Medicine;
Active Staff, Magee-Womens Hospital
Pittsburgh, Pennsylvania

William Oh, M.D.
Professor of Pediatrics and Obstetrics
Section of Reproductive and Developmental Medicine
Brown University Program in Medicine;
Pediatrician-in-Chief
Women and Infants Hospital of Rhode Island
Providence, Rhode Island

Robert Bryan Roberts, M.D., F.F.A.R.C.S. (Eng.)
Professor and Chairman, Department of Anesthesiology; and
Professor of Pharmacology
Wright State University School of Medicine,
Dayton, Ohio

Foreword

In the past two decades, anesthesia for obstetrics has achieved the distinction of a scientific and professional subspeciality. This achievement has come about largely as a result of relatively few individuals devoting their full-time clinical, teaching and research efforts to this field. Dr. Abouleish is one of these dedicated pioneers and this excellent text embodies much of his vast experience, wealth of information and his devotion to obstetric anesthesia.

From a teaching point of view, the volume is beautifully organized. The anatomic, physiologic, pharmacologic and psychologic bases for the safe practice of obstetric anesthesia are first presented in an easy-to-read, step-by-step fashion. With this background, the anesthetic care of the woman in labor and her newborn is described in a clear, concise and authoritative style. Based on many years' experience and sound physiologic principles, the author describes how he personally administers anesthesia and explains the basis for these decisions. The generous use of illustrations greatly enhances the teaching value of the text. Highlights of this monograph are the excellent chapters on Aspiration and Am-

niotic Fluid Embolism, subjects that have long been of special interest to Dr. Abouleish.

The author has oriented this presentation to the practitioner and student of anesthesia. At the same time, comprehensive coverage by his collaborators will make this volume appeal to obstetricians, pediatricians, nurses and, indeed, all persons involved in the care of the parturient and neonate. Skillful application of the information in this volume will help one provide optimal care for the mother and her newborn.

The author is to be complimented for making available a monograph that deals with all aspects of obstetric anesthesia so clearly, succinctly and conclusively. This is an important contribution to the scientific literature and will serve as a valuable source of knowledge in this field for a long time.

FRANK MOYA, M.D.
Chairman, Department of Anesthesiology and Director, Pain Center, Mount Sinai Medical Center; Clinical Professor, Department of Anesthesiology University of Miami School of Medicine Miami, Florida

Preface

After 23 years of clinical experience in anesthesiology, both in the United States and abroad, I realized the need for a book on obstetrical anesthesia that would be comprehensive yet easy to read, a book that would recognize the importance of the basic sciences and at the same time be both comprehensive and specific in regard to clinical procedures. This book is the final result of that realization. Its theme relates quite simply to the physician's duty to relieve the parturient's pain and to support her both physically and mentally in the course of the delivery.

Most of Part One is concerned with fundamental considerations in anatomy, physiology, psychology and pharmacology. Since local anesthetic drugs and the vertebral blocks, namely epidural, caudal, and spinal, are widely used in any modern obstetrical unit, the pharmacology of these drugs and the effects of these blocks are described in detail. Two chapters are devoted to certain special causes of maternal death which are aspiration pneumonitis, amniotic fluid embolism, and disseminated intravascular coagulopathy. The remainder of the first part deals with evaluation of the fetal condition before and during parturition, and the effects of anesthetic drugs used at term on the fetus and the neonate.

Part Two describes the various techniques available for obstetrical analgesia and anesthesia, including "prepared childbirth," hypnosis, and acupuncture. This section has been complemented by detailed drawings showing each technical step.

Part Three addresses itself to the postpartum period. It includes neonatal resuscitation which may be conducted by anesthesia, obstetric or pediatric personnel, depending on the circumstances and the policy of the given institution. The organization and management of the neonatal intensive care unit is also described in this section. The final chapter deals with postpartum tubal ligation, an increasingly requested operation. It describes the various techniques, including laparoscopic tubal ligation, which causes important physiologic derangements of the respiratory and cardiovascular systems as if it were a sudden full-term pregnancy.

I hope that my colleagues in the fields of anesthesia, obstetrics, and neonatology will benefit from and enjoy reading the subject as presented, and I hope, too, that as members of one team we may increasingly be aware of our interdependency as we care for the woman in labor and for the newborn.

Ezzat Abouleish, M.D.

Acknowledgments

To the eminent contributors, my colleagues and friends, Dr. Steve N. Caritis, Dr. Sofronio B. de la Vega, Dr. Daniel Edelstone, Dr. Ray McKenzie, Dr. Eberhard Mueller-Heubach, Dr. William Oh and Dr. Robert Bryan Roberts, I extend my sincere gratitude for the precious time they generously gave in preparing their invaluable chapters. I should also like to express my appreciation to Mr. Ronald Filer of the Medical Art Division, University of Pittsburgh School of Medicine, for the illustrations in Chapter 1, and to Mr. Ronald Kubiak, Director of the Medical Art Division at Magee-Womens Hospital, for his patience in bringing to life my raw sketches. Without the help and reassurance of my wife, Atiya, who perused and edited every line in the thirteen chapters I wrote, I should not have been able to finish this book. My appreciation is extended to Mrs. Beverly Tamburino for her always painstaking secretarial work. I should like to thank also my colleagues, Dr. Murray Blair and Dr. Ronald Gilcher, for their help in revising the manuscripts of Chapters 4 and 9. I wish to express my acknowledgment to the authors and editors of medical journals and books for their permission to reproduce illustrations and tables from their published scientific data. Special thanks must be expressed to *Pennsylvania Medicine* for allowing me to quote extensively in Chapters 3 and 8 from our articles of Volumes 77 (1974) and 78 (1975). My cordial thanks are extended to Mr. Stuart Freeman, Senior Editor, Medical Books, of the J. B. Lippincott Company, for his high recommendation, invaluable support, continuous encouragement and constructive criticism.

EZZAT ABOULEISH, M.D.

Contents

Part Three: The Postpartum Period

Part One

Basis of Obstetric Anesthesia and Analgesia

1

Pain of Parturition: Anatomy, Physiology, and Psychology

Ezzat Abouleish, M.D.

Before scientific and intelligent management of the obstetric patient can be accomplished, the following basic sciences should be well comprehended: (1) the *anatomy* of the nerve supply of the uterus and the birth canal; (2) the *physiology* of pain; and (3) the *psychologic effects* of pain on the parturient as well as the effects of her psychologic background on reaction to pain.

ANATOMY AND OBSTETRIC PAIN

THE NERVE SUPPLY OF THE UTERUS

The nerves supplying the uterus are autonomic in origin and are divided into sympathetic and parasympathetic (Fig. 1-1). The *sympathetic* nerve supply of the uterus is divided into efferent and afferent nerve supplies. The *efferent* sympathetic nerve supply to the uterus arises from T5 to L2 inclusive.[8] Its exact role during labor is not clear. It is related to the uterine motor activity as well as to the regulation of the blood supply. According to Greene,[21] the motor nerve fibers supplying the uterus probably arise from T5 to T10 segments. The exact localization of the motor fibers of the uterus in humans has yet to be determined.

There are three sites for neurons in the sympathetic efferent system (Fig. 1-2A).

The first sympathetic neuron lies in the hypothalamus. The second lies in the lateral gray mass of the spinal cord. From there, the preganglionic nerve fibers leave the spinal cord with the anterior nerve root, continue in the mixed nerve, and then come out as the white rami communicantes of the paravertebral sympathetic ganglia where they usually relay in the third neuron. The postganglionic fibers arise from the third neuron and continue within the sympathetic chain, ultimately reaching the uterus. Sometimes these third neurons are located outside the paravertebral sympathetic chain close to the uterus.

The *afferent* sympathetic nerve supply of the uterus, adnexa, and ligaments reaches T10 to L1 segments inclusive.[2,3,13,20,53,54] The pain sensation of labor, which is one type of visceral pain,[24] is carried by means of the afferent sympathetic system. For any painful nerve impulse, three sites of neurons are involved (Fig. 1-2A). The first neuron site for uterine pain lies in the posterior nerve root ganglion. The second neuron site is found in the spinal cord itself in the posterior gray matter. The third neuron site is located in the thalamus. If the anterior nerve root is divided, the efferent sympathetic impulses to the uterus are severed but not the afferent stimuli carrying uterine pain. These pain stimuli

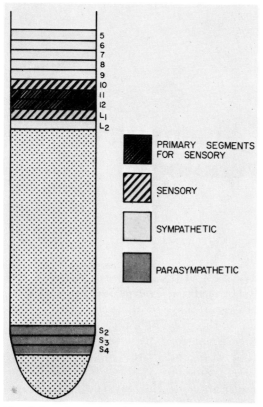

Fig. 1-1. Nerve supply of the uterus (segmental distribution).

are interrupted if the posterior nerve roots are damaged. However, if a paravertebral block is performed at the sympathetic chain, impulses in both the efferent and afferent sympathetic nerves are blocked.

The *parasympathetic* nerve supply of the uterus arises from S2 to S4. It is carried by the nervi erigentes. Its role in labor is not clear.

PAIN IMPULSES DURING LABOR

Impulses to the Spinal Cord

Pain impulses to the spinal cord during labor are carried by the sympathetic afferent nerve fibers in the body of the uterus, in the cervix, adnexa, and ligaments (Fig. 1-3). These nerve fibers communicate with other autonomic nerves around the cervix and uterus, forming what is called the inferior hypogastric plexus. From this plexus, the fibers continue along the iliac

vessels as the right and left hypogastric nerves. Reaching the bifurcation of the aorta, these nerves communicate with the superior hypogastric plexus. Continuing either by way of the sympathetic chain directly or first by the aortic plexus and then to the sympathetic chain, they proceed to the posterior nerve roots and from there to the spinal cord. Some of the fibers, coming from the ovaries, uterine ligaments, fallopian tubes and the uterus, are carried by the ovarian nerves to the aortic plexus, then laterally to the sympathetic chain, to the posterior nerve roots, and finally to the spinal cord.[20] The final termination of all these nerve fibers is in the posterior nerve root ganglia.

Impulses in the Spinal Cord

From neurons in the posterior root ganglia, the nerve fibers enter the spinal cord to form the tract of Lissauer. They then relay to neurons of the posterior horn of the spinal cord (see Fig. 1-2A).[61] From these neurons, nerve fibers cross into the spinal cord to the other side anterior to the central canal to form part of the lateral spinothalamic tract. If there is dilatation of the central canal, interruption of these nerve fibers carrying sensations of pain and of temperature may occur. Other sensations, such as those that have to do with muscle-joint position and vibration, remain intact because they are carried to the posterior white matter without crossing at the spinal level. Touch sensation is carried by both means and thus is still preserved, although it might be impaired.[14] This is why, in syringomyelia, loss of the sensations of pain and temperature occurs without loss of the sensation of touch or of vibration, or that related to muscle-joint position—so-called dissociated anesthesia.

Details of Pain Nerve Fibers and Neuron Connections in the Spinal Cord. In the posterior root ganglion there are neurons of different sizes (see Fig. 1-2B).[57] The *large neurons* give rise to thickly myelinated nerve fibers (A-fibers), referred to for simplicity as the large fibers. Primarily,

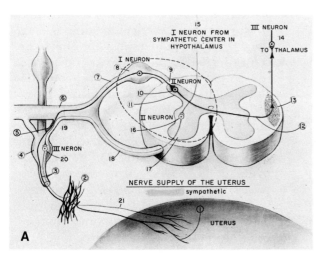

Fig. 1-2. *A.* Nerve supply of the uterus. Pain (sensory or afferent sympathetic: (1) = uterus; (2) = autonomic plexuses; (3) = sympathetic chain; (4) = sympathetic ganglion; (5) = white ramus communicans; (6) = mixed nerve; (7) = posterior nerve root; (8) = posterior root ganglion (location of primary neuron); (9) = tracts of Lissauer; (10) = posterior horn neurons; (11) = posterior horn; (12) = crossing pain fibers; (13) = lateral spinothalamic tract; (14) = tertiary neurons in the thalamus. Efferent sympathetic: (15) = primary neurons in sympathetic center in hypothalamus; (16) = secondary neurons in lateral horn from which arise preganglionic fibers; (17) = anterior horn; (18) = anterior nerve root proceeding to the junction with the mixed nerve (6); (19) = white ramus communicans approaching the sympathetic ganglion (5); (20) = sympathetic ganglion from which arise postganglionic nerve fibers (21) which supply uterus; (21) = postganglionic nerve fibers. *B.* Details of connections of pain fibers and neurons in the spinal cord. (1) = medial bundle; (2) and (3) = lateral bundle; T.L. = tract of Lissauer; H.C. = higher centers; S.G. = substantia gelatinosa; S.P.N. = sympathetic preganglionic neuron; L.S.T.T. = lateral spinothalamic tract; S.M.N. = somatic motor neuron; A.R. = anterior root.

they carry sensations of vibration, proprioception, and, to a certain extent, touch. The *medium neurons* give rise to thinly myelinated nerve fibers (A-delta fibers). The *small neurons* give rise to unmyelinated nerve fibers (C-fibers). The thinly myelinated and unmyelinated nerve fibers carry sensations of pain, temperature, and part of touch. They are referred to for simplicity as the small fibers.

Within the posterior root, the nerve fibers arrange themselves as they approach the spinal cord into a medial and a lateral bundle. The large fibers constitute the medial bundle, while the small fibers form the lateral bundle.

On entering the spinal cord, the fibers of the lateral bundle ascend or descend for a short distance in the tract of Lissauer be-

fore they synapse with posterior horn neurons.

The Spinal Cord Neurons. Brot Rexed,[45] a Swedish anatomist, was the first to observe that the spinal gray matter resembles multilaminated cerebral cortex. Rexed described such lamination in cats,[45-47] and this was confirmed in man by Truex and coworkers.[57,58]

Lamina I caps the surface of the posterior horn and bends around its margin. It contains numerous cells, including the nucleus posteromarginalis.[57] The small nerve fibers probably give connections to these neurons which subsequently influence the neurons of the substantia gelatinosa.

Lamina II (substantia gelatinosa of Rolando) contains numerous small neu-

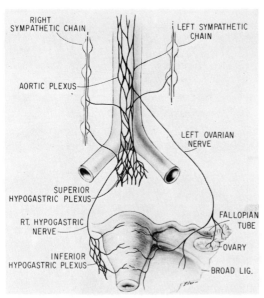

Fig. 1-3. Sympathetic nerve supply of the uterus (pelvic and abdominal distribution). Uterine nerves arise from (1) the upper part of the uterus (upper uterine segment), the contraction of which contributes to pain; (2) the lower part of the uterus (lower uterine segment), the distention of which contributes to labor pain; and (3) the cervix, the dilatation of which contributes to pain. Ovarian nerve supplies the ovary, fallopian tube, broad ligament, round ligament, and the side of the uterus, and communicates with the uterine plexus. Note that both sympathetic efferent and afferent fibers are shown together.

rons with short axons. These neurons of the substantia gelatinosa are connected with each other, with substantia gelatinosa neurons of other spinal segments, and probably with neurons of laminae I and V.

The function of the substantia gelatinosa is not yet well determined. According to Melzack and Wall,[42] the substantia gelatinosa neurons modulate the pain impulses entering the central nervous system. The substantia gelatinosa neurons, by acting on interneurons located in deeper laminae, can control pain impulses leaving those interneurons to other spinal nerve cells. Originally the interneurons were thought to be in lamina IV,[42] but now they are believed to be in lamina V.[32] From interneurons, pain impulses relay in neurons of

laminae VI, VII, and VIII. The latter neurons give rise to the lateral spinothalamic tract nerve fibers that cross anterior to the central canal to the anterolateral part of the spinal cord. The interneurons also send impulses to sympathetic preganglionic neurons in lamina VII. These latter neurons send out preganglionic sympathetic nerve fibers that leave the spinal cord with the anterior nerve root. Sympathetic reflex activity secondary to pain (e.g., vasoconstriction) can therefore occur. However, this is not the only mechanism for these autonomic changes. Central impulses from the hypothalamus also play an important role in the production of these effects. Impulses from interneurons extend also to the *large somatic motor neurons of lamina IX.* The latter neurons send motor impulses to striated muscle fibers through the anterior nerve root. This explains the reflex muscle spasm that accompanies pain. The tissue ischemia produced by the reflex vasospasm and muscle spasm perpetuates the pain cycle (see Fig. 1-12).

Gate Control Theory of Pain. The substantia gelatinosa neuron has an inhibitory effect on the interneuron. Each nerve fiber entering the spinal cord has both a direct and an indirect effect on the interneuron (see Fig. 1-2B). The indirect effect is caused by changing the inhibitory tone of the substantia gelatinosa on the interneuron. The net result depends on the balance between these two effects.

A large fiber, for example, stimulates both substantia gelatinosa and interneuron. Since stimulation of the substantia gelatinosa increases the inhibitory effect on the interneuron, the ultimate result is inhibition of the interneuron (called a *negative feedback* effect). This inhibition will prevent pain impulses from being conveyed to the other deeper nuclei (i.e., the gate for pain is closed). It is important to note that ascending large fibers also lead to central inhibition of pain impulses. On the other hand, impulses carried by a small nerve fiber stimulate the interneuron and inhibit the substantia gelatinosa through a preliminary connection with neurons, probably in lamina I. Inhibition of the substantia gelatinosa relieves its inhibitory effect on the interneuron and in a way increases the interneuron's response to stimulation (a phenomenon called *positive feedback*). In other words, the interneuron becomes more responsive to painful stimuli and the gate for pain is now opened.

It is important to note that the substantia gelatinosa neuron, or this gate system, is constantly under the influence of impulses from higher centers as well. The balance between these various peripheral and central stimuli determines the degree of opening of the gate and consequently the sensation and severity of pain (Fig. 1-4).

This one-gate control theory,[42] the two-gate theory,[40] and the multi-gate theory at different levels of the central nervous system can help one to understand pain, acupuncture, and the action of anesthetics and analgesics.[33] There is still much more to be learned before such subjects can be completely comprehended.

Impulses in the Brain Stem

The sensory pain fibers continue up the spinal cord, as the lateral spinothalamic tract, to reach the brain stem and send numerous impulses to (1) the reticular formation, stimulating the whole central nervous system (Fig. 1-5), and (2) the tegmental tract, which is important because through it impulses ascend to the thalamus and hypothalamus and descend to the spinal cord to inhibit pain. The tegmental tract forms a balance that regulates the number of impulses reaching the brain. With destruction of this tract, the number of impulses and the subsequent reaction to pain become excessive.[23]

In the brain stem, the lateral spinothalamic tract gives off the central gray pathway.

Impulses at the Thalamus

Both the spinothalamic and the central gray pathway tracts end in the ventral posterolateral nucleus of the thalamus; therefore, if one of these tracts is damaged, the thalamus still can receive painful stimuli through the other tract. It is of importance to know that the pain nerve fibers

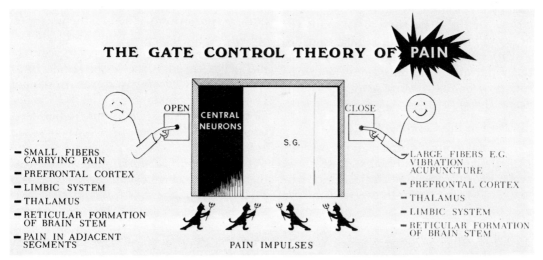

Fig. 1-4. The gate control theory of pain. The substantia gelatinosa of Rolando (S.G.) is constantly under the influence of descending and peripheral sensory inputs. The balance between the various stimuli determines the degree of opening of the gate and consequently the sensation and severity of pain.

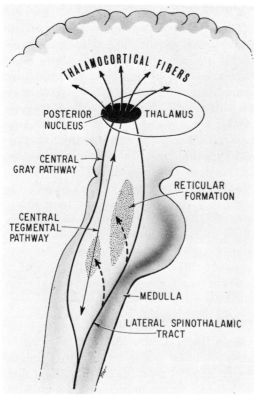

Fig. 1-5.   Pain fibers in the brain stem.

send impulses also to the intralaminar thalamic nuclei. The ventral posterolateral nucleus of the thalamus is important for the sensation of pain with regard to its localization and severity, while the intralaminar nuclei are important for the affective component of pain (e.g., its unpleasantness).

Impulses at the Cerebral Cortex

From the ventral posterolateral nucleus of the thalamus, nerve fibers radiate to the cerebral cortex, forming the thalamocortical fibers which relay into two parts of the cerebral cortex. One is the postcentral gyrus, which is Sensory Area I (Fig. 1-6). The other, which is called Sensory Area II, lies posterior to the inferior part of the postcentral gyrus and above the lateral fissure. If the cerebral cortex is removed, the sensation of pain is felt only crudely; it is not localized and cannot be differentiated with regard to intensity, since the cerebral cortex is important for localization and discrimination of pain. Sensory Area I is mainly for localization of pain, and Sensory Area II is mainly for discrimination of pain.[23] From Sensory Areas I and II there are connections with the prefrontal cortex and the limbic system to regulate the affective component of pain.

THE NERVE SUPPLY OF THE PERINEUM

During the second stage of labor, there is a somatic pain due to stretching and dilatation of the perineum in addition to the visceral pain caused by uterine contraction. The five nerves that supply the perineum and external genital organs are discussed below (Fig. 1-7).

The Pudendal Nerve

The pudendal nerve is the main nerve supplying the perineal structures and external genitalia (Fig. 1-8). It arises from the sacral plexus, S2 to S4,[20] and leaves the pelvis through the greater sciatic foramen to pass behind the junction of the ischial spine with the sacrospinous ligament. Lateral and posterior to it lie first the posterior cutaneous nerve of the thigh and then the sciatic nerve. The pudendal nerve reenters the pelvis through the lesser sciatic foramen. It then accompanies the pudendal vessels in the pudendal canal, which lies along the lateral wall of the ischiorectal fossa.[19] It divides into three branches (see below).

The inferior hemorrhoidal nerve (inferior rectal nerve) usually arises from the pudendal nerve just before the latter enters the pudendal canal. However, sometimes it arises higher up or even separately from the sacral plexus.[20] This independent course may occur in as often as 50 per cent of the cases,[34] and may explain some of the cases of failure of analgesia of the perineum following pudendal nerve block.

Fig. 1-6. Cortical representation of pain.

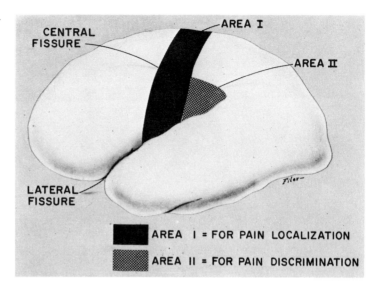

CENTRAL FISSURE

AREA I

AREA II

LATERAL FISSURE

AREA I = FOR PAIN LOCALIZATION

AREA II = FOR PAIN DISCRIMINATION

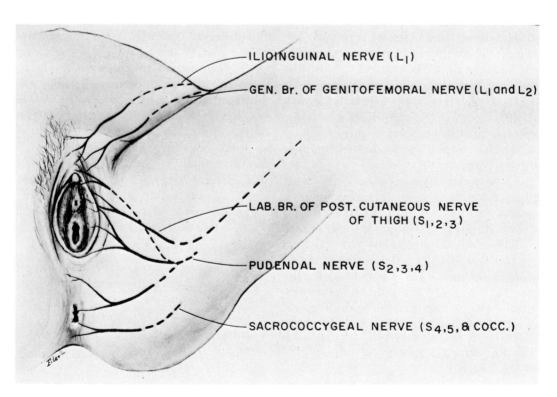

ILIOINGUINAL NERVE (L_1)

GEN. Br. OF GENITOFEMORAL NERVE $(L_1$ and $L_2)$

LAB. BR. OF POST. CUTANEOUS NERVE OF THIGH $(S_{1,2,3})$

PUDENDAL NERVE $(S_{2,3,4})$

SACROCOCCYGEAL NERVE $(S_{4,5,}$ & COCC.)

Fig. 1-7. Nerve supply of the perineum.

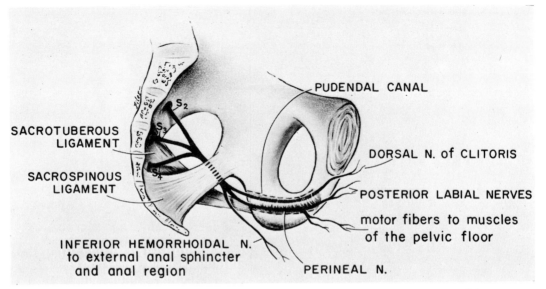

SACROTUBEROUS LIGAMENT

SACROSPINOUS LIGAMENT

INFERIOR HEMORRHOIDAL N. to external anal sphincter and anal region

PUDENDAL CANAL

DORSAL N. of CLITORIS

POSTERIOR LABIAL NERVES

motor fibers to muscles of the pelvic floor

PERINEAL N.

Fig. 1-8. The pudendal nerve and its branches. Note that the inferior hemorrhoidal nerve can arise higher up from the pudendal nerve or separately from the sacral plexus.

For this reason, after depositing the local anesthetic at the expected site of the pudendal nerve behind the sacrospinous ligament, the needle is advanced further, and the local anesthetic is injected to block the inferior hemorrhoidal nerve in case it arises separately. The inferior hemorrhoidal nerve carries motor fibers to the external anal sphincter muscle in addition to sensory nerve fibers to the perineum in the anal region.

The perineal nerve carries motor fibers to the muscles of the pelvic floor as well as sensory fibers to the perineum and the corresponding labia majus and minus.

The dorsal nerve of the clitoris courses forward along the ramus of the ischium and then runs ventrally along the inferior margin of the pubic bone to supply the clitoris and the corresponding corpus cavernosum.

The Posterior Cutaneous Nerve of the Thigh

The posterior cutaneous nerve of the thigh arises from S1 to S3 and leaves the pelvis with the sciatic nerve through the greater sciatic foramen, to be distributed to the posterior aspect of the thigh, knee, and upper part of the leg. It gives rise to the perineal branches, which run medially toward the groove between the thigh and perineum to supply the skin of the labium and the adjacent proximal medial surface of the thigh.[20] After performing a transvaginal block of the pudendal and inferior hemorrhoidal nerves, the needle is advanced for 1 to 2 cm., and the local anesthetic is injected to block the posterior cutaneous nerve of the thigh as well.

The Sacrococcygeal Nerve

The sacrococcygeal nerve (S4, S5 and the coccygeal nerve) supplies the skin behind the anus in the anococcygeal region.

The Ilioinguinal Nerve

The ilioinguinal nerve (L1) accompanies the round ligament in the inguinal canal and ends by supplying the skin of the mons pubis and upper part of the labium majus.

The Genital Branch of the Genitofemoral Nerve

The genital branch of the genitofemoral nerve (L1 and L2) passes through the inguinal canal to take part in the nerve supply of the anterior part of the perineum and the adjacent inguinal region.

In conclusion, although the main nerve supply of the perineum is the pudendal nerve, other nerves are involved. Therefore, to get adequate perineal analgesia for episiotomy, vaginal delivery, and repair, local infiltration of the line of incision, pudendal nerve block, and transvaginal block of the inferior hemorrhoidal nerve and the posterior cutaneous nerve of the thigh, are all required.

PHYSIOLOGY OF OBSTETRIC PAIN

ETIOLOGY

Each organ in the body is made to respond to a specific stimulus in the form of pain. The skin, for example, is a protective surface. Because the skin is constantly exposed to temperature changes, if it is exposed to extreme cold or heat, pain is experienced. However, because the cervix is not usually exposed to changes in temperatures, nature did not make it sensitive to cold or heat, but rather to stretching and dilation. Cutting of the uterus or burning of the cervix is not painful. On the other hand, dilatation of the cervix (e.g., secondary to uterine contractions) can be painful. There are no special receptors for pain in the body of uterus or the cervix, but there are nerve fibers among their tissues.

Factors Involved in the Pain of Uterine Contractions

1. **Stretching of the Cervix.** Strong uterine contractions lead to stretching of the cervix and subsequent pain sensation.

2. **Distention of the Lower Uterine Segment.** Sometimes the cervix does not dilate (e.g., when a patient has had a Shirodkar operation in which the cervix is closed with a suture), but the uterine contractions are still painful because of distention of the lower uterine segment.

3. **Relative Ischemia of the Muscle Fibers and Accumulation of Metabolites.** As the muscle contracts, it consumes more energy and at the same time interferes with its blood supply. The net result is relative ischemia of the muscle fibers and accumulation of metabolites, causing pain.

4. **Traction on the Ligaments.** The uterus is suspended by ligaments, and each time the uterus contracts, it moves forward and pulls on the ligaments. This also can cause pain during labor.

Braxton-Hicks Contractions. During pregnancy, the mother has uterine contractions, called Braxton-Hicks contractions, which are usually not painful. They are physiologic and beneficial because they allow the mixing of blood into the intervillous spaces of the placenta. It is only when uterine contractions reach a certain threshold and the intrauterine pressure reaches a certain level that these contractions are felt as pain. This threshold of intrauterine pressure varies from one patient to another, but usually it is about 25 torr. Contractions during pregnancy are normally below this threshold level.

MECHANISM OF REFERRED PAIN

There are many explanations for the referred-pain mechanism.[37,39] One explanation is that both the uterus and certain somatic structures, such as the lower abdominal wall, share the same neuron pool (Fig. 1-9).[50,55] The impulses from the uterus reach their own neurons as well as those neurons receiving impulses from the abdominal wall. When the stimulus from the uterus is sufficiently strong, these neurons receiving impulses from the abdominal wall are also stimulated. The brain, therefore, interprets the pain as if it were arising in the referred area. The sharing of

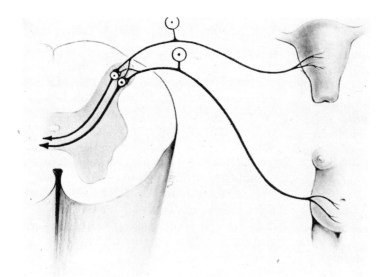

Fig. 1-9. Mechanism of referred pain. Nerve impulses arising from the uterus stimulate the neurons of the abdominal wall as well as those of the uterus.

neurons between the uterus and the area of referred pain can happen at the spinal cord or the thalamus.[23]

The pain of uterine contraction is referred to ligaments, muscles, and skin of the abdominal wall (Fig. 1-10).

The referred pain of uterine contraction is usually distributed in the lower abdomen, on the lateral side of the body from the iliac crest to the greater trochanter (Fig. 1-11A), from the umbilicus downward to the groin (Fig. 1-11B), and in the lower back (Fig. 1-11C). The nerve supply of these areas reflects, therefore, the nerve supply of the uterus.[57] The area around the umbilical region is supplied by T10. Below that region the area is supplied by T11 and T12, where pain is maximum anteriorly. The hypogastric region is supplied by the iliohypogastric nerve which arises from L1. The mons pubis and the region of the labia are supplied by the ilioinguinal nerve (L1) and the genital branch of the genitofemoral nerve (L1 and L2). The area from the iliac crest downward to the greater trochanter of the femur is supplied by the lateral cutaneous branch of the 12th (subcostal) nerve, where maximum pain is felt laterally. Behind that area the skin is supplied by the

lateral branch of the iliohypogastric nerve (L1). Posteriorly, the mother feels pain in the lower back. The areas opposite the 3rd, 4th, and 5th lumbar spines are supplied by the posterior primary rami of T10, T11, and T12, and the area opposite the upper part of the sacrum is supplied by L1. During parturition, pain is referred to these areas.

Anatomically, early in labor, the pain is localized to the areas supplied by segments T11 and T12.[11] As labor progresses, other segments inside the spinal cord are involved, most probably by radiation (e.g., to segments T10, L1 and L2; see Fig. 1-12).

The parasympathetic uterine nerve supply (the nervi erigentes) and the pudendal nerve arise from S2, S3, and S4, and it is thought that the former is responsible for carrying labor pain which is felt in the back.[15] However, we believe that this is not the case because, on an anatomical basis, the area of referred pain is supplied by the thoracic and L1 segments, as previously described. On a clinical basis, during the first stage of labor, relief of both abdominal and back pain is obtained by a segmental epidural block of T10 to L1. Moreover, during the second stage of labor, a true saddle block where sacral

Fig. 1-10. Somatosensory distribution of a spinal nerve to the structures to which uterine pain is referred.

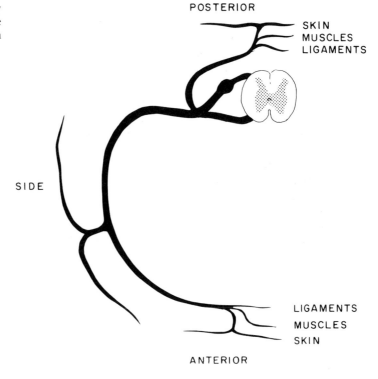

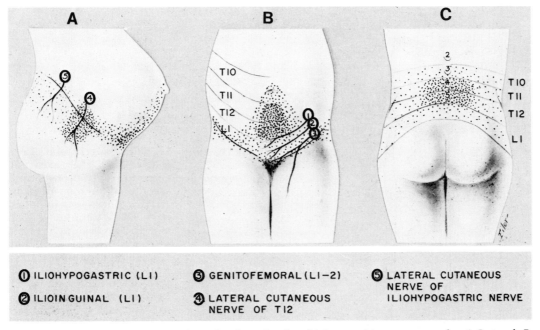

① ILIOHYPOGASTRIC (L1)	③ GENITOFEMORAL (L1-2)	⑤ LATERAL CUTANEOUS NERVE OF ILIOHYPOGASTRIC NERVE
② ILIOINGUINAL (L1)	④ LATERAL CUTANEOUS NERVE OF T12	

Fig. 1-11. The area of distribution of referred pain of labor and its nerve supply: *A.* Lateral. *B.* Anterior. *C.* Posterior; 2, 3, 4, 5 are lumbar spinous processes.

roots only are affected does not relieve the abdominal or the back pain of labor. The use of midforceps in these cases is not welcomed by the patient, and manual removal of the placenta is a painful experience for the mother. In these situations, the sacral segments are blocked, and in spite of this there is inadequacy of analgesia. Furthermore, in nonpregnant females or during early pregnancy, if spinal block is performed for dilatation and curettage and does not reach at least T11, the patient experiences pain during cervical dilatation in spite of the complete blockade of the nervi erigentes arising from the sacral segments.

During the second stage of labor, an added source of pain is the stretching of the perineum by the advancing fetal part. The perineum is supplied mainly by the pudendal nerve, but other nerve roots and structures can add to the pain due to direct pressure by the fetus.

In summary, we believe that the sacral segments are not involved in the referred pain of labor caused by contraction of the uterus or dilatation of the cervix. They are only involved if there is direct pressure by the fetus on adjacent organs and nerves, such as the sciatic nerve, or if there is stretching of somatic structures, such as the sacroiliac joint and perineum.

EFFECTS OF PAIN

Effects at the Segmental Level

Reflex vasoconstriction and reflex spasm of the somatic muscles occur as a result of pain.[6] If these becomes excessive, there will

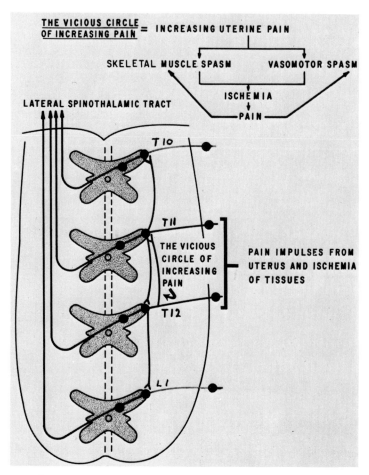

Fig. 1-12. Mechanism of extension of the area of referred pain with increasing severity or duration of pain. As pain increases, impulses from dorsal neurons of T11 and T12 are sent to adjacent segmental neurons (T10 and L1). These impulses ultimately inhibit the neurons of the substantia gelatinosa of Rolando. Consequently, the gate for pain is opened, and this leads to stimulation of interneurons in segments T10 and L1.

be hypoxia of the tissues which will perpetuate pain, and a vicious circle is set up (Fig. 1-12).[5]

Effects at the Suprasegmental Level

Stimulation of the autonomic nervous system occurs as a result of pain.

Cardiovascular System. An increase in the cardiac output results from the pain itself. This increase could amount to 60 per cent of the original level. Tachycardia and arrhythmias can occur. If the pain is prolonged and excessive, not necessarily due to labor but to any other cause, cardiac arrest and death can occur.

Respiration. Rapid, shallow breathing, tachypnea, breath-holding, or hyperventilation can result from painful stimuli. Carbon dioxide can reach a very low level if hyperventilation occurs, especially in unpremedicated patients.[9] Such respiratory alkalosis can be harmful to the fetus. Maternal alkalosis causes fetal hypoxia by producing a shift in the maternal oxygen dissociation curve to the left.[38,44]

Sweating. Profound diaphoresis may occur in both conscious and inadequately anesthetized patients.

Decrease in Uterine Blood Flow. The uterine blood vessels are especially sensitive to the sympathetic tone. Stressful stimuli, such as pain, have been shown to reduce uterine blood flow in ewes.[54a] Such a mechanism, which can be harmful especially to a compromised fetus, can occur in humans if pain is severe. It has also been proven that exogenous administration of catecholamines markedly reduces uterine blood flow by redistribution of cardiac output.[48] Such a mechanism can occur in women during painful labor, due to release of endogenous catecholamines.

Effects at the Higher Centers Level

The affective component of pain depends upon many factors, including previous experiences, physical and psychologic conditions, culture, and religious beliefs.[56] The affective component of pain is a complex reaction controlled by many centers in the brain (Fig. 1-13). Through afferent impulses, these centers gather information about the nature of pain. Depending upon the circumstances of the present condition, past experiences, knowledge of similar situations, and probability of outcome of different response strategies, these centers send impulses to other parts of the central nervous system that conduct the reaction to pain.

PSYCHOLOGY OF OBSTETRIC PAIN

Depending upon the *physical* condition of the patient, pain may be exaggerated, for instance, if the patient is exhausted or has fever. Depending upon the *psychological* condition of the mother, her report of pain may be an expression of fear, a sense of insecurity, a cry for help, a demand for attention, or an attempt to control others.[10] Hospital personnel should exercise care when talking in front of a patient who is in labor because they may frighten her unintentionally.

Expectation, either from suggestion or from previous experiences, plays an important role in the attitude of the patient toward pain. An easy, atraumatic, previous labor is reflected in the relaxed behavior of the patient. On the other hand, if the patient has had a bad experience, she is apprehensive, and this raises her pain reaction. Expectation as a result of suggestion, such as in natural childbirth (better called prepared childbirth), hypnosis, and acupuncture, can control the parturient's attitude toward pain and her report of pain sensation; whether she experiences less pain is another issue. In one study of acupuncture in obstetrics,[1] feeling of pinprick was not less intense in the lower abdomen than in other parts of the body (e.g., the shoulder). In spite of this, 63 per cent of patients reported 66 per cent of pain relief with acupuncture.

Distraction increases the pain threshold, such as in prepared childbirth where the

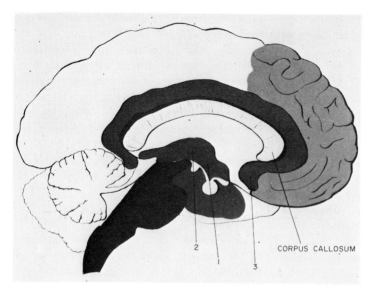

Fig. 1-13. Brain centers controlling the affective component of pain.

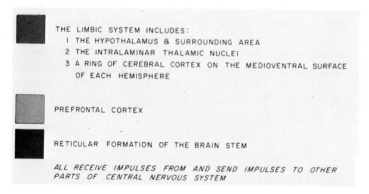

THE LIMBIC SYSTEM INCLUDES:
1 THE HYPOTHALAMUS & SURROUNDING AREA
2 THE INTRALAMINAR THALAMIC NUCLEI
3 A RING OF CEREBRAL CORTEX ON THE MEDIOVENTRAL SURFACE
OF EACH HEMISPHERE

PREFRONTAL CORTEX

RETICULAR FORMATION OF THE BRAIN STEM

ALL RECEIVE IMPULSES FROM AND SEND IMPULSES TO OTHER
PARTS OF CENTRAL NERVOUS SYSTEM

mother concentrates on breathing, in acupuncture where the patient concentrates on needle vibrations, and in hypnosis where the patient concentrates on the hypnotist's voice. Developing *conditioned reflexes* to benefit the mother during childbirth can also increase the pain threshold (e.g., if the mother feels Braxton-Hicks contractions during pregnancy and breathes deeply and slowly, a conditioned reflex is built where such rhythm of breathing is associated with painless contractions). If acupuncture needles are inserted in a suitable patient and vibrated during pregnancy and the patient feels Braxton-Hicks contractions, a similar conditioned reflex can be built. The same applies to hypnosis, substituting the voice of the hypnotist for the acupuncture needles or respiratory exercises.

If mothers-to-be are coached to tolerate pain (without recourse to pain-relieving drugs), they can be highly *motivated* and tend to please their coaches by suppressing and not reporting pain sensation.

On the whole, psychologic methods of analgesia for childbirth, such as prepared childbirth, hypnosis, and acupuncture, have common factors that raise the patient's pain threshold and change her reaction to pain sensation. Such factors include suggestion, motivation, distraction, and conditioned reflex. If these are combined with *education* about the process of childbirth and if the patient is *properly selected*, psychologic methods can be quite beneficial.

Cultural factors are important determinants of reaction to pain, since people of different cultures react differently. In some African tribes, if the wife screams during childbirth, it is considered a sign of illegitimate pregnancy. Therefore, she bites on a stone and suppresses her pain expression. Reaction to pain can be modified by *religious beliefs*. This is of importance in certain parts of the world. Some Mediterranean women are taught to scream during childbirth to keep away evil spirits. Thus some hospitals are provided with sound-proof rooms for their labor.

APPLIED METHODS OF PAIN RELIEF DURING CHILDBIRTH

There are numerous methods of pain relief which vary according to the stage of labor, the condition of the mother, the condition of the fetus, the experience of the anesthesiologist, and the experience of the obstetric team. If an obstetrician is not familiar with a certain anesthetic technique, it is advisable not to force such a new technique on him in an emergency situation. On the other hand, there should be a place for new techniques that can improve relief of pain and anesthetic safety.

In the first stage of labor, pain can be relieved in many ways, such as by paracervical block,[43,49,52,59] paravertebral block,[11] epidural block,[18,31] and spinal block.[17] Block of the higher senses can be produced by psychologic methods, by intramuscular or intravenous analgesics such as meperidine, or by inhalation analgesics such as nitrous oxide, trichlorethylene, methoxyflurane, cyclopropane, ether, or halothane (Fig. 1-14A). These anesthetics, in analgesic concentration, have no harmful effects on mother or fetus.[8] In the early part of the first stage of labor, meperidine and chlorpromazine are usually sufficient. In the second part of the first stage, the preferred method of pain relief varies

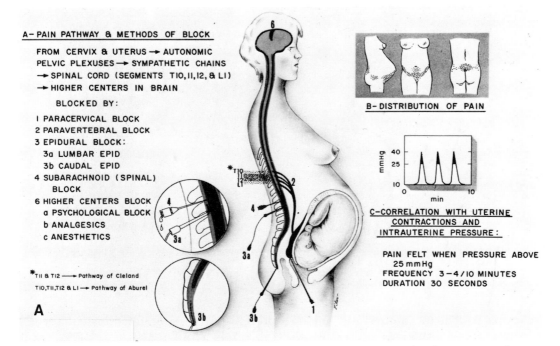

Fig. 1-14. Obstetric anesthesia and analgesia: *A*. First stage. *(Continued on next page.)*

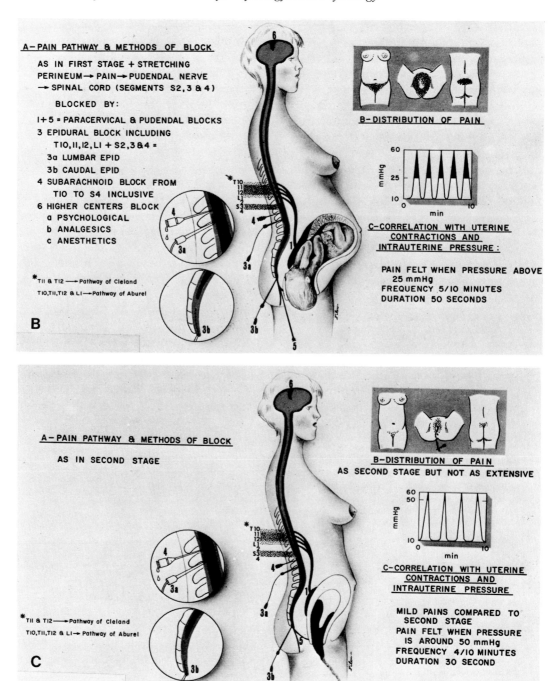

A—PAIN PATHWAY & METHODS OF BLOCK

AS IN FIRST STAGE + STRETCHING
PERINEUM → PAIN → PUDENDAL NERVE
→ SPINAL CORD (SEGMENTS S2,3 & 4)

BLOCKED BY:

1+5 = PARACERVICAL & PUDENDAL BLOCKS
3 EPIDURAL BLOCK INCLUDING
    T10,11,12,L1 + S2,3&4 =
    3a LUMBAR EPID
    3b CAUDAL EPID
4 SUBARACHNOID BLOCK FROM
    T10 TO S4 INCLUSIVE
6 HIGHER CENTERS BLOCK
    a PSYCHOLOGICAL
    b ANALGESICS
    c ANESTHETICS

*T11 & T12 —→ Pathway of Cleland
T10,T11,T12 & L1 —→ Pathway of Aburel

B—DISTRIBUTION OF PAIN

**C—CORRELATION WITH UTERINE
CONTRACTIONS AND
INTRAUTERINE PRESSURE :**

PAIN FELT WHEN PRESSURE ABOVE
    25 mmHg
FREQUENCY 5/10 MINUTES
DURATION 50 SECONDS

B

A—PAIN PATHWAY & METHODS OF BLOCK

AS IN SECOND STAGE

*T11 & T12 —→ Pathway of Cleland
T10,T11,T12 & L1 → Pathway of Aburel

**B—DISTRIBUTION OF PAIN
AS SECOND STAGE BUT NOT AS EXTENSIVE**

**C—CORRELATION WITH UTERINE
CONTRACTIONS AND
INTRAUTERINE PRESSURE**

MILD PAINS COMPARED TO
    SECOND STAGE
PAIN FELT WHEN PRESSURE
    IS AROUND 50 mmHg
FREQUENCY 4/10 MINUTES
DURATION 30 SECOND

C

Fig. 1-14 *(Continued)*. *B*. Second stage. *C*. Third stage.

from one patient to another and among hospitals. Some physicians prefer to administer a paracervical block, while others prefer epidural or caudal analgesia when the cervix is dilated 5 to 7 cm.[25-30] Still others start with epidural and then give a caudal block when the patient reaches the second stage of labor. This is called the double-catheter technique of Cleland.[12]

When the second stage of labor begins, and the mother has had continuous epidural, caudal, or spinal block, these techniques may be continued, provided that the analgesia extends to include the sacral and coccygeal segments (Fig. 1-14B). If the mother has had paracervical block, pudendal nerve block may be administered as well to provide adequate relief of pain.[36] The pudendal nerve can be blocked transvaginally, through the perineum or from the back through the sacral foramina. The most common method of pudendal nerve block is performed transvaginally, injecting the anesthetic drug at the ischial spine behind the sacrospinous ligament. However, pudendal nerve block by itself without paracervical block is inadequate. Pudendal nerve block can relieve pain in the perineum,[4,16,22,34-36,51,60] but not in the lower abdomen or the back, and high or mid-forceps application in such a condition can be quite traumatic to the patient's psyche.

In the third stage of labor, although the uterine contractions are strong, pain is slight. This is because the birth canal is already dilated and stretched, and the passage of the soft placenta is much easier than the passage of the fetal head (Fig. 1-14C). Usually the mother does not require relief of pain during this stage. If she does (e.g., for manual removal of the placenta), the methods of relief for the second stage can be used.

REFERENCES

1. Abouleish, E., and Depp, R.: Acupuncture in obstetrics. Anesth. Analg., *54*:83, 1975.
2. Aburel, E.: Accouchement sans douleurs, l'action de la rachianesthésie sur l'utérus en travail; au chlorhydrate de diéthyléne diamide de l'acide a-butyloxy cinchoniminque. Bull. Soc. Obstet. Gynecol. de Paris, pp 1–2, 1938.
3. ———: L'analgésie dermo-corticale dans les douleurs de l'accouchement. Hommage a la Memoire du Professeur Al Slátineau, Instit. de Arte Grafice, Brawo, JASI, pp. 3–12, 1939.
4. Apgar, V.: Pudendal block. Anesth. Analg., *36*:77, 1957.
5. Bonica, J. J.: The Management of Pain. Philadelphia, Lea & Febiger, 1953.
6. ———: Clinical Application of Diagnostic and therapeutic Nerve Block. Springfield, Ill., Charles C Thomas, 1958.
7. ———: An atlas on mechanisms and pathways of pain in labor. What's New, *217*:16, 1960.
8. ———: Principles and Practice of Obstetric Analgesia and Anesthesia. Ed. 1. Philadelphia, F. A. Davis, 1967.
9. ———: Recent developments in obstetrical anesthesia. Lecture presented to the American Society of Anesthesiologists, 1971.
10. Clark, W. C.: Pain sensitivity and the report of pain: an introduction to sensory decision theory. Anesthesiology, *40*:272, 1974.
11. Cleland, J. G. P.: Paravertebral anesthesia in obstetrics. Surg. Gynecol. Obstet., *57*:51, 1933.
12. ———: Continuous peridural and caudal analgesia in obstetrics. Anesth. Analg., *28*:61, 1949.
13. Crawford, J. S.: Anaesthesia for obstetric emergencies. Br. J. Anaesth., *43*:864, 1971.
14. Davidson, S.: The Principles and Practice of Medicine. Ed. 8. Edinburgh and London, E. & S. Livingstone, 1967.
15. Doughty, A.: Practical considerations in childbirth. *In* Wylie, W. D. and Churchill-Davidson, H. C. (eds.): A practice of Anaesthesia. Ed. 3, chap. 51, pp. 1388-1468. London, Lloyd-Luke, 1972.
16. Dugger, J. H., Kegel, E. E., and Buckley, J. J.: Transvaginal pudendal block. The safe anesthesia in obstetrics. Obstet. Gynecol., 1956.
17. Elam, J. O.: Catheter subarachnoid block for labor and delivery. Anesth. Analg., *49*:1007, 1970.
18. Flowers, C. E., Hellman, L. M., and Hingson, R. A.: Continuous peridural anesthesia and analgesia for labor, delivery and cesarean section. Anesth. Analg., *28*:181, 1949.
19. Grant, B.: Grant's Atlas of Anatomy. Ed. 5. Baltimore, Williams & Wilkins, 1962.
20. Gray, A.: *In* Goss, C. M. (ed.): Anatomy of the Human Body. Ed. 28, chap. 12, pp. 911-1038. Philadelphia, Lea & Febiger, 1967.
21. Greene, N. M.: Physiology of Spinal Anesthesia. Baltimore, Williams & Wilkins, 1969.
22. Greenhill, S. P.: Obstetrics. Ed. 13. Philadelphia, W. B. Saunders, 1965.
23. Guyton, A. C.: Textbook of Medical Physiology. Philadelpia, W. B. Saunders, 1967.
24. Haugen, F. P.: The autonomic neurons system and pain. Anesthesiology, *29*:785, 1968.
25. Hingson, R. A.: Continuous caudal analgesia in obstetrics, surgery and therapeutics. Br. Med. J., *1*:2777, 1949.
26. Hingson, R. A., and Cull, W. A.: Conduction anesthesia and analgesia for obstetrics. Clin. Obstet. Gynecol., *4*:87, 1961.
27. Hingson, R. A., Cull, W. A., and Benzinger, M.: Continuous caudal analgesia in obstetrics. Anesth. Analg., *40*:119, 1961.

28. Hingson, R. A., and Edwards, W. B.: Continuous caudal anesthesia during labor and delivery. Anesth. Analg., *21*:301, 1942.

29. ———: Comprehensive review of continuous analgesia for anesthetists. Anesthesiology, *4*:181, 1943.

30. ———: An analysis of the first ten thousand confinements managed with continuous caudal analgesia with a report of the authors' first one thousand cases. J.A.M.A., *123*:538, 1943.

31. Hingson, R. A., and Southworth, J. L.: Continuous peridural anesthesia. Anesth. Analg., *28*:215, 1944.

32. Kitahata, L., Taub, A., and Kosaka, Y.: Lamina-specific suppression of dorsal-horn unit activity by ketamine hydrochloride. Anesthesiology, *38*:4, 1973.

33. Kitahata, L. M., *et al.*: Lamina-specific suppression of dorsal-horn unit activity by morphine sulfate. Anesthesiology, *41*:39, 1974.

34. Klink. E. W.: Perineal nerve block. An anatomic and clinical study in the female. Obstet. Gynecol., *1*:137, 1953.

35. Kobak, A. J., Evans, E. F., and Johnson, G. R.: Transvaginal pudendal nerve block. Am. J. Obstet. Gynecol., *71*:981, 1956.

36. Kobak, A. J., Sadove, M. S., and Kobak, A. J., Jr.: Childbirth pain relieved by combined paracervical and pudendal nerve blocks. J.A.M.A., *183*:931, 1963.

37. Lennander, K. G.: Observations on the Sensitivity of the Abdominal Cavity. Trans. by A. E. Baker. London, J. Bale, Sons & Danielson, 1903.

38. Levinson, G., Shnider, S. M., de Lorimier, A. A., and Steffenson, J. L.: Effects of maternal hyperventilation on uterine blood flow and fetal oxygenation and acid-base status. Anesthesiology, *40*:340, 1974.

39. Mackenzie, J.: Symptoms and Their Interpretations. Ed. 2. London, Shaw & Sons, 1920.

40. Man, P. L., and Chen, C. H.: Acupuncture "anesthesia"—a new theory and clinical study. Curr. Ther. Res., *14*:390, 1972.

41. Melzack, R., and Casey, K. L.: Sensory, motivational and central control determinants of pain, a new conceptual model. *In* International Symposium on the Skin Senses. Pp. 423–443. Springfield, Ill., Charles C Thomas, 1968.

42. Melzack, R., and Wall, P. D.: Pain mechanisms: a new theory. Science, *150*:971, 1965.

43. Page, E. P., Kamm, M. L., and Chappel, C. C.: Usefulness of paracervical block in obstetrics. Am. J. Obstet. Gynecol., *81*:1094, 1961.

44. Ralston, D. H., Shnider, S. M., and de Lorimier, A. A.: Uterine blood flow and fetal acid-base changes after bicarbonate administration to the pregnant ewe. Anesthesiology, *40*,348, 1974.

45. Rexed, B.: The cyto-architectonic organization of the spinal cord in the cat. J. Comp. Neurol., *96*:415, 1952.

46. ———: A cyto-architectonic atlas of the spinal cord in the cat. J. Comp. Neurol., *100*:297, 1954.

47. ———: Some aspects of the cyto-architectonics and synaptology of the spinal cord. Prog. Brain Res., *11*:58, 1964.

48. Rosenfeld, C. R., Barton, M. D., Meschia, G.: Effects of epinephrine on distribution of blood flow in the pregnant ewe. Am. J. Obstet. Gynecol., *124*:156, 1976.

49. Rosenfeld, S. S.: Paracervical anesthesia for relief of labor pains. Am. J. Obstet. Gynecol., *50*:527, 1945.

50. Ruch, T. C.: Visceral sensations and referred pain. *In* Fulton, J. F. (ed.): A Textbook of Physiology. Ed. 16. Philadelphia, W. B. Saunders, 1947.

51. Sahay, P. A.: Pudendal nerve block. Br. Med. J., *1*:759, 1959.

52. Sandmire, H. F., and Stephen, D. A.: Paracervical block in obstetrics. J.A.M.A., *187*:775, 1945.

53. Shnider, S. M.: Obstetrical Anesthesia. Current Concepts and Practice. Baltimore, Williams & Wilkins, 1970.

54. ———: The use of regional anesthesia in obstetrics. The mother and newborn—recent advances. Gainesville, Ninth Annual Postgraduate Seminar, University of Florida, 1972.

54a. ———: Unpublished data.

55. Sinclair, D. C., Weddell, G., and Feindel, W. H.: Referred pain and associated phenomena. Brain, *71*:184, 1948.

56. Szasz, T. S.: Pain and Pleasure. New York, Basic Books, 1957.

57. Truex, R. C., and Carpenter, M. B.: Human Neuroanatomy. Ed. 6. Baltimore, Williams & Wilkins, 1971.

58. Truex, R. C., and Taylor, M.: Gray matter lamination of the human spinal cord. Anat. Rec., *160*:502, 1968.

59. White, C. A., and Pitkin, R. M.: Paracervical block anesthesia in obstetrics. Postgrad. Med., *33*:585, 1963.

60. Wilds. P. L.: Transvaginal pudendal nerve block. Obstet. Gyncol., *8*:385, 1956.

61. Wrights, S.: Applied Physiology. Ed. 11. London, Oxford University Press, 1967.

2

Changes in Maternal Physiology During Pregnancy, Parturition, and the Puerperium

Daniel Edelstone, M.D.

CHANGES IN BLOOD VOLUME
ANTEPARTUM CHANGES

During pregnancy an increase in the total maternal blood volume occurs as a result of an absolute increase in plasma volume as well as red and white blood cell volumes.[44] The plasma volume begins to increase during the sixth week of gestation and rapidly enlarges during the second and early third trimesters. A more gradual rise is observed during the last several weeks prior to the onset of labor (Fig. 2-1). The fall in maternal plasma volume which has been reported near term[29] represents a supine postural effect. When studies are performed with the patient in the lateral recumbent position, a distinct decrease in plasma volume during late pregnancy is not observed.[44]

The total increase in plasma volume by the end of pregnancy is approximately 1000 to 1500 ml. over prepregnancy values, representing an increase of approximately 40 to 50 per cent.[36] The mechanisms responsible for the increase in plasma volume during pregnancy remain unclear. Alterations in the renin-angiotensin-aldosterone system and in estrogen and progesterone concentrations,

and the effect of the placenta as a functional arteriovenous shunt have all been suggested as etiologic factors.

The volume of red blood cells increases progressively albeit slowly throughout gestation (see Fig. 2-1). On the average, an amount of about 250 to 450 ml. of red blood cells has been added to the maternal circulation at term. There are some indications that an increase in erythropoietin is responsible for the augmentation of red blood cell mass rather than an increase in red blood cell survival.[9]

The disproportionate increase in plasma volume compared to red cell mass results in hemodilution which is most obvious during the second trimester. The phrase "physiologic anemia of pregnancy" has been applied to this phenomenon but is an inaccurate description since anemia refers to a true deficiency of hemoglobin or red blood cells. Blood viscosity is decreased approximately 20 per cent as a consequence of hemodilution. Therefore, resistance to flow and the cardiac force required to circulate the blood are decreased.

The hypervolemia induced by pregnancy serves several functions. It enables the increased circulatory and metabolic

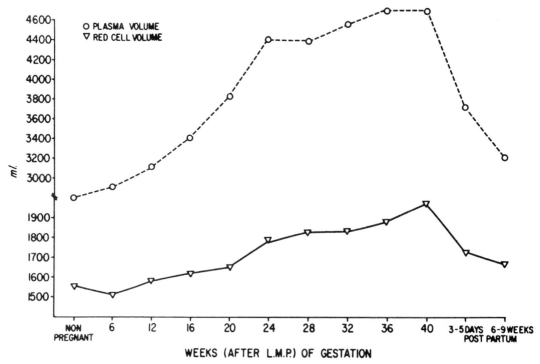

Fig. 2-1.   Plasma and red blood cell volumes during normal pregnancy and the puerperium. (Lund, C. J., and Donovan, J. C.: Blood volume during pregnancy. Am. J. Obstet. Gynecol., *98*:393, 1967)

needs of the uterus and fetoplacental structures to be met. Expansion of the blood volume serves to fill the greatly increased venous reservoir of the uterus and lower extremities during pregnancy, and provides a reserve against the sequestration of blood in the lower extremities. Consequently, protection from systemic hypotension (supine hypotensive syndrome) is afforded when the patient sits or is supine. Additionally, hypervolemia acts as a buffer against the potentially harmful effects of pregnancy-related hemorrhage.

INTRA- AND POSTPARTUM CHANGES

In uncomplicated vaginal deliveries, approximately 500 ml. of whole blood is lost during parturition and the first three hours of the puerperium. In cases of elec-

tive cesarean section, approximately 900 ml. of whole blood is lost. When cesarean hysterectomy is performed, total blood loss increases to approximately 1450 ml. Visual estimates of blood loss at delivery are frequently 50 to 75 per cent below the actual amount of blood lost.[44]

The pattern of response to significant puerperal blood loss differs from the response to blood loss seen in nonpregnant women. Significant blood loss by normal nonpregnant women results primarily in changes of hematocrit rather than blood volume.[44] However, when healthy normal puerperal women lose 20 to 25 per cent of their predelivery blood volume, postpartum blood volume decreases, while hematocrit does not change (Fig. 2-2). Not all women tolerate a large blood loss during parturition. Small women are much less capable of withstanding large puerperal blood loss since the degree of

Fig. 2-2. Blood volume and hematocrit changes following normal vaginal delivery. (Ueland, K., and Hansen, J. M.: Maternal cardiovascular dynamics. III. Labor and delivery under local and caudal analgesia. Am. J. Obstet. Gynecol., *103*:8, 1969)

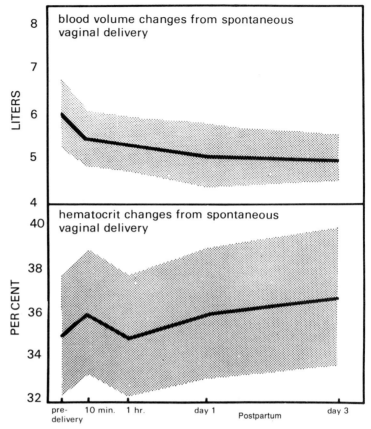

pregnancy-induced hypervolemia is generally related to maternal body size.

The hematocrit at 5 to 7 days postpartum is higher by 1 to 4 per cent than the predelivery value. Plasma volume gradually returns to nonpregnant values over the following 2 to 3 weeks (See Fig. 2-1).[43] Red blood cells that are added to the circulation during pregnancy but not lost at delivery disappear from the vascular space through the process of normal red cell senescence. The decrease in red blood cell volume is associated with a temporary depression of erythropoiesis which is probably due to a suppression of erythropoietin.[9] There is currently no evidence to support increased red cell destruction during the puerperium. By 8 weeks postpartum, all blood volume variables approximate prepregnancy values.

PATHOPHYSIOLOGY

In preeclampsia and eclampsia a reduction in plasma volume below normal pregnancy values is observed somewhat in proportion to the severity of the disease. Intravascular volume may be decreased by as much as 40 per cent, while the volume of red blood cells remains unchanged. The decrease in whole blood volume reduces the reserve against pregnancy-related hemorrhage and may partially explain the clinical observation that eclamptic women are particularly susceptible to intrapartum and puerperal shock. Blood viscosity also is greater in preeclamptic patients, increasing the resistance to flow in the microcirculation and perhaps contributing to the cardiac failure which is associated with two-thirds of eclamptic deaths.[9]

In the toxemias of pregnancy, an elevation of the hemoglobin concentration and hematocrit value occurs subsequent to contraction of the plasma volume. Therefore, an apparently "normal" hemoglobin concentration or hematocrit value in such patients may actually reflect a considerable red blood cell deficit in addition to a severely contracted plasma volume. In the puerperium, hemodilution is expected to occur in association with clinical improvement of the toxemia.

The contracted blood volume in pre-eclampsia is associated with vasoconstriction rather than extracellular volume depletion. Therefore, rapid expansion of the vascular volume does not correct the underlying pathophysiologic state and is contraindicated in the presence of hypertension.[18] Pulmonary edema, salt retention, or peripheral edema may be induced by the injudicious administration of electrolyte solutions or large volumes of fluid.

CHANGES IN CARDIAC FUNCTION

ANTEPARTUM CHANGES

Cardiac output rises 30 to 40 per cent early in gestation, reaching a peak by 20 to 24 weeks.[34] It is maintained at this high level through 32 weeks and thereafter slowly declines. By 38 to 40 weeks, resting cardiac output is approximately 15 per cent above nonpregnant values. Heart rate increases 10 to 15 beats per minute to a maximum at 28 to 32 weeks and remains at that rate until parturition. The initial rise in cardiac output is produced by an increased stroke volume since the change in heart rate occurs much later in pregnancy. As gestation progresses, stroke volume gradually returns to normal nonpregnant values (Fig. 2-3).[57] It appears unlikely that alterations in cardiac output and stroke volume result from fetal nutritional requirements since the timing and magnitude of the increases precede and exceed, respectively, the demands of the fetus.[34]

Resting cardiac output varies considerably, depending on gestational age and the position of the mother at the time of measurement.[30,34,57] The variation in cardiac output reflects alterations in diastolic filling due to changes in venous return from the lower extremities. In the supine position the term-size uterus can partially

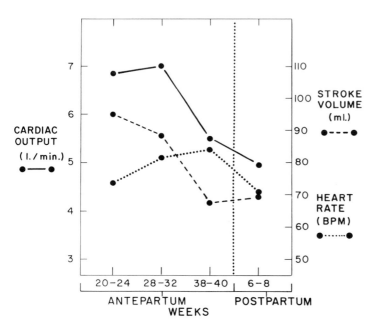

Fig. 2-3. Effect of gestational age and the puerperium on cardiac output, stroke volume, and heart rate measured in the lateral position. (Adapted from Ueland, K., Novy, M. J., Peterson, E. N., and Metcalfe, J.: Maternal cardiovascular dynamics. IV. The influence of gestational age on the maternal cardiovascular response to posture and exercise. Am. J. Obstet. Gynecol., *104*:856, 1969)

or completely occlude the inferior vena cava, decreasing venous return to the heart. Assumption of the lithotomy position exaggerates this effect.[58] Both positional changes can lead to the supine hypotension syndrome.

INTRA- AND POSTPARTUM CHANGES

During labor several changes occur in the maternal hemodynamic state (Fig. 2-4). A progressive increase in cardiac output is observed such that by the end of labor it exceeds by 50 per cent those values measured prior to the onset of labor. Heart rate decreases in the first stage of labor. However, a persistent, slight elevation to approximately 90 beats per minute is encountered during the second stage, and continues until 10 minutes postpartum. Stroke volume increases slowly during labor and reaches a maximum shortly after delivery.[54]

Uterine contractions produce varying hemodynamic responses, depending on maternal position.[53] During each uterine contraction, with the patient in the supine position, cardiac output increases 15 to 25 per cent above the levels observed between contractions, heart rate decreases 7 to 15 per cent, and stroke volume increases 21 to 33 per cent.[1,26,52,53] However, when patients are studied in the lateral position, uterine contractions produce an increase of only 7 per cent in cardiac output and stroke volume and do not alter the heart rate. Aortic and inferior vena caval compression, which occurs in the supine position, is responsible to a large degree for these discrepancies.[1,53] Consideration of the differences induced by positional changes is important in the management of pregnant cardiac patients during labor.

In the immediate puerperium (prior to delivery of the placenta) cardiac output increases markedly to a peak of 9 l./min. (approximately 80% above prelabor values

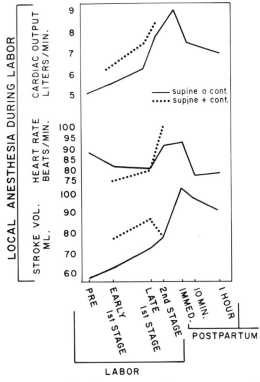

Fig. 2-4. Cardiac output, heart rate, and stroke volume during normal labor (local analgesia). (Ueland, K., and Hansen, J. M.: Maternal cardiovascular dynamics. III. Labor and delivery under local and caudal analgesia. Am. J. Obstet. Gynecol., *103*:8, 1969)

and 100% above normal nonpregnant levels (see Fig. 2-4). The elevated heart rate of late labor persists until 10 minutes postpartum when it decreases to approximately 75 beats per minute. Stroke volume, which reached a maximum at delivery, slowly falls thereafter.

Following delivery of the placenta, puerperal blood loss results in decreased central blood volume, decreased venous return to the heart, and decreased stroke volume. Since heart rate does not change during the remainder of the first hour of the puerperium, cardiac output also falls. Within 24 to 72 hours postpartum, cardiac output, heart rate, and stroke volume approximate those of early labor and return to normal nonpregnant values by 6 to 8 weeks after delivery (see Fig. 2-3).[54,57]

PATHOPHYSIOLOGY

In pregnant women with mild symptomatic valvular heart disease, cardiac output and oxygen consumption are lower than in normal pregnancy.[55] However, the increase in circulating blood volume is similar to that seen in the noncardiac patient. The average arteriovenous oxygen difference throughout pregnancy and the postpartum period is greater in patients with mitral valvular heart disease.[56] Tissue demands for oxygen are met by an increasing extraction of oxygen from circulating blood. When increases in cardiac output, blood volume, or stroke volume exceed the maximum capacity of the patient's diseased heart, dyspnea, palpitations, and frank congestive heart failure can develop. Maternal death due to cardiac decompensation frequently occurs between 14 and 18 gestational weeks,[20] correlating well with the predictable physiologic burden on the heart. Decompensation occurring later in pregnancy is usually precipitated by additional increases in cardiac output due to physical activity. Therefore, definite periods of rest are mandatory in patients with significant heart disease.

Serious complications may also develop during parturition and the early postpartum period in the pregnant cardiac patient. As many as two-thirds of all maternal deaths due to heart disease occur during the peripartum period.[15] During labor, cardiac output increases markedly, thus increasing the burden on the heart. Adequate analgesia and assumption of the lateral position during the first and second stages of labor are essential in minimizing the magnitude of the hemodynamic alterations.[54] Care in the use of intravenous fluids is necessary to avoid circulatory overload.

CHANGES IN PERIPHERAL CIRCULATION

ANTEPARTUM CHANGES

There is general agreement that systolic arterial blood pressure does not change significantly during normal pregnancy. Diastolic pressure falls by 10 to 15 torr, and therefore pulse pressure widens by similar increment. The decrease in mean arterial blood pressure results from a marked decrease in systemic vascular resistance.[2] The major factor contributing to the fall in systemic resistance is the addition of the placental circulation. The maximal fall in peripheral vascular resistance occurs between 14 and 24 weeks of pregnancy.

Central and upper extremity venous blood pressures are not altered during normal gestation. In the lower extremities venous pressure increases progressively, irrespective of maternal position, and reaches a peak at term.[41] The elevation in pressure has been attributed to mechanical obstruction by the gravid uterus,[30] but humorally related alterations in venous distensibility may also contribute to the changes.[40] Concomitantly, femoral venous blood flow is markedly decreased during normal pregnancy.[60]

The increased cardiac output of pregnancy is distributed to several organs.[28] Principal among these are the uterus, kidneys, and skin. Uteroplacental blood flow gradually increases from 50 ml./min. at 10 weeks gestation to approximately 600 to 700 ml./min. at term. A 90 per cent reduction in uterine vascular resistance is largely responsible for this increase. Renal blood flow is elevated soon after conception and remains so throughout pregnancy, reaching values of 900 to 1000 ml./min. at term. The increased blood flow to the skin is of the same order of magnitude as that to the kidneys.

The mechanisms controlling changes in regional blood flow and blood pressure are multifactorial. Endogenous estrogens play an important role, as do fundamental changes in vessel sensitivity to autonomic nervous system control.[4,48] A significant vasodilatory response to estrogen occurs in all major uterine tissues (i.e., myometrium, endometrium, and cotyledons), but the pattern and magnitude of the response through gestation are different for each tissue.[48] In late ovine pregnancy, for example, placental blood flow increases 25 per cent with estradiol-17β stimulation, while myometrial and endometrial flows increase by 100 per cent and 350 per cent respectively. Systemic infusion of estradiol-17β also produces significant vasodilation in the skin, adrenal glands, myocardium, and liver; skeletal muscle is the only tissue in which estrogen administration results in a decrease in blood flow.

INTRA- AND POSTPARTUM CHANGES

There are no significant changes in systolic or diastolic blood pressure during the first stage of labor. However, during the second stage, blood pressure rises 15 to 20 torr and remains elevated until 10 minutes postpartum (Fig. 2-5) At 1 hour postpartum, both systolic and diastolic blood pressures have returned to prelabor values. The changes in arterial blood pressure which occur with labor and delivery are less pronounced when regional analgesia is administered to reduce painful stimuli.[54] Central venous pressure rises progressively throughout labor, with an additional 50 per cent increment occurring immediately postpartum. By 1 hour following delivery, central venous pressure has declined to 7 cm. H_2O. During a uterine

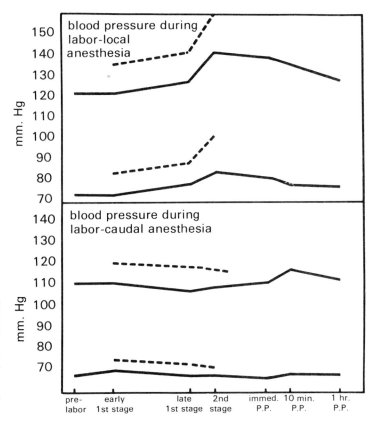

Fig. 2-5. Systolic and diastolic blood pressure during labor with local or caudal analgesia. (Ueland, K., and Hansen, J. M.: Maternal cardiovascular dynamics. III. Labor and delivery under local and caudal analgesia. Am. J. Obstet. Gynecol., *103*:8, 1969)

contraction, arterial blood pressure and central venous pressure increase 10 torr and 4 cm. H_2O respectively.[1] With parturition, femoral venous pressure falls [41] and femoral venous flow increases [60] in response to alleviation of the mechanical obstruction by the gravid uterus.

Because of peripheral venous dilatation and alterations in lower body blood flow and pressure, venous stasis with thrombosis is a recognized complication in antepartum patients. Since the hemodynamic changes occurring in the immediate postpartum period are especially dramatic, thrombosis is also a likely complication at this time.[42]

Regional blood flow studies during labor have focused on the changes which occur in the uteroplacental circulation. Uterine blood flow decreases with each uterine contraction but returns to baseline values with myometrial relaxation. The periodic reduction in uterine blood flow is associated with concomitant periodic increases in systemic blood volume, central venous pressure, cardiac output, and arterial blood pressure.[1] It is of clinical importance that the uterine circulation may lack the capability of autoregulation.[7,22] Therefore, any reduction in the arterial perfusing pressure, such as might occur during regional anesthesia or with peripartum blood loss, may compromise uteroplacental perfusion.

With delivery of the fetus and placenta, uterine perfusion falls abruptly, further accentuating changes in cardiac output and blood volume. As was discussed previously, these alterations can contribute to postpartum complications in patients with heart disease, preeclampsia, or eclampsia.

CHANGES IN RESPIRATORY FUNCTION

ANTEPARTUM CHANGES

Changes in the size of the maternal lung compartments begin as early as the fourth week of gestation. Progressive increases in vital capacity, tidal volume, and inspiratory capacity occur as pregnancy advances, with peak values obtained near term (Fig. 2-6).[32] Vital capacity increases from 3.3 l. in the nonpregnant state to 3.5 l. at term and is explained by the more favorable conditions under which the muscles of respiration function (i.e., increased stretching is imposed by the increased abdominal volume). Tidal volume increases from 0.37 to 0.65 l., while inspiratory capacity increases from 2.1 to 2.5 l. by term.

Functional residual capacity, expiratory reserve volume, and residual volume decrease as term approaches. Each of the latter two decreases approximately 20 per cent by term, to 1.0 and 1.3 l. respectively. The decrease in functional residual capacity is associated with changes in the balance between the elastic recoil of the lung and the combined elastic recoil of the chest wall in addition to the gravitational effects of the intra-abdominal contents.[32] Total lung capacity (the sum of inspiratory and functional residual capacities) remains constant at 4.8 l. throughout gestation. Since functional residual capacity decreases progressively, an increase in the inspiratory capacity must occur.

Minute ventilation increases in proportion to the increase in tidal volume. The increase in minute ventilation of 42 per cent at term is not associated with a significant increase in respiratory rate.[16,32] Since tidal volume increases while anatomic dead space remains unchanged, alveolar ventilation is greatly augmented. Changes in minute and alveolar ventilation are noted as early as the first trimester and are related to improvements in ventilation-perfusion relationships. Elevation in progesterone during pregnancy decreases the threshold of the medullary respiratory center to carbon dioxide.[28] The mild respiratory alkalosis which results from hyperventilation is compensated by renal excretion of bicarbonate. While blood hydrogen ion concentration remains within the normal range,[45] the alkali reserve is reduced

Fig. 2-6. Lung compartment volumes in late pregnancy compared with normal nonpregnancy. (Adapted from data of Knuttgen, H. G., and Emerson, K., Jr.: Physiological response to pregnancy at rest and during exercise. J. Appl. Physiol., *36*:549, 1974)

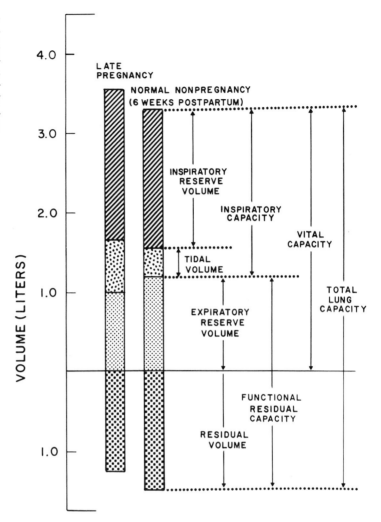

during pregnancy; thus the patient may more easily develop metabolic acidosis.

Diaphragmatic breathing assumes a more important role during pregnancy because of alterations in the mechanics of respiration. The change in the subcostal angle from 68 degrees to 103 degrees results in additional strength during the expiratory phase of respiration. The resultant altered position of the diaphragm, with an increase in length and a decrease in radius of curvature, might result in a more effective force of contraction.[32] While lung compliance (volume change induced per unit of pressure change) is unaltered dur-

ing pregnancy, total pulmonary resistance (airway resistance plus lung tissue resistance) is reduced by approximately 50 per cent. The bulk of the reduction is due to a decrease in airway resistance attributed to progesterone-induced changes in bronchiolar smooth muscle tone.[19] There is, however, some increase in vascular congestion of the upper airway; therefore nasal intubation can be traumatic and should be avoided if possible.

The dynamics of respiration appear not to be affected by normal gestation. Determinations of timed vital capacity and peak flow rate (as measured by peak flowmeter) show no changes with pregnancy, suggesting that the dynamic efficiency of ventilation is unchanged.

INTRA- AND POSTPARTUM CHANGES

During the intrapartum period, increased alveolar ventilation occurs. Early in labor, little change in ventilation or carbon dioxide tension ($PaCO_2$) is noted, but by the end of the first stage of labor, hyperventilation is pronounced and is accompanied by a fall in $PaCO_2$ to values as low as 18 torr. The second stage of labor is associated with frequent breath-holding during bearing-down efforts and results in small increases in $PaCO_2$ to approximately 25 torr.[46] The increased metabolic work and oxygen debt of labor produce lactic acidemia.[37] By 1 hour postpartum, buffering of fixed acids occurs and a compensated nonacidemic state exists. However, the carbon dioxide-hydrogen ion sensitivity of the central nervous system medullary chemoreceptors usually persists for several days to weeks postpartum, and $PaCO_2$ may remain below normal during that time.[5]

The mechanics of respiration are minimally altered during labor but change dramatically immediately following delivery. Diaphragmatic excursion does not return to normal prepregnancy values until the fourth to sixth week of the puerperium. Thoracic cage movements are less impaired during the postpartum period, owing to the decreased size of the uterus. The intercostal musculature is responsible for a larger share of the work of breathing.[23] Lung compliance is not altered prior to and during parturition, but both chest wall and total lung compliance are markedly decreased.[38] Immediately postpartum, total lung compliance and chest wall compliance rapidly approach normal nonpregnant values. This becomes important when a pressure ventilator is used during general anesthesia for delivery, because the sudden postpartum increase in compliance results in the delivery of a much greater tidal volume. This necessitates prompt adjustment of the ventilator to avoid significant reductions in $PaCO_2$, alkalosis, and circulatory alterations.[38]

In the early puerperium (first and second weeks), both vital capacity and total lung capacity are significantly reduced; by 6 to 12 weeks postpartum, both have usually returned to nonpregnant levels.[16] Tidal volume and inspiratory capacity decrease, while functional residual capacity, expiratory reserve volume, and residual volume increase to nonpregnant values by the sixth postpartum week (See Fig. 2-6).[32] Since serial studies at frequent intervals after delivery have not been performed, the time when each of these variables returns to normal prepregnancy values is unknown.

Studies of dynamic lung function in the early puerperium may reveal significant alteration.[16] Maximal breathing capacity is decreased, most likely as a result of poor maximal voluntary performance by the patient in the first several days after delivery. Normal test values are generally obtained by the sixth postpartum week. Forced expiratory volume and timed vital capacity, which depend less on subjective cooperation of the patient than the maximal breathing capacity, remain within the normal range throughout the puerperium.[32] These findings suggest that there is neither significant impairment of muscular efficiency nor airway obstruction following delivery.

PATHOPHYSIOLOGY

In patients with chronic obstructive pulmonary disease, the increased ventilation during pregnancy consumes considerable energy since the usually passive expiratory phase of breathing requires active muscular effort. Tidal volume cannot easily be increased. Women with obstructive disease who demonstrate hypoxemia and carbon dioxide retention at rest do not tolerate pregnancy well since pulmonary hypertension is usually present. Such women respond poorly to the additional demands of labor and often deteriorate postpartum,[43] most probably due to pulmonary congestion and a subsequent decrease in the ventilation-perfusion ratio. The association of pulmonary hypertension of any etiology with pregnancy is not favorable and is associated with maternal mortality rates as high as 53 per cent.[39]

CHANGES IN RENAL FUNCTION
ANTEPARTUM CHANGES

Renal plasma flow begins to rise early in the first trimester. A concomitant increase in glomerular filtration rate also is observed.[17,50] Because of the augmented filtration rate during normal pregnancy, plasma concentrations of urea nitrogen and creatinine are reduced.[50] The increases in renal plasma flow and glomerular filtration rate remain proportional until late in pregnancy, so that the filtration fraction (glomerular filtration rate/renal plasma flow) remains constant. Near-term renal plasma flow remains at an elevated value of 800 ml./min.[11] Early studies have suggested that flow falls as term approaches.[50] However, these reported changes are most likely positional since renal function can be significantly impaired late in pregnancy when measurements are made in either the supine or standing position.[3,11] Glomerular filtration rate increases in late gestation to values as high as 180 ml./min.[11] This increment late in pregnancy is most likely due to a decline in serum protein concentration;[47] the resultant fall in plasma oncotic pressure increases glomerular filtration and the filtration fraction.[6]

In order to maintain glomerular-tubular balance, an increase in glomerular filtration must be accompanied by an equal increase in the reabsorptive capacity of the renal tubules. Balance is essential for the maintenance of extracellular volume stability and sodium homeostasis.[8] The increase in exchangeable sodium which occurs during pregnancy is entirely accounted for by the products of conception and expanded plasma volume.[21] Extracellular water accumulation (approximately 6 l.) is evenly divided between the fetoplacental unit (fetus, amniotic fluid,and placenta) and maternal compartment (plasma volume, breasts, and uterus). Normal pregnancy is not associated with significant overhydration of maternal tissues.[12]

The tubular reabsorption of glucose and amino acids is not as efficient as that of sodium. Glycosuria (without hyperglycemia) or aminoaciduria may develop in normal gestation.[13,59] Serum uric acid values are decreased, owing to an increase in urate clearance.[24]

Anatomical alterations in the urinary tract during normal gestation are produced as a result of hormonal factors. The renal collecting structures are dilated, and muscle tone and rhythmic peristalsis of the ureter decrease as term approaches. An increase in the volume of urine contained within the renal pelvis and collecting system has been described.[35] These collective changes may present problems in obtaining valid clearance studies, particularly during periods of low urinary flow. The anatomical changes are an important factor in the increased frequency of urinary tract infections during pregnancy.

INTRA- AND POSTPARTUM CHANGES

In the early weeks of puerperium, renal plasma flow decreases rapidly, at a rate greater than plasma volume and cardiac output, and may be significantly below normal nonpregnant values for up to 25 weeks postpartum in some cases. Glomerular filtration rate slowly returns to normal nonpregnant values by the sixth postpartum week. The filtration fraction remains elevated for a variable length of time because of the abnormally low renal plasma flow. Plasma urea nitrogen and creatinine concentrations reach normal values in parallel with the decreases in glomerular filtration rate.[50]

Glomerular-tubular balance is maintained as precisely in the puerperium as during the antepartum period. In normal women the proportion of exchangeable sodium remains unchanged during the first 7 days postpartum[12] and gradually falls to normal nonpregnant levels by 6 weeks after delivery. The postpartum diuresis that regularly occurs between the second and fifth days rarely exceeds 2 l. of urine per day. Occasionally higher urine outputs are observed, but these are balanced by augmented fluid intakes.[27] Proteinuria during the first 24 hours and glycosuria within the first week of the puerperium may be present following a normal delivery; the sugar is lactose and is nonreducing in test systems utilizing glucose oxidase. Acetonuria is especially prominent following a prolonged and difficult labor. Serum uric acid concentration rises during labor, remains elevated in the early puerperium, and returns to normal within 7 to 10 days after delivery because of augmented uric acid clearance.[25]

Pregnancy-induced dilatation of the upper urinary tract is accentuated by mechanical factors associated with labor and delivery, and disappears by the end of the second to fourth postpartum weeks. Alterations in the lower urinary tract, including an increased bladder capacity and decreased muscle tone, frequently result in incomplete emptying of the bladder. Urinary retention occurs in approximately one-third of all puerperal women and is associated with an increased frequency of urinary tract infections.

PATHOPHYSIOLOGY

Renal function is impaired in pregnancies complicated by preeclampsia and eclampsia. Renal plasma flow and glomerular filtration rate are decreased 20 per cent and 33 per cent respectively in toxemic patients near term.[10] Creatinine and uric acid clearances are markedly reduced antepartum (approximately 20% and 50% respectively), but return to normal values as early as 6 days postpartum.[25] The most dramatic changes in preeclampsia and eclampsia involve sodium and water balance. Large increases in total body sodium and extravascular water occur prior to delivery in spite of a markedly contracted plasma volume.[10] Oliguria or anuria may be present throughout labor and during the first 24 hours of the puerperium, making the toxemic patient particularly susceptible to pulmonary edema and cardiac failure from iatrogenic fluid overload. Improvement in renal function is usually observed by 12 hours postpartum. Brisk diuresis usually ensues by 24 to 48 hours and appears to be proportional to the severity of the disease. Persistent oliguria, anuria, and the development of pulmonary edema indicate a grave prognosis.

CHANGES IN GASTROINTESTINAL, HEPATIC, AND GALLBLADDER FUNCTION

Gastrointestinal function is altered in several ways during gestation, parturition, and the early postpartum period. Gastric emptying time is delayed and gastric secretion is reduced prior to delivery.[28] During the immediate puerperium, tone and motility decrease even further. The delayed emptying time of the stomach is exaggerated by the administration of analgesic agents.[33] Vomiting and regurgitation with pulmonary aspiration may occur, especially with general anesthesia. Pulmonary aspiration of gastric contents continues to account for a high incidence of maternal morbidity and mortality. The administration of antacids prior to general anesthesia for delivery reduces the risk of chemical pneumonitis by raising the gastric pH above the critical level of 2.5.[51]

The decrease of muscle tone in all gastrointestinal structures is consistent with a generalized smooth muscle relaxation which is especially prominent in the uterus and peripheral blood vessels prior to delivery.[28] With delivery of the fetus and placenta, progesterone production decreases and the smooth muscle tone rapidly returns to normal.

Liver function is not significantly altered during the course of normal pregnancy and the puerperium. Hepatic arterial blood flow remains unchanged despite the antepartum augmentation of cardiac output and blood volume. Therefore, a smaller proportion of the cardiac output reaches the liver.[14] With a few exceptions, liver function tests remain unchanged from values found in nonpregnant women.[31] Serum concentrations of several hepatic enzymes (e.g., alkaline phosphatase) normally rise during the third trimester (as a result of increasing placental enzyme synthesis and excretion) and therefore are not necessarily indicative of maternal liver dysfunction.[14] These enzyme activities return to normal values early in the puerperium. The activity of serum cholinesterase falls during late pregnancy and remains low through labor and the first several days of the puerperium,[49] leading to a decrease in the required dose of succinylcholine. The paralyzing agent is safe to use during labor, provided the dose is titrated to the patient's need.

Gallbladder function is also impaired because of the pregnancy-related decrease in smooth muscle tone. Emptying is slowed and bile tends to concentrate; there is some evidence that pregnancy predisposes to gallstones.[28]

REFERENCES

1. Adams, J. Q., and Alexander, A. M.: Alterations in cardiovascular physiology during labor. Obstet. Gynecol., *12*:542, 1958.
2. Assali, N. S., and Brinkman, C. R., III: Disorders of maternal circulation and respiratory adjustments. *In* Assali, N. S. (ed.): Pathophysiology of Gestation. New York, Academic Press, 1972.
3. Assali, N. S., Dignam, W. J., and Dasgupta, K.: Renal function in human pregnancy. II. Effects of venous pooling on renal hemodynamics and water, electrolyte, and aldosterone excretion during normal gestation. J. Lab. Clin. Med., *54*:394, 1959.
4. Assali, N. S., and Prystowsky, H.: Studies on autonomic blockade. I. Comparison between the effects of tetraethylammonium chloride (TEAC) and high selective spinal anesthesia on blood pressure of normal and toxemic pregnancy. J. Clin. Invest., *29*:1354, 1950.
5. Bouterline-Young, H., and Bouterline-Young, E.: Alveolar carbon dioxide levels in pregnant, parturient and lactating subjects. J. Obstet. Gynaecol. Br. Emp., *63*:509, 1956.
6. Brenner, B. M., *et al.*: Dynamics of glomerular ultrafiltration in the rat. II. Plasma-flow dependence of GFR. Am. J. Physiol., *223*:1184, 1972.
7. Bruce, N. W., and Abdul-Karim, R. W.: Mechanisms controlling maternal placental circulation. Clin. Obstet. Gynecol., *17*:135, 1974.
8. Chesley, L. C.: Renal function in pregnancy. Bull. N.Y. Acad. Med., *41*:811, 1965.
9. ———: Plasma and red cell volumes during pregnancy. Am. J. Obstet. Gynecol., *112*:440, 1972.
10. ———: Disorders of the kidney, fluids and electrolytes. *In* Assali, N. S. (ed.): Pathophysiology of Gestation. New York, Academic Press, 1972.
11. Chesley, L. C., and Sloan, D. M.: The effect of posture on renal function in pregnancy. Am. J. Obstet. Gynecol., *89*:754, 1964.
12. Chesley, L. C., Valenti, C., and Uichanco, L.: Alterations in body fluid compartments and exchangeable sodium in the early puerperium. Am. J. Obstet. Gynecol., *77*:1054, 1959.
13. Christensen, P. J., *et al.*: Amino acids in blood plasma and urine during pregnancy. Scand. J. Clin. Lab. Invest., *9*:54, 1957.
14. Combes, B., and Adams, R. H.: Disorders of the liver in pregnancy. *In* Assali, N. S. (ed.): Pathophysiology of Gestation. New York, Academic Press, 1972.
15. Conradsson, T. B., and Werko, L.: Management of heart disease in pregnancy. Prog. Cardiovasc. Dis., *16*:407, 1974.
16. Cugell, D. W., *et al.*: Pulmonary function in pregnancy. I. Serial observations in normal women. Am. Rev. Tuberc., *67*:568, 1953.
17. Dignam, W. J., Titus, P., and Assali, N. S.: Renal function in human pregnancy. I. Changes in glomerular filtration rate and renal plasma flow. Proc. Soc. Exp. Biol. Med., *97*:512, 1958.
18. Ferris, T. F.: Toxemia and hypertension. *In* Burrow, G. N., and Ferris, T. F. (eds.): Medical Complications During Pregnancy. Philadelphia, W. B. Saunders, 1975.
19. Gee, J. B. L., *et al.*: Pulmonary mechanics during pregnancy. J. Clin. Invest., *46*:945, 1967.
20. Gordon, C. A.: Heart disease as a cause of maternal disease. Am. J. Obstet. Gynecol., *69*:701, 1955.
21. Gray, M. J., and Plentl. A. A.: The variations of

the sodium space and the total exchangeable sodium during pregnancy. Am. J. Obstet. Gynecol., *71*:1165, 1956.

22. Greiss, F. C., Jr.: A clinical concept of uterine blood flow during pregnancy. Obstet. Gynecol., *30*:595, 1967.

23. Grenville-Mathers, R., and Trenchard, H. J.: The diaphragm in the puerperium. J. Obstet. Gynaecol. Br. Emp., *60*:825, 1953.

24. Hayashi, T. T.: Uric acid and endogenous creatinine clearances during normal and toxemic pregnancy. Am. J. Obstet. Gynecol., *71*:859, 1956.

25. ———: Uric acid and endogenous creatinine clearances after normal and toxemic pregnancy. Am. J. Obstet. Gynecol., *73*:23, 1957.

26. Hendricks, C. H., and Quilligan, E. J.: Cardiac output during labor. Am. J. Obstet. Gynecol., *71*:953, 1956.

27. Hutchinson, D. L., Plentl, A. A., and Taylor, H. C.: The total body water and the water turnover in pregnancy studied with deuterium oxide as isotopic water. J. Clin. Invest., *33*:235, 1954.

28. Hytten, F. E., and Leitch, I.: The Physiology of Human Pregnancy. Philadelphia, F. A. Davis, 1971.

29. Hytten, F. E., and Paintin, D. B.: Increase in plasma volume during normal pregnancy. J. Obstet. Gynaecol. Br. Commonw., *70*:402, 1963.

30. Kerr, M. G.: The mechanical effects of the gravid uterus in late pregnancy. J. Obstet. Gynaecol. Br. Commonw., *72*:513, 1965.

31. Kessler, W. B., and Andros, G. J.: Hepatic function during pregnancy and puerperium. Obstet. Gynecol., *23*:372, 1964.

32. Knuttgen, H. G., and Emerson, K., Jr.: Physiological response to pregnancy at rest and during exercise. J. Appl. Physiol., *36*:549, 1974.

33. La Salvia, L. A., and Steffen, E. A.: Delayed gastric emptying time in labor. Am. J. Obstet. Gynecol., *59*:1075, 1950.

34. Lees, M. M., *et al.*: A study of cardiac output at rest throughout pregnancy. J. Obstet. Gynaecol. Br. Commonw., *74*:319, 1967.

35. Longo, L. D., and Assali, N. S.: Renal function in human pregnancy. IV. The urinary tract "dead space" during normal gestation. Am. J. Obstet. Gynecol., *80*:495, 1960.

36. Lund, C. J., and Donovan, J. C.: Blood volume during pregnancy. Am. J. Obstet. Gynecol., *98*:393, 1967.

37. Marx, G. F., and Greene, N. M.: Maternal lactate, pyruvate, and excess lactate production during labor and delivery. Am. J. Obstet. Gynecol., *90*:786, 1964.

38. Marx, G. F., Murthy, P. K., and Orkin, L. R.: Static compliance before and after vaginal delivery. Br. J. Anaesth., *42*:1100, 1972.

39. McCaffrey, R. M., and Dunn, L. J.: Primary pulmonary hypertension in pregnancy. Obstet. Gynecol. Surv., *19*:567, 1964.,

40. McCausland, A. M., *et al.*: Venous distensibility during pregnancy. Am. J. Obstet. Gynecol., *81*:472, 1961.

41. McClennan, C. E.: Antecubital and femoral venous pressure in normal and toxemic pregnancy. Am. J. Obstet. Gynecol., *45*:568, 1943.

42. Montaldo, N. J., *et al.*: Post-partum thrombophlebitis of the ovarian vein. Obstet. Gynecol., *34*:867, 1969.

43. Novy, M. J., and Edwards, M. J.: Respiratory problems in pregnancy. Am. J. Obstet. Gynecol., *99*:1024, 1967.

44. Pritchard, J. A.: Changes in the blood volume during pregnancy and delivery. Anesthesiology, *26*:393, 1965.

45. Prowse, C. M., and Gaensler, E. A.: Respiratory and acid-base changes during pregnancy. Anesthesiology, *26*:381, 1965.

46. Reid, D. H. S.: Respiratory changes in labour. Lancet, *1*:784, 1966.

47. Robertson, E. G.: Increased erythrocyte fragility in association with osmotic changes in pregnancy serum. J. Reprod. Fertil., *16*:323, 1968.

48. Rosenfeld, C. R., *et al.*: Effect of estradiol-17β on blood flow to reproductive and nonreproductive tissues in pregnant ewes. Am. J. Obstet. Gynecol., *124*:618, 1976.

49. Shnider, S. M.: Serum cholinesterase activity during pregnancy, labor, and the puerperium. Anesthesiology, *26*:335, 1965.

50. Sims, E. A. H., and Krantz, K. E.: Serial studies of renal function during pregnancy and the puerperium in normal women. J. Clin. Invest., *37*:1764, 1958.

51. Taylor, C., and Pryse-Davies, J.: The prophylactic use of antacids in the prevention of the acid-pulmonary-aspiration syndrome (Mendelson's syndrome). Lancet, *1*:288, 1966.

52. Ueland, K., Gills, R. E., and Hansen, J. M.: Maternal cardiovascular dynamics. I. Cesarean section under subarachnoid block anesthesia. Am. J. Obstet. Gynecol., *100*:42, 1968.

53. Ueland, K., and Hansen, J. M.: Maternal cardiovascular dynamics. II. Posture and uterine contractions. Am. J. Obstet. Gynecol., *103*:1, 1969.

54. ———: Maternal cardiovascular dynamics. III. Labor and delivery under local and caudal analgesia. Am. J. Obstet. Gynecol., *103*:8, 1969.

55. Ueland, K., Novy, M. J., and Metcalfe, J.: Hemodynamic responses of patients with heart disease to pregnancy and exercise. Am. J. Obstet. Gynecol., *113*:47, 1972.

56. ———: Cardiorespiratory responses to pregnancy and exercise in normal women and patients with heart disease. Am. J. Obstet. Gynecol., *115*:4, 1973.

57. Ueland, K., *et al.*: Maternal cardiovascular dynamics. IV. The influence of gestational age on the maternal cardiovascular response to posture and exercise. Am. J. Obstet. Gynecol., *104*:856, 1969.

58. Vorys, N., Ullery, J. C., and Hanusek, G. E.: The cardiac output changes in various positions in pregnancy. Am. J. Obstet. Gynecol., *81*:1312, 1961.

59. Welsh, G. W., and Sims, E. A. H.: The mechanisms of renal glycosuria in pregnancy Diabetes, *9*:363, 1960.

60. Wright, P., Osborn, S. B., and Edmonds, D. G.: Changes in the rate of flow of venous blood in the leg during pregnancy, measured with radioactive sodium. Surg. Gynecol. Obstet., *90*:481, 1950.

3

The Placenta and Placental Transfer of Drugs at Term

Ezzat Abouleish, M.D.

UTEROPLACENTAL CIRCULATION

The placenta has two sides—maternal and fetal. The fetal and maternal circulations are separate and independent of each other.

MATERNAL CIRCULATION OF THE PLACENTA

Nutrients and oxygen are carried to the placenta by the uterine and ovarian blood vessels. In the nonpregnant state, the uterine blood flow is about 100 ml./min.; during pregnancy it gradually increases to about 500 to 700 ml./min. The majority of the uterine blood flow reaches the placenta (400–600 ml./min.), and only a small fraction is used by the uterine muscle.[22] Fifty ml./min. of the placenta blood flow provides nutrients to the placental tissue; the remainder (350–550 ml./min.) reaches the intervillous space for metabolic and other exchanges with the fetal circulation (Table 3-1).

Table 3-1. Distribution of Uterine Blood Flow at Full Term

Uterine Blood Flow	ml./min.
Total uterine flow	500–700
To myometrium	100
To placenta	400–600
To placental tissue	50
To intervillous space	350–550

Increased total blood volume and cardiac output during pregnancy permit increased uterine blood flow without compromising perfusion of other maternal organs (i.e., liver and brain blood flows are not altered during pregnancy).

Blood reaches the placenta from the mother through the uterine arterioles, called spiral arterioles, which open directly into the intervillous space (Fig. 3-1). In the mature placenta there are approximately 60 to 100 arteriolar openings at its base.[25] These arterioles act independently of each other so that not all are patent and discharging simultaneously.[135] Blood leaves these arteriolar openings in fountain like spurts, entering the intervillous space with a pressure of 60 to 70 torr (Table 3-2). Pressure gradually drops as the blood passes through the intervillous space. Pressure in the intervillous space during uterine relaxation is about 10 torr, and pressure in the uteroplacental veins is 5 torr. In contrast to other organ tissues in the body, there is no capillary network between the spiral arterioles and the corresponding veins. Blood flow in the intervillous space is affected by the number of patent arterioles, the pressure in these arterioles, and the pattern and frequency of uterine contractions. The perfusion pressure depends on the difference be-

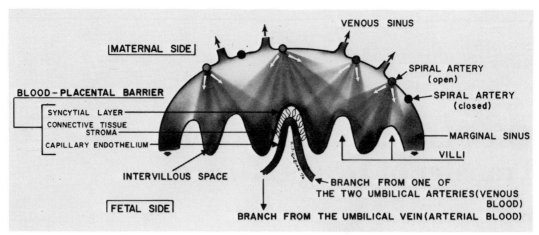

Fig. 3-1.   Schematic of the mature utero-placental circulation. (Abouleish, E.: Placenta transfer of drugs. Diagnostica, *in press.*)

Table 3-2. Human Maternal and Fetal Blood Pressures

	Site	torr
Maternal:	Spiral artery	70–80
	Intervillous space	10
	Venous sinuses	5
Fetal:	Umbilical artery	68
	Umbilical vein	28

tween the arteriolar and venous pressures. To allow adequate blood flow through the intervillous space, the perfusion pressure should be maintained. The high pressure at the arteriolar end of the intervillous space is a safeguard against increases in the venous pressure due to inferior vena caval compression. The blood flow in the intervillous space is nonhomogenous, and this is an important factor in delaying the equilibrium in drug levels between maternal and fetal blood. The autonomic innervation of uterine blood vessels, including the spiral arteries, is similar to that of other abdominal viscera which contain numerous terminals of sympathetic nerves located in the media. The relative distribution of alpha- and beta-adrenergic receptors for this vascular bed has not been determined. Preliminary information suggests that there are few beta-adrenergic receptors, and most of the receptors are alpha-adrenergic. Thus the uterine blood vessels are very sensitive to the sympathetic tone. Positive pressure ventilation, catecholamines,[3] and hypovolemia cause decreased uterine blood flow even in the absence of changes in the systemic blood pressure.

The capacity of the intervillous space in humans near term is 150 ml. The amount of oxygen contained in this reservoir is sufficient for a fetal consumption of only 1.5 to 2 minutes. In some pathologic states, this volume may be considerably reduced. The flow rate of blood through the intervillous space is very slow compared to the flow rate in other parts of the body (e.g., the mean flow velocity through the spiral artery is 300 mm./sec., while that of intervillous space is between 0.1 and 10 mm./sec.). The slowness of the blood flow in the intervillous space delays the transfer of drugs from mother to fetus; on the other hand, it tends to bring fetal and maternal blood levels of the drug into equilibrium if administered for a prolonged period of time.[5]

The villi have an extensive surface area to allow for the maternal-fetal exchanges.

The total length of these villi is 30 miles, providing a surface area of 15 square meters.[152] After bathing the villi, the maternal blood returns to the pelvic veins by way of the uteroplacental veins accompanying the spiral arterioles and at the margin of the placenta by the marginal sinus. During uterine contractions, blood flow through the uteroplacental circulation is impeded and outflow through the uteroplacental veins stops. A uterine contraction that raises the intrauterine pressure to 20 torr has a minimal effect on the intervillous circulation. If this pressure rises to 30 torr, the intervillous circulation decreases by as much as 50 per cent. Contractions leading to an intrauterine pressure of 40 torr or more completely stop the intervillous perfusion; the fetus becomes isolated from its mother and must live on the reserve it has. If this reserve is compromised, or if the uterine contractions become tetanic, fetal asphyxia occurs.

FETAL CIRCULATION OF THE PLACENTA

Within the umbilical cord there are three vessels: one umbilical vein carries arterial blood from the placenta to the inferior vena cava of the fetus, and two umbilical arteries carry venous blood from the internal iliac arteries of the fetus to the placenta. Each villus has two vessels—one artery and one vein. The arterial branch divides into a network of capillaries which drain into the corresponding venule. There are no arteriovenous shunts in the villi, which is a safety factor to allow oxygenation of blood as it passes through the capillary network before it reaches the venous side.[164] Umbilical flow increases as the fetus grows, and it reaches a rate of 250 ml./min. at term. Therefore, the fetal-maternal blood flow ratio is 1:1.5.[22] In spite of this difference in the flow rate, the placental exchange is enhanced by the countercurrent flow of maternal and fetal blood.[106] This arrangement, used frequently in engineering, is highly efficient in establishing chemical equilibrium between two bloodstreams and exists in sheep and rabbits. In a primate placenta, a counterflow pattern, as described in 1946 in an article by Barcroft and Barron,[15] is not seen.[164] Fetal blood flow makes a complete circle in each villus. Maternal blood flow, on the other hand, is arterial at the arteriolar orifices, venous at the outflow orifices, and intermediate elsewhere in the intervillous space. Uneven distribution of maternal to fetal blood flow would increase the net transplacental difference in oxygen tension and drug concentrations in the same way as ventilation-perfusion inequality in the lung increases the alveolar-arterial PO_2 difference.[98]

THE BLOOD-PLACENTAL BARRIER

The blood-placental barrier consists of those tissues separating fetal and maternal blood. At term these tissues consist of three layers (See Fig. 3-1): (1) syncytial layer, (2) stroma of connective tissue, and (3) fetal capillary endothelium. The barrier is about 2 to 6 μ in thickness,[178] and any substance in the maternal blood must cross this barrier before reaching the fetal blood and vice versa.

TRANSFER OF DRUGS ACROSS THE PLACENTA

It was formerly believed that the placenta is a semipermeable membrane which allows water and crystalloids to pass through but prevents the passing through of colloids and large molecules. This simple concept has been replaced by a more complex but still poorly understood one according to which the placenta selectively controls the rate of transfer of a wide variety of materials.[119] For all practical purposes, the blood-placental barrier resembles the blood-brain barrier, and therefore, factors affecting drug transfer are also similar.

It is now believed that any substance found in the maternal or fetal blood should be able to cross the placenta to some extent, unless it is destroyed or altered during passage. However, a very low degree of permeability may slow the entry, thereby rendering some drugs physiologically inactive and pharmacologically undetectable. The important questions are not only whether a substance does or does not pass the blood-placental barrier, but also the mechanism of transfer, the rate of transfer, the ultimate quantity of the substance transferred, and the effect on the fetus and newborn.[53] For all practical purposes, the drugs used in relation to obstetric anesthesia and analgesia cross the placental barrier almost by simple diffusion from the side of higher concentration to that of lesser concentration.

INFLUENCING FACTORS IN DRUG TRANSFER

The transfer to, and ultimate distribution of drugs in the fetus depends on three sets of factors (Table 3-3): (1) factors inherent in the drug itself, (2) maternal factors, and (3) fetal factors.

Drug Factors

The blood-placental barrier can be considered as a membrane made of lipoproteins which has small pores and an electrically charged surface. Therefore, the rate of transfer of a drug will vary according to the following considerations:

Lipid Solubility. Fat-soluble substances, such as barbiturates, can easily pass through the membrane.[117]

Molecular Weight. A substance with a molecular weight of less than 100, such as nitrous oxide, passes readily through the pores of the barrier in spite of its fat insolubility. Substances with a molecular weight of between 100 and 600 pass at a rate controlled by their size. Substances with a molecular weight of between 600 and 1,000 pass through the placental barrier at a rate controlled by their fat solubility and degree of ionization. Substances with a molecular weight of more than 1,000, such as dextrose, require a carrier system to pass through the barrier.

Degree of Ionization. Ions carrying the same charge as the placental membrane are repelled. On the other hand, substances carrying an opposite charge to the membrane will be held in the membrane.

Table 3-3. Factors Influencing Transfer of Drugs Across the Placenta

Drug Factors	Maternal Factors	Fetal Factors
1. Lipid solubility	1. Elimination of drug from maternal circulation	1. Fetal liver
2. Molecular weight		2. Progressive dilution of blood en route to fetal brain
3. Degree of ionization	2. Nonhomogenicity of blood in intervillous space	
4. Concentration gradient across the membrane	3. Separation of maternal from fetal circulation	3. Extensive shunting in fetal circulation
5. Binding to plasma proteins and red cells	4. Uterine contractions	4. Immaturity of the brain
6. Method of administration	5. Maternal blood volume	5. Enzymatic systems
7. Drug interaction	6. Uteroplacental blood flow	6. Fetal plasma, red cells, and pH
8. Drug metabolites		7. Compression of umbilical cord during delivery
9. Tissue binding		

Hence, ionization makes passing more difficult, since particles and substances are transferred in their undissociated or nonionized form.[48] The dissociation constant of a substance (pKa) is the pH at which 50 per cent of the substance is ionizable. Therefore, the closer the pKa of a substance to the pH of the maternal blood, the more the substance becomes ionized and subsequently less transferable across the membrane.

Concentration Gradient Across the Membrane. With a high maternal drug concentration relative to that of the fetus, a drug will pass easily to the fetus. This is an important factor applying to volatile as well as nonvolatile agents.

Binding of the Drug to the Plasma Proteins and Red Cells. Macromolecules and, therefore, drugs bound to macromolecules cross biologic membranes only with difficulty. Thus, the binding of a drug to the maternal plasma proteins constitutes an important factor controlling the transmission of the drug across the placenta.[48] An example is bupivacaine, which has a high binding capacity to the maternal plasma proteins.[170] Therefore, less of the drug is available for crossing to the fetus, which explains the lower ratio of umbilical to maternal level of bupivacaine as compared with lidocaine or mepivacaine.[171] At a higher total plasma drug concentration, the proportion of free drug will be higher, thus the amount transferable to the fetus will be increased.[171] This explains why with a higher maternal dose of the same drug not only the level of the drug in the umbilical blood will be more elevated but also the umbilical to maternal blood level ratio is higher.

Method of Administration. When a drug is given intravenously, it is carried around the body in a bolus form for one or two circulations.[125] Therefore, the drug presents itself at the placental site in a highly concentrated form. This leads to a high pressure gradient across the placental membrane and increased transfer of the drug to the fetus. This is particularly important in nonlipid, ionizable substances that pass across the blood-placental barrier with difficulty, such as muscle relaxants.[167] Slow intravenous injection of a drug into the mother decreases its transmission to the fetus and, therefore, adds to the safety of the infant.[97,167] Moreover, the amount of any drug transferred to the fetus can be decreased by injecting it at the beginning of a uterine contraction. By the time the bolus of the drug goes through the maternal circulation into the uterine arteries, the uterine contraction would be at its peak, and intervillous perfusion is arrested so that little or no drug can be transferred during this first circulation time.[55] Intramuscular injection produces a steady trickle in the maternal circulation. Therefore, the maternal blood level will not be as high as following the intravenous injection. Consequently, the gradient across the placenta and the transmission of the drug to the fetus will be less following intramuscular injection than after intravenous injection of the same dose.

The pharmacokinetics of inhalation anesthetics, such as halothane, differ from intravenous anesthetics, such as thiopental, or local anesthetics, such as lidocaine. In contrast to the latter two agents, which are usually given by single or intermittent injections, halothane is administered continuously to the mother. Therefore, the blood and tissue time concentration curves of halothane show a generally rising course[64] in contrast to the falling course encountered with thiopental[89] and lidocaine.[154]

Drug Interaction. This is an important factor which one should bear in mind, because competition between different drugs for plasma- or tissue-binding sites may affect the course of transmission of these drugs to the fetus and their toxicity.[66]

Drug Metabolites. Fetal depression may be due to the metabolites of a drug rather than to the drug itself. Therefore, in studying the placental transmission and the effects of drug on the fetus, the investigation is incomplete unless the drug's metabolites are also considered.

Tissue Binding. Following epidural injection of equal doses of bupivacaine, lidocaine, and mepivacaine, the maternal blood level is lowest with the first and highest with the last drug.[137] An important reason for such a difference is that bupivacaine has a greater binding capacity to the tissues of the epidural space than the other two drugs.

Maternal Factors

Elimination of the Drug From the Maternal Circulation. This is achieved by the drug leaving the intravascular bed and entering the extravascular compartments, by its excretion, and its metabolism. The elimination of a drug from the maternal blood will affect the balance across the placental membrane. If no elimination occurs, sooner or later equilibrium is reached, and the blood levels of the drug will be equal in the mother, umbilical vein, and umbilical artery. If elimination of the drug from the maternal circulation is faster than elimination of the drug from the fetal circulation, the maternal level will fall below the fetal level, and the passage of the drug will be reversed. In such a case the drug level in the umbilical artery will be higher than in the umbilical vein (e.g., with diazepam).[146]

Nonhomogenicity of the Blood in the Intervillous Space. Transmission to the fetus of a drug such as thiobarbiturate is delayed for about 2 minutes, owing to the nonhomogenicity of the blood in the intervillous space.

Separation of Maternal From Fetal Circulation. Thus, there is no instantaneous exchange between mother and fetus. This factor and the fact that the blood in the intervillous space is nonhomogenous are responsible for the delay in transmission of drugs (e.g., nitrous oxide and thiobarbital) from mother to fetus.

Uterine Contractions. During active labor and delivery, each time the uterus contracts, the fetus is isolated from the mother, and placental blood flow (as well as drug transmission) stops.

Maternal Blood Volume. In cases of hypovolemia, a given dose of a drug will be less diluted and thus reaches a higher concentration in maternal blood. The pressure gradient across the placental membrane becomes higher, allowing for more transmission of the drug to the fetus.

Uteroplacental Blood Flow. Uteroplacental blood flow affects equilibrium of drugs across the blood-placental barrier in a way similar to that of ventilation on the transmission of gases across the alveolar membrane. Accordingly, hypoperfusion of the placenta or hypoventilation of the lung delays the transmission of drugs or gases respectively.

Fetal Factors

Fetal Liver. The exact amount of umbilical vein blood flow that perfuses the human fetal liver is still controversial.[14,23,41] It has been estimated that in the human fetus the amount that bypasses the liver through the ductus venosus is from one-third to two-thirds of the placental venous return. Perfusion experiments in stillborn infants give similar results.[160] Therefore, a large portion of any drug crossing the placenta is immediately brought to the liver. In the human fetus, the left lobe of the liver receives blood mostly from the umbilical vein while the right lobe is supplied mostly by blood from the portal vein.[69,139] This explains the findings of Finster and coworkers[56] namely, that the concentration of thiopental in the left lobe of the human fetus is higher than in the right lobe, and both concentrations are higher than the maternal blood level (Table 3-4). However, following repeated maternal injections of thiopental, the two lobes of the fetal liver contained almost equal concentrations of the drug. This is due to the prolonged exposure of the fetus to thiopental and the recirculation of the drug within the fetal body, which pro-

Table 3-4. Average Thiopental Concentration in Two Anencephalic Human Babies After Injection into the Mothers*

Tissue		Concentration
Maternal	Venous blood	19 µg./ml.
Fetal	Subcutaneous fat	65 µg./g.
	Liver	
	Left lobe	53 µg./g.
	Right lobe	48 µg./g.
	Lungs	20 µg./g.
	Heart	10 µg./g.
	Muscle	9 µg./g.

*Developed from data by Finster, M., *et al.*: Tissue thiopental concentrations in the fetus and newborn. Anesthesiology, *36*:155, 1972.

duced nearly identical drug concentrations in all fetal vessels. The high thiopental uptake by the liver could be due not only to the pattern of fetal circulation, but also to the presence of two cytoplasmic protein fractions (Y and Z proteins) in the hepatic cells, which appear to be important in the uptake of organic anions from the plasma.[95]

The strategic position of the liver in the fetal circulation is important for extracting substantial amounts of the drugs entering the fetus and thus protecting the fetal brain.[54,56] Table 3-5 shows that following the injection of thiopental into the umbilical vein of guinea pigs, the concentration of the drug in the liver is 100 times higher than in the brain. The high uptake of drugs by the liver has been demonstrated

Table 3-5. Tissue Concentrations of Thiopental in Guinea Pig Fetus After Injection into Umbilical Vein*†

Tissue	Average Concentration (µg./g.)
Liver (middle lobe)	913
Brain	9
Spinal cord	14

*Developed from data by Finster, M. *et al.*: Tissue thiopental concentrations in the fetus and newborn. Anesthesiology, *36*:155, 1972.

†n=6.

with thiopental,[56] halothane,[64] lidocaine,[54] and cyclamate.[127] At all times the concentration of each drug is higher in the liver of the fetus than in the mother.

Progressive Dilution of Blood en Route to the Fetal Brain. Blood in the umbilical vein becomes diluted with blood from the gastrointestinal tract and lower limbs before it is shunted through the foramen ovale of the heart and then to the brain.[24] This dilution decreases the concentration of any drug that traversed the placenta.

Extensive Shunting in the Fetal Circulation. Fifty-seven per cent of the combined cardiac output of the lamb fetus (and presumably a similar amount in the human) returns to the placenta without perfusing fetal tissues. This is due to extensive shunting by way of the foramen ovale and the ductus arteriosus. Hence the fetal tissues are not exposed to over half of the absorbed quantity of the drug during each circulation.

Immaturity of the Brain of the Fetus and Young Neonate. The brain of the fetus and newborn has been found to be deficient in myelin.[164] This may explain the fact that newborns are more sensitive to the action of depressant drugs than are adults of the same species.[117]

Enzymatic Systems. Neonates are known to have poorly developed enzymatic systems. Therefore, some drugs, such as barbiturates and anilide-type local anesthetics (e.g., lidocaine and mepivacaine), are not readily metabolized by the newborn.

Fetal Plasma, Red Cells and pH. In the fetus these are different from those in the mother. Therefore, the extent of binding and ionization will be different on either side of the placental membrane.[171] There is, for example, a lower binding of amide-type local anesthetics in umbilical plasma than in maternal plasma. On the other hand, there is a possibility of greater binding of diazepam to fetal plasma proteins and fetal red cells. These differences in binding properties across the placenta will affect the gradient of the free, unbound portion of the drug and, therefore, the direction and rate of its transfer.

Compression of the Umbilical Cord During Delivery. Compression of the umbilical cord occurs to some extent in about one-third of vaginal deliveries.[83] This cord compression interferes with the transmission of drugs to and from the fetus.[104]

Protective Processes. The fetal liver, the progressive dilution of blood en route to the fetal brain, and the extensive shunting in the fetal circulation are all at least temporary protective factors tending to decrease the concentration of drug reaching the fetal brain. However, with time, the umbilical artery concentration approaches the umbilical vein concentration of the drug, and the quantity of the drug reaching the brain is high. Subsequently, continued redistribution of the drug within the fetus results in diminution of the drug concentration in the fetal brain. Meanwhile, in the case of a single dose, drug levels in maternal blood continue to decline, tending to establish a reverse gradient from the fetus outward. Thus, with time, both these factors contribute to lessening the effect of a bolus of a drug administered intravenously to the mother. This explains the maximum fetal depression between 3 and 7 minutes after intravenous injection of 8 mg./kg. of thiobarbiturate to the mother.[89] Before 3 minutes, delay in transmission to the fetus, the fetal liver uptake, and the progressive dilution and shunting in the fetus tend to protect the fetal brain. After 7 minutes, the progressive redistribution in the fetus and the fall in the maternal blood concentration tend to lower the brain level of thiobarbiturate, subsequently diminishing the fetal depression.[89] On the other hand, if the drug is repeatedly administered, the maternal blood concentration of the drug is sustained at a high level, and there is a tendency to "load" the fetus, despite the protective processes already mentioned.

TRANSFER OF SPECIFIC DRUGS RELATED TO OBSTETRIC ANESTHESIA AND ANALGESIA

Barbiturates

Barbiturates consist of highly lipid-soluble molecules which pass freely through the lipid membranes, such as the blood-brain, blood-placental, and other blood-tissue barriers. The slow-acting barbiturates, such as phenobarbital (Luminal), and the intermediate-acting barbiturates, such as amobarbital (Amytal), have been shown to traverse the blood-placental barrier rapidly and achieve equilibrium in 5 to 20 minutes. The fast-acting barbiturates, such as pentobarbital (Nembutal) and secobarbital (Seconal), can be detected in fetal blood within 1 minute of intravenous administration to the mother, and equilibrium is established between the mother and infant within 3 to 5 minutes. The initial studies of the placental transfer of the ultrafast-acting barbiturates, such as thiopental sodium (Pentothal), suggested that only minute amounts of the drug were found in the newborn infant during the first 5 to 7 minutes, and equilibrium between maternal and fetal blood was reached only after 10 to 12 minutes.[74] On the basis of this data, the misconception developed among clinicians that thiopental could be given to the mother without affecting the fetus if delivery were achieved within 8 minutes. However, subsequent studies showed that the drug passes the membrane within 45 seconds, achieving the highest concentration in the umbilical vein blood within 2 to 3 minutes after injection; then both maternal and fetal plasma concentrations of the drug fall exponentially (Fig. 3-2).[38,89] Since the metabolism of thiopental is slow (10–15% per hour), the fall in plasma concentration is mainly due to redistribution. In obstetrics, thiobarbiturate in a single dose of 4 mg./kg. is associated with the delivery of neonates of good Apgar score (7 or more)

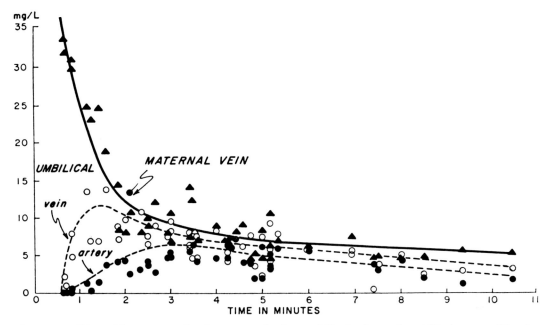

Fig. 3-2.   Thiamylal concentration in maternal vein, umbilical vein, and umbilical artery. (Kosaka, Y., Takahashi, T., and Mark, L. C.: Intravenous thiobarbiturate anesthesia for cesarean section. Anesthesiology, *31*:489, 1969)

in 90.0 per cent of cases. With a large dose (8 mg./kg.), marked neonatal depression can occur, since only 57.1 per cent of newborns had good Apgar scores. This is due to the associated high maternal and fetal blood levels of the drug. These neonates remain drowsy for many hours after delivery.[173] Repeated administration of small increments following the initial dose of thiobarbiturate has an intermediate effect. Therefore, in obstetrics, when a thiobarbiturate is to be used, the recommended dose is 4 mg./kg., administered once. Thiamylal and thiopental, both thiobarbiturates, have the same effect on the baby.[89]

Propanidid

Propanidid is a nonbarbiturate intravenous anesthetic. It is rapidly hydrolyzed in the body by esterases to pharmacologically inert products. Both maternal and fetal blood levels of propanidid are negligible within 3 to 4 minutes after intravenous injection.

Cholinesterase is present in large quantities in placental tissues and could play a part in breaking down propanidid, thus minimizing the concentration reaching the fetus.[39] This can explain the lower incidence of neonatal depression following propanidid induction (500 mg.) versus thiopental (250 mg.) for elective cesarean section.[13,27] However, the high incidence of maternal awareness and postoperative nausea and vomiting[44] are important disadvantages of propanidid.

In the author's opinion, if a thiobarbiturate dose is kept at or below 4 mg./kg., propanidid does not offer a practical advantage over the former drug.

Narcotics and Their Antagonists

Narcotics. There is extensive evidence in the literature that narcotics cross the blood-placental barrier.[7,22,109,119,153] This was suspected as early as 1885.[132] Narcotics are capable of causing fetal and neonatal depression. Fetal depression can be indicated by the onset of bradycardia (an average drop of 17 beats per minute) following maternal administration of morphine.[68] Neonatal depression is evidenced by respiratory depression, myosis, absence of reflexes, and hypotonia. It is advisable to avoid administration of narcotics to the mother when delivery is expected between 1 and 4 hours following their intramuscular administration. It is our policy to use narcotics only in the early part of the first stage of labor. If delivery occurs rapidly and unexpectedly after administration of a narcotic to the mother, naloxone (Narcan) can be injected into the umbilical vein postpartum. Synthetic narcotics are relatively safe for the fetus because they do not traverse the fetal brain barrier as easily as morphine.[101] Two of the commonly used narcotics in obstetrics, namely meperidine and pentazocine, require a more detailed discussion.

Meperidine rapidly crosses the blood-placental barrier.[26] After intravenous administration to the mother, the umbilical vein level reaches 70 per cent of the maternal level in 30 seconds. This is then maintained for 5 to 10 minutes, to be followed by a rapid decay.[23] Meperidine concentration is higher in the umbilical vein than in the umbilical artery for the first 3 to 5 minutes, but thereafter the levels virtually equalize. The maternal metabolites of meperidine also cross the placenta. Most studies have shown no correlation of the Apgar scores and the clinical condition of the infant with the level of meperidine in the plasma. However, there is always the possibility of neonatal depression following meperidine administration to the mother,[26] particularly when it is given shortly before delivery. With the use of continuous regional analgesia, the need for narcotics and the subsequent fetal depression are diminished.

Pentazocine (Talwin), a member of the benzomorphan series, is a potent analgesic; 40 mg. of pentazocine has an analgesic effect equal to 100 mg. of meperidine.[109] It has a low abuse liability and, therefore, it is not subject to narcotic control. Moreover, pentazocine has less emetic effect than meperidine.[115] With regard to its effects on the fetus, animal experiments have demonstrated no teratogenic or embryotoxic results.[177] However, the safety of its use during pregnancy is still uncertain.

During labor, pentazocine has proved to be a satisfactory analgesic drug,[46] crossing the placenta to a lesser degree than meperidine.[19] It causes no significant change in fetal heart rate.[4,52,107,109] Following its administration to the mother, the incidence of neonatal depression is not significant. Moore, Carson, and Hunter[109] found that following pentazocine administration to mothers within 4 hours before delivery, 2.6 per cent of the neonates were depressed, as compared with 6.8 per cent following administration of meperidine. However, Mowat, and Garney[115] found no significant difference between the two drugs in regard to neonatal depression.

Premixed Solutions of Narcotics. It is claimed that administration of premixed narcotic solutions can produce analgesia in the mother without fetal or maternal depression. Unfortunately, these claims have not been borne out by careful clinical trials. On the contrary, the premixed solutions provide less analgesia and have more side effects in the mother and fetus, and their use is not advised.[23]

Narcotic Antagonists. Narcotic antagonists, such as nalorphine, levallorphan, and naloxone (Narcan), also have been found to cross the placental membrane rapidly. This is not unexpected since they represent only slight modifications in the molecular structure of narcotics. The best available narcotic antagonist is naloxone. This is because it is effective and will not depress the newborn if the cause of depression is other than narcotics. Moreover, naloxone does not cause respiratory depression, even with overdosage. It can be administered to the mother intravenously (0.01 mg./kg.), in the adult injection form (0.4 mg./ml.), 10 to 15 minutes before delivery. Alternatively, it can be injected into the umbilical vein immediately after delivery, in which case its action is apparent in 30 to 90 seconds, or injected intramuscularly to the newborn, in which case the onset of action occurs in 3 to 5 minutes. The umbilical vein route is, if feasible, the route of choice. The dose is 0.01 mg./kg., available in neonatal injection form (0.02 mg./ml.) It is advisable to wait for 1 minute after injection and then to clamp the cord and separate the fetus. In this way the narcotic is antagonized in the fetus without depriving the mother of the analgesic and sedative effects of the narcotic. The fetal depression that follows neuroleptanalgesia in obstetrics can be corrected in the same way.

Tranquilizers

Chlorpromazine (Thorazine), promethazine (Phenergan), and promazine (Sparine) can be found in the umbilical vein blood within 1.5 to 2 minutes after intravenous administration to the mother, with a maximum fetal concentration occurring during the ensuing 2 to 3 minutes.[38] Most studies have shown that the concentration of the drug in the fetal blood is lower than that in the maternal blood. A significantly greater proportion of these drugs is passed to the fetus after intravenous administration to the mother than after intramuscular administration.

Diazepam (Valium). Diazepam is a drug which has only recently been used in obstetrics for its anticonvulsing, muscle-relaxing, amnesic, and tranquilizing actions. It has also been found to potentiate the analgesic effect of meperidine.[59] It rapidly crosses the placenta to the fetus. After intravenous administration to the mother during labor, it appears within 10 minutes in the fetal blood.[146] After intramuscular administration to the mother, diazepam reaches its peak in the maternal blood in 30 minutes and in the fetal blood

in 60 minutes.[81] The level of diazepam in the fetal blood is at least equal to,[42] if not higher than, the level in the maternal blood.[146] This can be due to more binding of diazepam to fetal blood cells and plasma proteins.[81] Diazepam concentrates in the fetal liver, which metabolizes the drug at a much slower rate than the adult liver (1:10).[81]

With regard to the effects of diazepam on the fetus, Flowers and coworkers[59] found that a significantly higher percentage of infants whose mothers had received diazepam were depressed as compared with those whose mothers had received no diazepam. The depressed neonates were characteristically hypotonic. The depressant effect of diazepam on the fetus was also manifested by loss of the normal beat-to-beat variation and periodic oscillations in the fetal heart rate,[46] which followed a relatively large intravenous dose (20 mg.) to mothers in labor. This cardiac action of diazepam can be due to sleepiness of the fetus, to the depressant effect of the drug on the cardiac reflex centers in the brain, or both.[18] However, this effect on the fetal heart rate is temporary and not associated with fetal acidosis.

In our experience, small intravenous doses of diazepam (2.5 mg. at a time, to a maximum of 10 mg.) usually have no fetal side effects during labor and delivery. In the uncooperative apprehensive patient, one or two of these increment doses are quite helpful for epidural or subarachnoid block, causing her sedation and relaxation during the procedure. Doses of 10 mg. are rarely exceeded in obstetrics, except as a treatment of convulsions.

Hydroxyzine Hydrochloride (Vistaril). Hydroxyzine hydrochloride is a tranquilizer that has been used in obstetrics without clinical ill effects on the fetus.[16,20,82] However, no data are available as yet regarding its transmission to the fetus.

Muscle Relaxants

Muscle relaxants possess a low degree of

fat solubility and are highly ionized at normal pH range. Because of these properties, they pass the blood-brain barrier and the blood-placental barrier with great difficulty. Usual clinical doses have no demonstrable effect on the newborn. If massive doses of these drugs (10 times the therapeutic dose, or more) are injected into the maternal circulation, the gradient across the placenta becomes so high that the relaxant is detected in appreciable amounts in the fetal blood and can have clinical effects on the newborn. Some of the commonly used muscle relaxants are discussed below.

Curare. The transplacental transmission of curare has interested many investigators for almost a century. Animal experiments have been widely performed since 1885.[132] Curare is one of the few drugs whose transplacental transmission has been tested from mother to fetus and vice versa. With regard to its transmission from mother to fetus in experimental animals, Preyer[132] and Harroun and Fisher[71] found no harmful effects on the fetus, provided the mother was well ventilated. Pittinger and Morris,[128] using dogs, injected huge amounts of curare into the uterine artery of the mother. This resulted in partially curarized pups. With regard to transmission from fetus to mother, Preyer[132] and Buller and Young[28] found that the drug can pass the placental barrier and cause maternal paralysis if injected into the fetal blood in massive doses.

Quantitative estimations of curare in the fetus after maternal administration have been performed.[32,40,130] The results indicate that after intravenous administration of the drug to the mother, the drug is transmitted to the fetus, but in such minute traces that it has no harmful effect on the fetus or newborn. These laboratory results were in accordance with the safe clinical use of the drug in obstetrics.[32,40,67,130,174,175]

The transmission of curare to, and its distribution in, the human fetus during the first trimester was recently studied using ^{14}C-dimethyltubocurarine.[88] The results show that ^{14}C-dimethyltubocurarine concentration in fetal plasma was about one-tenth of the maternal plasma concentration. ^{14}C-dimethyltubocurarine is transmitted to the fetus mainly in the intact form. Only a small part of its metabolites passes the placental barrier. Of the fetal tissues, the lungs and the liver showed the highest concentration. As expected, a markedly lower concentration was found in the brain tissue. The fetal brain concentration was about one-tenth per gram the fetal plasma concentration per milliliter and, since the fetal plasma concentration is about one-tenth the maternal plasma concentration, the similarity between the blood-brain barrier and the blood-placental barrier becomes evident. In summary, curare is safe to use in obstetric anesthesia in a dose of 0.4 mg./kg., provided the mother is adequately ventilated.

Gallamine Triethiodide (Flaxedil). Schwarz[147] determined the iodide concentration in the fetal blood at the time of delivery after maternal administration of gallamine. He found that 6 to 9 minutes after the injection of 80 mg. of gallamine triethiodide, significant increases in the concentration of iodide occurred in the neonate. Schwarz interpreted this as evidence that gallamine had crossed the placenta. This is why many anesthesiologists refrain from using it. However, since gallamine triethiodide is a quaternary ammonium salt, it is completely ionized in aqueous solution, and consequently, the transport of the triethylgallamine ion and the iodide ion through the body membranes will be independent of each other. Hence, iodide concentrations gave no indication of triethylgallamine concentrations. This explains the discrepancy between the clinical effects on the newborn and the laboratory findings. Based on the clinical effects on the fetus, Pittinger and Morris[129] found gallamine to be less transmissible than D-tubocurarine across the dog placenta. In humans, Crawford and Gardiner[40] found that, although gallamine in appreciable concentrations was detected in the fetal cord blood, none of the infants was depressed. Based on clinical results, Thomas and Gibson [166] and Bakhoum and Abouleish,[11] found gallamine safe in obstetrics. Therefore, further studies are required to clarify the placental transmission of gallamine and its effect on the fetus and newborn.

Succinylcholine. The transfer of succinylcholine has been examined by Moya[116] and Kvisselgaard,[118] who found that the drug did not pass from mother to fetus following normal clinical doses, but that low fetal plasma concentrations could be detected following a 300-mg. dose to the mother. Since the usual dose of succinylcholine is 1 mg./kg., this dose (300 mg. as a bolus) is several times the therapeutic dose. However, using ^{14}C succinyldicholine in monkeys, Drabkova and coworkers[45] found that succinylcholine in doses of 2 to 3 mg./kg., and in repeated doses of 1.2 mg./kg. injected intravenously, is rapidly transmitted to the fetus. The fetal level of succinylcholine slightly affected the electromyograph, with no depressant effect on the fetal respiration. Succinylcholine has been extensively used as a muscle relaxant in obstetrics, particularly for cesarean section. It has proved to be satisfactory and safe.

Alcuronium. Recently introduced as a safe, nondepolarizing muscle relaxant, alcuronium has also been used with favorable results in obstetrics.[37,148,163,167] Like most muscle relaxants, it crosses the placenta to the fetus in minute quantities without ill effects on the newborn.[168] When 10 to 15 mg. was injected slowly intravenously over a period of 2 to 6 minutes, it did not cross the placenta. This signifies the importance of the rate of injection as a factor for drug transmission to the fetus.

Pancuronium. Although no evidence is available in man, animal experiments suggest that in normal dosage pancuronium does not cross the placental barrier.[179] It has been used in cesarean section without ill effect on the newborn.[23,93] The dose is usually 0.065 mg./kg. Pancuronium has certain advantages over curare; pancuronium does not cause hypotension or histamine release. It is rapidly gaining an eminent place as a muscle relaxant in obstetrics.[122]

Belladonna Drugs

Belladonna drugs pass the blood-placental barrier; 1 mg. of atropine intravenously administered to the mother produces fetal tachycardia[75] and neonatal mydriasis.[132] Administration of atropine to the mother can prevent fetal bradycardia that occurs with maternal hemorrhage but will not correct the associated fetal hypoxia.[21] Thus, in acute fetal distress, atropine should not be used as a therapeutic measure to improve the fetal condition because, even if the fetal heart rate increases, fetal acidosis still persists. Scopolamine administered to the mother not only has a potentially depressant effect on the fetus,[58] but also it frequently causes agitation of the parturient. At one time, scopolamine was frequently used for its amnesic effect. Its combination with morphine, the so-called "twilight sleep," is only mentioned to be condemned and has no place in modern obstetrics because it predisposes to fetal and maternal depression, agitation, and inadequacy of pain relief. The loss of fetal beat-to-beat variability as a result of maternal administration of belladonna alkaloids may interfere with interpretation of fetal heart rate tracings. To reverse this effect, 2 to 5 mg. of physostigmine in 1-mg. increments is injected intravenously into the maternal circulation.[50]

Catecholamines

Rapid transfer of the catecholamines, norepinephrine, and isoproterenol from the maternal to the fetal side of the placenta has been demonstrated *in vitro* in the human placenta and *in vivo* in the guinea pig.[111] There are certain clinical implications in these findings. Isoproterenol is widely employed in the treatment of asthma in both pregnant and nonpregnant patients. While deleterious effects on the fetus have not, to date, been reported, these findings should alert obstetricians to the possible consequences should this powerful drug gain access to the fetal circulation. The ability of the placental monamine oxidases to deaminate catecholamines is limited to normal physiologic levels.[101]

Magnesium

Parenterally administered magnesium sulfate has been extensively used, at least in the United States, as an integral part of treatment of toxemias of pregnancy.[76] Therefore, the transplacental transmission of this drug and its effect on the fetus are important. Magnesium sulfate readily crosses the blood-placental barrier, and the fetal blood level of the drug rapidly reaches that of the mother.[134] The effect of Mg^{++} on the fetus is still debatable. Hutchinson and coworkers[79] and Stone and Pritchard[162] found no evidence of the adverse action of Mg^{++} on the infant. On the other hand, Lipsitz and English[96] found that Mg^{++} can cause fetal depression. Their findings showed that the clinical manifestations in the newborn with hypermagnesemia were similar to those in the adult—namely, hypotonia, hyporeflexia, hypotension, and respiratory depression. These symptoms should be looked for in newborns delivered from mothers who have had magnesium sulfate prior to delivery. The effects of excess magnesium or other central nervous system depressants on the already compromised newborn of a toxemic mother can be serious. Therefore, it is advisable to have the personnel and equipment ready for neonatal resuscitation whenever a toxemic mother is in labor.

Local Anesthetics

Local anesthetic drugs cross the placenta from mother to fetus[61,113,154] and from fetus to mother.[112] When these drugs are administered for regional analgesia in obstetrics, they are rapidly absorbed into the maternal blood and transmitted across the placenta.[10,57,65,113,154] Except in the case of spinal analgesia, relatively large doses are necessary, and these occasionally result in a high blood level of the drug in the fetus and neonatal depression.[105,113]

In discussing transmission of local anesthetics across the placental membrane and their effect and distribution in the fetus, two aspects of the subject have to be considered: (1) the drug used and (2) the regional technique applied.

Choice of Local Anesthetic Drug.
Ester-type drugs, such as procaine, chloroprocaine, and tetracaine, are broken down by esterases in maternal and fetal plasma and placenta. Moreover, since procaine is highly ionizable at normal maternal pH, it will not cross the placenta readily.[179]

Amide-type drugs have different pKa values and lipid solubility, and some have vasoconstrictor or vasodilator effects. Therefore, if administered epidurally in equal doses, they attain different maternal blood values; the ratio of mepivacaine to lidocaine to bupivacaine is 3:2:1.[137] For the same reasons, they cross the placental barrier to a different extent and the fetal-maternal ratio varies with the anesthetic drug. The umbilical venous plasma level is on the average 30 per cent of the maternal venous plasma level for bupivacaine,[171] 55 per cent for lidocaine,[138] and 70 per cent for mepivacaine.[113]

In contrast to findings with lidocaine, mepivacaine, and bupivacaine, data obtained from a study involving epidural administration of prilocaine suggested net reverse transfer of this drug across the placenta in about 50 minutes after administration. This is evidenced by concentration ratios of drugs in the umbilical artery to drug in the umbilical vein greater than unity.[131] Umbilical levels of prilocaine slightly in excess of corresponding maternal levels have also been reported.[72,131] The fact that prilocaine is less bound to maternal plasma than other amide drugs[51] may help to explain these findings.

In epidural analgesia, epinephrine added to the local anesthetic lowers the maternal blood level of the local anesthetic and therefore, by decreasing the threshold across the placental membrane, decreases the level in the fetus. This is evident with local anesthetics such as lidocaine.[61] However, with bupivacaine, the addition of epinephrine did not significantly alter the fetal blood level of the local anesthetic.[137] This is probably due to the initially low level of maternal bupivacaine, the minor effect of epinephrine on the maternal level, the inherent vasoconstrictor effect of bupivacaine, and the change of the pH of the solution by the addition of epinephrine. Therefore, when bupivacaine is used for epidural analgesia, the addition of epinephrine does not add to the fetal protection and can even prolong the course of labor[70] or cause hypotension,[172] both these results being undesirable. Moreover, epinephrine may reduce uterine blood flow either by redistribution of the cardiac output or by direct action on the uterine blood vessels. In conclusion, with the use of bupivacaine, the addition of epinephrine to the local anesthetic in obstetrics has been discontinued (see Chap. 4).

Of the amide-type agents, the drug of choice for epidural analgesia is bupivacaine, not only because it has the longest analgesic action, but also because it reaches the lowest maternal level and is the least transmitted to the fetus.[80] The least recommended drug for regional anesthesia is prilocaine, because of its high fetal transmission and its tendency to cause methemoglobinemia in the mother and fetus.[9,131]

Choice of Regional Technique. The following regional anesthetic techniques are presented in the order of increasing transmission of the local anesthetic and its effect on the fetus and newborn:

1. *Spinal.* The spinal technique makes use of the lowest dosage of local anesthetic. Thus there is no evidence that fetal depression can be due to the local anesthetic *per se* when used for the subarachnoid block.

2. *Lumbar Epidural and Caudal.* It is widely believed that little of the local anesthetic agent administered into the epidural space of the mother reaches the fetus.[61,154,171] The infants are usually vigorous at birth, provided there have been no maternal complications, such as maternal hypotension or convulsions.[72,133]

3. *Paracervical Block.* This is the only regional analgesic technique in obstetrics that exposes the fetus to the risk of overdosage (see Chap. 16). Following paracervical block, the high level of the local anesthetic in the fetal blood leads to myocardial depression, bradycardia, and fetal acidosis.[10,62,65,140,152,155,165] Furthermore, a number of cases of perinatal deaths have been ascribed to local anesthetic intoxication of the fetus following paracervical block.[49,124,143,165]

Fetal Distribution of Local Anesthetics. Finster and coworkers[57] have studied the distribution of lidocaine in pregnant guinea pigs. Following intravenous injection of lidocaine to the mother (10 mg./kg.), fetal levels of the drug in the blood and most parenchymatous organs were found to be consistently lower than maternal levels. The only parenchymatous organ exhibiting higher fetal than maternal levels of lidocaine was the liver. This was attributed to the strategic position of the liver in the fetal circulation as well as to the deficiency of drug-metabolizing enzymes in the fetal and newborn liver.[60]

On the whole, compared with general anesthesia, regional analgesia has been associated with excellent Apgar scores,[77,100,119] and, in the author's opinion, it is the best and safest method of control of obstetric pain in most cases of labor, delivery, and cesarean section.

Dissociative Anesthetics

Ketamine, a phenocyclidine derivative, will be discussed as an example of a dissociative anesthetic. Ketamine has recently been used in obstetrics.[6,29,91,97,99,110] It has the following *advantages*:

1. Rapid induction
2. Intense analgesia. Therefore, 100 per cent oxygen can be used until the fetus is delivered[99]
3. Strong uterine contractions[84,97] with the decreased possibility of postpartum bleeding
4. Rise of blood pressure, making it a suitable induction agent in cases of antepartum hemorrhage and hypotensive conditions of the mother
5. Easy airway maintenance and less obtundation of the protective pharyngeal and laryngeal reflexes than other induction agents
6. Minimal respiratory depression with slow injection of low doses required for light anesthesia. This is advantageous because it abolishes the hyperventilation and respiratory alkalosis associated with labor
7. A bronchodilator effect, making it suitable for patients with asthmatic disease.[35]

Ketamine has the following *disadvantages* for the mother:

1. Hallucinations and unpleasant dreams. These can be reduced, but not eliminated, by proper use of adjuvant drugs such as droperidol.[145]
2. Rise of blood pressure. Therefore, it is not a suitable anesthetic for mothers with hypertensive disease (e.g., preeclampsia).
3. Possibility of aspiration. Although ketamine causes minimal obtundation of the upper airway reflexes, cases of aspiration have been reported following its administration.[126]
4. Respiratory depression. With excessive speed of administration and/or excessive dosage, maternal respiratory depression and apnea occur.[97] This apnea is accompanied in both mother and fetus by a relatively stiff chest that makes effective controlled respiration difficult.[151]
5. Increase of uterine tone. This may decrease the placental perfusion, thus contributing to fetal depression.[63]
6. Excessive salivation, nausea, and vomiting. These undesirable side effects occur in two-thirds of obstetric cases.[97]

During labor, ketamine and one of its two metabolites cross the blood-placental barrier.[97] The maternal level is always higher than the fetal level. The maternal to fetal ratio reaches a steady level in as little as 5 minutes with little subsequent variation. The clinical effects of ketamine transmission on the fetus and newborn are still debatable. Some authors consider it to have no harmful effect.[29,91,99] However, others found that it caused lowering of the fetal pH and increased P_{CO_2} with a variable effect on P_{aO_2}.[97] These changes were reflected by increased fetal depression, as indicated by low Apgar scores at 1 minute (avg. 4–6).[97,110] Endotracheal intubation for resuscitation was required in a number of cases but was difficult because of excessive muscle tone.[110] After the initial depression, all infants returned rapidly to normal, as evidenced by the high Apgar scores at 5 minutes (avg. 8) and 10 minutes (avg. 9). The ketamine fetal depression is proportionate to the dose given to the mother. Recently, it has been found that with a low intravenous dose of 0.2 to 0.4 mg./kg. and a dosage limit of 100 mg., fetal and maternal side effects are minimal.[6] The action of ketamine on the EEG and on a potential epileptic character are still controversial.[34,176] Its safe use in preeclamptic and eclamptic patients has yet to be documented.

Whether ketamine offers advantages over other available drugs used in obstetrics and whether its use is safer for the fetus and neonate await further studies. Until these are completed, the author does not recommend ketamine in obstetrics except as an induction agent in emergency hypotensive conditions or in the asthmatic mother.

Inhalation Anesthetics

All inhalation anesthetic gases or vapors pass through the placental membrane rapidly. Their high speed of transfer is related to their rapid rate of diffusion, relatively high fat solubility, and usual low molecular weight. Administered in analgesic concentration with the mother awake, oriented, and cooperative, no significant depression of the newborn is seen, regardless of duration of administration and agent used.[23] However, when administered in anesthetic concentrations, the degree of neonatal depression is proportionate to the depth and duration of maternal anesthesia.

Nitrous Oxide. Nitrous oxide, having a small molecular size, is rapidly transmitted from the mother to the fetus. Earlier studies[32,158] indicated that the fetal blood levels of nitrous oxide were 50 to 65 per cent of the maternal levels. However, recent studies using more refined techniques of measurement show that the fetal to maternal ratio averages 80 per cent after anesthesia has exceeded 3 minutes.[104] Uptake of the agent by fetal tissues is also rapid, with the umbilical artery to umbilical vein blood nitrous oxide concentration ratio increasing progressively with the duration of anesthesia.[104] Thus the difference between umbilical vein and umbilical artery levels is decreased with time. Increasing the duration of anesthesia from 3 to 19 minutes raises the level of nitrous oxide in the umbilical artery from 34 to 90 per cent of the umbilical vein level and from 23 to 78 per cent of the maternal arterial level.[104] This

fetal transmission of nitrous oxide is unrelated to maternal carbon dioxide tension or pH and occurs in both vaginal delivery and cesarean section. The increase of nitrous oxide in fetal tissues with time leads to the buildup of the anesthetic drug in the fetal brain, with subsequent fetal depression proportionate to the induction-delivery time.

The conclusion is that the increased incidence of neonatal depression following nitrous oxide anesthesia exceeding 15 minutes may represent fetal narcosis. In addition, diffusion hypoxia plays an important role as a cause of neonatal depression. Rapid diffusion of nitrous oxide from pulmonary capillary blood to alveoli commences with the first breath of life, and this process reduces oxygen partial pressure in the alveoli, resulting in hypoxemia and neonatal depression.[33,136] *Therefore, it is our policy that every newborn delivered after nitrous oxide anesthesia to the mother should receive oxygen by face mask for at least a few minutes, irrespective of its Apgar score.*

Methoxyflurane. Methoxyflurane and its metabolites cross the blood-placental barrier rapidly, with the potential effect of fetal and neonatal depression.[149,169] However, the acid-base status of infants delivered under methoxyflurane anesthesia is normal.[30,36] There is considerable fetal uptake of methoxyflurane, whether the latter is used for analgesia or anesthesia. This is indicated by the higher level of umbilical vein concentration than that of the umbilical artery.[92] Clark and coworkers[30] found a correlation between the methoxyflurane level in the umbilical vein and artery and fetal depression. They set critical levels of methoxyflurane in the fetus beyond which fetal depression is liable to occur. The critical level in the umbilical vein is 6 mg./100 ml. and in the umbilical artery is 3 mg./100 ml. However, no such correlation was found by other investigators.[93,156] In analgesic concentrations, methoxyflurane does not depress the fetus.[31,93] In anesthetic concentrations it can depress the fetus, depending on duration of anesthesia and concentration used, as evidenced by the following studies:

1. When methoxyflurane was used for short periods of time (1–15 minutes), as for vaginal delivery, the maternal blood level was high (4.25 mg./100 ml.). However, the mean umbilical vein and artery levels were low (1.99 mg./100 ml. and 0.85 mg./100 ml. respectively), and the neonates were not depressed.[31] The shortness of the time during which the mothers were exposed to the anesthetic apparently prevented high levels of the anesthetic from occurring in these infants.

2. When methoxyflurane was used intermittently as an analgesic for labor, and then as an anesthetic for the actual delivery, the mean methoxyflurane level in the maternal venous blood was higher (5.4 mg./100 ml.). The mean blood levels in umbilical vein and artery were higher (3.68 mg./100 ml. and 1.69 mg./100 ml. respectively), and about one-sixth of the neonates were depressed.[31]

3. When 0.1 per cent methoxyflurane was used to supplement nitrous oxide and oxygen muscle-relaxant anesthesia for cesarean section, there was no fetal depression related to methoxyflurane.[93] The mean maternal artery level at delivery was low (1.72 mg./100 ml.), and the mean umbilical vein level was even lower (0.54 mg./ 100 ml.). The low concentration of methoxyflurane used here (0.1%) in contrast to the higher concentrations in the other methods mentioned above (avg. 0.5%) explains the lower levels of the drug in both the mother and fetus and the better conditions of the neonates.

Halothane. Halothane has been used in obstetric anesthesia.[17,43,87,108,161] However, halothane can cause maternal hypotension and relaxation of the uterus with the possibility of postpartum hemorrhage.[120,121] Moreover, it rapidly crosses the blood-placental barrier,[150] with the potentiality of neonatal depression. Some anesthesiologists use a small concentration of halothane to supplement nitrous oxide and oxygen for cesarean section. Moir[108] found the use of muscle relaxants and nitrous oxide and oxygen (70:30) was accompanied by more depressed newborns than was the case when using muscle relaxants and nitrous oxide and oxygen (50:50) supplemented by 0.5 per cent halothane. The administration of 0.5 per cent halothane to the mother did not cause neonatal depression. By allowing an increase in the percentage of oxygen in the nitrous oxide-oxygen mixture, and probably by slightly relaxing the uterine muscle, the condition of the newborns was better. This was in agreement with the work of Rorke and coworkers,[141] who found that, as the maternal PaO_2 rose toward 300 mm. Hg, fetal oxygenation and neonatal Apgar scores improved. Halothane (0.5%) did not lead to maternal hypotension or increase in the postpartum hemorrhage. The incidence of awareness of the mother during general anesthesia was 0.0 per cent with halothane addition, as compared with 2 per cent when only nitrous oxide and oxygen were administered.[108] However, the use of 0.7 per cent halothane was accompanied by maternal hypotension, excessive bleeding, and more fetal depression, therefore, it is not advisable. Therefore, the safety of halothane is limited. Its safe use in toxemic patients where liver dysfunction is common has yet to be proven. Many anesthesiologists believe that halothane has little place in obstetric anesthesia unless intrauterine manipulations are required (e.g., internal podalic version).

Cyclopropane. Like all other inhalation anesthetics, cyclopropane has no depressant effect on the fetus in analgesic doses. In anesthetic doses it does depress the fetus. The fetal depression is proportionate to the duration of anesthesia and the concentration of cyclopropane in the anesthetic mixture. Fetal transmission has been studied by many investigators.[8,78,144,157] Cycloproprane can be detected in the umbilical cord blood within 1.5 minutes of its administration to the mother. Subsequently, both the fetal and maternal blood levels of cyclopropane rise with increased duration of anesthesia. Fetal blood level usually reaches 80 per cent of maternal blood level.

Diethyl Ether. Ether is rapidly transmitted to the fetus. The level in fetal blood is proportionate to duration of anesthesia and ether concentration. Fetal blood concentration can reach 96 per cent of maternal blood concentration within 15 minutes.[159]

Trichloroethylene. Owing to its high lipid solubility, trichloroethylene is very rapidly transmitted to the fetus, and fetal blood level can exceed maternal blood level in 16 minutes.[73] This is due to the greater affinity of the drug for fetal than for maternal blood.

Chloroform. Chloroform has low molecular weight and high fat solubility. Therefore, as expected, it passes rapidly to the fetus. In analgesic concentrations, it has no more depressant effect on the newborn than nitrous oxide; in anesthetic concentrations, it consistently depresses the neonate.[116]

Other New Anesthetics. Many new anesthetic drugs have been introduced to anesthesia (e.g., Ethrane, fluroxene, and forane). Of these, the most recommended drug is fluroxene because of its rapid onset of action, good analgesic properties, increase of cardiac output, and peripheral vasodilatation. This is why it is recommended for anesthesia for patients with sickle cell disease.[102] Fluroxene is readily transmitted through the placenta to the fetus.[103] The fetal to maternal concentration ratio is increased with increasing duration of anesthesia and concentration of the anesthetic. However, significant fetal depression has not been attributed to fluroxene. Fluroxene has a depressant action on uterine contractions, which is dose-related.[180] It is also a halogenated compound which does not seem to be free of the problems associated with other halogenated compounds in use—chiefly, the possibility of liver damage.

TRANSFER OF OXYGEN TO THE FETUS

To discuss the various factors influencing the fetal oxygenation, the oxygen transport from the maternal alveoli to the fetus is followed. Each step tends to facilitate this process.

Maternal Factors

Hyperventilation Plus Decreased Dead Space During Pregnancy. This leads to a higher maternal arterial Po_2 than in the nonpregnant state (see Chap. 2).

Increased Cell Mass. During pregnancy, hormonal factors, such as placental lactogen, play an important role in augmenting the erythyropoietin secretion by the kidneys.[85] This leads to bone marrow stimulation, resulting in an increase of the red cell mass by about 500 ml.

Increased Cardiac Output. The cardiac output is gradually increased with pregnancy, reaching 30 to 40 per cent above the nonpregnant state.[94] The increase in cardiac output facilitates the transport of oxygen to the placenta.

Decreased Blood Viscosity. During pregnancy the maternal blood viscosity is decreased, owing to the relatively higher increase in the plasma volume than in the cell mass. This decreased viscosity allows for better perfusion of the intervillous space. Conditions associated with increased viscosity (e.g., active sickling of the red cells), can jeopardize the fetus.

Decreased Vascular Resistance at the Uterine Arterioles. At full term, the uterine arterioles are considered maximally dilated, leading to optimum perfusion of the intervillous space. Diseases or factors that increase the uterine vascular resistance can lead to fetal hypoxia.

Maternal Hemoglobin Oxygen Dissociation Curve. The female is naturally adapted for delivering oxygen to the fetus. The blood of normal nonpregnant women releases more oxygen under standard conditions than that of normal men, and the female hemoglobin-oxygen dissociation curve is shifted to the right.[47] The increased concentration of 2,3-diphosphoglycerate (2,3-DPG) is probably the cause. With pregnancy, there is further increase in 2,3-DPG, especially in the latter half of gestation.[142] The increase in this factor weakens the attachment of oxygen to the Hb molecule, and thus oxygen is readily released. The increase in 2,3-DPG is therefore said to cause a shift in the hemoglobin-oxygen dissociation curve to the right (i.e., more oxygen is released at a certain pressure). Owing to the hyperventilation during pregnancy, there is associated respiratory alkalosis which tends to shift the Hb-O_2 dissociation curve to the

left (i.e., making it difficult for oxygen to be released at the intervillous space). However, the increase in 2,3-DPG overcompensates for the respiratory alkalosis, resulting in an overall shift in the Hb-O_2 dissociation curve to the right.

In the intervillous space, the maternal blood not only gives oxygen, but also gains CO_2, thus becoming more acidotic. Acidosis weakens the O_2-Hb attachment, and the oxygen release is therefore more than with alkaline blood at the same pressure; the Hb-O_2 dissociation curve is said to be shifted to the right (Fig. 3-3A). This displacement is called the Bohr effect. On the fetal side, the blood circulating through the umbilical arteries is more acidic and, as it passes through the umbilical capillary, it loses CO_2 and becomes more alkaline (Table 3-6). Thus the Hb-O_2 binding becomes stronger, and more oxy-

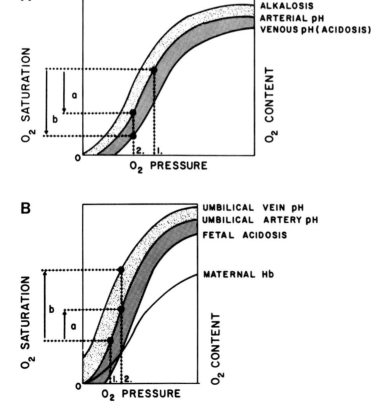

Fig. 3.3 Hemoglobin-oxygen dissociation curves of mother and fetus at the intervillous space. *A.* Oxygen given by mother. The oxygen liberated by the decrease in oxygen tension from 1 to 2 is "a" if the pH of the blood remains the same. However, owing to CO_2 uptake by the maternal blood the pH of the blood decreases, thus, the O_2 liberated increases to "b." *B.* Oxygen taken by fetus. As the fetal blood releases CO_2, it becomes more alkaline, thus the amount of O_2 carried is increased from "a" to "b."

Table 3-6. Normal Fetal pH and Blood Gases*

Site	Po_2 (torr)	Pco_2 (torr)	pH
Umbilical vein	23–32	40–50	7.3–7.35
Umbilical artery	15–23	45–65	7.2–7.3

*Mother spontaneously breathing room air.

gen can be carried by the fetal Hb (Fig. 3-3B). The Bohr effect at the placenta, by acting both on the maternal and fetal blood, enhances the transport of oxygen from the mother to the fetus.

Placental Factors

Owing to their small molecules, oxygen and carbon dioxide cross the placenta by simple diffusion. The maternal PaO_2 is always much higher than the fetal Po_2 and the difference increases as the former rises. On breathing room air, for example, the maternal PaO_2 is about 104 torr, while the fetal O_2 in the umbilical vein is about 30 torr. Increasing the maternal PaO_2 to 300 torr causes an increase in fetal Po_2 to only 45 torr.[12,105] Further increase in maternal PaO_2 does not result in an increase in fetal Po_2.

Not only is hyperoxygenation of the mother and fetus not harmful, but also the neonatal condition is better with high fetal oxygen. That is why it is advantageous to administer oxygen to the mother with a compromised fetus and in cases of cesarean section. However, the rise in fetal oxygen levels following administration of O_2 to the mother is not as significant with a diseased placenta as with normal conditions.

The marked gradient between maternal and fetal Po_2 is due to two factors:

1. The thickness of the tissues separating the maternal from the fetal blood. In the lungs, the oxygen in the air sacs is separated only by two thin layers of epithelium, the alveolar and capillary membranes. In the placenta the fetal capillary is separated from the intervillous spaced by the wall of the villi, which varies considerably in its thickness in different locations and at different stages of fetal development. It is thinnest near term to provide the least resistance to diffusion of oxygen and other needed materials. However, the thickness of a mature human placenta varies from 3 to 30 μ.

2. Nonhomogenicity of the blood in the intervillous space. The Po_2 in the intervillous space varies between 100 and 40 torr. Thus the villi exposed to the maternal blood of low Po_2 do not have a good chance of taking a large amount of oxygen.

In spite of these difficulties, the placenta has favorable characteristics for oxygen transport, such as the extensive surface area of the villi and the slow rate of flow, allowing better equilibrium between the two sides.

Fetal Factors

Increased Red Cell Mass and Higher Hb Concentration. In the fetus there is polycythemia in order to carry oxygen more efficiently. This is the most important fetal factor in the oxygen transport.

Fetal Hemoglobin. Fetal hemoglobin has more affinity to oxygen than maternal hemoglobin; in other words, its Hb-O_2 dissociation curve is shifted more to the left (see Fig. 3-3B).[123] It is also characterized by the fact that its dissociation curve is steeper, especially at O_2 pressures from 15 to 30 torr (i.e., slight increase in pressure results in marked oxygen-carrying capacity). This might be due to the reduced 2,3-DPG in fetal blood.[86] However, fetal Hb is not essential for fetal survival since intrauterine transfusion with adult erythrocytes has been successful.

Increased Cardiac Output. Normally, the fetal heart rate is fast (120–150 beats/min.) This helps to transfer oxygen from the placenta to the fetal tissues.

On the whole, it should be considered that normally the fetus is adequately oxygenated, and not present in a hypoxic atmosphere. The low fetal Po_2 is compensated for by the other fetal factors, mainly increased hemoglobin. The result is that, under normal circumstances, oxygen supply to the fetus allows for both the maintenance of fetal life and fetal growth.

TRANSFER OF CARBON DIOXIDE FROM THE FETUS

The transport of CO_2 follows the opposite pathway to that of oxygen and is much easier, owing to the better diffusion of CO_2 (CO_2 diffusion rate is twenty times that of O_2).

REFERENCES

1. Abouleish, E.: The placenta and placenta transfer of drugs a term. Pa. Med., *78*:56, 1975.
2. ———: Placenta transfer of drugs. Diagnostica, *in press.*
3. Adamsons, K., Mueller-Heubach, E., and Myers, R. E.: Production of fetal asphyxia in the rhesus monkey by administration of catecholamines to the mother. Am. J. Obstet. Gynecol., *109*:248, 1971.
4. Adriani, J., and Robinson, E. W.: Pain relieving drugs: the new versus the old. J. La. State Med. Soc., *116*:385, 1964.
5. Aherne, W., and Dunnill, M. S.: Quantitative aspects of placental structure. J. Pathol., *91*:123, 1966.
6. Akamatsu, T. J., *et al.*: Experiences with the use of ketamine for parturition. I. Primary anesthetic for vaginal delivery. Anesth. Analg., *53*:284, 1974.
7. Apgar, V., *et al.*: The transmission of meperidine across the human placenta. Am. J. Obstet. Gynecol., *64*:1368, 1952.
8. ———: Comparison of regional and general anesthesia in obstetrics with special reference to transmission of cyclopropane across the placenta. J.A.M.A., *165*:2155, 1957.
9. Arens, J. F., and Carrera, A. E.: Methemoglobin levels following peridural anesthesia with prilocaine for vaginal deliveries. Anesth. Analg., *49*:219, 1970.
10. Asling, J. H., *et al.*: Paracervical block anesthesia in obstetrics. II. Etiology of fetal bradycardia following paracervical block anesthesia. Am. J. Obstet. Gynecol., *107*:626, 1970.
11. Bakhoum, W., and Aboul-Eish, E.: General anesthesia in cesarean section. Anesth. Analg., *36*:35, 1957.
12. Baraka, A.: Correlation between maternal and foetal P_{O_2} and P_{CO_2} during caesarean section. Br. J. Anaesth., *42*:434, 1970.
13. Baraka, A., *et al.*: Propanidid versus thiopentone for induction of general anaesthesia in elective caesarean section. Br. J. Anaesth., *43*:609, 1971.
14. Barclay, A. E., Franklin, K. J., and Prichard, M. M. L.: The Foetal Circulation and Cardiovascular System, and the Changes They Undergo at Birth. Springfield, Ill., Charles C Thomas, 1944.
15. Barcroft, J., and Barron, D. H.: Blood pressure and pulse rate in the foetal sheep. J. Exp. Biol., *22*:63, 1946.
16. Bare, W. W.: Double-blind evaluation of hydroxyzine hydrochloride for labor and delivery. Am. J. Obstet. Gynecol., *83*:18, 1962.
17. Batt, B.: Is halothane safe for surgical removal of retained products of conception? Anesth. Analg., *48*:338, 1969.
18. Beard, R. W., *et al.*: The significance of the changes in the continuous fetal heart rate in the first stage of labour. J. Obstet. Gynaecol. Br. Commonw., *78*:865, 1971.
19. Beckett, A. H., and Taylor, J. F.: Blood concentrations of pethidine and pentazocine in mother and infant at time of birth. J. Pharm. Pharmacol., *19*[Suppl.]:50S, 1967.
20. Benson, C., and Benson, R. C.: Hydroxyzine-meperidine analgesia and neonatal response. Am. J. Obstet. Gynecol., *84*:37, 1962.
21. Boba, A., Plotz, E. J., and Linkie, D. M.: Effect of atropine on fetal bradycardia and arterial oxygenation: experimental study in the dog during graded hemorrhage and following vasopressor administration. Surgery, *58*:267, 1965.
22. Bonica, J. J.: Effects of analgesia and anesthesia on the fetus and newborn. In Caldeyro-Barcia, R. (ed.): Effects of Labor and Delivery on the Fetus and Newborn. New York, Pergamon Press, 1967.
23. ———: Obstetric Analgesia and Anesthesia. New York, Springer-Verlag, 1972.
24. Born, G. V. R., *et al.*: Changes in the heart and lungs at birth. Cold Spring Harbor Symp. Quant. Biol., *19*:102, 1954.
25. Boyd, J. D., and Hamilton, J. W.: Development and structure of the human placenta from the end of the third month of gestation. J. Obstet. Gynaecol. Br. Commonw., *74*:161, 1967.
26. Brackbill, Y., Kane, J., and Manniello, R. L.: Obstetric meperidine usage and assessment of neonatal status. Anesthesiology, *40*:116, 1974.
27. Bradford, E. M. W., and Moir, D. D.: Anaesthesia for caesarean section: comparison of thiopentone and propanidid. Br. J. Anaesth., *41*:274, 1969.
28. Buller, A. J., and Young, I. M.: Action of d-tubocurarine chloride on foetal neuromuscular transmission and placental transfer of this drug in rabbits. J. Physiol., *109*:412, 1949.
29. Chodoff, P., and Stella, J. G.: Use of C1-581, a phencyclidine derivative for obstetric anesthesia. Anesth. Analg., *45*:527, 1966.
30. Clark, R. B., *et al.*: An evaluation of methoxyflurane analgesia and anesthesia for obstetrics. South. Med. J., *61*:687, 1968.
31. ———: The effect of methoxyflurane on the foetus. Br. J. Anaesth., *42*:286, 1971.
32. Cohen, E. N., *et al.*: Thiopental, curare, and

nitrous oxide anesthesia for cesarean section with studies on placental transmission. Surg. Gynecol. Obstet., *97*:456, 1953.

33. Coleman, A. J., *et al.*: Some implications of nitrous oxide in obstetric practice—a preliminary report. S. Afr. J. Obstet. Gynaecol., *10*:31, 1972.

34. Corssen, G., Little, S. C., and Tavakoli, M.: Ketamine and epilepsy. Anesth. Analg., *53*:319, 1974.

35. Corssen, G., *et al.*: Ketamine in the anesthetic management of asthmatic patients. Anesth. Analg., *51*:588, 1972.

36. Cosmi, E. V., and Marx, G. F.: Acid-base status and clinical condition of mother and foetus following methoxyflurane anaesthesia for vaginal delivery. Br. J. Anaesth., *40*:94, 1968.

37. Coulter, R. L.: The use of the relaxant diallytoxiferine in caesarean section. N.Z. Med. J., *65*:373,1966.

38. Crawford, J. S.: Some aspects of obstetric anaesthesia. Br. J. Anaesth., *28*:146, 1956.

39. ———: Studies of Epontol. Br. J. Anaesth., *40*:713, 1968.

40. Crawford, J. S., and Gardiner, J. E.: Some aspects of obstetric anaesthesia. Part II. The use of relaxant drugs. Br. J. Anaesth., *38*:154, 1956.

41. Dawes, G. S.: Foetal and Neonatal Physiology. A Comparative Study of the Changes at Birth. Chicago, Year Book Medical Publishers, 1968.

42. DeSilva, J. A. F., D'Anconte, L., and Kaplan, J.: The determination of blood levels and the placental transfer of diazepam in humans. Curr. Ther. Res., *6*:115, 1964.

43. Dixon, D. G., and Matheson, D. I.: Fluothane and other nonexplosive halogenated hydrocarbons in obstetric anaesthesia. Can. Med. Assoc. J., *79*:365, 1958.

44. Downing, J. W., Coleman, A. J., and Meer, F. M.: An intravenous method of anaesthesia for caesarean section. Part I. Propanidid. Br. J. Anaesth., *44*:1069, 1972.

45. Drabkova, J., Crul, J. F., and Van Der Kleijn, E.: Placental transfer of ^{14}C-labelled syccinylcholine in near-term Macaca mulatta monkeys. Br. J. Anaesth., *45*:1087, 1973.

46. Duncan, S. L. B., Ginsburg, J., and Morris, N. F.: Comparison of pentazocine and pethidine in normal labor. Am. J. Obstet. Gynecol., *105*:197, 1969.

47. Eaton, J. W., *et al.*: Variation in 2,3-diphosphoglycerate and ATP levels in human erythrocytes and effects on oxygen transport, red cell metabolism, and function. *In* Brewer, G. J. (ed.): Red Cell Metabolism and Function. Pp. 21–38. New York, Plenum Press, 1970.

48. Editorial: Placental transmission of anaesthetic agents. Br. J. Anaesth., *41*:799, 1969.

49. ———: Paracervical block in labour. Br. J. Anaesth., *42*:657, 1970.

50. Egilmez, A., Boehm, F. H., and Smith, B. E.: Placental transfer and transplacental fetal pharmacology of physostigmine. Sixth World Congress of Anesthesiology, Abstracts of Papers. Pp. 120–121. Excerpa Medica, 1976.

51. Eriksson, E.: Prilocaine, an experimental study in man of a new local anaesthetic with special regards to efficacy, toxicity and excretion. Acta Chir. Scand. [Suppl.], *358*:1, 1966.

52. Filler, W., Jr., and Filler, N. W.: Effect of a potent non-narcotic analgesic agent (pentazocine) on uterine contractility and fetal heart rate. Obstet. Gynecol., *28*:224, 1966.

53. Finster, M.: The placental transfer of drugs. The mother and newborn, recent advances. Ninth Annual Postgraduate Seminar Proceedings, University of Miami School of Medicine, Department of Anesthesiology, Miami, Florida, and University of Florida College of Medicine, Divison of Anesthesiology, Gainesville, Florida, 9, 1972.

54. Finster, M., Perel, J. M., and Papper, E. M.: Uptake of thiopental by fetal tissues and the placenta. [Abstract] Fed. Proc., *27*:706, 1958.

55. Finster, M., *et al.*: Plasma thiopental concentrations in the newborn following delivery under thiopental-nitrous oxide anesthesia. Am. J. Obstet. Gynecol., *95*:621, 1966.

56. ———: Tissue thiopental concentrations in the fetus and newborn. Anesthesiology, *36*:155, 1972.

57. ———: The placental transfer of lidocaine and its uptake by fetal tissues. Anesthesiology, *36*:159, 1972.

58. Flowers, C. E., Jr., Littlejohn, T. W., and Wells, H. B.: Pharmacologic and hypnoid analgesia. Obstet. Gynecol., *16*:210, 1960.

59. Flowers, C. E., Rudolph, A. J., and Desmond, M. M.: Diazepam (Valium) as an adjunct in obstetric analgesia. Obstet. Gynecol., *34*:68, 1969.

60. Fouts, J. R., and Hart, L. G.: Hepatic drug metabolism during the perinatal period. Ann. N.Y. Acad. Sci., *123*:245, 1965.

61. Fox, G. S., and Houle, G. L.: Transmission of lidocaine hydrochloride across the placenta during caesarean section. Can. Anaesth. Soc. J., *16*:136, 1969.

62. Freeman, R. K., *et al.*: Fetal cardiac response to paracervical block anesthesia. Part 1. Am. J. Obstet. Gynecol., *113*:583, 1972.

63. Galloon, S.: Ketamine for obstetric delivery. Anesthesiology, *44*:522, 1976.

64. Geddes, I. C., *et al.*: Distribution of halothane-^{82}Br in maternal and foetal guinea pig tissues. Br. J. Anaesth., *44*:542, 1972.

65. Gordon, H. R.: Fetal bradycardia after paracervical block: correlation with fetal and maternal blood levels of local anesthetic (mepivacaine). N. Engl. J. Med., *279*:910, 1968.

66. Gravenstein, J. S.: Mechanisms of drug interactions. Audio-Digest, *14*(14):16, 1972.

67. Gray, T. C.: d-Tubocurarine in caesarean section. Br. Med. J., *1*:444, 1947.

68. Grimwade, J., Walker, D., and Wood, C.: Morphine and the fetal heart rate. Br. Med. J., *3*:373, 1971.

69. Gruenwald, P.: Degenerative changes in right half of liver resulting from intra-uterine anoxia. Am. J. Clin. Pathol., *19*:801, 1949.

70. Gunther, R. E., and Bellville, J. W.: Obstetrical caudal anesthesia. II. A randomized study comparing 1 per cent mepivacaine with 1 per cent mepivacaine plus epinephrine. Anesthesiology, 37:288, 1972.

71. Harroun, P., and Fisher, C. W.: Physiological effects of curare; its failure to pass placental membrane or inhibit uterine contractions. Surg. Gynecol. Obstet., 89:73, 1949.

72. Hehre, F. W., Hook, R., and Hon, E. H.: Continuous lumbar peridural anesthesia in obstetrics. VI. The fetal effects of transplacental passage of local anesthetic agents. Anesth. Analg., 48:909, 1969.

73. Helliwell, P. J., and Hutton, A. M.: Thrichlorethylene anesthesia. Anaesthesia, 5:4, 1950.

74. Hellman, L. M., et al.: Sodium pentothal anesthesia in obstetrics. Am. J. Obstet. Gynecol., 48:851, 1944.

75. ———: Some factors affecting the fetal heart rate. Am. J. Obstet. Gynecol., 82:1055, 1961.

76. Hibbard, B. M., and Rosen, M.: The management of severe pre-eclampsia and eclampsia. Br. J. Anaesth., 49:3, 1977.

77. Hingson, R. A.: Lumbar epidural anesthesia. Physicians Bull., Pp. 117–120, December, 1946.

78. Hingson, R. A., and Hellman, L. M.: Anesthesia for Obstetrics. Philadelphia, J. B. Lippincott, 1956.

79. Hutchinson, H. T., et al.: Effects of magnesium sulfate on uterine contractility, intrauterine fetus, and infant. Am. J. Obstet. Gynecol., 88:747, 1964.

80. Hyman, M. D., and Shnider, S. M.: Maternal and neonatal blood concentrations of bupivacaine associated with obstetrical conduction anesthesia. Anesthesiology, 34:81, 1971.

81. Idänpään-Heikkilä, J. E., et al.: Placental transfer and fetal metabolism of diazepam in early human pregnancy. Am. J. Obstet. Gynecol., 109:1011, 1971.

82. Inmon, W. B., and Kitchings, J. T.: A study of the effect of meprobamate on labor and delivery. Am. J. Obstet. Gynecol., 79:1139, 1960.

83. James, L. S.: The effect of pain relief for labor and delivery on the fetus and newborn. Anesthesiology, 21:405, 1960.

84. Jawalekar, K. S., Jawalekar, S. R., and Mathur, V. P.: Effect of ketamine on isolated murine myometrial activity. Anesth. Analg., 51:685, 1972.

85. Jepson, J. H.: Endocrine control of maternal and fetal erythropoiesis. Can. Med. Assoc. J., 98:844, 1968.

86. ———: Factors influencing oxygenation in mother and fetus. Obstet. Gynecol., 44:906, 1974.

87. Johnstone, M., and Breen, P. J.: Halothane in obstetrics: elective caesarean section. Br. J. Anaesth., 48:386, 1966.

88. Kivalo, I., and Saarikoski, S.: Placental transmission and foetal uptake of ^{14}C-dimethyltubocurarine. Br. J. Anaesth., 44:557, 1972.

89. Kosaka, Y., Takahashi, T., and Mark, L. C.: Intravenous thiobarbiturate anesthesia for cesarean section. Anesthesiology, 31:489, 1969.

90. Kvisselgaard, N., and Moya, F.: Investigation of placental thresholds to succinylcholine. Anesthesiology, 22:7, 1961.

91. Langrehr, D.: Clinical and experimental experience in 1600 anesthesias with ketamine, with special consideration of its use in risk patients and in obstetrics. Paper presented to the International Symposium L'anesthesia vigile et subvigile. Ostende, Belgium, April 17–20, 1969.

92. Latto, I. P., Rosen, M., and Molloy, M. J.: Absence of accumulation of methoxyflurane during intermittent self-administration of pain relief in labour. Br. J. Anaesth., 44:391, 1972.

93. Latto, I. P., and Wainwright, A. C.: Anaesthesia for caesarean section: analysis of blood concentrations of methoxyflurane using 0.0 per cent methoxyflurane and 40 per cent oxygen. Br. J. Anaesth., 44:1050, 1972.

94. Lees, M. M., et al.: A study of cardiac output at rest throughout pregnancy. J. Obstet. Gynaecol. Br. Commonw., 74:319, 1967.

95. Levi, A. J., Gatmaitan, Z., and Arias, I. M.: Two hepatic cytoplasmic protein fractions, Y and Z, and their possible role in the hepatic uptake of bilirubin, sulfobromophthalein, and other anions. J. Clin. Invest., 48:2156, 1969.

96. Lipsitz, P. J., and English, I. C.: Hypermagnesemia in the newborn infant. Pediatrics, 40:856, 1967.

97. Little, B., et al.: Study of ketamine as an obstetric anesthetic agent. Am. J. Obstet. Gynecol., 113:247, 1972.

98. Lumley, J., Walker, A., and Wood, C.: Placental oxygen tensions: differences between veins. Am. J. Obstet. Gynecol., 13:846, 1972.

99. McDonald, J. S., Mateo, C. V., and Reed, E. C.: Modified nitrous oxide for ketamine hydrochloride for cesarean section. Anesth. Analg., 51:975, 1972.

100. Marx, G. F.: Placental transfer and drugs used in anesthesia. Anesthesiology, 22:294, 1961.

101. ———: Placental transfer of anesthetic agents. Anesthesia Rounds by Ayerst Laboratories, 4:1, 1973.

102. ———: Obstetric anesthesia in the presence of medical complications. Clin. Obstet. Gynecol., 17:165, 1974.

103. Marx, G. F., Eckstein, K. L., and Halevy, S.: Placental transmission and maternal and neonatal elimination of fluroxene. Anesth. Analg., 52:654, 1973.

104. Marx, G. F., Joshi, C. W., and Orkin, L. R.: Placental transmission of nitrous oxide. Anesthesiology, 32:429, 1970.

105. Marx, F. G., and Mateo, C.: Effects of different oxygen concentrations during general anaesthesia for elective caesarean section. Can. Anaesth. Soc. J., 18:587, 1971.

106. Metcalfe, J., Bartels, H., and Moll, W.: Gas exchange in the pregnant uterus. Physiol. Rev., 47:782, 1967.

107. Mitchell, M. T.: Evaluation of a new non-narcotic analgesic in obstetrics. Minn. Med., *46*:1230, 1963.

108. Moir, D. D.: Anaesthesia for caesarean section: an evaluation of a method using low concentrations of halothane and 50 per cent of oxygen. Br. J. Anaesth., *42*:136, 1970.

109. Moore, J., Carson, R. M., and Hunter, R. J.: A comparison of the effects of pentazocine and pethidine administered during labour. J. Obstet. Gynaecol. Br. Commonw., *77*:830, 1970.

110. Moore, J., McNabb, T. G., and Dundee, J. W.: Preliminary report on ketamine in obstetrics. Br. J. Anaesth., *43*:779, 1971.

111. Morgan, C. D., Sandler, M., and Panigel, M.: Placental transfer of catecholamines in vitro and in vivo. Am. J. Obstet. Gynecol., *112*:1068, 1972.

112. Morishima, H. O., and Adamsons, K.: Placental clearance of mepivacaine following administration to the guinea pig fetus. Anesthesiology, *28*:343, 1967.

113. Morishima, H. O., *et al.*: Transmission of mepivacaine hydrochloride (Carbocaine) across the human placenta. Anesthesiology, *27*:147, 1966.

114. Morrison, J. C., *et al.*: Metabolites of meperidine related to fetal depression. Am. J. Obstet. Gynecol., *115*:1132, 1973.

115. Mowat, J., and Garrey, M. M.: Comparison of pentazocine and pethidine in labour. Br. Med. J., *2*:757, 1970.

116. Moya, F.: Use of chloroform inhaler in obstetrics. N.Y. J. Med., *61*:421, 1961.

117. ———: Mechanisms of drug transfer across the placenta with particular reference to chemotherapeutic agents. Antimicrob. Agents Chemother., *5*:1051, 1965.

118. Moya, F., and Kvisselgaard, N.: The placental transmission of succinylcholine. Anesthesiology, *22*:1, 1961.

119. Moya, F., and Thorndike, V.: Passage of drugs across the placenta. Am. J. Obstet. Gynecol., *84*:1778, 1962.

120. Munson, E. S., and Embro, W. J.: Enflurane, isoflurane and halothane and isolated human uterine muscle. Anesthesiology, *46*:11, 1977.

121. Naftalin, N. J., *et al.*: The effects of halothane on pregnant and nonpregnant human myometrium. Anesthesiology, *46*:15, 1977.

122. Neeld, J. B., Jr., *et al.*: A clinical comparison of pancuronium and tubocurarine for cesarean section anesthesia. Anesth. Analg., *53*:7, 1974.

123. Novy, M. J.: Alterations in blood oxygen affinity during fetal and neonatal life. *In* Astrup, P., and Rorth, M. (eds.): Oxygen affinity of Hemoglobin and Red Cell Acid Base Status. Pp. 696–712. New York, Academic Press, 1972.

124. Nyirjesy, I., *et al.*: Hazards of the use of paracervical block anesthesia in obstetrics. Am. J. Obstet. Gynecol., *87*:231, 1963.

125. Paton, W. D.: The principles of drug action. Proc. R. Soc. Med., *53*:815, 1960.

126. Penrose, B. H.: Aspiration pneumonitis following ketamine induction for general anesthesia. Anesth. Analg., *51*:41, 1972.

127. Pitkin, R. M., Reynolds, W. A., and Filer, L. J., Jr.: Placental transmission and fetal distribution of cyclamate in early human pregnancy. Am. J. Obstet. Gynecol., *108*:1043, 1970.

128. Pittinger, C. B., and Morris, L. E.: Placental transmission of d-tubocurarine chloride from maternal to fetal circulation in dogs. Anesthesiology, *14*:238, 1953.

129. ———: Observations of the placental transmission of gallamine triethiodide (flaxedil), succinylcholine chloride (anectine), and decamethonium bromide (syncurine) in dogs. Anesth. Analg., *34*:107, 1955.

130. Pittinger, C. B., Morris, L. E., and Keettel, W. C.: Vaginal deliveries during profound curarization. Am. J. Obstet. Gynecol., *65*:635, 1953.

131. Poppers, P. J., and Finster, M.: The use of prilocaine hydrochloride (Citanest) for epidural analgesia in obstetrics. Anesthesiology, *29*:1134, 1968.

132. Preyer, W.: Spezielle Physiologie des Embryo. Leipzig, T. Grieben, 1885.

133. Printz, J. L., and McMaster, R. H.: Continuous monitoring of fetal heart rate and uterine contractions in patients under epidural anesthesia. Anesth. Analg., *51*:876, 1972.

134. Pritchard, J. A.: Use of magnesium ion in the management of eclamptogenic toxemias. Surg. Gynecol. Obstet., *100*:131, 1955.

135. Ramsey, E. M., Corner, G. W., Jr., and Donner, M. W.: Serial and cineradioangiographic visualization of maternal circulation in the primate (hemochorial) placenta. Am. J. Obstet. Gynecol., *86*:213, 1963.

136. Reid, D. H. S.: Diffusion anoxia at birth. Lancet, *2*:757, 1968.

137. Reynolds, F.: The influence of adrenaline on maternal and neonatal blood levels of local analgesic drugs. *In* Proceedings of the Symposium on Epidural Analgesia in Obstetrics. Pp. 31–40. Kingston Hospital, Kingston-upon-Thames, England, March 18, 1971.

138. Reynolds, F., and Taylor, G.: Maternal and neonatal blood concentrations of bupivacaine. A comparison with lignocaine during continuous extradural analgesia. Anaesthesia, *25*:14, 1970.

139. Robinson, G. J. B.: Thiopental and the fetal liver. [Correspondence] Anesthesiology, *37*:570, 1972.

140. Roger, K. F., *et al.*: Fetal cardiac response to paracervical block anesthesia. Part 1. Am. J. Obstet. Gynecol., *113*:583, 1972.

141. Rorke, M. J., Davey, D. A., and Du Toit, H. J.: Foetal oxygenation during caesarean section. Anaesthesia, *23*:585, 1968.

142. Rorth, M., and Bille Brathe, N. E.: 2,3-DPG in human pregnancy. *In* Astrup, P., and Rorth, M. (eds.): Oxygen Affinity of Hemoglobin and Red Cell Acid Base Status. Pp. 692–695. New York, Academic Press, 1972.

143. Rosefsky, J. B., and Petersiel, M. E.: Perinatal

deaths associated with mepivacaine paracervical block anesthesia in labor. N. Engl. J. Med., *278*:530, 1968.

144. Rovenstine, E. A., Adriani, J., and Studdiford, W. E.: Gas changes in maternal and fetal blood during cyclopropane obstetric anesthesia. Calif. West. Med. J., *53*:59, 1940.

145. Sadove, M. S., *et al.*: Clinical study of droperidol in the prevention of the side-effects of ketamine anesthesia: a progress report. Anesth. Analg., *50*:526, 1971.

146. Scher, J., Hailey, D. M., and Beard, R. W.: The effects of diazepam on the fetus. J. Obstet. Gynaecol. Br. Commonw., 79:635, 1972.

147. Schwarz, R.: Chemische Untersuchungen zur displacentaren Passage von Gallamin. Anaesthetist, 7:299, 1958.

148. Shaw, H. A., and Hunt, S. R.: The use of diallylnortoxiferine in anaesthesia. N.Z. Med. J., *65*:371, 1966.

149. Shen, W., Taves, D. R., and Donald, R.: Fluoride concentrations in the human placenta and maternal and cord blood. Am. J. Obstet. Gynecol., *119*:205, 1974.

150. Sheridan, C. A., and Robson, J. G.: Fluothane in obstetrical anaesthesia. Can. Anaesth. Soc. J., 6:365, 1959.

151. Sherline, D. M.: Discussion. Am. J. Obstet. Gynecol., *113*:258, 1972.

152. Shnider, S. M.: Obstetrical Anesthesia. Current Concepts and Practice. Baltimore, Williams & Wilkins, 1970.

153. Shnider, S. M., and Moya, F.: Effects of meperidine on the newborn infant. Am. J. Obstet. Gynecol., 89:1009, 1964.

154. Shnider, S. M., and Way, E. L.: The kinetics of transfer of lidocaine (Xylocaine) across the human placenta. Anesthesiology, 29:944, 1968.

155. Shnider, S. M., *et al.*: Paracervical block in anesthesia in obstetrics. I. Fetal complications and neonatal morbidity. Am. J. Obstet. Gynecol., *107*:619, 1970.

156. Siker, E. J., *et al.*: Placental transfer of methoxyflurane. Br. J. Anaesth., *40*:588, 1968.

157. Smith, C. A.: Effect of obstetrical anesthesia upon oxygenation of maternal and fetal blood with particular reference to cyclopropane. Surg. Gynecol. Obstet., *69*:584, 1939.

158. ———: Effect of nitrous oxide oxygen ether anesthesia upon oxygenation of maternal and fetal blood at delivery. Surg. Gynecol. Obstet., 70:787, 1940.

159. Smith, C. A., and Barker, R. H.: Ether in blood of newborn infant: quantitative study. Am. J. Obstet. Gynecol., *43*:763, 1942.

160. Stave, U.: Physiology of the Perinatal Period. Vol. 1, New York, Appleton-Century-Crofts, 1970.

161. Stoelting, V. K.: Fluothane in obstetric anesthesia. Anesth. Analg., *43*:243, 1964.

162. Stone, S. R., and Pritchard, J. A.: Effect of maternally administered magnesium sulfate on the neonate. Obstet. Gynecol., *35*:574, 1970.

163. Tay, G.: Diallylnortoxiferine—a new relaxant. Singapore Med. J., *4*:90, 1963.

164. Taylor, G.: Placental circulation. *In* Schurr, C., and Feldman, S. A. (eds.): Scientific Foundations of Anesthesia. Ed. 1. Philadelphia, F. A. Davis, 1970.

165. Teramo, K., and Widholm, O.: Studies of the effect of anaesthetics on the foetus. Part I. The effect of paracervical block with mepivacaine upon foetal acid-base values. Acta Obstet. Gynecol. Scand. [Suppl.], *46*:2, 1967.

166. Thomas, B. E., and Gibson, J.: Relaxant drugs in obstetric anaesthesia. J. Obstet. Gynaecol. Br. Emp., *60*:378, 1953.

167. Thomas, J., Climie, C. R., and Mather, L. E.: The placental transfer of alcuronium: a preliminary report. Br. J. Anaesth., *41*:297, 1969.

168. ———: Placental transfer of alcuronium. [Correspondence] Br. J. Anaesth., *41*:641, 1969.

169. Try, B. W., Taves, D. R., and Donald, R.: Maternal and fetal flurometabolite concentrations after exposure to methoxyflurane. Am. J. Obstet. Gynecol., *119*:199, 1974.

170. Tucker, G. T., *et al.*: Binding of anilide-type local anesthetics in human plasma: I. Relationships between binding, physicochemical properties, and anesthetic activity. Anesthesiology, *33*:287, 1970.

171. ———: Binding of anilide-type local anesthetics in human plasma. II. Implications in vivo, with special reference to transplacental distribution. Anesthesiology, *33*:304, 1970.

172. Ueland, K., *et al.*: Maternal cardiovascular dynamics. VI. Cesarean section under epidural anesthesia without epinephrine. Am. J. Obstet. Gynecol., *114*:775, 1972.

173. Villee, C. A.: Placental transfer of drugs. Ann. N.Y. Acad. Sci., *123*:237, 1965.

174. Whitacre, R. J.: Curare in cesarean section. Anesth. Analg., *27*:164, 1948.

175. Whitacre, R. J., and Fisher, A. J.: Clinical observations on the use of curare in anesthesia. Anesthesiology, *6*:124, 1945.

176. Winters, W.: Epilepsie or anesthesia with ketamine. Anesthesiology, *36*:309, 1972.

177. Winthrop Laboratories: Talwin, Brand of Pentazocine. TW-109F, 1969.

178. Wisloski, G. B.: Introductory remarks. *In* Flexner, L. B. (ed.): Gestation. Transactions of the First Conference. New York, Josiah Macy, Jr., Foundation, 1954.

179. Wylie, W. D., and Churchill-Davidson, H. C.: A practice of anaesthesia. Ed. 3. Chicago, Year Book Medical Publishers, 1972.

180. Zargham, I., Leviss, S., and Marx, G. F.: Uterine pressures during fluroxene anesthesia. Anesth. Analg., *53*:568, 1974.

4

Local Anesthetic Drugs

Ezzat Abouleish, M.D.

Local anesthetics are the main drugs utilized in obstetric anesthesia. Therefore, detailed considerations of the anatomy, physiology, physics, chemistry, mechanisms of action, pharmacokinetics, and pharmacology, all are required for proper, safe, and intelligent use of these drugs.

ANATOMY AND PHYSIOLOGY OF NERVE FIBERS

THE NEURON

The term neuron is used to describe the nerve cell and its processes, namely the dendrites and the axon.

THE AXON

The axon is also called the axis cylinder or nerve fiber. It varies in length in different species from a few microns to a few meters; in man it can reach a length of as long as 90 cm. It varies in thickness from 0.5 to 20 μ.* The thicker fibers are called *myelinated (medullated) nerve fibers*, which consist of the following structures, starting from within the nerve fiber outward (see Fig. 4-1):

The Axoplasm

The axoplasm is the central core of the nerve fiber and is composed of a semifluid material which flows from the cell body.

*One micron (μ) is $^1/_{1000}$ of a millimeter.

The Nerve Membrane

The nerve membrane separates the axoplasm from the extracellular compartment. Its structure and function are discussed in detail below.

The Myelin Sheath

The myelin sheath surrounds the nerve membrane in the myelinated nerve fiber. It consists of a specialized set of *Schwann cells* wrapped around the axon. A *node of Ranvier*, where the myelin sheath is absent, indicates the junction of two Schwann cells. The nodes of Ranvier are regularly spaced at intervals of 0.5 to 2 mm. The distance between two nodes is proportionate to the diameter of the axon by a factor of roughly one hundred. Each node is 0.5 μ in length and its surface is 4 μ^2.[34] At these nodes, the nerve membrane is exposed to the surrounding medium and ionic exchanges necessary for nerve excitation take place. Cocaine, for instance, is only effective in blocking nerve conduction when applied at nodes of Ranvier and not in between.[34] The neurilemma, underneath which lies the cell nucleus, is the outermost cell membrane of the Schwann cell.

The myelin sheath is composed of alternating layers of lipids and proteins and bears a relation to the size of the axon, i.e., the diameter of the axon is always one-half that of the entire myelinated fiber. The myelin's insulating properties enable the

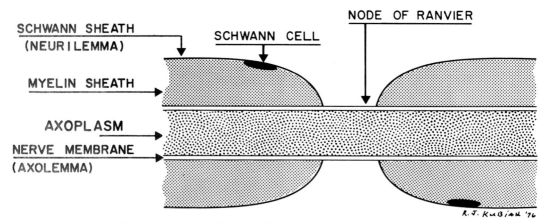

Fig. 4-1.   Longitudinal section of a myelinated nerve fiber.

fiber to conduct an impulse much faster due to the reduction of current loss through direct and capacitive leakage.

In unmyelinated nerve fibers, the myelin sheath is absent because the Schwann cell does not spin around the axon, but just encircles it once. (Fig. 4-2). The axon is never completely engulfed or isolated from the outside by the Schwann cell.

Postganglionic autonomic fibers and somatic fibers less than 1 μ in diameter are unmyelinated (C-fibers); the rest of the nerve fibers are myelinated (Table 4-1).

Enclosing Layers

Enclosing layers vary in composition and thickness according to the location of the nerves. For instance, a local anesthetic injected into the subarachnoid space acts rapidly because the nerves there are covered by one thin layer which is an extension of the pia mater. When a local anesthetic is injected epidurally, it has to diffuse through the much thicker extension sheaths from the dura and arachnoid, as well as the one from the pia. When injected into a peripheral nerve, e.g., the sciatic nerve, the local anesthetic has to transverse the barriers which are now called epineurium, perineurium, and endoneurium, plus the nerve sheath which surrounds the nerve roots forming the sciatic nerve.

THE NERVE MEMBRANE

The nerve membrane surrounds the axoplasm and has a thickness of 70 to 80

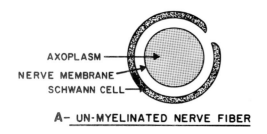

A– UN-MYELINATED NERVE FIBER

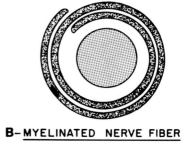

B–MYELINATED   NERVE FIBER

Fig. 4-2.   Cross sections of unmyelinated and myelinated nerve fibers. *A.* In the unmyelinated nerve fiber, the Schwann cell surrounds the nerve fiber. *B.* In the myelinated nerve fiber the Schwann cell spins around the nerve fiber and forms the myelin sheath.

Table 4-1. Types, Sizes, and Functions of Nerve Fibers

Type	*Myelination*	*Diameter* *(μ)*	*Conduction Velocity* *(m./sec.)*	Function
A-fibers	Yes	2–20	10–120	Somatic nerves
α β		Largest		Carry motor, proprioception, and touch impulses
γ				Carry efferent impulses to muscle spindle
δ		Smallest		Carry pain and temperature sensations, transmit sharp pain sensations; faster rate than C-fibers
B-fibers	Yes	3	10–20	Autonomic preganglionic (blocked easier and recover faster than pain fibers although they have larger diameter)
C-fibers	No	0.5–1μ	0.5–2	Postganglionic autonomic; carry pain and temperature sensations (responsible for the dull ache)

Å*. It is the most important structure for nerve conduction as well as the one most often affected by local anesthetic drugs. It is composed mainly of lipids and proteins, but also contains small amounts of sugars, electrolytes, and other chemicals.[84] The nerve membrane is regarded as being essentially impermeable to cations except at special regions where pores or channels exist through which cations move. This concept that local anesthetics act only at certain receptors in the membrane may give the false impression that the membrane is in a rigid state. On the contrary, all of its components are in a fluid condition.

ELECTROCHEMICAL CHANGES ACCOMPANYING NERVE STIMULATION

The stimulation of a nerve and the firing of an impulse are accompanied by impor-

---

*One Ångström unit (Å) = $^1/_{1000}$ micron; or 10^{-10} meter; or 0.1 nanometer (millimicron).

tant electrical changes as well as ionic exchanges across the nerve membrane.

Electrical Changes

During the resting state, the nerve membrane has a high electrical resistance, about 50 times greater than that of the surrounding intra- and extracellular fluids. There is a negative electrical potential, called *the resting potential*, of approximately −70 mv. between the interior and exterior of the nerve fiber (Fig. 4-3).[27]

Following stimulation of the nerve, a relatively slow phase of depolarization occurs during which the electrical potential within the nerve becomes progressively less negative. When the difference in electrical potential between the internal and external surface of the nerve membrane reaches a critical level, called the *threshold of firing level*, usually at −55 mv., a rapid phase of depolarization occurs which ultimately reverses the electrical potential across the cell membrane.

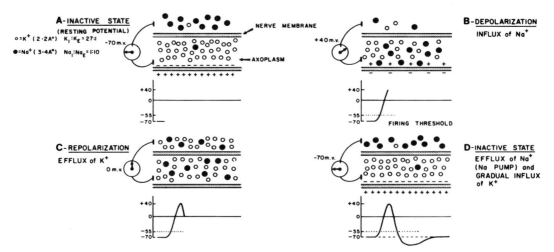

Fig. 4-3.   Electrochemical changes occurring during nerve stimulation.

At the peak of the depolarization phase, the interior of the nerve has a positive electrical potential of approximately +40 mv. compared to its exterior.

After completion of the depolarization phase, *repolarization* begins, during which the electrical potential within the nerve becomes progressively less positive and ultimately negative compared to its exterior. This continues and the membrane potential overshoots to reach −80 mv. for a short period, then gradually reaches the original level of −70 mv. The membrane is now considered to be in the *resting state* once more, and is ready for another impulse.

Ionic Exchanges

During the resting state the concentration of K^+ inside the nerve is higher and that of Na^+ is lower than in the surrounding extracellular fluid. The ratio of K^+ inside the nerve membrane to K^+ outside the nerve membrane ($K_I:K_E$) is 27:1 while the ratio of Na^+ ($Na_I:Na_E$) is 1:10 (Fig. 4-3). During the resting state ionic movements across the membrane are quite limited. However, K^+ moves 50 to 100 times more freely than Na^+. This may be related to the size of the hydrated ions in comparison to the pores that exist in the nerve membrane. The radius of these *channels* is estimated to be

about 2 Å, while the radius of hydrated Na^+ is 3.4 Å, and that of hydrated K^+ is 2.2 Å.[115] The number of Na^+ channels in the nerve membrane is extremely small; for example, in the rabbit vagus nerve there are about 30 Na^+ channels per μ^2.[98] There are separate pores for K^+ exchange which are about 50 times more numerous than those for Na^+.[61]

During excitation of the nerve, there is an increased permeability to ions across the nerve membrane. This is probably due to an increase in the size of the pores resulting from contracture of the membrane. This increased permeability is manifested by rapid influx of Na^+ into the nerve,[60,61] which is a passive process not requiring energy because of the concentration gradient. During nerve stimulation Na^+ move 10 times faster than K^+.[63]

When the nerve is maximally depolarized, the permeability to Na^+ decreases, and increased efflux of K^+ occurs, leading to *repolarization* of the nerve membrane. This is also a passive process not requiring energy because the K ions are moving in the direction of their concentration gradient.

The net result following nerve stimulation is, therefore, an increased Na^+ concentration inside and an increased K^+ concentration outside the nerve membrane. To restore the original concentrations of ions across the nerve membrane, Na^+ has to be pumped outside the nerve, by what is called a *sodium pump,* and K^+ has to gain access into the nerve. This is an active process requiring energy because ions are moved against their concentration gradient. However, the influx of K^+ does not require as much energy as the efflux of Na^+ because the former ions are moving with the electrical gradient across the nerve membrane; the influx of K^+ helps to bring up the membrane potential from -80 to -70 mv., that is, to its original resting state.

THE NERVE IMPULSE

Once the nerve is sufficiently stimulated, it fires and a nerve impulse is formed which propagates away from that point. Impulses traveling along a nerve are equal in amplitude and duration irrespective of the stimulus. Despite current loss through leakage and the capacitative nature of the nerve membrane, the potential in the adjacent nerve membrane is easily lowered to threshold value. The following depolarization restores the current and subsequently the adjacent portion of the nerve membrane becomes stimulated to the threshold, leading to firing and further propagation of the nerve impulse. Along the nerve membrane the Na^+ pores, by allowing ionic exchange, help to restore the current during the propagation of the nerve impulse.

Conduction Velocity of Nerve Impulses

Conduction velocity is the speed of conduction of a nerve impulse along a nerve, resulting from the propagation of electrochemical changes along the nerve membrane. The conduction velocity is usually expressed in meters per second (m./sec.). The velocity of propagation in vertebrates is usually from 1 to 100 m./sec., depending on the size of the nerve fibers,

the presence of the myelin sheath, or both. The larger the diameter of the nerve fiber the faster its conductivity. Myelinated nerve fibers have a higher conduction velocity than unmyelinated fibers of the same size.

There is a critical level of conductance velocity below which conduction completely fails and nerve block occurs.[63]

Refractory Periods

During the depolarization stage the nerve is completely refractory to any nerve stimulus. This period is called the *absolute refractory period.* During the stage of repolarization, only a strong stimulus can be effective. This period is called the *relative refractory period.*

The refractory periods determine the frequency of firing of a nerve fiber. Motor fibers have a higher frequency firing capacity than pain fibers. *The selectivity of the blocking action of local anesthetic drugs* varies.[25] Some local anesthetic drugs mainly affect high-frequency nerve fibers, others low-frequency nerve fibers, and a third group blocks nerve fibers equally independent of their firing frequency. This may explain the difference in preferential blockade by the local anesthetics bupivacaine and etidocaine, where the latter drug causes more motor than sensory blockade in spite of the fact that motor fibers are much thicker than sensory fibers.

Blocking of Nerve Impulses

Nerve conduction can be inhibited by physical as well as chemical means. Chemical blockade can be produced by many agents, such as local anesthetics, and a variety of chemical irritants, such as alcohol and phenol. In clinical practice a transient, reversible block is sought which is best achieved by local anesthetic drugs.

Local anesthetics do not interfere with the resting potential of the nerve membrane. However, they block the depolarization process by interfering with ionic exchange across the membrane. Blocking of

Na^+ flux is more important than blocking of K^+ for the production of nerve block. Initially some Na^+ channels are blocked, leading to increase of the excitation threshold, prolongation of the refractory periods, decrease of the action potential, and reduction of the conductance velocity. Ultimately the action potential and conduction become less than the critical levels, and the nerve impulse generation and propagation stop. The critical level of the number of Na^+ pores across the nerve membrane below which conduction fails was calculated to be $25/\mu^2$.[63]

Hyponatremia increases the potency of local anesthetics,[72] and progressive hyponatremia itself may produce a differential block. The effect of a reduced sodium concentration is to decrease the nerve action potential by decreasing the number of sodium ions available for diffusion through sodium channels. Of course, this parallels the effect of local anesthetics to reduce the number of functioning sodium channels.[101]

The Role of Calcium Ions

Changes in Ca^{++} modify the effect of local anesthetics. For instance, an increase in Ca^{++} concentration reverses the effect of procaine on the nerve fiber,[13] and a decrease in Ca^{++} has the opposite effect.[27] Calcium ions also play an important role in Na^+ exchange. At rest, they are concentrated at the orifice of the sodium channels and help to keep them closed.[44] On nerve stimulation, the discharge of the Ca^{++} aids in opening the Na^+ pores, thus allowing the Na^+ flux.

THE SIZES OF NERVE FIBERS
TYPES OF NERVE FIBERS

Nerve fibers are classified into A-, B-, and C-fibers (Table 4-1). A-fibers are the thickest, and C-fibers are the thinnest. Both A- and B-fibers are myelinated, and C-fibers are unmyelinated.

A-fibers are subdivided according to their diameter into A-alpha (A-α), A-beta (A-β), A-gamma (A-γ), and A-delta (A-δ) fibers; A-α fibers have the largest diameter.

Both A-α and A-β fibers carry motor, proprioceptive, and touch impulses. A-γ fibers carry efferent impulses to muscle spindle and aid in the regulation of muscle tone. Being smaller than α and β fibers they are blocked earlier, and with a smaller concentration of local anesthetic drugs. This explains the good abdominal relaxation during surgery under epidural analgesia despite the adequate respiratory functions. A-δ fibers, the smallest A-fibers, carry pain and temperature sensations. B-fibers constitute the preganglionic autonomic fibers. When they are blocked during spinal or epidural analgesia, hypotension may occur because of interruption of sympathetic impulses and subsequent decrease in the peripheral resistance.

C-fibers constitute the postganglionic autonomic nerve fibers as well as those carrying sensations of pain and temperature. *Man apparently processes two separate conducting systems that carry impulses related to pain:* one system is moderately fast by way of the myelinated A-δ fibers, and the other is slow by way of the C-fibers. The initial sharp pain sensation is carried by A-δ fibers, while the following sensation of dull ache is conducted by the C-fibers.

THE DIAMETER OF THE NERVE FIBER AND ITS SUSCEPTIBILITY TO BLOCKADE

The influence of the diameter of the nerve fiber on its susceptibility to blockade depends on the factor producing the block.

Blockade Caused by Local Anesthetics

The thinner a nerve fiber is, the smaller its volume relative to its surface, and the fewer the local anesthetic molecules required to produce a block. Therefore, in general, the thinner the nerve fiber, the more susceptible it becomes to local anesthetic drugs. An exception to this rule is B-fibers which, although larger than C-fibers, are blocked earlier and with a smaller concentration of local anesthetic drugs.[104] The reason for this is probably the difference in conduction between the B-fibers which are myelinated and the C-fibers which are unmyelinated. In myelinated nerve fibers the action potential currently generated at one node of Ranvier must be sufficient to depolarize the next node to the threshold; such a conduction method is called *saltatory*. In unmyelinated nerve fibers the conduction is not in "lapses," but continuous, i.e., the nerve impulse generated at one point is propagated *continuously* to the adjacent points, and therefore more difficult to block than in the case of myelinated nerve fibers of the same or even larger size.

Blockade Caused by Hypoxia

Hypoxia also has a greater blocking effect on small nerve fibers which have a wider surface area relative to their energy sources.

Physical Methods of Blockade

Blocking of nerve impulses can be produced by *pressure*, but this method is difficult to control and not always reversible. *By lowering the temperature of the nerve to 1 or 2°C.*, reversible nerve block can be obtained, but this method of nerve block is unselective since all nerves exposed to low temperature are blocked.

Spinal and epidural analgesia cause blockade of the preganglionic sympathetic fibers (B-fibers), thereby limiting the safety of these techniques. It is highly desirable to find a local anesthetic that selectively blocks sensory impulses while having no effect on B-fibers. Unfortunately both ester- and amide-linked local anesthetic drugs block B-fibers easier than other fibers.[104] However, the use of *electric current* to produce selective blockade, called anodal block, has been tried, is promising, and may be used in the future as an alternative or a substitute for local anesthetic drugs.[125] When a nerve is stimulated electrically with bipolar electrodes and the anode lies in the direction of the impulse propagation, some of the faster fibers activated at the cathode are blocked by the brief flow of current from the anode.

THE SHAPE OF NERVE FIBERS

With increasing activity there is an expansion of the nerve fiber, due in part to the exchange of Na^+ for K^+ internally.[63] Nerve fibers do not have a circular shape but tend to be ellipsoidal. An increase in volume following activity can thus be tolerated without mechanical strain on the surface membrane.

THE BLOCK PATTERN IN A PERIPHERAL NERVE

Since the initial anesthetic concentration is higher outside the nerve than inside the nerve, conduction block proceeds from mantle (outer) to core (inner) nerve bundles.[34] Because mantle fibers supply the proximal part of the body while core fibers supply the distal regions, the nerve block proceeds peripherally (i.e., in a brachial plexus block the upper arm becomes anesthetized before the hand). During recovery, the local anesthetic diffuses from the nerve to the surrounding tissues. Therefore, the drug supply of the mantle is depleted first and sensation is first regained in the corresponding area (i.e., in the upper arm). If anesthesia is to be maintained, smaller doses of the drug are required for maintenance than were required for the initial block because the nerve, especially the core, still contains an appreciable amount of the local anesthetic. However, in case of continuous epidural or caudal analgesia the refill doses are only slightly different from the initial dose because a certain volume of the anesthetic is required to reach the furthermost segments (e.g., for continuous caudal analgesia, to reach the T10 segment, the initial dose may be 20 ml. while the subsequent doses are 17 or 18 ml.).

PHYSICS AND CHEMISTRY OF LOCAL ANESTHETIC DRUGS
STRUCTURE OF LOCAL ANESTHETICS

There are many diverse compounds which possess local anesthetic properties. Therefore, it is difficult to define precisely the relationship between chemical structure and etiologic activity in regard to local anesthetic properties. In general, compounds that are clinically used for local anesthesia are *tertiary amines* (N-H$_3$), where each hydrogen ion is replaced by an organic group. They possess the following structure (Fig. 4-4): aromatic portion—intermediate chain—amine portion. Alterations in any portion of this chemical scheme will modify the anesthetic properties of the compound. For example, increase in the molecular weight of a local anesthetic drug, to a certain extent, prolongs its duration of action, improves its potency, and increases its toxicity.

The aromatic portion of the molecule determines the lipid solubility of the compound, the intermediate chain decides the metabolic pathway, and the amine portion controls the water solubility. There should be a fine balance between the lipophilic (fat-soluble) and the hydrophilic (water-

soluble) portions of the local anesthetic drug. If the molecule is too lipophilic, it becomes insoluble in water and therefore clinically useless. If it is too hydrophilic, there will be no un-ionized portion to penetrate the nerve membrane and thus no anesthetic activity. Thus alterations in either the aromatic or amine portion will affect the lipid-water distribution coefficient of the compound, called the *partition coefficient*. In addition, the drug's character can be altered by changes in either end of the molecule. For example, the replacement of the methyl group (CH$_3$) by a butyl group (C$_4$H$_9$) in the amine portion of the mepivacaine molecule results in an increase in the partition coefficient, protein binding, potency, toxicity, and duration of action (Tables 4-2 and 4-3; Fig. 4-5). The new drug formed is bupivacaine. Similarly, the addition of a butyl group to the aromatic portion of the procaine molecule is associated with an increase in partition coefficient, protein binding, potency, duration of action, and toxicity (Fig. 4-5). The compound thus formed is tetracaine.

The chain linking the aromatic and amine portions of the molecule can be either an ester- or amide-type. If it is an ester-type, the local anesthetic is said to belong to the *ester-linked group* and is hydrolyzed by the plasma cholinesterase. If the intermediate chain is an amide-type, the local anesthetic is said to belong to the *amide-linked group* and is mainly metabolized by the liver.

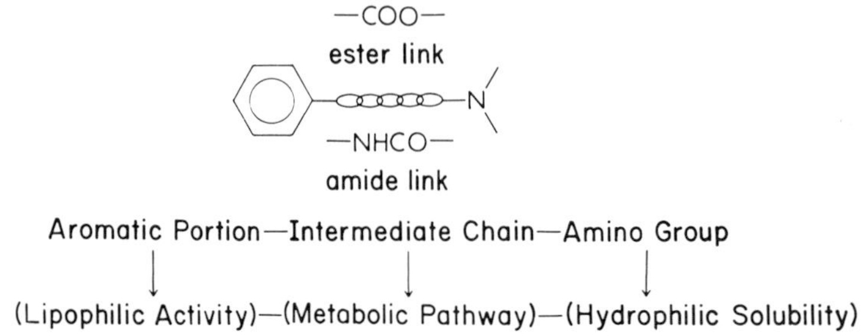

Fig. 4-4. General structure of local anesthetics.

Table 4-2. Characteristics of Amide-Type Local Anesthetics*

Agent	Molecular Weight	Partition Coefficient	pKa	Potency	Toxicity	Plasma Protein Binding (%)	Fetal to Maternal Ratio (Epidural)
Lidocaine	234	12	7.87	1	1	71	0.50
Mepivacaine	282	4	7.69	1	1	82	0.70
Bupivacaine	324	130	8.05	4	4	92	0.30
Etidocaine	276	190	7.74	3	4	94	0.20

*See references 57, 74, 90 and 119.

Table 4-3. Factors Influencing the Plasma Concentration of a Local Anesthetic Drug

I. Drug Dosage
   A. Single
   B. Multiple
II. Access of Drug to Bloodstream
   A. Direct intravenous injection: rate of injection
   B. Absorption from site of application
III. Type of Drug
   A. Degree of ionization
   B. Protein-binding capacity
   C. Vasoactivity
   D. Use of vasoconstrictors with drug
IV. Clearance of Drug
   A. Distribution
   B. Metabolism
     1. Ester
     2. Amide
   C. Excretion

PHYSIOCHEMICAL PROPERTIES OF LOCAL ANESTHETICS

Stability

The amides are very stable drugs and can withstand multiple sterilizations by heat. Autoclaving sterilization of ampules containing bupivacaine plus epinephrine does not lead to decrease in potency of either drug. However, the solution turns light yellow in color and emits a foul-smelling odor similar to rotten eggs or burnt rubber.[39] This is due to the breakdown of one of the preservatives added to the drug, leading to formation of hydrogen sulfide. It is recommended that ampules containing bupivacaine with epinephrine should not be autoclaved.

The esters are less stable than the amides.[73] The expiration date marked on the tetracaine (Pontocaine) ampule should be checked before using the drug for subarachnoid block. Tetracaine tolerates autoclaving well and can even be repeatedly autoclaved.[35]

In the United States, chloroprocaine hydrochloride is available commercially in two forms:

1. *Nesacaine.* This form is supplied in multi-dose vials containing a preservative (methylparaben and sodium sulphite) and is recommended for blocks other than epidural, caudal, or spinal.

2. *Nesacaine-CE.* This form is supplied in single-dose vials containing no preservative and can be used for any form of local anesthesia. Any unused portion of the vial should be discarded.

Chloroprocaine vials should not be autoclaved since this results in hydrolysis of the solution and loss of potency. The vials should be stored in the carton containers since chloroprocaine is sensitive to light. Discolored solution should be discarded. There is no need to store chloroprocaine vials in the refrigerator. On the other hand, if refrigerated, it may precipitate in the form of crystals that dissolve again at room temperature without loss of action.

Procaine loses activity by autoclaving.[35]

Molecular Weight

The commonly used local anesthetic drugs have molecular weights ranging from 230 to 350.

Salts of Local Anesthetics

Local anesthetics are weak bases. The commonly used salts of local anesthetics

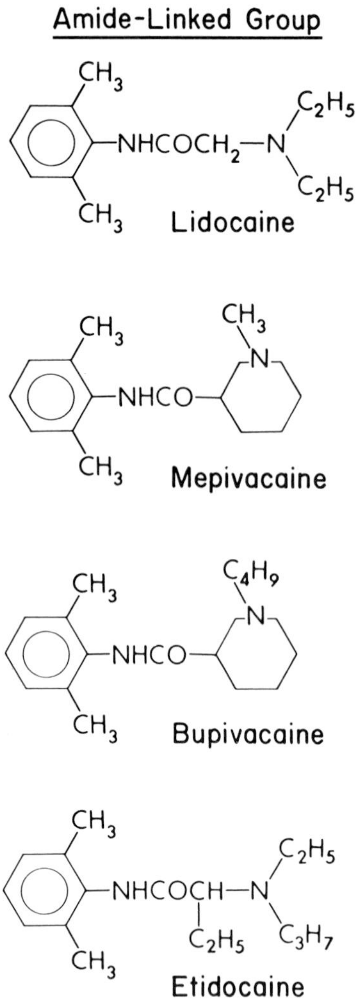

Amide-Linked Group

Lidocaine

Mepivacaine

Bupivacaine

Etidocaine

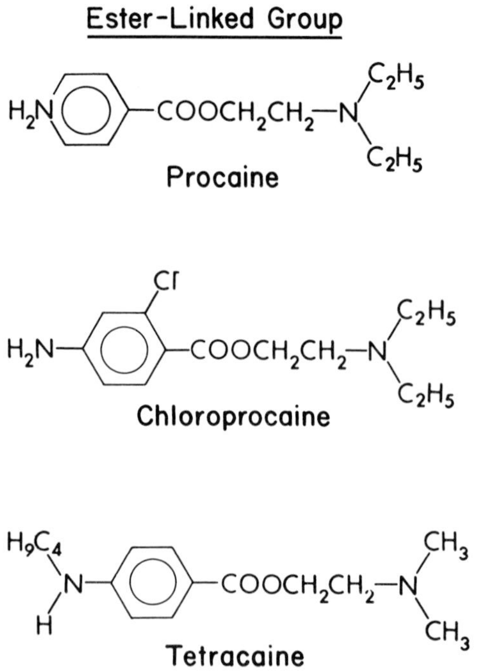

Ester-Linked Group

Procaine

Chloroprocaine

Tetracaine

Fig. 4-5.   Structures of some commonly used local anesthetic drugs.

are the chlorides. Being the salt of a strong acid and a weak base, such solutions are acidic (pH 4 to 5), although many commercial preparations are adjusted to pH 6 to 7. The buffering capacity of most tissues, as well as the blood perfusing them, is usually sufficient to rapidly restore the pH of the injected solution to near normal, thus allowing for better penetration of the nerve membrane.[101] An exception is the mucous membranes, where high concentrations of local anesthetics are required to compensate for deficiency of the buffering capacity. Commercial solutions containing epinephrine have a pH of 3 to 4 because

the acid sodium bisulfite is added to the mixture to prevent epinephrine oxidation. This may lower the tissue pH, interfere with the liberation of adequate quantities of the un-ionized form, and contribute to tachyphylaxis. On the other hand, the addition of concentrated epinephrine from ampules containing 1 mg./ml. to the local anesthetic preparation just prior to its administration does not lower the pH of the solution. If epinephrine is required, it is recommended that it be added to the local anesthetics just before injection. The ideal concentration of epinephrine in the mixture is 1:200,000.

CLASSIFICATION AND MECHANISMS OF ACTION OF LOCAL ANESTHETIC DRUGS

CLASSIFICATION ACCORDING TO CHEMICAL STRUCTURE

As described previously, local anesthetic drugs can be divided into ester- and amide-linked groups.

CLASSIFICATION ACCORDING TO MECHANISM OF ACTION

Modern classification of local anesthetics is according to mechanism of action and serves the purpose of searching for new local anesthetic drugs which are devoid of toxic action on the cardiovascular and central nervous systems.[110] Since conduction of the nerve impulse can be blocked by a wide variety of drugs, including local anesthetics, general anesthetics, and biotoxins, more than one mechanism is involved in the production of nerve block.[98]

There are four main mechanisms, and subsequently four classes of local anesthetics (Fig. 4-6).

Class I: Compounds Acting at the External Orifice of the Na Channel

Class I compounds cannot penetrate the nerve membrane and have no effect when applied internally into the axoplasm. Examples of this group are the biotoxins. Their lack of penetration and their specific external action are important characteristics of this group. These characteristics differentiate them from ordinary local anesthetic agents which can penetrate tissue barriers and thus produce toxic reactions.

Examples of biotoxins are saxitoxin and tetrodotoxin. According to Hille,[60] the external opening of the sodium channel is 5 Å long and 3 Å wide; tetrodotoxin, a puffer fish toxin, plugs this hole.

These biotoxins have a highly specific action and are effective in minute quantities. Indeed, the uptake of these toxins by nervous tissue has been used to determine the number of sodium channels. Usually, the local anesthetic drugs used in practice do not affect the binding of these biotoxins to the nerve membrane because of a different site of action. However, a variety of cations acting on the outside of the mem-

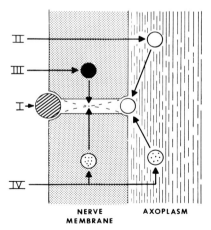

NERVE MEMBRANE   AXOPLASM

Ⅰ ▨ = PLUGGING THE EXTERNAL OPENING OF SODIUM CHANNEL

Ⅱ ◯ = PLUGGING THE INTERNAL OPENING OF SODIUM CHANNEL

Ⅲ ● = EXPANDING THE NERVE MEMBRANE, THUS CLOSING THE SODIUM CHANNEL

Ⅳ ⦿ = BOTH EXPANDING THE NERVE MEMBRANE, AND PLUGGING THE INTERNAL OPENING OF SODIUM CHANNEL

Fig. 4-6. Classification of local anesthetics according to their mode of action.

brane, such as Ca^{++}, do interfere with the toxin binding.

The fact that these biotoxins are highly specific, have a long duration of action, and act in minute quantities, has excited interest in the possibility of clinically using them or their derivatives as local anesthetics. Because of lack of penetration, they would be devoid of the systemic toxic reaction of the conventional local anesthetic drugs.

Class II: Compounds Acting at the Internal Orifice of the Na Channel

Class II compounds are highly ionizable, positively charged, quaternary compounds. They can easily block nerve impulses when internally applied but not when externally applied to the nerve membrane. Examples of this group are local anesthetic derivatives such as N-methyl or ethyl lidocaine.

Class III: Compounds Acting by Penetrating the Nerve Membrane, Causing Its Expansion, and Subsequently Closing or Distorting the Na Channel

These compounds, contrary to Class II compounds, are poorly ionizable and have high lipid solubility. An example of this group is benzocaine.

Class IV: Compounds Acting Both at the Internal Orifice of the Na Channel and in the Nerve Membrane, Causing Its Expansion

Class IV compounds act by the second and third mechanisms (Class II and Class III mechanisms) to block Na^+ exchange. Except for the topical local anesthetic benzocaine, mentioned under Class III, almost all drugs used clinically for local anesthesia belong to this group.

pH AND LOCAL ANESTHETIC ACTIVITY

The majority of local anesthetics are bases with a dissociation constant, pKa, ranging between 7 and 10. They exist in aqueous solution as a mixture of two forms, the un-ionized and the ionized forms, depending on the hydrogen ion concentration of the solution according to this equation:

$$B + H^+ \rightleftharpoons BH^+$$

where B is the un-ionized form, BH^+ is the ionized form, and H^+ is the hydrogen ion.

The relative concentration of each form depends on the pKa of the drug and the pH of the medium. At a pH of 7.4, the medium is relatively acidic to bupivacaine which has a higher pKa than lidocaine or mepivacaine (Table 4-2); therefore, there is a shift in the equation to the right and less B portion of bupivacaine is formed than with lidocaine or mepivacaine. Accordingly, at a pH of 7.4 the percentage of un-ionized portions of bupivacaine, lidocaine, and mepivacaine are 17, 24, and 39 respectively; with acidosis (pH 7) the percentages are 7.4, 11, and 20 respectively.[71] On the whole, if the medium is acidic, there is a shift of the equation to the right, and thus a more ionized fraction is formed. The B portion acts like compounds of Class III, i.e., by expanding the cell membrane. The BH^+ acts like compounds of Class II, i.e., by blocking the internal orifice of the Na^+ channel.

Local anesthetics were found to be more effective at a higher pH. It was therefore thought that the action of the local anesthetic drugs depended on the B form of the anesthetic.[116] However, recently it was found that the BH^+ form plays a more important role in nerve blocking once it reaches the axoplasm,[99] and is responsible for the major part of the blocking activity of the commonly used local anesthetic drugs.[91] The B form, being un-ionizable and fat-soluble, is responsible for the penetrating power of the local anesthetic drug. Hence, the augmented effectiveness of local anesthetic drugs with the rise in pH is due to enhanced penetration secondary to an increase in the un-ionized form.

The ionized form of the local anesthetic does not easily penetrate membranes, and therefore becomes "trapped" if there is intracellular acidosis.[107] This explains the increased toxicity of the local anesthetic with respiratory and metabolic acidosis.[126] The worst combination associated with local anesthetic drug toxicity is extracellular alkalosis where the B form of a local anesthetic exists and can easily diffuse into the cells,[43] combined with intracellular acidosis where more BH^+ type is formed and "trapped," producing a toxic reaction.

If a local anesthetic is injected into an infected area, the low pH of the environment causes a shift in the equation to the right and leads to marked reduction in the B form. This may preclude any local anesthetic effect.[122]

ACTIONS OF THE CARBONATED SOLUTIONS OF LOCAL ANESTHETICS

By raising the pH of the anesthetic solution, there is better penetration and more rapid onset of action. Moreover, carbonated solutions dissociate rapidly and liberate CO_2 which diffuses quickly into the nerve fiber and lowers the pH of the axoplasm. Therefore, more BH^+ is formed inside the nerve fiber, thus enhancing the blocking activity. This explains the finding that carbonated solutions of Class IV local anesthetics produce faster, more intense, and more prolonged analgesia than the chloride solutions.[20,21,26] The actions of compounds of Class I which do not penetrate, and of compounds of Class III which are poorly ionizable, are not affected by the addition of CO_2.

PHARMACOKINETICS OF LOCAL ANESTHETICS

The plasma and whole blood concentrations of local anesthetics are not necessarily interchangeable, neither are the arterial and venous concentrations.[118] For example, the peak maternal arterial level of bupivacaine which is reached in 15 to 30 minutes after epidural or caudal injection is 20 to 40 per cent higher than the level in the venous blood, and 90 per cent of the drug is in the plasma while only 10 per cent is in the erythrocytes.[87] Moreover, the compensatory vasoconstriction above the block increases the gradient between the arterial and venous levels of the drug in the area of vasoconstriction.

FACTORS INVOLVED IN THE PLASMA CONCENTRATION OF A DRUG

The plasma concentration of a drug depends on many factors summarized in Table 4-3. These factors are:

DOSAGE OF THE DRUG

The larger the dose injected, the higher the plasma level of the drug. The injection of the same dosage of local anesthetic, irrespective of the volume or concentration, produces the same plasma level. For example, in dogs following intramuscular injection, a change in the concentration of lidocaine from 2 to 64 per cent resulted in the same plasma level provided the dose was constant.[28]

With continuous techniques, the repeated administration of a drug leads to a cumulative effect.[16] The long intervals between injections with bupivacaine are an important factor causing less rise of the plasma level compared to mepivacaine.[87]

ACCESS OF THE DRUG TO THE BLOODSTREAM

Direct Intravenous Injection

The rate of intravenous injection plays an important role in determining the height of the drug level and the time of its occurrence. Assuming that a local anesthetic drug has a distribution half-life of 2 minutes, an intravenous bolus will produce the highest peak immediately following the end of injection. If the injection time is prolonged to 1 minute, the peak concentration will be reduced to 85 per cent of the bolus value. If the intravenous injection is prolonged to 2 minutes, the peak value reaches only 70 per cent of the bolus value.[80] Also, the peak value is reached later with a slower injection than with a bolus.

With extradural block the rate of injection also plays an important role in determining the height of the anesthetic level in the plasma; e.g., a 15-second injection produces a higher plasma concentration than a 60-second injection. Therefore, there is a good reason for slower rather than faster injection of local anesthetic drugs.

Absorption of Drug From the Site of Application

When a local anesthetic is administered, the plasma level of the drug depends on the rate of absorption from the site of application. If the area has a rich blood supply, the drug will be rapidly absorbed and transported, leading to a fast increase in plasma concentration. Very rapid absorption follows application of local anesthetics to the airway mucosa (Fig. 4-7). There are significantly higher levels of these drugs after intercostal regional block than following epidural block.[18] Following paracervical block, the maternal and fetal blood levels rise very quickly to levels many times higher than after epidural block. The rate of fall is also faster with paracervical block.[55,88] Following injection of the same dose of local anesthetics into the lumbar epidural space, the plasma level of the patient is about 100 per cent higher than following injection of the same dose through the caudal canal.[82] This may balance the higher volume of local anesthetics required to reach the same thoracic segment in the caudal as compared to the lumbar route.

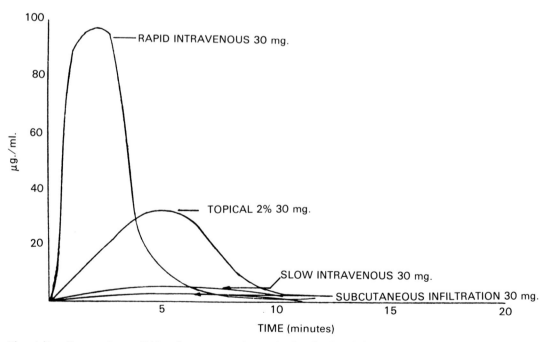

Fig. 4-7.   Comparison of blood concentrations obtained after injecting 30 mg. of tetracaine in dogs intravenously and rapidly over a 30- to 60-second interval; after application topically to the pharyngeal mucous membranes; after slow intravenous infusion; and after subcutaneous infiltration. (Adriani, J., and Campbell, B.: Fatalities following topical application of local anesthetics to mucous membranes. J. Am. Med. Assoc., *162*:1527, 1956)

TYPE OF DRUG USED

The plasma level of a drug depends on:

Degree of Ionization

Infusion of equal amounts of ^{3}H-labeled bupivacaine in rabbits showed a high plasma level of the drug in acidotic animals.[107] The reason for this is increased ionization of bupivacaine in the acidic blood, therefore, less diffusion into tissues, leading to increased plasma concentrations.

Protein-Binding Capacity

Local anesthetic drugs have different binding capacities to either the plasma proteins or erythrocytes. The unbound fraction of an agent increases with increase in the total blood drug concentration because the binding sites approach saturation. (Fig. 4-8). The ratio between the unbound and total drug varies in different individuals and in various pathophysiologic states. There is also species difference in the protein-binding capacity of local anesthetics,[65] and caution must be taken when applying results obtained in experimental animals to man.

The protein-binding capacities of the amide-type local anesthetics are in this order: etidocaine, bupivacaine, mepivacaine, lidocaine, and, the least, prilocaine. The relative binding capacity of these drugs does not correlate with their lipid solubility or their pKa.

The pharmacologic activity of a drug is related to its free or unbound fraction.[117] Moreover, the rate of disappearance of a drug from the bloodstream, by metabolism and tissue distribution, is dependent upon the concentration gradient of the unbound portion of the drug. When the concentration of the unbound molecule decreases, the drug molecules will dissociate from the plasma-protein complex. The rate of this process can be extremely high (i.e., milli- or microsecond).

Strong plasma-protein binding limits the transference of the local anesthetics across the placenta to the fetus. Only the *free* unbound drug crosses the blood-placental barrier, and for the free portion of the drug there is complete fetal/maternal equi-

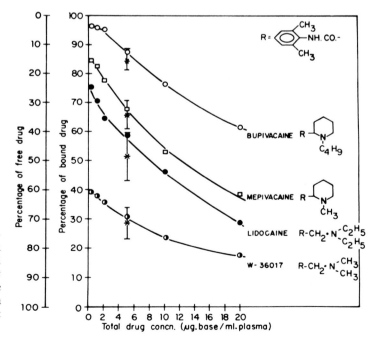

Fig. 4-8. Concentration dependence of human plasma binding of anilide-type local anesthetics. (Tucker, G. T., *et al.*: Binding of anilide-type local anesthetics in human plasma. Anesthesiology, *33*: 287, 1970)

librium (Fig. 4-9). On the other hand, the protein-bound portion of the drug in the maternal or fetal plasma determines to a large extent the total quantities of local anesthetics present on either side of the placenta.

The main factor in the fetal/maternal difference in regard to binding of the amide local anesthetics is the relative absence of the alpha globulins in the fetus. The binding of these drugs is mainly to the lipid-rich globulins, mainly alpha 1 and alpha 2 globulins.[79] Although these globulins have a low capacity for binding, they are still not saturated within the clinical range. After they become saturated, albumin would then bind to enormous amounts of local anesthetics.

A drug with high protein binding may be harmful to the neonate with hyperbilirubinemia. It may displace bilirubin from the binding site, subsequently, the free bilirubin penetrates the central nervous system and produces kernicterus.[70] However, bilirubin is bound to the albumin fraction of the fetal plasma protein, and the local anesthetic is mainly bound to the globulin fraction. Therefore, such a theoretical competition for the same plasma-protein site is unlikely.

Strong plasma-protein binding is also responsible for the slow clearance of the local anesthetic by the liver because the tissue/blood partition coefficient is decreased.

The order of the binding capacities of lidocaine, mepivacaine, and bupivacaine to the *red blood cells* is similar to the order of their binding capacities to plasma proteins.[119]

The affinity of local anesthetics to *tissue binding* is also parallel to their affinity to plasma proteins.[118] This explains the find-

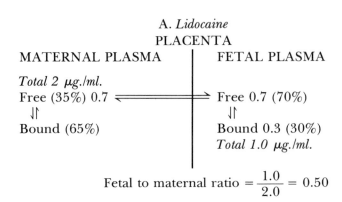

A. *Lidocaine*
PLACENTA

MATERNAL PLASMA | FETAL PLASMA

Total 2 μg./ml.
Free (35%) 0.7 ⇌ Free 0.7 (70%)
  ↓↑   ↓↑
Bound (65%) | Bound 0.3 (30%)
                           Total 1.0 μg./ml.

$$\text{Fetal to maternal ratio} = \frac{1.0}{2.0} = 0.50$$

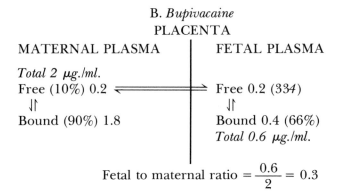

B. *Bupivacaine*
PLACENTA

MATERNAL PLASMA | FETAL PLASMA

Total 2 μg./ml.
Free (10%) 0.2 ⇌ Free 0.2 (334)
  ↓↑   ↓↑
Bound (90%) 1.8 | Bound 0.4 (66%)
                           Total 0.6 μg./ml.

$$\text{Fetal to maternal ratio} = \frac{0.6}{2} = 0.3$$

Fig. 4-9. Schematic representation of distribution of lidocaine and bupivacaine on either side of the placenta. (Abouleish, E.: Placenta transfer of drugs. Diagnostica, *in press*)

ing that the blood levels of the amide local anesthetics after epidural injection of equivalent doses are different, being in this order: bupivacaine, lidocaine, and, the highest, mepivacaine (Fig. 4-10).[96] This increase in tissue binding is partially responsible for the prolonged action of bupivacaine compared to lidocaine. *Moreover, due to increased affinity to lipids,* bupivacaine is taken up by the fatty areolar tissues of the epidural space, and this delays its absorption. Therefore, its persistence at sites near the nerve membrane prolongs its anesthetic effect and lowers its plasma level compared to lidocaine or mepivacaine.

In summary, following epidural analgesia, the neonatal level of bupivacaine is about one-tenth that of lidocaine[96] for the following reasons: (1) bupivacaine is administered in a dosage equivalent to one-fourth that of lidocaine; (2) bupivacaine is more bound to the epidural tissues, including fat, and thus the maternal blood level is lower than with lidocaine; (3) bupivacaine is more attached to the maternal plasma proteins than lidocaine, and thus its free portion amenable to fetal transmission is reduced; and (4) bupivacaine has a much longer duration of action than lidocaine; thus, the need for repeated administration is less.

Vasoactivity

Recently, the direct vasoconstrictor effect of some synthetic local anesthetic drugs has been investigated and will be discussed with the pharmacologic action of local anesthetic drugs. For example, the well known vasoconstrictive effect of cocaine plays an important role in delaying its absorption from the site of injection.

Use of Vasoconstrictors With Local Anesthetic Drugs

Epinephrine potentiates the action of local anesthetic drugs, prolongs their duration, and lowers maternal blood levels. These effects are attributed to: (1) decreased absorption of the local anesthetic due to vasoconstriction; and (2) decreased local blood flow and increased cellular metabolism leading to tissue acidosis. This effect occurs after the local anesthetic has penetrated into the nervous tissues. Reduction of pH decreases the un-ionized portion, and therefore prevents diffusion of the local anesthetic from the nerves and prolongs its duration of action.

These beneficial effects of epinephrine are apparent with lidocaine, mepiva-

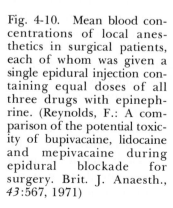

Fig. 4-10. Mean blood concentrations of local anesthetics in surgical patients, each of whom was given a single epidural injection containing equal doses of all three drugs with epinephrine. (Reynolds, F.: A comparison of the potential toxicity of bupivacaine, lidocaine and mepivacaine during epidural blockade for surgery. Brit. J. Anaesth., *43*:567, 1971)

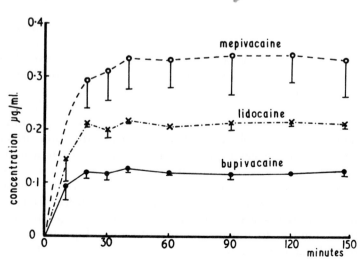

caine,[18,41] and etidocaine,[1,103] but not with bupivacaine.[96,118]

CLEARANCE OF THE DRUG FROM THE BLOODSTREAM

The plasma level of a drug depends not only on the dosage, accessibility to the circulation, and the drug type, but also on the clearance of the drug from the bloodstream which is affected by distribution, metabolism, and excretion.

Drug Distribution

Immediately after reaching the venous side of the circulation, about 30 per cent of the drug is taken by the lungs for 1 minute.[101] This temporary sequestration of the drug tends to momentarily lower its arterial level but may not be sufficient to prevent central nervous system toxicity in case of inadvertent intravenous injection. The vessel-rich tissues receive a large proportion of the drug and retain it for about 10 minutes.[67] By 15 minutes an appreciable amount of the local anesthetic is taken by the muscle group, not because the muscles have a specific affinity for local anesthetics, but due to their high vascular blood supply.[67] After prolonged administration, storage in the body fat plays an important role in maintaining the plasma level, especially with highly lipid-soluble drugs.

In conditions associated with poor tissue perfusion, such as heart failure or shock, distribution of the local anesthetic to muscle and fat is limited.[101] Furthermore, the reduced hepatic and renal blood flows decrease the elimination of the drug through metabolism and excretion. These factors tend to raise the blood level of the drug and restrict a greater proportion of it to the vessel-rich tissue group, including the brain and heart. This may explain in part the poor tolerance of patients with myocardial disease, especially those in heart failure, to intraveneously administered local anesthetics.[114]

Drug Metabolism

Local anesthetic drugs are not metabolized in the epidural or subarachnoid space. They have to be absorbed first and carried by the azygos veins to the vena cava and the heart, then distributed to the whole body, including the liver.[118]

Biotransformation of the local anesthetic drugs renders them less toxic and changes them into more soluble products that can be easily excreted.[35] There is marked species difference in the metabolism of local anesthetics, and one should not extrapolate experimental animal data to man. For example, procaine is hydrolyzed in human plasma at a rate of 4 to 20 times faster than in the plasma of laboratory animals.[50]

The metabolic pathway depends on the type of local anesthetic agent.

Ester-Linked Local Anesthetic Drugs. In man ester-linked local anesthetics are chiefly hydrolyzed by cholinesterases of the plasma, and probably of the placenta as well.[106] This hydrolysis occurs at the ester linkage. The aromatic portion of the drug is then excreted unchanged in the urine, while the amide portion may undergo further metabolic changes. The rate of hydrolysis occurs in this order: chloroprocaine, procaine, and, the least, tetracaine.[50] Chloroprocaine is hydrolyzed 4 times faster than procaine.[8]

The anesthetic quality and potential toxicity of the ester-type agents appear to bear an inverse correlation to the rate of hydrolysis.[28] Thus, chloroprocaine with the shortest duration of action and the least toxicity is the most rapidly hydrolyzed. The use of anticholinesterases, such as neostigmine, inhibits the hydrolysis of the ester-linked local anesthetics.[50]

If an obstetric patient or one of her relatives has a history of prolonged succinylcholine apnea, the ester-type local anesthetic drugs are contraindicated. The danger in such a case is that a sustained high level of the local anesthetic may occur, leading not only to maternal but also to fetal toxicity. The absence of a history of apnea following succinylcholine in the parents does not exclude them as possible carriers for abnormal pseudocholinesterase which is inherited as an autosomal recessive trait. Consequently the fetus may not be able to hydrolyze the ester-linked drug that reaches its circulation. This is very rare (1:200,000), but should be borne in mind.[124]

Cocaine, which is also an ester-linked drug, is rarely used in clinical practice today because of its addiction liability and restrictions by the Bureau of Narcotics. It is metabolized mainly in the plasma while one-fifth is excreted in the urine.[35]

Amide-Linked Local Anesthetic Drugs. The amide-type local anesthetic drugs are mainly metabolized by the liver and the products are then excreted by the kidneys.[6,109] For example, lidocaine is metabolized by liver microsomes but not by brain, kidney, or placental homogenates.[53] The precise metabolic pathway of the amides varies with each drug and the animal species. In rats, hepatectomy resulted in substantially higher tissue levels of lidocaine and an increase in the anesthetic activity and duration of toxic symptoms produced by this agent.[28] In addition, the rate of disappearance of lidocaine from blood was decreased in hepatectomized dogs and in patients whose liver had been removed during the course of liver transplantation.[6] For this reason, in patients with hepatic disease the dose of amide-linked local anesthetics should be reduced lest a toxic reaction occur.[105]

Clearance of the amide-linked local anesthetics by the liver depends mainly on the hepatic blood flow. In case of marked hypotension or heart failure, there is prolonged clearance of these drugs.

Prilocaine is the only clinically used amide-linked local anesthetic that is metabolized by both the kidney and liver, although the latter appears to be the prime site of metabolism.[52]

Enzyme induction can affect the bio-transformation of local anesthetics by the liver. For instance, pretreatment with phenobarbital accelerates the metabolism of procaine, lidocaine, and mepivacaine in rodents.[58] On the other hand, a monoamine oxidase inhibitor, such as iproniazid, slows the biotransformation of lidocaine and mepivacaine and prolongs their toxic effects. Perhaps epileptic patients under phenobarbital treatment metabolize local anesthetics faster than normal patients;[42] this was not noted with lidocaine in patients under phenobarbital treatment.[59]

Drug Excretion

In the mother, renal excretion of the unchanged drug accounts for a negligible proportion of the amide local anesthetics. For example, only 10 per cent of bupivacaine[81] and 2 to 11 per cent of lidocaine[9,17,109] are excreted by the kidney, while the rest is metabolized in the body. The percentages of the different metabolites excreted by the kidneys vary considerably with different species, depending on biliary recycling and further degradation by the liver prior to their excretion.[17]

Clearance of local anesthetics increases in the following order: bupivacaine, mepivacaine, lidocaine, and etidocaine.[118] However, their fat solubility increases in this order: mepivacaine, lidocaine, bupivacaine, and etidocaine.[19,119] Therefore, clearance of these drugs has no correlation with their fat solubility.

Following epidural injection of bupivacaine or etidocaine, the clearance curve of the drugs from the bloodstream is biphasic.[73] There is an initial rapid fall in drug concentration to 50 per cent, called *the initial half-life of the drug*, which occurs within 25 to 35 minutes. Following this there is a gradual fall to 50 per cent of the new level, called *the late half-life of the drug*, which occurs within 2 to 4 hours (Fig. 4-11). The initial clearance is due to the rapid drug distribution; the late fall is due to the slow metabolism by the liver.

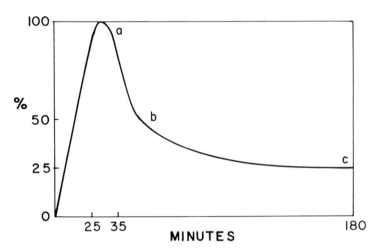

Fig. 4-11. Clearance curve of bupivacaine or etidocaine following epidural block. Segment a-b = the initial half-life of the drug; segment b-c = the late half-life of the drug. (Adapted from Lund, P. C., Cwik, J. C., and Pagdanganan, R. T.: Etidocaine—a new long-acting anesthetic agent: a clinical evaluation. Anesth. Analg., 52:482, 1973)

When bupivacaine is used for continuous epidural analgesia, the maximum plasma level of the drug reached after prolonged analgesia (8 hours) is not significantly higher than the peak reached after the initial dose.[113] This indicates that the rate of clearance of bupivacaine is approximately the same as the rate of its administration for providing analgesia. The maximum plasma concentration of bupivacaine is usually 0.68 µg./ml. which is much lower than the toxic level (> 4 µg./ml.).[113] This is an important advantage of bupivacaine over other amide drugs.

In the neonate, owing to the inadequate enzymatic metabolism by the liver, renal excretion is a very important route for clearance of the amide-type local anesthetics (e.g., 90% of mepivacaine is excreted unchanged in 24 hours).[83]

TACHYPHYLAXIS TO LOCAL ANESTHETICS

Tachyphylaxis to a local anesthetic drug must be considered when a progressive increase in the maintenance dose is required to assure adequate analgesia. This particularly occurs when the block has been allowed to relapse into complete functional recovery.

The mechanism of tachyphylaxis is probably due to a progressive decline in the pH of the epidural space due to repeated administration of the local anesthetic salts, usually chlorides. Subsequently, there is reduction of the un-ionized form and a decrease in the penetrative power of the local anesthetic.[23] There is a correlation between the rate of development of tachyphylaxis and the pKa of the local anesthetic agent, i.e., tolerance occurs more rapidly to agents with a lower pKa. To prevent tachyphylaxis, drugs of long duration of action and with a high pKa should be used (i.e., bupivacaine is preferred to mepivacaine or lidocaine). A buffer to increase the pH within the epidural space and the carbonated solutions of local anesthetics rather than the chloride salts have been used to avoid tachyphylaxis. However, the combination of epinephrine and carbonated solutions increases tachyphylaxis.[85]

A statement that a patient has developed tachyphylaxis should not be used as a "cover-up" for inadequacy of drug dosage or technique, such as faulty position of the catheter. Such causes of inadequate analgesia should be excluded and corrected if present before considering tachyphylaxis as the cause.

The author has not encountered tachyphylaxis with the use of bupivacaine. This is due to:

1. The inherent properties of the drug

itself (i.e., its high pKa and long duration of action)

2. The use of a higher concentration of the drug (e.g., 0.375% to 0.5% rather than 0.125%)

3. The administration of a larger volume of the local anesthetic solution to obtain a rather wide margin of block. As analgesia wears off, the area of blockade becomes retracted. If one or two segments on each side of the required segmental block are also included, the duration of block is prolonged and aberrant anatomical variations can be compensated for.

4. Injection of the "refill" doses at the proper time. Repeated injections of local anesthetics at specific times are not advisable because the duration of action of drugs varies in different individuals. On the other hand, as soon as the patient starts to feel uncomfortable a refill dose should be injected.

DRUG POTENCY

To produce the same degree and extent of block, the required dosages of anes-thetic drugs are inversely proportionate to their potency. Lidocaine is slightly less potent than mepivacaine. Bupivacaine is about 3 to 4 times as potent as either lidocaine or mepivacaine (Table 4-4).[87] Therefore, 0.5 per cent bupivacaine is equivalent to 1.5 to 2 per cent lidocaine or mepivacaine. Without epinephrine, 0.75 per cent bupivacaine has a longer duration of action and more intense analgesia than 1 per cent etidocaine with or without epinephrine.[1]

GENERAL PHARMACOLOGIC AND TOXIC EFFECTS OF LOCAL ANESTHETICS

Local anesthetic drugs have an effect on almost every system in the body.

EFFECTS ON THE CARDIOVASCULAR SYSTEM

The hemodynamic effects of local anes-thetics are complex. They may be due to direct action on the cardiovascular system, central stimulation of the autonomic centers, peripheral sympathetic blockade, and

Table 4-4. Actions of Local Anesthetic Drugs Without Epinephrine During Epidural Analgesia*

Drug	Conc.	Onset (min.)	Sensory Effects (Average) Maximum (min.)	Regression† (hours)	Duration (hours)	Onset (min.)	Motor Effects (Average) Maximum (min.)	Duration (hours)
Lidocaine	1%	7	20	1.25	1.75	—	—	—
	2%	5	19	1.5	2	9	25	1.75
Mepivacaine	1%	8	22	1.5	2	—	—	—
	2%	7	20	1.75	3	13	25	2.25
Bupivacaine	0.25%	5	20	2.5	4	—	—	—
	0.5%	4	19	2.75	5	10	30	4
	0.75%	4	17	3.5	7	10	20	5
Etidocaine	0.5%	4	17	2.5	4	10	18	4.75
	1%	4	16	3	4.5	9	16	5.5
Chloroprocaine	2%	3	10	0.75	1.25	10	15	1
	3%	3	8	1.25	1.5	7	12	1.25

*References 19, 48, 73, 74, and 87.
†Regression refers to the time between last injection and regression of the maximum anesthetic level by 2 dermatomes.

indirect effect due to hypoxia if it occurs secondary to convulsions or an extensive intravertebral block.

Cardiac Actions of Local Anesthetics

Recently, lidocaine has been successfully used as an antiarrhythmic drug. This has led to great expansion of knowledge of its cardiac effects, which are:

Electrophysiologic Effects[11,31]

At Therapeutic Concentrations. The mechanism of ventricular arrhythmias is illustrated in Figure 4-12A. Due to a diseased Purkinje fiber, there is unidirectional block of the electrical wave impulse, preventing its propagation forward to, but not from, the ventricular muscle. Therefore, the impulse has to reach the corresponding ventricular muscle by way of the adjacent muscle supplied by a healthy Purkinje fiber. The impulse is then conducted back to the healthy Purkinje fiber and a circus movement is created leading to an ectopic focus. Lidocaine, by improving the conductivity of the diseased Purkinje fiber,

abolishes the block and the ventricular muscles are simultaneously stimulated (Fig. 4-12B). Therefore the circus movement disappears, and subsequently the arrhythmia vanishes.

At Toxic Doses. Local anesthetics depress the rate of depolarization of both the conductive tissue and the ventricular muscle itself, leading to various kinds and degrees of heart blocks.

Effects on the Contractile Force of the Heart

At Therapeutic Doses. With a plasma level of 4 to 8 μg./ml. lidocaine, there is an increase in the mean arterial blood pressure due to enhancement of the cardiac output.[16,65] The same effect was found with other local anesthetics such as chloroprocaine[49] or mepivacaine.[65] This increase in cardiac output is mainly due to a rise in the heart rate, caused by increased activity of the central sympathetic system whose inhibition is reduced by the depressant action of lidocaine on the higher centers.

The interaction of lidocaine with anes-

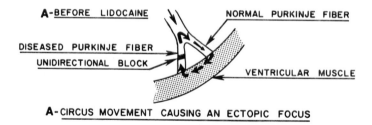

A-CIRCUS MOVEMENT CAUSING AN ECTOPIC FOCUS

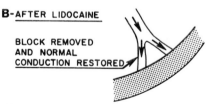

B-SIMULTANEOUS STIMULATION OF THE VENTRICULAR MUSCLE

Fig. 4-12. Mechanism of the antiarrhythmic action of lidocaine.

thetics such as barbiturates or halothane causes cardiovascular depression which is not seen with lidocaine alone.[77]

At Toxic Doses. Local anesthetics ultimately depress the myocardium, leading to hypotension and cardiac arrest.

VASCULAR ACTIONS OF LOCAL ANESTHETICS

After intravenous infusion, lidocaine and mepivacaine increase the tone of the *veins* which represent the capacitance vessels.[56,66] This increases the venous return to the heart and contributes to the rise in the cardiac output and the mean arterial blood pressure.

On the arterial side of the circulation where most of the peripheral resistance is encountered, local anesthetics, including lidocaine, bupivacaine, and etidocaine, have a vasodilating effect and, therefore, decrease the peripheral resistance.[12,41] However, in experimental animals, local anesthetics may directly increase the vascular tone and the peripheral resistance.[2] This *in vivo* vasoconstricting property of the local anesthetics is supported by the *in vitro* studies on spontaneously contractible vascular tissue such as the rat portal vein.[2,12] Both the myogenic tone and the rate of the spontaneous contractions of the portal vein are initially increased, then inhibited, by the increasing dosage of local anesthetic drugs. This direct effect can be due to drug actions on the cytoplasmic Ca^{++} and its exchange with the extracellular compartment.

In conclusion, local anesthetic drugs have generally a vasodilating effect and a potential vasoconstricting action on certain vascular compartments (e.g., the veins) and at certain concentrations. Clinically, the overall effect is a decrease in peripheral resistance and an increase in venous return to the heart. However, if sympathetic blockade accompanies the administration of local anesthetics (e.g., during epidural or spinal block), the decrease in peripheral resistance becomes more man-

ifest,[16] and any direct venoconstricting effect below the block becomes suppressed by indirect vasodilating action. The only local anesthetic drug that appears to have a consistent vasoconstricting effect is cocaine. Its initial temporary vasodilation is followed by prolonged vasoconstriction.[92] Cocaine's vasoconstricting action is due to inhibition of the reuptake of catecholamines by the adrenergic nerve terminals resulting in a higher concentration of norepinephrine at the receptor site, thus prolonging vasoconstriction.[62,76]The direct vasoconstrictor effect of the local anesthetics may be responsible for the reduction of the uterine blood flow and fetal bradycardia following paracervical block.

At or below dosages that produce convulsions, the local anesthetics clinically used today do not depress the cardiovascular system unless the patient is hypoxic, acidotic, under the influence of circulatory depressant drugs, or has sympathetic blockade.[90]

CENTRAL NERVOUS SYSTEM EFFECTS

CENTRAL NERVOUS SYSTEM DEPRESSION CAUSED BY LOCAL ANESTHETICS

Local anesthetic drugs are central nervous system depressants. This is evidenced by the suppressive effects of local anesthetics against seizures produced by electric shock,[46] convulsive drugs such as pentylenetetrazol,[11] and epilepsy.[10] Local anesthetic drugs have been used to supplement general anesthesia.[120] They can also inhibit alcoholic withdrawal seizures in mice.[51]

Local anesthetic drugs, with the exception of cocaine, do not cause addiction.

CONVULSIVE EFFECTS OF LOCAL ANESTHETICS

Mechanism

The convulsive effect of local anesthetics is a continuation of their depressive effect on the central nervous system and is due to selective blockade of the inhibitory cortical synapses.[33] This allows the facilitatory neurons to function unopposed, thus leading to an increase in central nervous system excitation, ultimately manifested in convulsions. Further increase in dosage of the local anesthetics produces depression of both inhibitory and facilitatory neurons, leading to a generalized state of CNS depression, including apnea. The evidence for this theory is that when procaine is applied to the cortical neurons *in vitro*, only depression of the neurons is obtained.[54]

Seizure foci originate in the amygdala in cats and rabbits, but no specific foci were observed in rhesus monkeys.[90]

Hypoxia, hypercapnia, acidosis, and circulatory depression reduce the dose of the local anesthetics required to cause convulsions.[32,86,120]

Etiology

A local anesthetic can cause convulsions in the following conditions:

Inadvertent Intravenous Injection of Too Large a Dose. As previously stated, at 1 μg./ml. the degree of plasma binding of bupivacaine, mepivacaine, and lidocaine is 92 per cent, 82 per cent, and 71 per cent respectively. Expressing this data conversely, the relative concentration of the unbound drugs is 1:2.2:3.5 respectively. Although the physiologic effects of a drug depend on the free portion which diffuses through membranes, in acute toxicity the reaction depends on the total dose injected and will not follow the above ratios. This is because the plasma-protein binding sites of

the drug become overwhelmed by the sudden administration of a too large dose, so that the deciding factor will be the relative intrinsic toxicity of the drug. Therefore, the toxic dose of bupivacaine will be just one-fourth that of either lidocaine or mepivacaine.[119] An intravenous bolus dose of lidocaine in excess of 1.5 mg./kg. or an equivalent dose of the other drugs (See Table 4-2), exposes the patient to a toxic reaction (Table 4-7).

Slow intravenous injection raises the total amount of the local anesthetic drug that can be administered before the patient (or experimental animal) develops toxic manifestations. For example, with bupivacaine a 70-kg. patient convulses with an intravenous bolus of 50 mg. whereas the same patient tolerates 100 mg. without toxic reaction if the latter dose is infused over 20 minutes.[81] Using etidocaine, 236 mg. could be intravenously injected in man at 10 mg./min. before developing toxic manifestations, whereas only 161 mg. could be tolerated at 20 mg./min.[103] With bupivacaine, the dose tolerated at the same rate of infusion is less than that of etidocaine because etidocaine is more rapidly cleared from the plasma than bupivacaine. However, the tolerated plasma level for both drugs in man is the same, 2 μg./ml. of plasma.

There is a species difference in tolerance levels of these drugs. Dogs and monkeys, for instance, tolerate a high level.[65,90] The seizure threshold of bupivacaine or etidocaine in the rhesus monkey is 4 μg./ml. (Table 4-5). In the same species there is also a difference in tolerance.[90]

Table 4-5. Local Anesthetic Seizure Thresholds in Rhesus Monkey*

Drug	*Infusion Rate* (mg./kg./min.)	*Seizure Dose* (mg./kg.)	*Plasma Conc. at Onset of Seizures* (μg./ml.)
Bupivacaine	1	4.4 ± 1.2	4.4 ± 1.7
Etidocaine	1	5.4 ± 1.2	4.3 ± 1.4
Lidocaine	4	22.5 ± 4.4	18.2 ± 1.5

*Developed from data by Munson, E. S., *et al.*: Etidocaine, bupivacaine and lidocaine seizure thresholds in monkeys. Anesthesiology, *42*:471, 1975.

Exceeding the Maximum Permissible Dosages (Table 4-6). The plasma level of a drug can exceed the seizure threshold if excessive amounts of the drug are administered, especially with continuous techniques in which the blood concentrations of the drug are increased with each subsequent dose. This, as mentioned before, is particularly evident with lidocaine and mepivacaine while almost absent with bupivacaine because of the long intervals between doses with the latter drug. With the amide-linked local anesthetics, if the patient has severe liver disease, a toxic level may be reached with a therapeutic dose, especially if hypotension occurs. Hypotension reduces the liver perfusion, thus decreasing the clearance of the drug. With ester-linked local anesthetics, if the patient has abnormal pseudocholinesterase, a toxic level may be reached with a therapeutic dose.

Anaphylactic Reaction to the Drug. This is very rare. There should have been a history of reaction to the drug in the form of a skin rash, bronchial asthma, or laryngeal edema (see Allergic Reactions to Local Anesthetics, below).

Abnormal Susceptibility to the Drug. With abnormal susceptibility, a toxic rather than a therapeutic response follows the regular therapeutic dose. This is extremely rare and is usually used as a "cover-up" of a faulty technique (e.g., inadvertent intravenous injection).

SIGNS AND SYMPTOMS OF TOXIC REACTIONS TO LOCAL ANESTHETICS

Mild Toxic Reactions

Symptoms of a mild reaction usually follow the test dose of the drug. The patient senses a metallic taste and develops numbness of the face, tinnitus in the ears, vertigo, blurred vision, nausea and vomiting, slurred speech, and a change in the sensorium such as apprehension or irrational behavior.

Table 4-6. Maximum Permissible Doses of Local Anesthetic Drugs for Epidural or Caudal Analgesia

Drug	Without Epinephrine Adult mg./kg.	(70 kg.)	With Epinephrine Adult mg./kg.	(70 kg.)
Lidocaine	9	600	12	750
Mepivacaine	9	600	12	750
Bupivacaine	3	200	3.5	250
Etidocaine	4	300	5.5	400
Chloroprocaine	12	800	14	1000

Moderate Toxic Reactions

Following the previous mild manifestations, a moderate reaction to the local anesthetic may develop, in which case the patient stares, loses consciousness, and develops tremors and twitching especially of the facial muscles.

Severe Toxic Reactions

After the previous manifestations of mild and moderate toxic reactions which occur in a very rapid succession, in less

Table 4-7. Intravenous Lidocaine in Man*

Usual Therapeutic Doses and Levels	Should Not Exceed†
I. V. Bolus: 0.75 mg./kg. (Repeat if necessary up to 3 times.)	1.5 mg./kg.
Infusion: 25–50 µg./kg./min.	50 µg./kg./min.
2–4 mg./min. for 70-kg. adult	4 mg./min. for 70-kg. adult
100–200 mg./hour for 70-kg. adult	250 mg./hour for 70-kg. adult (no more than 8 hours)
Plasma Level: 2–8 µg./ml.	10 µg./ml.

*Developed from data by Usubiaga, J. E.: *In* Munson, E. S., *et al.*: Local anesthetic drug-induced seizures in rhesus monkeys [guest discussion]. Anesth. Analg., *49*:994, 1970, and Grace, W. J.: Protocol for the management of arrhythmias in acute myocardial infarction. Crit. Care. Med., 2:235, 1974.

†Doses should be reduced in liver disease, hypotension, and heart failure.

than 1 minute following the end of inadvertent intravenous injection, the patient convulses. The seizures are in the form of tonic, then clonic spasms, followed by apnea. Fortunately, with the clinically used local anesthetic drugs, the blood pressure and pulse rate show slight elevation. The acid-base state and the blood gases are normal until the onset of seizures.[89] The patient then becomes rapidly cyanotic because of the increased oxygen demand and the inability to breathe.

The main dangers of convulsions are respiratory inadequacy, respiratory obstruction, physical trauma, vomiting, regurgitation, and aspiration. These may lead to acute heart failure and arrest if not prevented or corrected at the proper time.

Accompanying the prodromal symptoms there is preseizure electrical activity of the brain characterized by diffuse slowing with large-amplitude spikes and slow-wave complexes (Fig. 4-13).[90] These preseizure EEG changes and the prodromal symptoms are especially evident with lidocaine and chloroprocaine. With etidocaine the preseizure changes are not so evident, while bupivacaine occupies an intermediate position.[90] However, the EEG changes accompanying the seizures are similar in all of these drugs. There are bursts of high-amplitude spikes lasting for 3 to 5 seconds, alternating with periods of electrical silence.[45] During these bursts of electrical activity the pupils in monkeys were found to dilate, then to reconstrict with the termination of the paroxysmal high-voltage activity.[24] Whether these pupillary changes are related to sympathetic discharge has yet to be determined.

Fortunately, the patient develops amnesia of the prodromal symptoms, the convulsive episode, and a certain period after the incident.

DIFFERENTIAL DIAGNOSIS OF THE CAUSE OF CONVULSIONS

There are many possible causes of convulsions in association with parturition other than toxic reaction to local anesthetics. These are:

Anesthetic-Related Causes

Hypertensive Crisis. Sudden severe hypertension may occur during parturition, leading to cerebral encephalopathy or cerebrovascular accident. This hypertensive episode can be due to:

1. *Epinephrine.* The pressor dose of epinephrine is 70 μg./min. Cerebral hemorrhage and a blood pressure above 300 mm. Hg can follow intravenous injection of 0.5 mg. of epinephrine.[54]

2. *Vasopressors.* The use of an excessive dose of a vasopressor, particularly of an alpha pressor, to counteract hypotension before or after delivery may lead to severe hypertension. This is particularly seen when the vasopressor is combined with an ergot preparation.[22]

3. *Ergot Alkaloids.* Even without a vasopressor, the intravenous or intramuscular ergot alkaloid injection can lead to severe hypertension and convulsions,[3] especially in a toxemic or hypertensive patient. Ergot should only be used to control a life-threatening hemorrhage when other methods have failed, and only by the intramuscular route.

4. *Ketamine Anesthesia.* Ketamine can cause a rise of blood pressure and carries a potential danger of a hypertensive crisis in a toxemic or hypertensive patient.

Marked Hypotension. A severe fall in blood pressure may lead to cerebral ischemia and convulsions. Major regional analgesia such as spinal, epidural, or caudal blocks can produce hypotension which, if severe and prolonged, causes convulsions and even permanent cerebral damage. It cannot be stressed enough that a patient under these blocks should be continuously monitored.

The intravenous administration of oxytocin in a hypovolemic patient can cause marked vasodilation and hypotension. Oxytocin should be administered by intravenous infusion or by intramuscular

Fig. 4-13. Electroencephalographic changes with convulsive doses of lidocaine and etidocaine. *A.* Electroencephalographic record before and during infusion of lidocaine, 4 mg./kg./min. to the onset of seizure. The seizure dosage of lidocaine was 18.8 mg./kg. The irregular pattern of large-amplitude spike and slow-wave complexes just prior to seizure is apparent in all EEG leads. SM COR indicates sensory motor cortex; HIPP, Hippocampus; CAUD, caudate nucleus; AMYG, amygdala; ECG, electrocardiogram; PG, pneumogram. *B.* Electroencephalographic record before and during infusion of etidocaine, 1 mg./kg./min. The seizure dosage of etidocaine was 4.5 mg./kg. This record and record *A* were obtained from the same animal. Note the relative absence of induced electrical changes with the exception of a few spike and slow-wave complexes in each EEG lead. The symbols are the same as in *A.* (Munson, E. S., *et al.*: Etidocaine, bupivacaine and lidocaine seizure thresholds in monkeys. Anesthesiology, *42*:471, 1975)

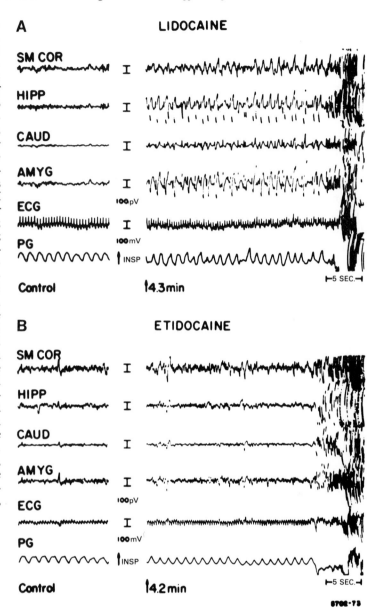

route, but never in a bolus exceeding 2 units.[123]

Hypoxia With or Without Hypercapnia. This may result from paralysis of the muscles of respiration under regional analgesia. Also, it can be due to respiratory insufficiency under general anesthesia. A particular danger to the parturient is aspiration of gastric contents which can occur with general anesthesia or extensive block, especially if the mother has been oversedated.

Obstetric-Related Causes

Eclampsia. This is a major but not the only, cause of convulsions in obstetrics.

The history of toxemia during the antenatal course, and the presence of signs such as hyper-reflexia, hypertension, and/or albuminuria before the onset of seizures, help to diagnose the case.

Embolism. Emboli usually reach the pulmonary circulation and lead to hypoxia and systemic hypotension. However, cerebral embolism can occur if there is associated valvular cardiac disease or a patent shunt through which the embolus bypasses the pulmonary circulation and directly reaches the systemic circulation. The most common source of embolism during parturition is the amniotic fluid. This should be kept in mind if the convulsing patient is hypotensive and cyanotic especially without having received general or local anesthesia.

Severe Hypotension Secondary to Bleeding. Hemorrhage is a major cause of maternal death[112] and may be preceded by convulsions due to cerebral ischemia.

1. Hemorrhage can occur during the *antenatal period* due to placenta previa or abruptio placentae.

2. It can occur *intrapartum* due to rupture of the uterus.

3. It can happen *postpartum* due to uterine atony, ruptured uterus, or lacerated cervix.

Hypovolemia should be adequately and promptly corrected not only for the immediate results, but also for the delayed effects on the parenchymatous organs, especially the kidneys and lungs, and the healing power of the body.

Associated Disease. Certain diseases associated with pregnancy may worsen with pregnancy and parturition, leading to convulsions. These include:

1. *Intracranial Hemorrhage.* This may be secondary to a ruptured berry aneurysm or a severe hypertensive attack.

2. *Heart Failure.* A cardiac patient, especially during the postpartum period, may develop acute heart failure, cerebral hypoxia, and convulsions.

3. *Hypoglycemia.* In a diabetic patient, excessive doses of insulin may lead to hypoglycemia and convulsions. The usual dosage of insulin may cause marked hypoglycemia during the postpartum period due to the removal of anti-insulin factors which were associated with the presence of the placenta. Therefore, the dosage of insulin during the day of parturition should be either omitted or markedly reduced. In the postpartum period the maternal blood sugar should be closely checked and intravenous glucose infusion administered.

Hyperventilation. In unpremedicated patients with severe pain, the $PaCO_2$ may be reduced to a markedly low level. This may be exaggerated if an attempt is made to reduce pain by hyperventilation leading to tetany which can be mistaken for convulsion. The treatment in such cases is to give analgesics or, better yet, to administer an epidural block.

Other Causes of Convulsions

Other causes, although unrelated to pregnancy and anesthesia, can produce seizures and be mistakenly diagnosed as a toxic reaction to a local anesthetic drug. These diseases include:

Associated Neurologic Disease.

1. *Epilepsy.* During the patient's antenatal visits any history of convulsions should be recorded. The epileptic patient's chart should be clearly marked, and, if under treatment, the drugs and dosages should be specified. This saves confusion and unnecessary treatment which could be dangerous if an epileptic convulses in the labor suite or delivery room.

2. *Brain Tumor.* The patient's medical history and previous investigations usually make such a cause quite evident.

Drug Withdrawal. If a patient is addicted to narcotics or barbiturates, withdrawal symptoms, including seizures, may occur. In these cases proper history and observation are important.

Hysteria. This can take any form, including convulsions, but such a diagnosis of hysteria should be considered only after excluding all other causes.

PROPHYLAXIS AGAINST TOXIC REACTIONS TO LOCAL ANESTHETICS

The use of local anesthetic drugs should be taken seriously. Before these drugs are used, whether for dentistry, surgery, or obstetrics, a thorough knowledge of their pharmacology and complications should be obtained, with attention to details. Drugs and equipment for cardiopulmonary resuscitation as well as anticonvulsant drugs such as diazepam should be readily available. Proper training and adequate experience with cardiopulmonary resuscitation are prerequisites for using local anesthetic drugs in any form and for any purpose.

In obstetrics, especially with continuous epidural or caudal analgesia, the injection of a test dose of the local anesthetic is mandatory before administering the therapeutic dose. Aspiration before, during, and after injection should be done. The absence of a bloody aspirate does not exclude the presence of the tip of the needle or catheter in a blood vessel. Injection of a local anesthetic should be done slowly. The blood pressure should be measured before and repeatedly after injection. Verbal contact with the patient should be continued throughout. An intravenous cannula must be inserted and securely taped in the parturient, especially before starting any anesthetic or analgesic technique. An assistant should be present in the room to help in case a complication occurs. Sometimes work in the delivery room tends to be rushed, but it should always be remembered that safety comes first.

Diphenylhydantoin (Dilantin) not only is ineffective in preventing local anesthetic seizures, it may even enhance them.[36] In cats, the intravenous injection of diazepam, 0.3 mg./kg., was found to prevent local anesthetic convulsions.[47] Diazepam is a better anticonvulsant drug than barbiturates.[36] In cats, alertness, gait, and especially coordination were much less affected by diazepam than by pentobarbital. EEG changes were minimal after diazepam administration, whereas those following pentobarbital administration were strikingly different from controls. Further, the barbiturate-lidocaine sequence caused more respiratory, circulatory, and central nervous system depression than after diazepam-lidocaine. Lastly, periods of electrical inactivity of the brain were briefer and the EEG returned to normal sooner after the diazepam-lidocaine sequence than following pentobarbital-lidocaine. *However, the use of these drugs in clinical practice before the administration of a local anesthetic drug is neither a guarantee against seizures nor a substitute for proper techniques.* Even intravenous doses of thiopental, sufficient to cause sleep (2 to 4 mg.), will not prevent convulsions; they will only increase the amount of local anesthetic drugs required to produce a convulsion.[120]

Diazepam has significant anticonvulsant actions without cardiovascular or respiratory depression.[36,47,90] The primary site of the antagonistic action of diazepam to local anesthetic-induced seizures is at the brain stem reticular formation.[47]

TREATMENT OF TOXIC REACTIONS TO LOCAL ANESTHETICS

TREATMENT OF MILD REACTIONS

Further injection of the local anesthetic drugs is stopped, the patient is reassured, and the site of injection or technique is changed.

TREATMENT OF MODERATE REACTIONS

Oxygen is administered by a face mask, and intravenous diazepam, 0.1 mg./kg., is injected.[90] Diazepam in such a dose rapidly aborts or terminates the convulsions without circulatory or respiratory depression, which is a major advantage over barbiturates.

TREATMENT OF SEVERE REACTIONS

Oxygen is administered by a face mask and diazepam is injected intravenously. If convulsions are not stopped or recur, cricoid pressure is applied, succinylcholine is injected, and intubation is performed using a cuffed endotracheal tube. (The use of a cuffed endotracheal tube is a safeguard against aspiration.) Respiration is then controlled using oxygen, and the situation is evaluated. The maternal pulse and blood pressure are measured and the fetal heart rate is computed. Usually the fetal heart rate is normal, but if slow, intrauterine resuscitation should be allowed if possible. By waiting rather than rushing the delivery, the drug level in the fetus will be reduced, and the fetal condition will improve by properly oxygenating and maintaining the maternal circulation. Proper ventilation is important to prevent both metabolic acidosis due to hypoxia and respiratory acidosis due to CO_2 accumulation. Both kinds of acidoses potentiate the convulsive effects of local anesthetic drugs.[45]

If severe hypotension, regurgitation, aspiration, or cardiac arrest develop, appropriate treatment should be instituted. The decision in these cases whether or not to deliver the baby and the delivery route will depend on the maternal and fetal conditions, the stage of labor, the type of drug, and the risks of waiting versus the risks involved in delivering a baby carrying a large dosage of a local anesthetic.

PROGNOSIS

If resuscitative equipment is available and the operator is experienced, the prognosis is usually good. Although convulsions increase the brain oxygen demand, both brain oxygenation and cerebral metabolic requirements remain satisfactory provided pulmonary ventilation is adequate and the arterial blood pressure is normal.[95] If respiratory arrest occurs, the airway is obstructed, or aspiration develops, hypoxia, especially of the brain and heart, supervenes, leading to cardiac arrest, cerebral damage, or death.

EPILEPTIC PATIENTS AND LOCAL ANESTHETIC DRUGS

There is no evidence of a greater susceptibility of epileptic patients to local anesthetics.[37] Lidocaine has even been successfully used to terminate seizures in cases with status epilepticus.[14] Therefore local anesthetic techniques, such as epidural, caudal, or subarachnoid block, should not be denied to epileptic patients.

LD$_{50}$ OF LOCAL ANESTHETICS

The LD_{50} of a drug is the dose that causes death in 50 per cent of the test subjects. The LD_{50} of local anesthetics varies markedly with different species and routes of administration. For example, the LD_{50} of intravenous lidocaine is from 15 to 62 mg./kg. depending on the animal species.[127] In mice the average LD_{50} of lidocaine is 34 mg./kg. intravenously, 142 mg./kg. intraperitoneally, and 425 mg./kg. subcutaneously, the ratio being 1:4:13 respectively. The LD_{50} is several times the convulsive dose, provided the airway is kept patent and ventilation is maintained.

ALLERGIC REACTIONS TO LOCAL ANESTHETICS

True allergic reactions to local anesthetic drugs are extremely rare, especially with the amide drugs.[15] Ester-type drugs, especially tetracaine, are associated with more allergic reactions than the amide group.[6]

An individual may develop cross-sensitization to drugs that are chemically related (i.e., if a patient becomes allergic to one drug in a chemical family, sensitization may develop to other drugs of the same family). For example, benzocaine, the ethyl ester of para-aminobenzoic acid, may induce an allergic state if used repeatedly on the skin or mucous membranes. Following sensitization to benzocaine, procaine, which is closely allied to benzocaine, may cause an allergic response when administered at a later date, even without any previous exposure.[57] On the other hand, lidocaine, which is an amide, will produce no allergic reaction.[97] Therefore, if there is a history of allergy to one ester drug, an amide should be administered, and most probably will prove safe to use.

Allergy may be due to the preservative added to the local anesthetic and not to the local anesthetic drug itself.[6] The preservative usually used is paraben or methylparaben, both of which are chemically related to p-aminobenzoate. Therefore, there may be cross-sensitization between the ester drugs and the preservative of the amide drugs; in these cases the amide drug without the preservative should be tested and, if no allergic reaction occurs, administered.

There may be a cross-sensitization between procaine and procaine penicillin if procaine is the allergen.[6]

Patients who have a history of multiple allergies are more prone to have allergic reactions to other drugs.[94]

In dogs, increasing doses of lidocaine up to 46 mg. per hour were administered without changing the gastric secretion. Thus lidocaine had no histaminelike or histamine-liberating action in dogs.[127] Moreover, it has antihistaminic effects in certain animals. It prevents the bronchospasm initiated by histamine aerosol in guinea pigs and the hypotension resulting from intravenous injection of histamines in anesthetized animals.[127]

Local anesthetic drugs are needed for obstetrics, dentistry, and minor and even major surgery. Moreover, lidocaine may be required to treat ventricular arrhythmias during surgery and cardiac catheterization, or following myocardial infarction. Therefore, owing to this extensive use of local anesthetic drugs and their increasing application, one should not easily accept without verification or challenge a statement that a patient is allergic to one or all local anesthetic drugs. *Denying a patient the use of local anesthesia based only on a shaky history is unfair and may be life-threatening.* Proper understanding of the clinical picture, differential diagnosis, and verification of allergy to local anesthetics are therefore important.

CLINICAL PICTURE OF ALLERGIC REACTIONS

The types of allergic reactions to local anesthetics are mild, moderate, or severe. A patient may suffer from one or more of these types.

Mild Allergic Reactions

Mild allergic reactions occur immediately following the administration of the local anesthetic. They manifest in the form of urticaria, conjunctivitis, rhinitis, and skin wheals.[5,75,93,102,121]

Moderate Allergic Reactions

Moderate reactions usually occur within a few hours. They are in the form of swelling at the site of application, and/or edema of the face, pharynx, uvula, and even the larynx. There may be an associated bronchospasm.

Severe Allergic Reactions

Severe allergic reactions occur suddenly and immediately following administration of the drug. The manifestations are described as anaphylactic shock. There is sudden cardiovascular collapse associated with severe bronchospasm. They can occur after the administration of only a minute quantity of the drug due to the liberation of huge quantities of histamine.

DIFFERENTIAL DIAGNOSIS OF ALLERGIC REACTIONS TO LOCAL ANESTHETICS

Before assuming that cardiovascular collapse, respiratory problems, convulsions, severe swelling of the area, and/or edema of the face are due to allergic reaction to the local anesthetic drug, the circumstances surrounding the incident, all the drugs used, and details of the surgical procedure should be evaluated.

The following conditions should be excluded first:

Overdosage of Local Anesthetic

This can be due to the administration of an excessive dosage, too rapid absorption, or inadvertent intravenous injection of the intended drug; it may also follow the use of another more toxic drug administered by mistake.

Overdosage of Epinephrine

Overdosage of epinephrine is the second most common cause of systemic reaction during or following local anesthesia.[75] Tachycardia, pallor, sweating, and hypertension are characteristics of epinephrine reaction.

Vasovagal Syncope

With vasovagal syncope, the patient may sweat, become pale, and faint even before injecting the local anesthetic drug. Fear and the sitting-up position are predisposing factors.

Allergic Reaction to Other Drugs or Metallic Alloys

All administered drugs should be known, and in dental cases any metallic alloys used should be confirmed[69] so that the cause of an allergic reaction may be determined.

Surgical Trauma

Swelling of the face and pharynx can be secondary to surgical trauma and not necessarily due to any drug reaction.

TESTS FOR ALLERGY TO LOCAL ANESTHETICS

There are many tests used to determine allergies.

The Skin Test

After sterilizing the skin with alcohol and allowing it to dry, using a tuberculin syringe, 0.01 ml. of the suspected solution is injected intradermally into the inner surface of one forearm.[7] A similar volume of normal saline, used as a control, is injected into the corresponding part of the other forearm. The test is read in 15 to 20 minutes:

0 = no sign other than the puncture

1 = flare or wheal with erythema more than 1 cm. in diameter.

2 = flare or wheal with erythema more than 2 cm. in diameter.

3 = flare or wheal with erythema more than 3 cm. in diameter.

The skin test has many pitfalls. *A false positive test* can result from:

1. Trauma by the needle or tissue distention causing histamine release

2. Change in skin osmolality

3. The preservative used in the injected solution

4. Skin allergy due to exposure to the drug or similar compounds, but absence of allergy of internal organs (e.g., the cardiovascular system, which is the important target in severe reactions).

On the other hand, the skin test may give a *false negative result* if allergy is not due to the drug itself, but due to a metabolite.

However, the skin test is simple and can be performed by the clinician in the office. If the result is negative, it means that the patient can most probably receive the anesthetic tested.[6] If the result is positive, it is better to avoid using this drug. Therefore, if a patient has a history of a reaction to a local anesthetic drug (e.g., procaine), a skin test using another drug which is different chemically (e.g., lidocaine) is performed and, if negative, the latter drug can be used. If the nature of the drug associated with a previous allergic reaction is unknown, skin testing of a drug from each group is performed.

The Intranasal-Ophthalmic Test

This test is used either to confirm the skin test or as a substitute for it. It is rarely used.

A drop of the test solution is instilled in the conjunctival sac of the patient.[5] A true positive reaction shows a chemical conjunctivitis within 20 minutes. If no change occurs, the patient is placed in the recumbent position, baselines of pulse and blood pressure are obtained, and equipment as well as drugs necessary for resuscitation are kept readily available. One drop of the test solution is instilled into one nostril. Several minutes are allowed to elapse while the blood pressure and pulse are determined. If no adverse response occurs, two more drops are placed in the nostril, the quantity instilled being doubled at succeeding 3-minute intervals until a dose of 2 ml. is reached. The patient is then closely observed for 24 hours to determine whether any delayed allergic reactions develop. The test is stopped if any abnormal effects appear at any time during the procedure.

The Intravenous Test

This method recommended by Steinhaus[108] is the surest test to prove that a patient will not develop any serious reaction to a given drug. It is usually applied following a negative skin test.

The patient is placed in the recumbent position in the delivery or operating room. An intravenous cannula is inserted into the hand or forearm and an intravenous infusion (e.g., 5% dextrose in water) is started. The pulse and blood pressure are measured and the ECG monitor is attached. Resuscitative equipment, such as the anesthesia machine with facilities for endotracheal intubation, drugs for cardiovascular stimulation such as epinephrine, metaraminol and mephentermine, and antihistaminics as well as hydrocortisone should be available in the room. An assistant should also be present. Small increasing increments of the local anesthetic drug are injected while the vital signs are monitored and verbal contact with the patient is continued. For example, in the case of lidocaine, increments of 5, 10, 20, and 30 mg. are intravenously injected at 5-minute intervals. If the patient's vital signs and sensorium do not show any significant changes, the use of the drug is considered safe.

The author has used this technique in 23 patients with a history of alleged reaction to local anesthetics. In 14 cases in which subarachnoid block was planned, lidocaine was tested and used for the block without sequelae. In 9 cases in which epidural analgesia was requested, bupivacaine in one-fourth the dosage of lidocaine was tested, and subsequently used for the block uneventfully. The patients appreciated not only the analgesia during parturition, but also the reassurance that they were not allergic to these drugs which, of course, can be used for purposes other than childbirth as well.

Tests *In Vitro*

These immunologic tests such as the lymphocyte transformation technique[69] can prove a patient's sensitivity to a certain drug. These are elaborate tests requiring special laboratory facilities, and appreciable time is consumed before the results are obtained.

TREATMENT OF ALLERGIC REACTIONS TO LOCAL ANESTHETICS

Mild or Moderate Allergic Reactions

To counteract the reaction, antihistaminic drugs (e.g., 50 mg. of promethazine) can be used by either the intravenous or intramuscular route. If the patient's response is inadequate, corticosteroids (e.g., 100 mg. of corticosterone acetate) can be intravenously administered.

Severe Allergic Reactions

Intravenous injection of corticosteroids, cardiovascular stimulants, and adequate ventilation with oxygen are applied to control the severe reactions.

ACTION OF LOCAL ANESTHETICS ON THE BLOOD

In low concentrations, local anesthetics as well as a variety of drugs such as steroids and tranquilizers protect cellular and subcellular membranes; in high concentrations, they have the opposite effects. Thus, *in vitro* the lysis of red cells when suspended in hypotonic solution is prevented by lidocaine.[100] However, the addition of lidocaine in various concentrations, ranging from 25 to 500 mg./l, to citrate-phosphate-dextrose solution (CPD) does not improve the preservative characteristic of the anticoagulant.[4] This study also showed no evidence that lidocaine, even in high concentrations, destroys red cells or prevents them from being gradually hemolysed or from leaking potassium with time.

In vitro, lidocaine inhibits phagocytosis by the white blood corpuscles and decreases their metabolic activity.[30] This is attributed to a decreased activity of the white blood corpuscles rather than to a toxic effect by lidocaine because there is no increased lysis of the white cells.[4]

Commonly used local anesthetics do not cause significant changes in either the blood coagulation mechanisms or its components.[127]

Prilocaine can cause methemoglobinemia in both the mother and neonate. This is due to o-toluidine, a metabolite of prilocaine. A dose-response relationship exists between the total dose of prilocaine and methemoglobinemia.[29] However, a sufficient degree of methemoglobinemia causing cyanosis of the neonate followed a dose as low as 200 mg. of prilocaine.[78] Hypoxia is proportionate to the degree of methemoglobinemia. If methemoglobin compromises 60 per cent of the hemoglobin, ataxia, prostration, and unconsciousness occur. If 80 per cent of hemoglobin becomes transformed into methemoglobin, death occurs. The treatment of methemoglobinemia is intravenous injection of 1 to 2 mg./kg. of methylene blue.

ACTION OF LOCAL ANESTHETICS ON BACTERIA

Chloroprocaine in concentrations of 0.1 per cent to 0.02 per cent has a marked bacteriostatic effect on cultures of *Aerobacter aerogens*. The effect is even more marked with cultures of *E. coli*.[48] With cultures of *Staphylococcus aureus* and *Staphylococcus albus*, only the higher concentrations are effective. Bupivacaine (0.25%) is bactericidal at 37°C., but not at room temperature, to *S. epidermidis* and *corynebacterium*.[64]

ACTION OF LOCAL ANESTHETICS ON THE MYONEURAL JUNCTION

Local anesthetics have a depressant action on the myoneural junction, probably by decreasing acetylcholine.[54] These effects are additive to those of curare and antagonistic to those of physostigmine.

ACTION OF LOCAL ANESTHETICS ON THE AUTONOMIC GANGLIA

Local anesthetic drugs have a ganglion-blocking action because they inhibit the stimulating effects of acetylcholine when added to the perfusing fluid. Moreover, they inhibit acetylcholine production in the ganglia in response to preganglionic stimulation.[54]

The effects of local anesthetics on the myoneural junction and autonomic ganglia are clinically insignificant when the drugs are administered alone.[68] However, when applied in the presence of other pharmacologic agents, these effects become clinically important. For example, the duration of apnea caused by a muscle relaxant can be considerably prolonged by lidocaine.[38]

TERATOGENIC EFFECTS OF LOCAL ANESTHETICS

The possibility of the teratogenic effects of most local anesthetic drugs has not yet been studied. Therefore their use during the first trimester should be avoided if possible, unless the potential benefits outweigh the unknown hazards. As a rule, during early pregnancy, spinal is preferred to epidural or caudal techniques owing to the limited dosage of local anesthetics needed for subarachnoid block.

PROPERTIES OF AN IDEAL LOCAL ANESTHETIC IN OBSTETRICS

The following properties are required for a drug to be an ideal local anesthetic in obstetrics:

Maternal Considerations

1. Does not cause damage to nervous tissue, i.e., its action is reversible

2. Does not cause damage to other tissues

3. Has a high therapeutic index, i.e., low toxicity and a wide margin of safety. In convulsive doses there is no depression of the cardiovascular system, thus allowing for better resuscitation

4. Has a wide range of effectiveness, whether for a nerve block or a major vertebral block

5. Has a rapid onset of action

6. Has an adequate analgesic property

7. Has an adequate duration of effectiveness. If used for continuous analgesia in labor or surgery, its action should be prolonged to minimize the need and risks of repeated "refills." If used for delivery only, its action should be short to minimize the period of the patient's stay in the recovery room

8. Has a controllable and predictable muscular relaxation

9. Is compatible with other local anesthetic drugs

10. Has a minimal effect on the uterine contractibility

11. Has no vasoconstriction of the uterine arteries.

Fetal Considerations

1. Has a minimal transmission to the fetus

2. Has a minimal effect on the fetus and newborn

3. Can be easily detoxified and/or excreted by the fetus and newborn if excessive amounts inadvertently reach it.

The ideal local anesthetic drug is yet to be discovered.

REFERENCES

1. Abdel-Salam, A., Vonwiller, J. B., and Scott, D. B.: Evaluation of etidocaine in extradural block. Br. J. Anaesth., *47*:1081, 1975.
2. Aberg, G.: Studies on Mepivacaine and Its Optically Active Isomers With Special Reference to Vasoactive Properties. Thesis from the Department of Pharmacology, School of Medicine, Lindhoping, Sweden, 1972.
3. Abouleish, E.: Postpartum hypertension and convulsion after oxytocic drugs. Anesth. Analg., *55*:813, 1976.
4. Abouleish, E., and Klionsky, B. L.: The use of lidocaine for blood storage. *Unpublished data.*
5. Adriani, J.: Comment. Evaluation of intracutaneous testing for investigations of allergy to local anesthetic agents. Anesth. Analg., *49*:182, 1970.
5a. Adriani, J., and Campbell, B.: Fatalities following topical application of local anesthetics to mucous membranes. J. Am. Med. Assoc., *162*:1527, 1956.
6. Aldrete, J. A., *et al.*: Effects of hepatectomy on the disappearance rate of lidocaine from blood in man and dog. Anesth. Analg., *49*:687, 1970.
7. Arora, S., and Aldrete, A.: Investigation of possible allergy to local anesthetic drugs. Anesth. Rev., *3*(7):13, July, 1976.
8. Aven, M., and Foldes, F. F.: The chemical kinetics of procaine and chloroprocaine hydrolysis. Science, *114*:206, 1951.
9. Beckett, A. H., Boyes, R. N., and Appleton, P. J.: The metabolism and excretion of lignocaine in man. J. Pharmacol. [Suppl.], p. 756, 1966.
10. Bernhard, C. G., and Bohm, E.: Local Anesthetics as Anticonvulsants: a Study on Experimental and Clinical Epilepsy. Stockholm, Almqvist & Wiksell, 1965.

11. Bigger, J. T., Jr., and Mandel, W. J.: Effect of lidocaine on the electrophysiological properties of ventricular muscle and Purkinje fibers. J. Clin. Invest., 49:63, 1970.

12. Blair, M. R.: Cardiovascular pharmacology of local anaesthetics. Br. J. Anaesth., 47:247, 1975.

13. Blaustein, M. P., and Goldman, D. E.: Competitive action of calcium and procaine on lobster axon: a study of the mechanism of action of certain local anesthetics. J. Gen. Physiol., 49:1043, 1966.

14. Bohm, E., Flodmark, S. M. L., and Petersen, I.: Effect of lidocaine (Xylocaine) on seizure and interseizure electroencephalograms in epileptics. Arch. Neurol. Psychiat., 81:550, 1959.

15. Bonica, J. J.: Testing for local anesthetic sensitivity. Audio-Digest, 15(5), 1973.

16. Bonica, J. J., Berges., P. U., and Morikawa, K.: Circulatory effects of peridural block. I. Effects of level of analgesia and dose of lidocaine. Anesthesiology, 33:619, 1970.

17. Boyes, R. N.: A review of the metabolism of amide local anaesthetic agents. Br. J. Anaesth., 47:225, 1975.

18. Braid, D. P., and Scott, D. B.: The systemic absorption of local analgesic drugs. Br. J. Anaesth., 37:394, 1965.

19. Bridenbaugh, P. O., et al.: Preliminary clinical evaluation of etidocaine (Duranest): a new long-acting local anaesthetic. Acta Anaesthesiol. Scand., 18:165, 1974.

20. Bromage, P. R.: A comparison of the hydrochloride and carbon dioxide salts of lignocaine and prilocaine in epidural analgesia. Acta Anaesthesiol. Scand., 16:55, 1965.

21. Bromage, P. R., et al.: Quality of epidural blockade. III: Carbonated local anaesthetic solutions. Br. J. Anaesth., 39:197, 1967.

22. Casady, G. M., Moore, D. C., and Bridenbaugh, D. L.: Postpartum hypertension after use of vasoconstrictor and oxytocin drugs. J.A.M.A., 172:101, 1960.

23. Cohen, E. N., et al.: The role of pH in the development of tachyphylaxis to local anesthetic agents. Anesthesiology, 29:994, 1968.

24. Cohn, M. L. et al.: The antagonism of some of the effects of lidocaine by thiamylal. Annual Meeting of the American Society of Anesthesiologists, 1971. Washington, D.C., Abstracts of Scientific Papers, p.s., 1971.

25. Courtney, K. R.: Frequency-Dependent Inhibition of Sodium Currents in Frog Myelinated Nerve by GEA-968, a New Lidocaine Derivative. Dissertation, University of Washington, Seattle, 1974.

26. Cousins, M. J., and Bromage, P. R.: A comparison of the hydrochloride and carbonated salts of lignocaine for caudal analgesia in outpatients. Br. J. Anaesth., 43:1149, 1971.

27. Covino, B. G.: Local anesthesia. 1. N. Engl. J. Med., 286:975, 1972.

28. ———. Local anesthesia. 2. N. Engl. J. Med., 286:1035, 1972.

29. Crawford, J. S.: Principles and Practice of Obstetric Anesthesia. Ed. 3, p. 88. Oxford, Blackwell Scientific Publications, 1972.

30. Cullen, B. F., and Haschke, R. A.: Local anes-

31. Davis, L.D., and Temete, J. V.: Electrophysiological actions of lidocaine on canine ventricular muscle and Purkinje fibers. Circ. Res., 24:639, 1969.

32. de Jong, R. H.: Effects of lidocaine on spontaneous cortical and subcortical electrical activity. Arch. Neurol., 18:277, 1968.

33. ———: Local anesthetic seizures. Anesthesiology, 30:5, 1969.

34. ———: Physiology and Pharmacology of Local Anesthesia. Springfield, Ill., Charles C Thomas, 1970.

35. ———: Biotransformation of local anesthetics: general concepts. International Anesthesia Clinics (Biotransformation of local anesthetics, adjuvants and adjunct agents), 13:(4):1, 1975.

36. de Jong, R. H., and Heavner, J. E.: Local anesthetic seizure prevention: diazepam versus phenobarbital. Anesthesiology, 36:449, 1972.

37. de Jong, R. H., and Walts, L. F.: Lidocaine-induced psychomotor seizures in man. Acta Anaesthesiol. Scand. [Suppl.], 23:598, 1966.

38. De Kornfeld, T. J., and Steinhaus, J. E.: The effect of intravenously administered lidocaine and succinylcholine on the respiratory activity of dogs. Anesth. Analg., 38:173, 1959.

39. de Leo, B. C., et al.: Instability of steam-autoclaved bupivacaine with epinephrine. Anesthesiology, 40:297, 1974.

40. Dhuner, K. G., et al.: Blood levels of mepivacaine after regional anaesthesia. Br. J. Anaesth., 37:746, 1965.

41. Dhuner, K. G., and Lewis, D. H.: Effect of local anaesthetics and vasoconstrictors upon regional blood flow. Acta Anaesthesiol. Scand. [Suppl.] 23:347, 1966.

42. DiFazio, C. A., and Brown, R. E.: Lidocaine metabolism in normal and phenobarbital pretreated dogs. Anesthesiology, 36:238, 1972.

43. Dodson, W. E., Hillman, R. E., and Hillman, L. S.: Brain tissue levels in a fatal case of neonatal mepivacaine (Carbocaine) poisoning. J. Pediatr., 86:624, 1975.

44. Eger, E. I., II.: Anesthetic Uptake and Action. P. 33. Baltimore, Williams & Wilkins, 1974.

45. Englesson, S., and Matousek, M.: Central nervous system effects of local anaesthetic agents. Br. J. Anaesth., 47:241, 1975.

46. Essman, W. B.: Anticonvulsive properties of Xylocaine in mice susceptible to audiogenic seizures. Arch. Int. Pharmacodyn. Ther., 164:376, 1966.

47. Feinstein, M. B., Lenard, W., and Mathias, J.: The antagonism of local anesthetic induced convulsions by the benzodiazepine derivative diazepam. Arch. Int. Pharmacodyn. Ther., 187:144, 1970.

48. Foldes, F. F., and McNall, P. G.: 2-Chloroprocaine: new local anesthetic agent. Anesthesiology, 13:287, 1952.

49. Foldes, F. F., et al.: Comparison of toxicity of intravenously given local anesthetic agents in man. J.A.M.A., 172:1493, 1960.

50. Foldes, F. F., et al.: The intravenous toxicity of

local anesthetic agents in man. Clin. Pharmacol. Ther., *6*:328, 1965.

51. Freund, G.: The prevention of ethanol withdrawal seizures in mice by lidocaine. Neurology, *23*:91, 1973.

52. Geddes, I. C.: Studies of the metabolism of Citanest C14. Acta Anaesthesiol. Scand. [Suppl.], *15*:37, 1965.

53. ———: Metabolism of local anesthetic agents. Int. Anesthesiol. Clin., *5*:525, 1967.

54. Goodman, L. S., and Gilman, A.: The Pharmacological Basis of Therapeutics. Ed. 5. New York, Macmillan, 1975.

55. Gordon, H. R.: Fetal bradycardia after paracervical block correlation with fetal and maternal blood levels of local anesthetic (mepivacaine). N. Engl. J. Med., *279*:910, 1968.

56. Groseth-Dittrich, M. F., Vyden, J. K., and Mandel, W. J.: Peripheral hemodynamic effects of lidocaine. Circulation, *46*[Suppl. II]: 639,1972.

57. Hanauer, A.: Gruppensensibilisierung gengenüber Anaesthetika, Chemotherapeutika und Antibiotika. Dtsch. Med. Wochenschr., *80*:1175, 1955.

58. Heinonen, J.: Influence of some drugs on toxicity and rate of metabolism of lidocaine and mepivacaine: experimental study on mice and rats. Ann. Med. Exp. Biol. Fenn., *44*[Suppl. 3]:1, 1966.

59. Heinonen, J., Takki, S., and Jarho, L.: Plasma lidocaine levels in patients treated with potential inducers of microsomal enzymes. Acta Anaesthesiol. Scand., *14*:89, 1970.

60. Hille, B.: The permeability of the sodium channel to metal cations in myelinated nerve. J. Gen. Physiol., *59*:637, 1972.

61. ———: Potassium channels in myelinated nerve. Selective permeability to small cations. J. Gen. Physiol., *61*:669, 1973.

62. Iversen, L. L.: Inhibition of noradrenaline uptake by drugs. J. Pharm., Pharmacol., *17*:62, 1965.

63. Jack, J. J. B.: Physiology of peripheral nerve fibres in relation to their size. Br. J. Anaesth., *47*:173, 1975.

64. James, F. M., III, *et al.*: Bacteriology of continuous epidural analgesia. Annual Meeting of the American Society of Anesthesiologists, 1975. Abstracts of Scientific Papers, pp. 3–4, 1975.

65. Jorfeldt, L. L., *et al.*: The effects of local anaesthetics on the central circulation and respiration in man and dog. Acta Anaesthesiol. Scand., *12*:153, 1968.

66. ———: The effects of mepivacaine and lidocaine on forearm resistance and capacitance vessels in man. Acta Anaesthesiol. Scand., *14*:183, 1970.

67. Katz, J.: The distribution of ^{14}C-labelled lidocaine injected intravenously in the rat. Anesthesiology, *29*:249, 1968.

68. Katz, R. L., and Gissen, A. J.: Effects of intravenous and intra-arterial procaine and lidocaine on neuromuscular transmission in man. Acta Anaesthesiol. Scand. [Suppl.], *36*:103, 1969.

69. Lehner, T.: Lignocaine hypersensitivity. [Letter] Lancet, *1*:1245, 1971.

70. Levinson, G., and Schnider, S. M.: Placental transfer of local anesthetics: clinical implications. Clin. Anesth. (Parturition and Perinatology) *10*(2):173, 1973.

71. Levy, R. H.: Local anesthetic structure, activity and mechanism of action. *In* Eger, E. I., II (ed.): Anesthetic Uptake and Action. Pp. 322–331. Baltimore, Williams & Wilkins, 1974.

72. Lorente de No, R.: On the effect of cocaine upon sodium-deficient frog nerve. J. Gen. Physiol., *35*:203, 1951.

73. Lund, P. C., Cwik, J. C., and Gannon, R. T.: Extradural anaesthesia: choice of local anaesthetic agents. Br. J. Anaesth., *47*:313, 1975.

74. Lund, P. C., Cwik, J. C., and Pagdanganan, R. T.: Etidocaine—a new long-acting anesthetic agent: a clinical evaluation. Anesth. Analg., *52*:482, 1973.

75. Lynas, R. F.: A suspected allergic reaction to lidocaine. Anesthesiology, *31*:380, 1969.

76. MacMillan, W. H.: A hypothesis concerning the effect of cocaine on the action of sympathomimetic amines. Br. J. Pharmacol., *14*:385, 1959.

77. McWhirter, W. R., Frederickson, E. L., and Steinhaus, J. E.: Interactions of lidocaine with general anesthetics. South. Med. J., *65*:796, 1972.

78. Marx, G. F.: Fetal arrhythmias during caudal block with prilocaine. Anesthesiology, *28*:222, 1967.

79. Mather, L.: Discussion: Effects of anaesthesia on blood flow. Br. J. Anaesth., *47*:240, 1975.

80. ———: Discussion: Clinical tolerance of anaesthetics. Br. J. Anaesth., *47*:333, 1975.

81. Mather, L. E., Long, G. J., and Thomas, J.: The intravenous toxicity and clearance of bupivacaine in man. Clin. Pharmacol. Ther., *12*:935, 1971.

82. Mazze, R. I., and Dunbar, R. W.: Plasma lidocaine concentrations after caudal, lumbar epidural, axillary block and intravenous regional anesthesia. Anesthesiology, *27*:574, 1966.

83. Meffin, P., Long, G. J., and Thomas, J.: Clearance and metabolism of mepivacaine in the human neonate. Clin. Pharmacol. Ther., *14*:218, 1973.

84. Meymaris, E.: Chemical anatomy of the nerve membrane. Br. J. Anaesth., *47*:164, 1975.

85. Moir, D. D., *et al.*: Extradural analgesia in obstetrics: a controlled trial of carbonated lignocaine and bupivacaine hydrochloride with or without adrenaline. Br. J. Anaesth., *48*:129, 1976.

86. Moore, D. C.: *In* Munson, E. S., Gutnick, M. J., and Wagman, I. H.: Local anesthetic drug-induced seizures in rhesus monkeys [audience participation]. Anesth. Analg., *49*:996, 1970.

87. Moore, D. C., *et al.*: Caudal and epidural blocks with bupivacaine for childbirth. Report of 657 parturients. Obstet. Gynecol., *37*:667, 1971.

88. Morishima, H. O., *et al.*: Transmission of mepivacaine hydrochloride (Carbocaine) across the human placenta. Anesthesiology, *27*:147, 1966.

89. Munson, E. S., Gutnick, M. J., and Wagman, I.

H.: Local anesthetic drug-induced seizures in rhesus monkeys. Anesth. Analg., *49*:986, 1970.

90. Munson, E. S., *et al.*: Etidocaine, bupivacaine and lidocaine seizure thresholds in monkeys. Anesthesiology, *42*:471, 1975.

91. Narahashi, T., and Frazier, D. T.: Site of action and active form of local anesthetics. Neurosci. Res., *4*:65, 1971.

92. Nishimura, N., *et al.*: Effects of local anesthetic agents on the peripheral vascular system. Anesth. Analg., *44*:135, 1965.

93. Noble, D. S., and Pierce, G. F.: Allergy to lidocaine. Lancet, *2*:1436, 1961.

94. Peters, G. A., and Marcoux, J. P.: Evaluation of intracutaneous testing of investigation of allergy to local anesthetic agents, comment. Anesth. Analg., *49*:181, 1970.

95. Plum, F., Posner, J. B., and Troy, B.: Cerebral metabolic and circulatory responses to induced convulsions in animals. Arch. Neurol., *18*:1, 1968.

96. Reynolds, F.: The influence of adrenaline on maternal and neonatal blood levels of local analgesic drugs. *In* Proceedings of the Symposium on Epidural Analgesia in Obstetrics, 1971. Pp. 31–40. London, H. K. Lewis, 1972.

96a. ———: A comparison of the potential toxicity of bupivacaine, lignocaine and mepivacaine during epidural blockade for surgery. Br. J. Anaesth., *43*:567, 1971.

97. Rickles, N. H.: Procaine allergy in dental patients: diagnosis and management: preliminary report. Oral Surg., *6*:375, 1953.

98. Ritchie, J. M.: Mechanism of action of local anaesthetic agents and biotoxins. Br. J. Anaesth., *47*:191, 1975.

99. Ritchie, J. M., and Greengard, P.: On the mode of action of local anesthetics. Annu. Rev. Pharmacol., *6*:405, 1966.

100. Roth, S., and Seeman, P.: All lipid-soluble anaesthetics protect red cells. Nature [New Biol.], 231, 1971.

101. Rowland, M.: Local anesthetic absorption, distribution and elimination. *In* Eger, E. I., II (ed.): Anesthetic Uptake and Action. Pp. 233–360. Baltimore, Williams & Wilkins, 1974.

102. Sadove, M. S., *et al.*: Classification and management of reactions to local anesthetic agents. J.A.M.A., *148*:17, 1952.

103. Scott, D. B.: Evaluation of clinical tolerance of local anaesthetic agents. Br. J. Anaesth., *47*:328, 1975.

104. Scurlock, J. E., Heavner, J. E., and de Jong, R. H.: Differential B and C fibre block by an amide- and an ester-linked local anaesthetic. Br. J. Anaesth., *47*:1135, 1975.

105. Selden, R., and Sasahara, A.: Central nervous system toxicity induced by lidocaine: report of a case in a patient with liver disease. J.A.M.A., *202*:908, 1967.

106. Shnider, S. M.: Personal communication, 1975.

107. Sjostrand, U., and Widman, B.: Distribution of bupivacaine in the rabbit under normal and acidotic conditions. Acta Anaesthesiol. Scand. [Suppl.], *50*:1, 1973.

108. Steinhaus, J. E.: Testing for local anesthetic sensitivity. Audio-Digest, 15 (5), 1973.

109. Sung, C. Y., and Truant, A. P.: Physiological disposition of lidocaine and its comparison in some respects with procaine. J. Pharmacol. Exp. Ther., *112*:432, 1954.

110. Takman, B.: The chemistry of local anaesthetic agents: classification of blocking agents. Br. J. Anaesth., *47*:183, 1975.

111. Tanaka, K.: Anticonvulsant properties of procaine, cocaine, adiphenine and related structures. Proc. Soc. Exp. Biol. Med., *90*:192, 1955.

112. Taylor, E. S.: Intrapartum and postpartum hemorrhage. Clin. Obstet. Gynecol., *3*:646, 1960.

113. Thomas, J., Climie, C. R., and Mather, L. E.: The maternal plasma levels and placental transfer of bupivacaine following epidural analgesia. Br. J. Anaesth., *41*:1035, 1969.

114. Thomson, P. D., *et al.*: Lidocaine pharmacokinetics in advanced heart failure, liver disease and renal failure in humans. Ann. Intern. Med., *78*:499, 1973.

115. Tower, D. B.: Molecular transport across neural and non-neural membranes. *In* Tower, D. B., Luse, S. A., and Grundfest, H. (eds.): Properties of Membranes and Diseases of the Nervous System. Chap. 1. New York, Springer-Verlag, 1962.

116. Trevan, J. W., and Boock, E.: The relation of hydrogen ion concentration to the action of the local anaesthetics. Br. J. Exp. Pathol., *8*:307, 1927.

117. Tucker, G. T.: Discussion: Clinical tolerance of anaesthetics. Br. J. Anaesth, *47*:332, 1975.

118. Tucker, G. T., and Mather, L. E.: Pharmacokinetics of local anaesthetic agents. Br. J. Anaesth., *47*:213, 1975.

119. Tucker, G. T., *et al.*: Binding of anilide-type local anesthetics in human placenta. 1. Relationships between binding, physiochemical properties, and anesthetic activity. Anesthesiology, *33*:287, 1970.

120. Usubiaga, J. E.: *In* Munson, E. S., Gutnick, M. J., and Wagman, I. H.: Local anesthetic drug-induced seizures in rhesus monkeys [guest discussion]. Anesth. Analg., *49*:994, 1970.

121. Walker, R. T.: Hypersensitivity reaction to lignocaine. J. R. Nav. Med. Serv., *57*:53, 1971.

122. Watson, P. J.: The mode of action of local anesthetics. J. Pharm. Pharmacol., *12*:257, 1960.

123. Weis, F. R., *et al.*: Cardiovascular effects of oxytocin. Obstet. Gynecol., *46*:211, 1975.

124. Wheeler, M.: Chloroprocaine and pseudocholinesterase deficiency. [Letter] J.A.M.A., *233*:770, 1975.

125. Whitwam, J. G., and Kidd, C.: The use of direct current to cause selective block of large fibres in peripheral nerves. Br. J. Anaesth., *47*:1123, 1975.

126. Widman, B.: Plasma concentration of local anaesthetic agents in regard to absorption, distribution and elimination, with special reference to bupivacaine. Br. J. Anaesth., *47*:231, 1975.

127. Wiedling, S.: Xylocaine: the Pharmacological Basis of Its Clinical Use. Ed. 2. Stockholm, Almqvist & Wiksell, 1964.

5

Effects of Vertebral Blocks on the Cardiovascular System

Sofronio B. de la Vega, M.D.

Regional anesthetic techniques that block a significant area of distribution of the sympathetic nervous system can cause cardiovascular changes of varying degrees.[6] Techniques that do not involve sympathetic blockade have no direct influence on cardiovascular performance unless significant amounts of the local anesthetic agents have gained access to the general circulation. For these reasons, the following discussions on the cardiovascular effects of vertebral block anesthesia will be focused on epidural, whether lumbar or caudal, and subarachnoid blocks.

MONITORING OF CARDIOVASCULAR CHANGES DURING VERTEBRAL BLOCK ANESTHESIA

The cardiovascular changes associated with vertebral blocks are dramatic events that can be monitored in many ways to assess the patient's well-being and to predict and anticipate measures to keep the patient in a sound physiologic state. Arterial blood pressure is the most readily accessible and commonly measured parameter during anesthesia. However, several authorities regard the blood pressure value *per se,* more so when taken indirectly by the commonly used Riva-Rocci method, as the least informative piece of information with regard to the well-being of the cells or organs of the body.[16,21,41] A normal or high blood pressure reading does not necessarily mean adequate tissue perfusion, and a low blood pressure value is not always associated with a hypoperfusion state. Also, there are many dynamic variables that interact and influence the blood pressure values. But be that as it may, blood pressure monitoring, because of its simplicity, will remain as one of the standard assessments for cardiovascular performance during the practice of clinical anesthesia. The heart rate and the quality of the peripheral pulse must also be frequently assessed.

A perplexing problem with arterial blood pressure monitoring is the question of what is an adequate level of blood pressure. How low can the blood pressure be maintained without significantly decreasing tissue perfusion? There is no one right answer to this question because there are many variables that influence the level of arterial blood pressure. In addition, there are many individual patient factors to consider before labeling a blood pressure value as adequate or inadequate for tissue perfusion. According to Greene,[28] the level of arterial blood pressure which is theoretically adequate for cellular respiration and metabolism in normal patients under spinal anesthesia is a mean arterial pressure of at least 30 to 35 torr. Obviously, this value is greatly modified in the presence of cardiovascular pathology or pregnancy where the environment of the fetus could be compromised.

In the clinical practice of obstetric vertebral block anesthesia, the minimum cardiovascular monitoring must include frequent determinations of arterial blood pressure and heart or pulse rate. These must be supplemented by hourly urinary output measurements and cerebral function assessment to evaluate the adequacy of organ perfusion and hydration. One can assess cerebral function by establishing verbal contact with the patient at all times while under block anesthesia. Fetal monitoring is necessary to appraise the uterine environment of the neonate during labor and delivery. The author feels that invasive and sophisticated cardiovascular monitoring is not warranted in the routine practice of clinical obstetric anesthesia.

FACTORS INFLUENCING CARDIOVASCULAR CHANGES DURING VERTEBRAL BLOCK ANESTHESIA

The cardiovascular changes that occur following spinal or epidural anesthesia are mainly due to preganglionic sympathetic blockade.[30] The manifestations of these changes are influenced *by the extent of the block* and *the period of time required to establish the block*. Spinal anesthesia is established in a few minutes whereas epidural anesthesia is much slower in onset. It must be realized that the circulatory derangements following vertebral block anesthesia depend on the level and extent of sympathetic block, not on the level and extent of analgesic block. In most instances the sympathetic block involves an average of two (but can involve as many as six) spinal segments beyond the boundaries of the sensory block.[29]

Another factor that influences the cardiovascular responses to major vertebral block anesthesia is the *direct systemic effect of the local anesthetic agent used.* Invariably the local anesthetic agents, whether administered epidurally or injected in the subarachnoid space, will gain access into the general circulation. The role of absorption and the total amount administered are critical issues in the cardiovascular responses and in the development of local anesthetic toxicity. The amount of local anesthetic agents used in spinal anesthesia is small and the slow rate of absorption in the subarachnoid space makes it unlikely that direct effects of the local anesthetics are significant.[28] The cardiovascular effects of spinal anesthesia are therefore solely related to the extent of sympathetic blockade. In epidural anesthesia, the circulatory effects are directly related to the extent of sympathetic blockade as well as the direct effects of the absorbed local anesthetic agents on the cardiovascular system.[13]

The practice of incorporating *vasoconstrictor drugs* in the anesthetic solution to produce local vasoconstriction at the injection site may cause cardiovascular changes during vertebral block anesthesia. Epinephrine has been the agent of choice for this purpose. Besides prolonging the duration of the sympathetic block when a vasoconstrictor is added, significant cardiovascular changes can occur when systemic absorption takes place.

The most important factor in the cardiovascular response to vertebral blocks is *the condition of the "receptor-effector system"*—the patient.[59] The main points to consider here are the presence of preexisting diseases, particularly of the cardiovascular system, the degree of sympathetic influence on the cardiovascular system, the blood volume, and the presence and nature of concurrent medications.

Numerous etiologic factors that were thought in the past to be operative have been clinically and experimentally disproven. For example, it was thought that circulatory changes were produced by skeletal muscle paralysis; however, neuromuscular blocking agents like curare, producing the same degree of skeletal muscle paralysis, have no significant effect on the circulation.[65] On the other hand, some degree of hypotension is not unusual in test subjects and patients with pain problems given sympathetic and somatic sensory block by differential spinal or epidural blocks in whom skeletal muscle paralysis is not appreciable. It was also thought that the local anesthetic agent introduced in the spinal subarachnoid space diffused into the cranial subarachnoid space, producing depression of vital centers in the brain stem and cerebral cortex. However, Greene[28] believes that in clinical practice the concentration of local anesthetic agent in the ventricular cerebrospinal fluid during spinal anesthesia is not strong enough to produce medullary and cortical depression. If respiratory arrest and cardiovascular collapse occur with high spinal anesthesia, they are usually due to inadequate medullary blood flow secondary to extreme arterial hypotension and not due to the direct action of the local anesthetic drug on the medullary centers. Deficiency of adrenal hormones has been considered as a result of sympathetic denervation of the adrenal gland, but the normal secretions of catecholamines[54] and adrenocortical hormones[15,43] have been shown not to be affected by sympathetic blockade. Ward and coworkers,[62] invoked a reflex mechanism causing a transient increase in vasomotor tone and cardiac output activated by increased extradural and cerebrospinal fluid pressure following epidural injections. However, Akamatsu and coworkers[1] demonstrated that epidural injection of 20 ml. of saline in patients known to be free of cardiovascular diseases did not produce cardiovascular alterations.

There are numerous studies available in the literature dealing with cardiovascular performance under different levels of vertebral block anesthesia. Conculsions derived from these studies do not always concur with one another because of the differences in experimental design. Some of the inherent differences are the utilization of different animal species as the test subjects and the differences in monitoring cardiovascular parameters. An obvious point of variation in the studies performed on human subjects is the employment in some studies of healthy human volunteers who are usually young and kept in a well-controlled laboratory environment as opposed to the clinical studies performed on sick, traumatized (surgery), and probably elderly patients who are under all kinds of stress.

PREGANGLIONIC SYMPATHETIC BLOCKADE

The common denominator that spinal and epidural analgesia share which greatly influences cardiovascular performance is the reversible preganglionic sympathetic blockade. The magnitude of these cardiovascular changes is seen as a function of the extent of the sympathetic blockade and the body's ability to compensate for hemodynamic changes. In spite of the distinct similarities between spinal and epidural anesthesia there are qualitative and quantitative differences in their cardiovascular physiology.

EFFECTS ON CARDIAC FUNCTION

Sympathetic denervation of the heart, as in upper thoracic epidural block, is associated with reduced cardiac performance. This is manifested by decreased cardiac output as a result of decreased stroke volume and bradycardia, even in the presence of elevated central venous pressure.[44] The bradycardia is due to the unopposed vagal slowing of the heart. When the sympathetic blockade is extended, as in total sympathetic blockade, venous pooling of blood occurs and venous return to the heart is decreased. This is manifested by a low central venous pressure (preload), significant bradycardia, and decreased cardiac output. The bradycardia in this instance is not only due to unopposed vagal slowing of the heart secondary to blockade of the cardiac accelerator nerve (T1 to T4 inclusive) but also due to low atrial filling pressure because of the diminished venous return to the heart (Bainbridge reflex). Greene[28] asserts that bradycardia during spinal anesthesia is related more to the development of arterial hypotension than to the height of the anesthesia. Cases of extreme sinus bradycardia that progressively developed to cardiac asystole after spinal[64] and epidural[9] blocks to the T5 to T4 sensory level have been reported. (The mechanism of bradycardia is also discussed in Chapter 15, Subarachnoid Block.)

The ability of the heart to eject blood per unit of time depends on the venous return (preload), myocardial contractility (inotropism), the resistance to flow or impedance (afterload), and the heart rate (chronotropism) [10] Kennedy and coworkers[38] have shown that spinal anesthesia does not directly affect myocardial contractility as long as the cardiac accelerator nerve remains functional. Under spinal anesthesia, the cardiac output is, within limits, directly related to the venous return (preload) and heart rate, and inversely related to the aortic-outflow impedance (afterload). The total peripheral resistance (afterload) is generally but only modestly decreased following spinal and epidural anesthesia without epinephrine.[62] Gorlin[26] pointed out that mechanisms reducing impedance usually cause a small but definite augmentation in cardiac output and not infrequently a reduction in filling pressure of the ventricles. Decreased peripheral resistance tends to counterbalance the effect of decreased venous return and bradycardia on cardiac output.

It appears then that the decrease in cardiac output after spinal and epidural block is mainly due to decreased venous return

(preload) with the associated bradycardia. As with other cardiovascular parameters, the magnitude of decrease in cardiac output is more under spinal block than under epidural block without epinephrine. Ward and coworkers[62] reported a 17.7 per cent decrease in cardiac output in healthy human volunteers under spinal anesthesia to the T5 sensory level. Bonica and coworkers[7] recorded an 8 per cent decrease at the same sensory level. With epidural anesthesia to the T5 level using plain lidocaine solution, Ward and coworkers[62] recorded only a 5.4 per cent decrease while Bonica and coworkers[7] reported no significant change in cardiac output. When epinephrine is added to the epidural anesthetic solution there is a marked increase of 30 per cent in cardiac output. The increase in cardiac output is due to an increase in stroke volume by 13 per cent and an increase in heart rate by 16 per cent.

The difference in the cardiovascular response between spinal and epidural anesthesia using plain local anesthetic solution could be ascribed to the short induction time of spinal anesthesia and on the larger amount of local anesthetic agent used in epidural anesthesia. The circulatory adjustments may not be as adequate in spinal anesthesia because of its rapid onset compared to the slower-acting epidural anesthesia.

EFFECTS ON PERIPHERAL RESISTANCE

The vascular resistance in the blocked areas of the body is decreased due to arteriolar, capillary, and venous dilatation.[54] The decrease in the local vascular resistance is independent of the existing vascular resistance elsewhere in the circulatory circuit. There is a marked increase in the blood flow to the lower extremities in subjects receiving a vertebral block. The involved extremities are hyperemic and warm to the touch.[51] A sharp contrast exists in the unblocked upper extremities when the extent of the sympathetic block is limited to T4 and below. The hands may appear pale and be cold to the touch because of extreme vasoconstriction. This compensatory vasoconstriction in the unblocked areas produces a local increase in the vascular resistance. The degree of compensatory vasoconstriction depends, among other factors, on the degree of vasodilation in the sympathectomized area.

The total peripheral resistance refers to the overall resistance of the whole circulatory system. The total *peripheral resistance* value is the algebraic sum of the resistances in the various regions of the body. In the presence of sympathetic blockade, the total peripheral resistance may be increased,[44] decreased,[6,8,62] or unchanged,[56,57,] depending upon the net effect of the vasodilatation in the blocked areas and the extent of the compensatory vasoconstriction in the unblocked areas. However, it is generally accepted that the total peripheral resistance is slightly decreased when the sympathetic block is at T4 and below. The maximum decrease in total peripheral resistance during complete sympathetic blockade is about 20 per cent.[65] In monkeys, Sivarajan and coworkers[57] did not find a significant change in total peripheral resistance even after T1 sensory block and a concomitant decrease of 22 per cent in mean arterial pressure. He postulated that the decrease in mean arterial pressure could have activated the renin-angiotensin mechanism in the kidneys. Renin release can occur in response to lowered mean arterial pressure even in nonsecreting denervated kidneys in adrenalectomized dogs.[4] Angiotensin has a direct vasoconstrictor effect on the denervated arterioles.

EFFECTS ON ARTERIAL BLOOD PRESSURE

There is general agreement, based on experimental as well as clinical evidence, that the arterial blood pressure decreases after sympathetic blockade. The mean arterial blood pressure is directly proportional to the cardiac output and total peripheral resistance, both of which can decrease during sympathetic blockade. In the nonpregnant state the incidence and degree of hypotension are generally related roughly to the extent of the sympathetic blockade and more precisely to the occurrence of bradycardia. Greene[28] made a critical analysis of the possible relationships between hypotension, bradycardia, and extent of sympathetic blockade. He concluded that the height of the block cannot be correlated either to changes in heart rate or to changes in arterial blood pressure. However, he asserted that there is a direct and almost precise relationship between the changes in arterial blood pressure and heart rate: the heart rate invariably falls when the blood pressure falls. Although the relationship between the height of the block and hypotension is not exact, the clinician is alerted to be prepared at all times to prevent, minimize, and treat hypotension when the block is unexpectedly high.

The incidence of arterial hypotension following spinal block has been reported to range from 3 per cent[49] to 85 per cent.[27] Under epidural anesthesia, the incidence ranges from 1.4 per cent[18] to 9.0 per cent.[48] Hypotension is decidedly more common in sick and obstetric patients. Different criteria have been used in classifying blood pressure values. In the obstetric anesthesia circle, hypotension exists when the systolic blood pressure is below 100 mm. Hg or when there is a fall in systolic blood pressure of more than 20 per cent.

The limitations of arterial blood pressure for clinical monitoring have been mentioned. During spinal or epidural anesthesia, changes in arterial blood pressure do not correlate with those of cardiac output.[53] Small decreases in arterial blood pressure are due predominantly to decreases in total peripheral resistance, with cardiac output alterations playing only a minor role. If the systolic blood pressure falls more than 20 per cent from the pre-block blood pressure value, decrease in cardiac output is a significant etiologic factor.

When hypotension occurs with spinal block it usually develops during the first 10 minutes after subarachnoid injection and will reach its lowest level in 15 minutes. With epidural block hypotension occurs within 20 minutes and reaches maximum within 30 minutes. The first half hour after the block is administered is a critical period in terms of cardiovascular alterations.

EFFECTS ON PERIPHERAL CIRCULATION

In the circulatory system, blood flow is directly related to the perfusion pressure and inversely related to the vascular resistance. The pressures within the aorta, large arteries, and main arterial branches are generally maintained at a constant value. Pressures in the resistance (arterioles) and capacitance (veins) vessels, however, are subject to physiologic regulation and pharmacodynamic responses, including the effects of sympathetic block.[53] In general the vasomotor tone of the arterioles is regulated mainly by local metabolic requirements and waste products and secondarily by sympathetic vasoconstrictor fibers. Sympathetic blockade results in relaxation of the smooth muscles in all the affected arterioles and precapillary sphincters, decreasing or eliminating vasomotion but increasing the number of open capillaries.[28] In accordance with Poiseuille's law, large alterations in vascular resistance and blood flow can occur with even small alterations in the radius of the arteries and arterioles. After sympathetic denervation there is increased capillary flow. Owing to the increased vascular bed there is a greater uptake of oxygen from blood, resulting in a decrease of the central venous oxygen content and saturation.[61]

The venous system acts as an active vascular reservoir for blood. It reacts to both neurogenic and humoral stimuli, resulting in alterations in cardiac output and arterial blood pressure. It is estimated that 70 per cent of the total blood volume is contained in the venous side of the circulation[53] and that the distensibility and contractility of the veins contribute decisively to the maintenance of adequate central blood volume.[54] After sympathetic blockade, venous pressure decreases irrespective of changes in arterial blood pressure.[28,44,61]

EFFECTS ON REGIONAL BLOOD FLOWS

After vertebral block there is redistribution of cardiac output to the different organs of the body. Generally there is a decrease in the absolute blood flow to the different organs as a result of decrease in mean arterial blood pressure and cardiac output. The autoregulation mechanisms in the body's vital organs, like the heart, brain, and kidneys, tend to minimize the changes resulting from decreased perfusion pressure. Renal blood flow decreases by about 10 per cent[39] when the block is at the T5 level. Hepatic blood flow is also decreased due to increased splanchnic vascular resistance and reduced mean arterial blood pressure when epinephrine is omitted in the epidural anesthetic solution.[40] Even in the presence of absolute decreases in blood flow to the heart and brain, the percentages of the cardiac output directed to them are not changed significantly.[56,57] However, the myocardial minute work (mean arterial blood pressure times cardiac output) proportionately decrease to the extent that perfusion relative to myocardial workload is adequate. The two regions that have consistently increased blood flow, both in absolute and percentage of cardiac output, are the lungs and the lower extremities.[56] The increased blood flow to the lungs promotes gas exchange which is beneficial, but the increased perfusion to the lower extremities is obviously inappropriate since the leg muscles are paralyzed and inactive.

The uterine blood flow studies done in pregnant ewes and pregnant women concur that the uterine blood flow generally decreases in proportion to the reduction in maternal arterial blood pressure. Uterine blood flow did not decrease without simultaneous maternal hypotension in laboring women managed by continuous segmental lumbar epidural anesthesia.[14] Pregnant ewes made hypotensive to 50 per cent of the original blood pressure by spinal block showed a 65 per cent reduction in uterine blood flow.[42] When near-term pregnant ewes were bled to 50 per cent of their original blood pressure values, uterine blood flow decreased proportionately, and uterine vascular resistance did not change significantly. When the perfusing pressure had fallen to about 50 torr, uterine blood flow decreased more than the perfusing pressure, suggesting uterine vasoconstriction or probably collapse of uterine vessels (critical closing pressure for the uterine vascular bed ranges from 40–50 torr.)[12]

The cardiovascular effects of local anesthetic agents are discussed in Chapter 4. In summary local anesthetic agents increase the cardiac output, may decrease the peripheral resistance, and increase the venous return to the heart. These effects are modified by sympathetic blockade.

CARDIOVASCULAR EFFECTS CAUSED BY VASOCONSTRICTOR DRUGS IN ANESTHETIC SOLUTIONS USED FOR VERTEBRAL BLOCKS

The usual rationale for incorporating vasoconstrictor drugs in the local anesthetic solutions is to:

1. Prolong the duration of action of the block
2. Enhance the intensity of the block
3. Minimize the incidence of unilateral or spotty block

4. Lower the concentration of local anesthetic agent in the blood to minimize systemic toxicity
5. Increase the cardiac output

Like the local anesthetic agent, the vasoconstrictor drugs incorporated in the solution to accomplish the above objectives will eventually find their way into the systemic circulation. Several reports are available in the literature dealing with the circulatory modifications by epinephrine-containing local anesthetic solutions.[2,7,9,11,13,39,46,59,60,62] All the reports agree that the cardiovascular changes are dose-dependent and reflect the β effects of epinephrine on the heart and vascular bed. In normal man there seems to be a synergistic action between epinephrine and vasomotor blockade. It was noted by Bonica and coworkers[8] that the decrease in total peripheral resistance was 50 per cent greater with peridural analgesia produced by lidocaine with epinephrine than the sum of the decreases in total peripheral resistance produced by lidocaine vasomotor block alone and epinephrine alone. The decrease in mean arterial blood pressure was modest (10%) because the marked diminution in total peripheral resistance (37%) was counteracted by the marked increase in cardiac output (47%).

The usual epinephrine dose in spinal anesthesia is small and its rate of absorption is slow so that no cardiovascular effect is detected apart from the changes associated with spinal sympathetic blockade. In epidural anestheia the usual amount of epinephrine employed ranges from 80 to 130 μg./dose. This amount of epinephrine produces a predominantly β-adrenergic stimulation. In the heart, the heart rate and stroke volume increase. This increase is usually more than offset by generalized peripheral vasodilation with marked decrease in total peripheral resistance resulting in a decrease in mean arterial blood pressure. Epinephrine "robs" the body of its compensatory vasoconstriction mechanism in the unblocked areas, an important homeostatic mechanism during vertebral sympathetic blockade.

Epinephrine stimulates β_1-adrenergic receptors in the heart at all dose levels, increasing heart rate and stroke volume. The β_1-adrenergic stimulation is independent of the alterations in cardiac function secondary to increased venous return and other peripheral effects. In the peripheral circulatory system, epinephrine is one of a number of drugs that have a dual or biphasic effect. The chief vascular action of epinephrine is exerted mainly on the smaller arterioles and precapillary sphincters, although veins and larger arteries also respond to the drug. Various vascular beds react differently, but at low dose levels β_2 receptors, being more sensitive, are activated, causing vasodilation and a fall in total peripheral resistance and mean arterial blood pressure. At larger dose levels the α-adrenergic receptors are also activated and vasoconstriction predominates, causing an increase in mean arterial blood pressure.[34] Arteriolar and capillary vasoconstriction are not usually encountered with epidural analgesia unless the drug is inadvertently injected intravenously. The α-adrenergic receptors responsible for venoconstriction are stimulated at lower dose levels,[59] thereby increasing venous tone and return. The increase in venous return (preload), myocardial contractility (inotropism) and heart rate (chronotropism) complemented by decrease in total peripheral resistance (afterload) is an ideal combination for increasing cardiac output.[10] Following epidural injection of epinephrine the cardiovascular effects occur within 5 minutes and peak in about 15 minutes. The peripheral effects may last for 1.5 to 2 hours depending upon the dose.[8]

In situations where the stimulation of β_1-adrenergic receptors causing tachycardia is not warranted, phenylephrine is the preferred drug. Phenylephrine is a powerful direct α-adrenergic receptor stimulant with very little effect on the β-adrenergic receptors of the heart.[34] The hemodynamic effects of phenylephrine in man are characterized by increase in blood pressure because of generalized vasoconstriction, reflex bradycardia, and decreased cardiac output despite an elevated central venous pressure. Because of phenylephrine's negative inotropic effects one must weigh the advantages against the disadvantages before using this drug. Phenylephrine does not have the myometrial-inhibiting effect characteristic of epinephrine.[59,60]

However, one must be cognizant of the fact that in animal studies[31,52] disturbing findings were noted when epinephrine and norepinephrine were infused into pregnant ewes at 0.2 to 0.5 μg./kg./min. Uterine vascular conductance decreased by 50 per cent while uterine arterial blood flow decreased by 39 per cent suggesting vasoconstriction. The decrease in uterine arterial blood flow occurred even in the absence of significant changes in systemic arterial pressure. At this dose level stimulation of beta receptors was evidenced by increase in heart rate, cardiac output, and skeletal muscle blood flow. The decrease in the uterine blood flow is most pronounced in the endometrium (-58.7 per cent ± 5.3), followed by the myometrium (-36.9 per cent ± 6.4) and the placental cotyledons (-34.5 per cent ± 4.7). The epinephrine-induced vasoconstriction in each component of the vascular bed of the pregnant uterus signified greater sensitivity of the reproductive tissues to the vasoconstrictive properties of epinephrine. On this basis Rosenfeld and coworkers[52] suggested that deleterious effects might occur in a pregnant woman exposed to relatively low arterial concentrations of epinephrine. Also the addition of epinephrine in the epidural anesthetic solution predictably produced diminution of uterine activity mainly by decreasing the intensity of uterine contractions and occasionally by reducing the frequency of uterine contractions.[47] The conclusion from these studies is that although the use of epinephrine is recommended with epidural analgesia for surgery, it is not advisable in obstetrics.

INFLUENCING FACTORS IN THE CONDITION OF THE PATIENT ("RECEPTOR-EFFECTOR SYSTEM") ON THE CARDIOVASCULAR RESPONSE TO VERTEBRAL BLOCKADE

The ultimate determinant that influences the cardiovascular response to vertebral blockade is the ability of the "receptor-effector system," the patient, to respond and mobilize numerous compensatory mechanisms to maintain cardiovascular homeostasis. Most of the changes mentioned so far are adjustments recorded from well-controlled experimental environments in animals and healthy volunteers. There is no question that any deviation from normal health will modify the nature and magnitude of the patient's response. The following discussions will focus on the more important factors that affect the ability of the patient to respond to spinal and epidural anesthesia.

Age

Younger patients are less prone to excessive cardiovascular changes after spinal or epidural block. Their cardiovascular and autonomic nervous systems are relatively free of disease so that they have a higher residual autonomous vascular tone in the blocked areas and a more active reflex homeostatic compensatory mechanism in the unblocked areas.

Blood Volume

Decreased circulating blood volume from any cause, be it hemorrhage or plain dehydration, accentuates the cardiovascular depression produced by sympathetic blockade.[9,38] Pooling of blood occurs in the anesthetized areas irrespective of the blood volume, so that relatively greater amounts of blood are "removed" from the effective circulating blood volume in hypovolemic compared to normovolemic individuals.

Hypovolemia is one of the contraindications of vertebral block anesthesia. If one has to give a block in a hypovolemic patient, extreme caution must be observed. The blood volume should be expanded as rapidly as possible before induction of the block, and sympathetic blockade should be confined to a very limited area appropriate to the contemplated surgical procedure.

Sympathetic Activity

The state of sympathetic activity before and after the block plays a major role in the cardiovascular responses to vertebral block anesthesia. Roughly, the magnitude of cardiovascular change is, to a certain extent, proportional to the sympathetic tone. In conditions caused by or associated with high sympathetic activity, more profound fall in blood pressure is expected after spinal or epidural block. Hemorrhage[17] and other causes of hypovolemia, fear and apprehension provoked by injury and disease, congestive heart failure, and hypertensive states with contracted plasma volume, including toxemias of pregnancy, are all associated with high sympathetic tone. Even in normal pregnancy the autonomic nervous system plays a large role in maintenance of arteriolar and, more importantly, venous tone.[25] Sympathetic blockade in these instances can precipitate cardiovascular instability that can be hazardous unless precautions are taken to minimize the expected hypotension.

On the other hand, an active sympathetic nervous system that has the capability to increase its tone in the unblocked areas usually adequately compensates for the lost activity in the blocked areas so that the total peripheral resistance is only modestly decreased.[6,62]

Other Medications

Central nervous system depressants (i.e., barbiturates, narcotics, and general anesthetics) have been demonstrated to accentuate the cardiovascular depression produced by the sympathetic blockade and the direct myocardial-depressant effect of local anesthetics.[19,45] Patients may not be able to mobilize compensatory mechanisms effectively when the circulatory homeostatic mechanisms are dampened by narcotics, barbiturates, and other central nervous system depressants. The central autonomic stimulant effect of local anesthetics on cardiac output is abolished by decerebration and vagotomy,[37] and presumably central nervous system depressants can also decrease cardiac function by depression of central autonomic control.

Another group of drugs are the antihypertensive agents. Diuretics decrease plasma volume and certain drugs like reserpine deplete the body catecholamine stores. Ganglionic blockers and specific adrenergic receptor blockers diminish or abolish sympathetic influences on the cardiovascular system. Cardiovascular depression could be magnified if vertebral block is undertaken in the presence of these drugs. The homeostatic mechanisms of the body are "handcuffed" so that very little or no circulatory compensatory adjustments may take place.

Pregnancy

Pregnancy imposes adjustments on the maternal cardiovascular system to meet the metabolic and excretory requirements of the growing fetus. By necessity, the cardiac output and the blood volume increase progressively and the total peripheral resistance decreases to meet the demands of the growing fetus with the least energy expenditure on the maternal circulatory system. Great care must be observed to avoid additional cardiac stress or cardiac depression during anesthesia so as not to compromise the mother and her baby.

Because of the weight and the anterior location of the uterus, all gravida at term experience some degree of aortocaval compression when the supine position is assumed. However, only about 15 per cent

of these women manifest signs and symptoms of supine hypotensive syndrome.[35] The clinical manifestations of the syndrome include hypotension, tachycardia, pallor, fainting spells with or without nausea and vomiting. The majority of pregnant women can compensate for the caval obstruction by initially increasing the sympathetic tone. Also, numerous vascular adjustments in and around the uterus take place to compensate for the systemic and placental circulation disturbances caused by aortocaval compression.[3] A decrease in resistance of the uterine and placental vascular bed as a consequence of selective dilatation of the arteries promotes maximal blood flow to the uterus. Whereas the supine hypotensive syndrome is the result of compressive obstruction of the inferior vena cava, in some instances the abdominal aorta is the vessel mainly affected. In this instance the brachial artery pressure is normal or even higher than normal but the femoral pressure is decreased.[22,63] In the supine position, the uterus may divide the maternal circulation into a hyperdynamic zone characterized by normal or increased aortic pressure above the point of obstruction and a low pressure system characterized by decreased arterial pressure, decreased blood flow, and increased venous pressure below the obstruction. Whereas there is some degree of compensation for a decreased venous return secondary to mild to moderate inferior vena caval compression, there is no compensation for decreased placental perfusion secondary to lower aortic obstruction unless ovarian-uterine arterial anastomosis develops around the site of obstruction. Any alterations in any one or all of these built-in circulatory adjustments can jeopardize the fetus. This must be kept in mind when providing anesthesia to parturient women.

THE MANAGEMENT OF HYPOTENSION IN OBSTETRICS

The authors consider a patient to have hypotension when the systolic blood pressure falls 20 per cent or more below the original value. In the pregnant woman, the original level of blood pressure is the reading obtained when she is on her side and not having a uterine contraction.

For the management of hypotension secondary to vertebral blocks, attention should be paid to the underlying cause. Measures must be directed toward insuring adequate venous return, maintenance of cardiac efficiency, and optimum total peripheral resistance. In treating hypotension it is preferable to apply therapeutic modalities which increase the perfusion of the vital organs with the least energy expenditure on the cardiovascular system. However, measures to prevent hypotension should be the primary goal.

PREVENTIVE MODALITIES

Proper Selection of Patients

This entails proper preoperative evaluation of patients. The adequacy of blood volume must be the primary consideration. In the presence of dehydration or hemorrhage, volume replacement should be accomplished before instituting the vertebral block. If this is not feasible because of the urgency of the situation, vertebral block should be abandoned and general anesthesia used instead. However, volume replacement must still be done during and after induction of general anesthesia. This point stresses the proper fluid maintenance of all obstetric patients.

Fluid Loading

Before the initiation of vertebral block, especially for cesarean section, the patient should have received at least 10 ml./kg. of electrolyte solution within 15 minutes before the block. This is more important with spinal block than with epidural analgesia because of the rapid cardiovascular changes with the former technique. While performing the block and following its induction, the intravenous infusion must continue at a rapid rate. In healthy parturients rapid infusion of up to 1 liter of electrolyte solutions has been demonstrated to be safe and effective in the prevention and treatment of hypotension following vertebral blocks.[66]

Lateral Position or Uterine Displacement

The pregnant woman at term should not be allowed to stay flat on her back for prolonged periods of time because of aortocaval compression and its attendant sequelae. The problem is magnified when the compensatory mechanisms cannot be activated due to the sympathetic blockade. It is only appropriate that the parturient should labor on her side at all times. When she has to be on her back for any reason (e.g., for ceasarean section) the uterus must be displaced from the great vessels irrespective of the brachial artery pressure. The uterus is displaced either manually, with a device (Colon-Marales; Kennedy), a wedge, or by tilting the operating table. The method of choice varies according to the preference of the anesthesiologist. Eckstein and Marx[22] found that 60 per cent of pregnant women in the supine position had significant femoral artery hypotension, while only 18 per cent developed significant brachial artery hypotension. This has been attributed to compression of the abdominal aorta by the gravid uterus. The uterus is usually displaced to the left; rarely when this fails to correct the supine hypotension, it is displaced to the right.

Elevation of the Legs or Slight Trendelenburg Position

This is done to enhance the venous return to the heart. The Trendelenburg position can be resorted to only after the stabilization of the vertebral block.

Constrictive Bandages Applied to the Lower Extremities

This is done before the vertebral block to prevent venous pooling in the lower extremities.

Limiting the Extent of the Vertebral Block Appropriate to the Contemplated Procedure

Segmental epidural block during labor and delivery, by limiting nerve blockade to the specific segments involved, will minimize the cardiovascular changes.

Prophylactic Vasopressors

Opinions are divided whether prophylactic vasopressors are necessary and beneficial[20,33] or potentially harmful and not required.[23] For good reasons the authors follow the latter school (for details see Chap.15)

The uterine blood flow decreases roughly in proportion to the decrease in maternal blood pressure[36] and fetal deterioration can occur.[24,55]

THERAPEUTIC MODALITIES

If hypotension occurs despite proper positioning and fluid administration, the following modalities are warranted:

Vasopressors

The judicious use of a vasopressor is sometimes required. In obstetrics, pressor agents with predominantly β-adrenergic receptor effects are preferred to predominantly α-adrenergic receptor stimulants. The reason for this is the fact that the uterine vasculature is almost maximally dilated[32] so that any vasconstrictor agent at any dose level can cause uterine vasoconstriction and probably a decrease in uterine blood flow. In addition, because of hormonal influences, the pregnant uterine vasculature is more sensitive to the effects of catecholamines.[52] The two vasopressor agents that have a rightful place in obstetric anesthesia are ephedrine and mephentermine (Wyamine). Both agents have predominantly β-adrenergic receptor effects causing increased heart rate and myocardial contractility and, to a lesser degree, a peripheral vasoconstriction. In ad-

dition, mephentermine causes a pronounced increase in venous return to the heart due to direct venoconstriction.[58] Early studies in hypotensive ewes have shown that both drugs restore the uterine blood flow up to 90 per cent of the prespinal levels.[36] More recent studies have shown that they do not significantly alter the uterine blood flow in normotensive ewes.[50] It would be interesting to remeasure the uterine blood flow following these vasopressors combined with a fluid preloading (10 ml./kg.) as practiced clinically.

Atropine Sulfate

The hypotension following vertebral block is invariably associated with bradycardia.[28] If the relative hypovolemia is being remedied by either rapid intravenous infusion and/or proper positioning, increasing the heart rate by intravenous atropine (0.01 mg./kg.) usually brings the blood pressure to acceptable levels. If a vasopressor is to follow atropine, the vasopressor dose should be halved. Atropine facilitates the positive inotropic and chronotropic action of the beta vasopressors.[36]

Oxygen Administration

Oxygen is administered in conjunction with other therapeutic modalities (i.e., blood volume expansion and vasopressors). However, one must be aware of the fact that merely increasing the maternal PaO_2 in the presence of uterine vasoconstriction does not necessarily improve fetal oxygenation.[5]

REFERENCES

1. Akamatsu, T. J., *et al.*: Cardiovascular response to increased epidural pressure in the elderly surgical patients. Pacif. Med. Surg., 75:160, 1967.
2. Amory, D. W., Sivarajan, M. D., and Lindbloom, L. E.: Blood flow changes during epidural anesthesia with epinephrine in the rhesus monkey. Abstracts of Scientific Papers. American Society of Anesthesiologists Annual Meeting, Chicago, 1975.
3. Bieniarz, J., *et al.*: Aortocaval compression by the

uterus in late human pregnancy: IV. Circulatory homeostasis by preferential perfusion of the placenta. Am. J. Obstet. Gynecol., *103*:19, 1969.

4. Blaine, E. H., Davis, J. O., and Prewitt, R. L.: Evidence for renal vascular receptor in control of renin secretion. Am. J. Physiol., *220*:1593, 1971.

5. Boba, A., Linkie, D. M., and Plotz, E. J.: Fetal effects of spinal hypotension. Observations in the dog at term of pregnancy. Obstet. Gynecol., *37*:247, 1971.

6. Bonica, J. J., Berges, P. U., and Morikawa, K.: Circulatory effects of peridural block: 1. Effects of level of analgesia and dose of lidocaine. Anesthesiology, *33*:619, 1970.

7. Bonica, J. E., *et al.*: A comparison of the effects of high subarachnoid and epidural anesthesia. Acta Anesthesiol. Scand. [Suppl.] , *23*:429, 1966.

8. ———: Circulatory effects of peridural block: II. Effects of epinephrine. Anesthesiology, *34*:514, 1971.

9. ———: Circulatory effects of peridural block: III. Effects of acute blood loss. Anesthesiology, *36*:219, 1972.

10. Braunwald, E.: Current concepts in cardiology: determinants and assessment of cardiac function. N. Engl. J. Med., *296*:86, 1977.

11. Bridenbaugh, P. O., *et al.*: Role of epinephrine in regional block anesthesia with etidocaine: a double-blind study. Anesth. Analg., *53*:430, 1974.

12. Brinkman, C. R. III, Mofid, M., and Assali, N. S.: Circulatory shock in pregnant sheep: III. Effects of hemorrhage on uteroplacental and fetal circulation and oxygenation. Am. J. Obstet. Gynecol., *118*:77, 1974.

13. Bromage, P. R.: Physiology and pharmacology of epidural anesthesia. Anesthesiology, *28*:592, 1967.

14. Brotanek, V., *et al.*: The influence of epidural anesthesia on uterine blood flow. Obstet. Gynecol., *42*:276, 1973.

15. Buchan, P. C., Milne, M. K., and Browning, M. C. K.: The effect of continuous epidural blockade on plasma 11-hydroxycorticosteroid concentrations in labour. J. Obstet. Gynaecol. Br. Commonw. 5 *80*:974, 1973.

16. Buchbinder, N., and Ganz, W.: Hemodynamic monitoring: invasive techniques. Anesthesiology, *45*:146, 1976.

17. Chien, S.: Role of the sympathetic nervous system in hemorrhage. Physiol. Rev., *47*:214, 1967.

18. Crawford, J. S.: Lumbar epidural block in labour: a clinical analysis. Br. J. Anaesth., *44*:66, 1972.

19. ———: Patient management during extradural anesthesia for obstetrics. Br. J. Anaesth., *47* [Suppl.]:273, 1975.

20. Cucchiara, R. F., and Restall, C. J.: Mephentermine and intravenous fluids for the prevention of hypotension associated with spinal anesthesia. Anesthesiology, *34*:109, 1973.

21. Dripps, R. D., Eckenhoff, J. E., and Vandam, L. D.: Introduction to Anesthesia: the Principles of Safe Practice. Ed. 4, pp. 84–98. Philadelphia, W. B. Saunders, 1972.

22. Eckstein, K. L., and Marx, G. F.: Aortocaval compression and uterine displacement. Anesthesiology, *40*:92, 1974.

23. Eng, M., *et al.*: The effects of methoxamine and ephedrine in normotensive pregnant primates. Anesthesiology, *35*:354, 1971.

24. ———: Spinal anesthesia and ephedrine in pregnant monkeys. Am. J. Obstet. Gynecol., *115*:1095, 1973.

25. Ferris, T. F.: Toxemia and hypertension. *In* Burrow, G. N., and Ferris, T. F., (eds): Medical Complications During Pregnancy. P. 55. Philadelphia, W. B. Saunders, 1975.

26. Gorlin, R.: Current concepts in cardiology: practical cardiac hemodynamics. N. Engl. J. Med., *296*:203, 1977.

27. Gottschalk, W.: Regional anesthesia. I. Spinal, lumbar epidural, and caudal anesthesia. Obstet. Gynecol., *3*:385, 1974.

28. Greene, N. M.: Physiology of Spinal Anesthesia. Ed. 2. Baltimore, Williams & Wilkins, 1969.

29. ———: Area of differential block in spinal anesthesia with hyperbaric tetracaine. Anesthesiology, *19*:45, 1958.

30. ———: Physiology of sympathetic denervation. Annu. Rev. Med., *13*:87, 1962.

31. Greiss, F. C.: The uterine vascular bed: effect of adrenergic stimulation. Obstet. Gynecol., *21*:295, 1963.

32. ———: Pressure-flow relationship in the gravid uterine vascular bed. Am. J. Obstet. Gynecol., *96*:41, 1966.

33. Gutsche, B. B.: Prophylactic ephedrine preceding spinal analgesia for cesarean section. Anesthesiology, *45*:462, 1976.

34. Innes, I. R., and Nickerson, M.: Norepinephrine, epinephrine, and the sympathomimetic amines. *In* Goodman, L. S., and Gilman, A. (eds.): The Pharmacologic Basis of Therapeutics. Ed. 5, pp. 477–492, 502–503, New York, Macmillan, 1975.

35. James, F. M., III: Maternal considerations in obstetrical anesthesia. Anesth. Rev., *3*:33, 1976.

36. James, F. M., III, Greiss, F. C., and Kemp, R. A.: An evaluation of vasopressor therapy for maternal hypotension during spinal anesthesia. Anesthesiology, *33*:25, 1970.

37. Kao, F. A., and Jalar, U. H.: The central action of lignocaine and its effect on cardiac output. Br. J. Pharmacol., *14*:522, 1959.

38. Kennedy, W. F., Jr., *et al.*: Cardiovascular and respiratory effects of subarachnoid block in the presence of acute blood loss. Anesthesiology, *29*:29, 1968.

39. ———: Systemic cardiovascular and renal hemodynamic alterations during peridural anesthesia in normal man. Anesthesiology, *31*:414, 1969.

40. ———: Simultaneous systemic and hepatic hemodynamic measurements during high peridural anesthesia in normal man. Anesth., Analg., *50*:1069, 1971.

41. Kessler, M., Hoper, J., and Krumme, B. A.: Monitoring of tissue perfusion and cellular function. Anesthesiology, *45*:184, 1976.

42. Lucas, W., Kirschbaum, T., and Assali, N. S.: Spinal shock and fetal oxygenation. Am. J. Obstet. Gynecol., *93*:583, 1965.

43. Lush, D., *et al.*: The effect of epidural analgesia on the adrenocortical response to surgery. Br. J. Anaesth., *44*:1169, 1972.

44. McClean, A. P., *et al.*: Hemodynamic alterations associated with epidural anesthesia. Surgery, *62*:79, 1967.

45. McWhirter, W., *et al.*: Cardiovascular effects of controlled lidocaine overdosage in dogs anesthetized with nitrous oxide. Anesthesiology, *39*:398, 1973.

46. Martin, W. E., *et al.*: A comparison between cardiovascular effects of sciatic-femoral block with bupivacaine and with lidocaine. Anesth. Analg., *52*:454, 1973.

47. Matadial, L., and Cibils, L. A.: The effect of epidural anesthesia on uterine activity and blood pressure. Am. J. Obstet. Gynecol., *125*:846, 1976.

48. Moir, D. D., and Willocks, J.: Epidural analgesia in British obstetrics. Br. J. Anaesth., *40*:129, 1968.

49. Phillips, O. C.: Clinical management of spinal anesthesia. *In* Hershey, S. G. (ed.): Refresher Courses in Anesthesiology. Vol. 4, p. 81. Philadelphia, J. B. Lippincott, 1976.

50. Ralston, D. H., Shnider, S. M. and deLorimier, A. A.: Effects of equipotent ephedrine, metaraminol, mephentermine, and methoxamine on uterine blood flow in the pregnant ewe. Anesthesiology, *40*:354, 1974.

51. Roe, C. F., and Cohn, F. L.: Sympathetic blockade during spinal anesthesia. Surg., Gynecol. Obstet., *136*:265, 1973.

52. Rosenfeld, C. R., Barton, M. D., and Meschia, G.: Effects of epinephrine on distribution of blood flow in the pregnant ewe. Am. J. Obstet. Gynecol., *124*:156, 1976.

53. Shimosato, S.: Circulatory adjustment under spinal anesthesia. *In* Massion, W. H., (ed.): Effects of Hemorrhage on Anesthetic Requirements. Int. Anesthesiol. Clin., *12*(1):127, 1974.

54. Shimosato, S., and Etsten, B. E.: The role of the venous system in cardiocirculatory dynamics during spinal and epidural anesthesia in man. Anesthesiology, *30*:619, 1969.

55. Shnider, S. M., *et al.*: Vasopressors in obstetrics. I. Correction of fetal acidosis with ephedrine during spinal hypotension. Am. J. Obstet. Gynecol., *102*:911, 1968.

56. Sivarajan, M., Amory, D. W., and Lindbloom, L. E.: Systemic and regional blood flow during epidural anesthesia without epinephrine in the rhesus monkey. Anesthesiology, *45*:300, 1976.

57. Sivarajan, M., *et al.*: Systemic and regional blood-flow changes during spinal anesthesia in the rhesus monkey. Anesthesiology, *43*:78, 1975.

58. Smith, N. T., and Corbascio, A. N.: The use or misuse of pressor agents. Anesthesiology, *33*: 58, 1970.

59. Stanton-Hicks, M. A.: Cardiovascular effects of extradural anaesthesia. Br. J. Anaesth., *47*[Suppl.]:253, 1975.

60. Stanton-Hicks, M., Berges, P. U., and Bonica, J. J.: Circulatory effects of peridural block: IV. Comparison of the effects of epinephrine and phenylephrine. Anesthesiology, *39*:308, 1973.

61. Stevens, W. C., Cain, W. E., and Hamilton, W. K.: Circulatory studies during spinal anesthesia: central and peripheral venous oxygen saturation before and after administration of vasopressors. Anesth., Analg., *47*:725, 1968.

62. Ward, R. J., *et al.*: Epidural and subarachnoid anesthesia. Cardiovascular and respiratory effects. J.A.M.A., *191*:275, 1965.

63. Weaver, J. B., Pearson, J. F., and Rosen, M.: Posture and epidural block in pregnant women at term. Effects on arterial blood pressure and limb blood flow. Anaesthesia, *30*:752, 1975.

64. Westone, D. L., and Wong, K. C.: Sinus bradycardia and asystole during spinal anesthesia. Anesthesiology, *41*:87, 1974.

65. Willenkin, R. L., and Greene, N. M.: Circulatory effects of spinal and epidural anesthesia. *In* Fabian, L. (ed.): Anesthesia and the Circulation. Clin. Anesth., *3*:109, 1964.

66. Wollman, S. B., and Marx, G. F.: Acute hydration for prevention of hypotension of spinal anesthesia in parturients. Anesthesiology, *29*:374, 1968.

6

Effects of Vertebral Blocks on the Respiratory System

Ezzat Abouleish, M.D.

Effects on the respiratory system during vertebral blocks may be due to the block of nerves caused by the technique or due to the direct action of drugs used to produce epidural analgesia, vasoconstriction, or sedation (Tables 6-1 and 6-2).

RESPIRATORY EFFECTS DUE TO NERVE BLOCKADE

Spinal and epidural techniques share the properties which result from paralysis of the various types of nerve fibers.

Table 6-1. Effects of Vertebral Blocks on the Respiratory System Caused by Blocking of Nerves

Type of Nerve	Effect
Motor	Therapeutic effect: expiration mainly affected Extensive effect: respiratory inadequacy
Sensory	Sense of dyspnea. Improving respiratory pattern
Autonomic	Hypotension; if excessive, causes respiratory arrest Improvement of ventilation in patients with pulmonary disease Bronchial dilatation

Table 6-2. Effects of Vertebral Blocks on the Respiratory System due to the Direct Action of Drugs

Type of Drug	Therapeutic Effect	Toxic Effect
Local anesthetic	Sedation; bronchodilatation	Convulsions → apnea
Vasoconstrictor (epinephrine)	Beta effect, e.g., bronchodilatation	Hypertension → pulmonary edema
Sedative or narcotic supplement	Relief of sense of dyspnea	Respiratory depression

EFFECTS OF MOTOR NERVE BLOCKADE

The muscles of respiration are either inspiratory or expiratory. The inspiratory muscles are mainly the diaphragm and the external intercostal muscles.[11] The diaphragm plays the major role in inspiration and is supplied by the thick phrenic nerve which arises from C3 to C5. On the other hand, the expiratory muscles, namely the abdominal muscles and the internal intercostals, are supplied only by the thoracic nerves. Therefore, a motor nerve blockade to the T1 segment will paralyze all the muscles of expiration while the diaphragm is spared. Consequently the forced ex-

113

piratory effort, as measured by the expiratory reserve volume, is lost while the inspiratory capacity is reduced only 20 per cent.[9] Earlier studies have found that as a result of paralysis of the intercostals the residual volume and the functional residual capacity are reduced.[9] However, recent studies have shown that the functional residual capacity, pulmonary gas distribution, and closing capacity are not significantly decreased with epidural analgesia.[14] Since during normal ventilation exhalation is passive and results from recoil of the expanded chest during inspiration, normal ventilation is not affected in spite of a block to the T1 level. Also, since inspiration is slightly affected, the remaining inspiratory capacity is still 3 to 6 times the average tidal volume.[9] In premedicated patients, the arterial oxygenation, evidenced by the PaO_2 and the alveolar-arterial oxygen gradient ($PAo_2 - Pao_2$), is not significantly changed by a high epidural block (to the T2 level).[14,18] However, total paralysis of the muscles of expiration can be harmful due to the abolishment of the power to cough. In such a case, if the patient regurgitates and the regurgitated material is not sucked out by the anesthesiologist, it will accumulate in the pharynx and above the vocal cords, the patient being unable to get rid of it by vomiting or coughing. Since the laryngeal reflex is intact the vocal cords will close, temporarily preventing aspiration. Ultimately, as a result of hypoxia and hypercapnia, the cords will open and aspiration occurs. Therefore a patient specially with such a high block should be carefully watched. Patients with pulmonary disease should clear their chests as much as possible before spinal or epidural block.

Fortunately, the motor nerve blockade under spinal or epidural analgesia is lower than the sensory nerve level.[10] Under spinal block, the motor blockade is two segments lower than the sensory blockade and four segments lower with epidural block. The reason for this is that motor fibers are thicker than sensory fibers and thus are more difficult to block. In subarachnoid block, progressive dilution of the local anesthetic by cerebrospinal fluid as it ascends from the lumbar region leads to more extensive sensory than motor blockade. In lumbar epidural block, the far segments are exposed to less drug than those close to the site of injection; therefore, the saturation of the motor nerve fibers is less complete than of the sensory nerve fibers. Moreover, under epidural analgesia motor paralysis is incomplete compared to spinal block. Therefore, with a high block to the T1 level there is less embarrassment of respiration with epidural block than with subarachnoid block. However, if the diaphragmatic movement is impeded due to a large tumor or pregnancy, *a too high motor block*, whether under spinal or epidural analgesia, may cause respiratory insufficiency; thus, under these circumstances, respiration should be assisted until the tumor is removed or the baby is delivered.

If the patient has a strong hand grip, it indicates that the block is below the T1 level, the phrenic nerves are intact, and the respiration is adequate. If the diaphragmatic movement is poor, the upper chest is retracting with inspiration, the alae nasae are working, tracheal tug is present, the patient's voice is weak or whispering, the hand grip is weak or absent, and the arms are limp, then the respiration has to be assisted or controlled with high FIO_2. If the patient is unconscious, correction of hypoxia and hypotension before intubation is essential. If the patient is conscious, the masseters and laryngeal muscles are intact because they are supplied by the cranial nerves. Under these circumstances, the best method to assist or control ventilation is by a mask and bag. An attempt to intubate would not only be difficult because of the intact masseters, but may be fatal because of initiating laryngospasm on top of the hypoxia and hypotension. If such a patient has to be intubated, ketamine induction, 1 mg./kg. is better than thiobarbiturate because of her cardiovascular instability. A muscle relaxant, ensuring relaxation of the masseters and larynx, makes intubation quick and atraumatic. Cricoid pressure should be applied to avoid regurgitation as a result of paralysis of the upper esophageal sphincter. Following intubation, artificial ventilation should be adequate without too much positive pressure which can decrease the venous return to the heart, subsequently reducing the cardiac output. The best posture for the patient is the horizontal position with the lower limbs elevated if possible. This ensures adequate venous return to the heart without the cerebral congestion which may result from the Trendelenburg position. Of course anti-Trendelenburg position is not advisable because of the associated vasomotor paralysis.

EFFECTS OF SENSORY NERVE BLOCKADE

Dyspnea

In unpremedicated or lightly sedated patients such as with cesarean section, the patient frequently feels short of breath. However, measurement of the blood gases shows signs of hyperventilation such as hyperoxygenation and hypocapnia (Fig. 6-1).[2] The causes of dyspnea, despite adequate respiration, are apprehension due to the sensory changes following the block plus the loss of the usual information reaching the respiratory centers from the stretch receptors in the intercostal muscles.[9] The respiratory centers, being uninformed of the degree of expansion of the chest wall, make the patient feel short of breath and tend to overact by hyperventilating. However, in any case of dyspnea under vertebral blocks, inadequate ventilation should be excluded. In cases of adequate ventilation, reassurance of the patient and/or cautious administration of a sedative is required.

Ventilation Pattern

During painful uterine contractions the patient tends to hyperventilate, predominantly by increasing the tidal volume while the respiratory frequency may decrease.[17] This hyperventilation is harmful to both the mother and fetus. In the mother it leads to increased oxygen consumption.[4] Although the oxygen cost of ventilation is 1 per cent of the total oxygen consumption with normal ventilation, it increases disproportionately as the minute ventilation rises because of the low efficiency of respiratory muscles.[1] This hyperventilation plus the vasoconstriction produced by pain lead to a steady increase in maternal lactate concentration,[5] diminished base excess, and metabolic acidosis.[8] Hyperventilation leads also to maternal hypocapnia which causes a shift in the oxygen dissociation curve to the left, i.e., rendering delivery of oxygen to the fetus more difficult.[13] Hypocapnia also increases blood shunts in the placenta and causes constriction of the umbilical vessels.[15] All of these plus the constriction of the uterine blood vessels due to the secretion of catecholamines as a result of pain lead to fetal acidosis. Elimi-

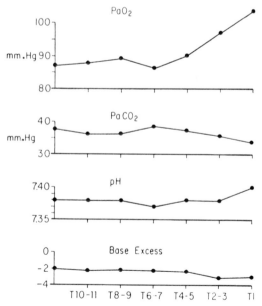

Fig. 6-1. Arterial blood gases and acid-base balances during various levels of peridural analgesia. (Bonica, J. J., Berges, P. U., and Morikawa, K.: Circulatory effects of peridural block: I. Effects of level of analgesia and dose of lidocaine. Anesthesiology, *33*:619, 1970)

nation of the hyperventilation associated with pain decreases the oxygen demand and corrects the maternal metabolic acidosis[17] and marked hypocapnia;[16] this explains the better metabolic status of both the mother and fetus under epidural analgesia compared to cases that had pudendal nerve block or no anesthesia.[20,21] The beneficial effects of epidural analgesia on oxygen consumption and acid-base status of the mother are absent in elective cesarean section because there is no associated labor pain.[17]

Following abdominal surgery, blocking of the pain sensory fibers improves ventilation, prevents atelectasis, and corrects the abnormal ventilation/perfusion ratio resulting from restricted respiratory movements.[3,6,7,9,10,18]

EFFECTS OF AUTONOMIC NERVE BLOCKADE

Effects on Vasomotor Fibers

The sympathetic nerve fibers are smaller than the sensory or the motor nerve fibers. Therefore, the sympathetic nerve blockade is almost two segments higher than the sensory nerve level. Extensive vasomotor paralysis leads to hypotension which is exaggerated in the pregnant woman due to the inferior vena caval compression by the gravid uterus. If hypotension is severe resulting in central nervous system ischemia, the respiratory centers become paralyzed and apnea occurs. In these cases, ventilation can be restored by correcting the hypotension. If during an attempted epidural block the drug is inadvertently injected into the subarachnoid space, the direct paralyzing effect of the local anesthetic on the respiratory center is an added factor to the effect of ischemia.

In patients with chronic obstructive pulmonary disease, blocking of the sympathetic nerve fibers is beneficial.[3] Due to systemic pooling of blood and decreased blood flow through the anastomotic vessels, sympathetic nerve blockade leads to reduction of the pulmonary pressure and the pulmonary blood volume. These effects result in a redistribution of the pulmonary blood flow and improvement of the ventilation/perfusion ratio. Moreover, paralysis of the expiratory muscles of respiration reduces the chance of air trapping and results in a better pattern of ventilation.[19]

Effects on Bronchodilator Fibers

Theoretically, interruption of the sympathetic nerve fibers (T1 through T4) leads to bronchoconstriction. However, epidural block causes bronchodilatation. This is due to interruption of the afferent sympathetic bronchoconstrictor impulses,[2a] hypotension causing reflex bronchodilatation,[2b] and a direct effect of the drug on the bronchial musculature.[19]

EFFECTS DUE TO THE ACTION OF DRUGS USED IN VERTEBRAL BLOCKS

Local Anesthetics

With subarachnoid block, the dose of the local anesthetic injected is so small that it has no direct effect on the respiratory centers.[12] Any effect of spinal block is due to hypotension and lack of perfusion of these centers. On the other hand, with epidural analgesia, the dose of the local anesthetic is about 10 times that used for subarachnoid block, and can have a direct effect on the respiratory centers.

In therapeutic doses, the local anesthetic is gradually absorbed from the epidural space, causing sedation and decrease in ventilation which is equivalent to sleeping conditions. It also produces relaxation of the smooth muscles of the bronchial tree.[19] *If the local anesthetic has been inadvertently injected intravascularly or an excessive dose has been administered*, convulsions followed by apnea occur. Respiratory insufficiency and cardiovascular collapse follow. Being unconscious, the patient is exposed to the dangers of aspiration pneumonitis.

Vasoconstrictors

If epinephrine is added to the local anesthetic, it will exert its own pharmacologic effects on the respiratory system. Its absorption from the epidural space produces a beta effect, i.e., causes bronchodilatation. However, if it is inadvertently injected intravenously it can produce severe hypertension and serious arrhythmias leading to acute pulmonary edema.

Sedative or Narcotic Supplement

In therapeutic doses these relieve the sense of dyspnea that occurs at the onset of the vertebral block. However, *excessive administration* of these drugs to compensate for inadequate anesthesia can lead to serious respiratory depression and offset the advantages of a vertebral block.

REFERENCES

1. Best, C. H., and Taylor, N. B.: The Physiological Basis of Medical Practice. Ed. 8, p. 1002. Baltimore, Williams & Wilkins, 1966.
2. Bonica, J. J., Berges, P. U., and Morikawa, K.: Circulatory effects of peridural block: I. Effects of level of analgesia and dose of lidocaine. Anesthesiology, *33*:619, 1970.
2a. Bromage, P. R.: Total respiratory compliance in anesthetized subjects and modifications produced by noxious stimuli. Clin. Sci., *17*:217, 1958.
2b. ———: Hypotension and vital capacity. Anaesthesia, *11*:39, 1956.
3. ———: Physiology and pharmacology of epidural analgesia. Anesthesiology, *28*:593, 1967.
4. Bryans, F. E., and Belither, A.: 17-Hydroxycorticosteroid levels in pregnancy. Am. J. Obstet. Gynecol., *82*:52, 1961.
5. Cain, S. M.: Diminution of lactate rise during hypoxia by P_{CO_2} and beta-adrenergic blockade. Am. J. Physiol., *217*:110, 1969.
6. Diament, M. L., and Palmer, K. N. V.: Postoperative changes in gas tensions of arterial blood and in ventilatory functions. Lancet, *2*:180, 1966.
7. ———:Venous/arterial pulmonary shunting as the principal cause of postoperative hypoxaemia. Lancet, *1*:15, 1967.
8. Eichenholze, A., *et al.*: Primary hypocapnia: a cause of metabolic acidosis. J. Appl. Physiol. *17*:283, 1962.
9. Freund, F. G.: Respiratory effects of subarachnoid and epidural block. *In* Bonica, J. J. (ed.): Regional Anesthesia: Recent Advances and Current Status. Pp. 98–107. Philadelphia, F. A. Davis, 1969.
10. Freund, F. G., *et al.*: Ventilatory reserve and level of motor block during high spinal and epidural anesthesia. Anesthesiology, *28*:834, 1967.
11. Ganong, F. N.: Review of Medical Physiology. Ed. 4, pp. 520–521. Los Altos, Cal., Lange Medical Publications, 1969.
12. Greene, N. M.: Physiology of Spinal Anesthesia. Ed. 2. Baltimore, Williams & Wilkins, 1969.
13. Levinson, G., *et al.*: Effects of maternal hyperventilation on uterine blood flow and fetal oxygenation and acid-base status. Anesthesiology, *40*:340, 1974.
14. McCarthy, G. S.: The effect of thoracic extradural analgesia on pulmonary gas distribution, functional residual capacity and airway closure. Br. J. Anaesth., *48*:243, 1976.
15. Motoyama, E. K., *et al.*: Adverse effect of maternal hyperventilation of the foetus. Lancet, *1*:286, 1966.
16. Pearson, J. F., and Davies, P.: The effect of continuous lumbar epidural analgesia on maternal acid-base balance and arterial lactate concentrations during the second stage of labour. J. Obstet. Gynaecol. Br. Commonw., *80*:225, 1973.
17. Sangoul, F., Fox, G. S., and Houle, G. L.: Effect of regional analgesia on maternal oxygen consumption during the first stage of labor. Am. J. Obstet. Gynecol., *121*:1080, 1975.
18. Sjogren, S., and Wright, B.: Respiratory changes during continuous epidural blockade. Acta Anaesth. Scand., *16*:27, 1972.
19. Wiedling, S.: Xylocaine: the Pharmacological Basis of Its Clinical Use, Ed. 2. Stockholm, Almqvist & Wiksell, 1964.
20. Zador, G., Lindmark, G., and Nilsson, B. A.: Pudendal block in normal vaginal delivery. Acta Obstet. Gynecol. Scand. [Suppl.], *34*:64, 1974.
21. Zador, G., and Nilsson, B. A.: Low dose intermittent epidural anaesthesia. II. Influence on labour and foetal acid-base. Acta Obstet. Gynecol. Scand. [Suppl.], *34*:17, 1974.

7

Effects of Vertebral Blocks on the Nervous System

Ezzat Abouleish, M.D.

NEUROLOGIC EFFECTS OF INTRAVERTEBRAL BLOCKS

The neurologic complications of intravertebral techniques require special consideration because of the many misconceptions concerning them which should be clarified (e.g., "Spinal anesthesia commonly causes permanent paralysis."). Although most of these misconceptions were formed more than 20 years ago and have been eliminated, they still exist in the minds of some of the medical profession and the public.

The complications of intravertebral techniques on the nervous system can be due to direct or indirect effects.

DIRECT EFFECTS

PROBLEMS PRODUCED BY DRUGS AND CHEMICALS

Neurolytic Reaction and Chemical Meningitis

Injection of a local anesthetic contaminated with a neurotoxic substance used for cold sterilization, such as phenol, or for cleansing syringes and needles, such as detergents, produces extensive paralysis and sensory loss.[50,62,87] Such a problem has been eliminated by avoiding these neurotoxic substances and using autoclav-

ing for sterilization. If ethylene oxide is used for sterilization, adequate aeration time should be allowed.

Nerve damage can also occur due to inadvertent injection of a wrong drug into the subarachnoid or epidural space. This complication can be avoided only by vigilance. Ampules containing different drugs may look alike, and the only way to avoid injecting the wrong drug is to read the label carefully. For example, there is a strong similarity between the ampules containing gallamine triethiodide (a nondepolarizing muscle relaxant) and the ampules containing cinchocaine (a local anesthetic used for spinal block). The inadvertent injection of the former in place of the latter into the subarachnoid space has produced convulsions and even death.[42] Also, the inadvertent epidural injection of thiopental can lead to serious neurologic complications as a result of irritation of nerves and spasm of blood vessels.[36] If such an accident occurs, the epidural injection of a local anesthetic reduces pain and relieves vascular spasm; irrigation of the epidural space using normal saline is beneficial, and the administration of steroids reduces the possibility of a chemical inflammatory reaction.

The excess of the cleansing solution applied to the patient's back should be removed before the spinal needle is introduced. Such a chemical is usually neurotoxic if it reaches the nerves in sufficient quantity. The use of an introducer before the spinal needle helps to prevent the contamination of the needle by any remains of the degerming solution.

Drug Overdosage

With spinal analgesia, the dose of local anesthetic injected is so small that its harmful effects on the central nervous system cannot be through the bloodstream, even if injected intravascularly. On the other hand, with epidural or caudal analgesia, the local anesthetic can produce convulsions if the dose is exceeded or injected intravenously (see Chap. 4).

Trauma by Needle or Catheter

Dural Tear

If the dura is punctured, a tear is produced proportionate to the size of the needle. This can lead to post-lumbar-puncture cephalgia, which is explained in detail later in this chapter. Cranial nerve palsy can occur if leakage of cerebrospinal fluid is excessive or prolonged. This was especially common in the past when continuous spinal analgesia was utilized by introducing a 16-gauge needle through which a catheter was advanced.[85]

Backache

The incidence of backache following subarachnoid block varies between 0.7 per cent[84] and 2.7 per cent.[68] When epidural analgesia is used the incidence is 2 per cent, whereas backache occurred in 7.6 per cent of cases after caudal analgesia.[24] The higher incidence with caudal than with epidural analgesia is probably due to the conditions for which the block has been used rather than to the anesthetic procedure itself.

Radicular Nerve Injury

Injury of a nerve root can be produced by the needle itself or by the drug.[68,69] If a patient feels paresthesia as the needle is introduced, the needle should be withdrawn and directed away from the affected site. One must make sure that there is a free flow of cerebrospinal fluid before injecting the drug and that the patient does not feel pain during injection. The cerebrospinal fluid osmotic pressure is 257 to 305 milliosmoles per liter.[40] The majority of the commonly used local anesthetic drugs are hyperosmotic, but once administered they are rapidly diluted by the large volume of the cerebrospinal fluid unless injected directly into a nerve root. Therefore, aspiration before injection not only verifies the position of the needle, but also ensures free mixing of the local anesthetic with the cerebrospinal fluid. Also, it is a golden rule to stop injection at any moment the patient experiences pain which can be attributed to the injected solution; the identity of the injected drug should be rechecked.

Spinal Cord Injury

If lumbar puncture is attempted above the termination of the spinal cord (2nd lumbar vertebra), there is a possibility of its direct injury by the needle. (The spinal cord extends more caudad in children than in adults, and therefore further caution is required in the former age group.) The use of continuous spinal technique carries with it the danger of spinal cord or nerve injury; the catheter can advance to reach the spinal cord and be in prolonged contact with it or with the bare nerve roots. This is one of the reasons why continuous spinal analgesia has fallen into disrepute. If epidural block is attempted above L2, the danger of damage to the spinal cord is less than with subarachnoid block because in epidural block the spinal cord is separated from the needle or catheter by the thick dura and the cerebrospinal fluid. However, if the epidural space is not properly identified, the needle could possibly be advanced too far, puncturing the dura and injuring the spinal cord. Therefore, thoracic or cervical epidural techniques are not to be performed by the novice.

Hematoma Formation

If intravertebral block is utilized in a patient who is under anticoagulant therapy, a hematoma may be produced causing compression of the spinal cord and subsequent paraplegia.[24,81]

INFECTION

An epidural abscess, causing compression of the spinal cord and irritation of the nerves, has been reported following epidural block both with and without the use of bacterial filters.[22,74] Epidural abscess or septic meningitis should not occur if aseptic techniques are followed. The routine use of bacterial filters is not necessary with continuous epidural analgesia for obstetrics.[1] Adhering, therefore, strictly to sterile techniques, utilizing a disposable blunt needle instead of a reusable adaptor at the end of the epidural catheter, and using a disposable syringe for each injection are important factors in reducing the incidence of contamination. The use of a bacterial filter is not a substitute for these rules. (See also Chaps. 13 and 14.)

INDIRECT EFFECTS

Vertebral blocks can produce nervous complications as a result of circulatory and respiratory insufficiencies.

EFFECTS DUE TO CIRCULATORY INSUFFICIENCY

Associated hypotension is usually the result of sympathetic blockade or the supine hypotensive syndrome, and rarely due to toxic action of the local anesthetic. If it is prolonged or severe, cerebral ischemia can occur, leading to various degrees of disabilities, from temporary paralysis to death. (See also Chap. 5.)

EFFECTS DUE TO RESPIRATORY INSUFFICIENCY

This can be due to *peripheral effect* (e.g., paralysis of the nerves supplying the muscles of respiration when the local anesthetic extends to the upper cervical region), or to *central effect* (e.g., paralysis or depression of the respiratory centers due to severe ischemia or a toxic reaction to the drug). Respiratory insufficiency can lead to asphyxia with subsequent temporary or permanent damage to the central nervous system. (See also Chap. 6.)

CONCLUSION

The most serious effects of the vertebral blocks that still occur are the indirect ones, namely, effects due to circulatory and/or respiratory insufficiency. Proper understanding of physiology and pharmacology and meticulous attention to details are the only safeguards against these complications. Both respiration and circulation should be well monitored and adequately maintained during any of these techniques.

With regard to the direct effects of vertebral blocks, lesions such as cauda equina syndromes, adhesive arachnoiditis, and septic or chemical meningitis should be of historic nature in the present era of sterile techniques, new drugs, better knowledge of basic sciences, and experienced hands. The occurrence of a neurologic manifestation, such as paralysis following spinal or epidural block, may be due to an associated or preexisting disease;[57,81,84] therefore, it is unfair to hold the anesthetic procedure responsible until all other possible causes are excluded.

In over 27,000 spinals performed in the last six years at Magee-Womens Hospital, there have been no cases of cranial nerve palsy. This is probably due to the use of fine needles (e.g., 24- to 26-gauge) and the proper management of post-lumbar-puncture cephalgia. Some patients reported weakness of the lower limbs, but when closely questioned they felt rather that their lower limbs were easily tired, and when examined they had no neurologic signs. A similar incidence of these complaints followed general anesthesia.[30] The only neurologic complications were spinal headache, backache, and radicular sensory changes in the lower limbs. Both the backache and the sensory changes could be due to softening of the ligaments and the lordosis accompanying pregnancy, to the parturition, or to the obstetrical interference. Fortunately, the sensory disturbances are usually temporary, lasting only 4 to 8 weeks, and the backache usually responds to physiotherapy. By far the most troublesome and most frequent complication is post-lumbar-puncture cephalgia which will be discussed in detail below.

POST-LUMBAR-PUNCTURE CEPHALGIA

PHYSIOLOGY OF THE CEREBROSPINAL FLUID

The cerebrospinal fluid (CSF) is mainly secreted by the choroid plexus. It also diffuses through central nervous system blood vessels and is formed by ependymal cells.[47]

The total volume of CSF is about 150 ml., of which 100 ml. surrounds the brain and 50 ml. surrounds the spinal cord. In different species including man, an amount of CSF equal to its total volume is produced every 4 hours.[70] Experimentally, the rate of CSF production has been found to remain constant between CSF pressures of −50 and +200 mm. H_2O. An increased rate of production does not seem to occur under physiologic conditions. However, in pathologic situations (e.g., hydrocephalus), CSF production can be 4 times the normal rate.[23] Its production is reduced with respiratory or metabolic alkalosis.[64] The rate of its secretion during pregnancy, when there is chronic respiratory alkalosis, is yet to be determined. Also, the rate of CSF secretion in cases with spinal headache is unknown.

The CSF pressure is determined by the balance between the rate of CSF production and its absorption. Normally it has a pressure of 100 to 150 mm. H_2O.

The CSF circulates from the lateral ventricles to the third ventricle through the foramina of Monro, then to the fourth ventricle through the aqueduct of Sylvius, then to the general subarachnoid space through the foramina of Luscha and Magendie (Fig. 7-1). It is absorbed by the arachnoid villi and granulations that are related to the cerebral venous sinuses and the spinal veins.

The specific gravity of CSF is about 1.007[89] compared to water at 37°C. Local anesthetic drugs used for spinal analgesia are made hyperbaric (having a specific gravity higher than CSF) by the addition of dextrose. For example, 5 per cent lidocaine in 7.5 per cent dextrose has a specific gravity of 1.032, and tetracaine in 5 per cent dextrose has a specific gravity of 1.018. The specific gravity of drugs used for epidural analgesia are hypobaric, e.g., 0.5 per cent bupivacaine has a specific gravity of 1.0059.[52] Therefore the patient should be in a horizontal position during the injection of the test dose of epidural or caudal block. If the patient is in a sitting position and the dura has been inadvertently punctured, the local anesthetic can spread cephalad to produce a total subarachnoid block.[52]

The CSF is a clear, colorless fluid which varies from the plasma in the following aspects:[70]

1. Glucose in the CSF is about two thirds of that in the plasma.

2. Proteins in the CSF are very low, about 15 to 45 mg. per cent.

3. Chlorides and sodium contents in CSF are slightly higher than in the plasma (Table 7-1).

4. The pH of the CSF is usually 7.34 and is affected by changes in the blood pH.[70]

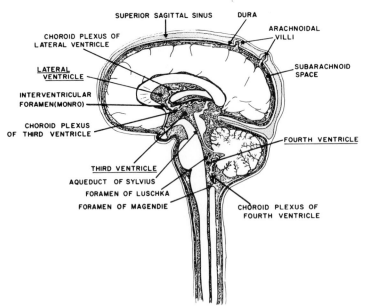

SUPERIOR SAGITTAL SINUS   DURA

CHOROID PLEXUS OF
LATERAL VENTRICLE

ARACHNOIDAL
VILLI

LATERAL
VENTRICLE

SUBARACHNOID
SPACE

INTERVENTRICULAR
FORAMEN(MONRO)

CHOROID PLEXUS
OF THIRD VENTRICLE

FOURTH VENTRICLE

THIRD VENTRICLE
AQUEDUCT OF SYLVIUS
FORAMEN OF LUSCHKA
FORAMEN OF MAGENDIE

CHOROID PLEXUS OF
FOURTH VENTRICLE

Fig. 7-1. Circulation of cerebrospinal fluid.

5. The CSF has few cells, usually 4 to 5 lymphocytes per ml.

The use of a urine test strip* is a guide method of identifying CSF in case of doubt.[8,71] Testing the temperature of the dripping fluid on the dorsum of the hand is unreliable. The pH of local anesthetics and of saline is acidic (about 5) compared to that of CSF which is alkaline. The glucose test in CSF is helpful but may be weak especially in a fasting patient. The protein test in CSF is weak due to low levels of proteins in CSF, but is relatively strong in local anesthetic solutions because the active nitrogen in the hydrophilic radical acts on the test indicator in a manner similar to the nitrogen protein. Therefore, the presence of a pH of 7 or more on the test strip, especially with a positive glucose, indicates the presence of CSF.

One of the main functions of the CSF is to act as a cushion for the brain within its solid vault.[47] Were it not for the CSF, any blow to the head would cause the brain to be juggled around and severely damaged.

*Ames Multistix, Division of Miles Laboratories, Elkhart, Indiana 46514.

Table 7-1. Composition of the Cerebrospinal Fluid

Constituent	Value
Glucose	40–80 mg.%
Proteins	15–45 mg.%
Chloride	120–130 mEq./l.
Sodium	140–150 mEq./l.
Bicarbonate	25–30 mEq./l.
pH	7.20–7.60

MECHANISM OF POST-LUMBAR-PUNCTURE CEPHALGIA

Post-lumbar-puncture cephalagia (PLPC) is as old as the discovery of subarachnoid block. In 1898, August Bier himself developed PLPC after the first attempt of subarachnoid block in man.[61] In 1902 Siccard postulated the leakage of CSF to be the cause of PLPC (Fig. 7-2), and since 1925 this has become the dominant theory to explain PLPC.

The Leakage Theory

There is leakage of CSF to the epidural space as a result of the dural puncture(s) used for a subarachnoid block or for diagnostic purposes.[80] Subsequently, the CSF pressure drops, the "cushion" effect of CSF is lost, and the brain sags, leading to traction on the intracranial sensitive structures, namely the blood vessels, nerves, and tentoria (Fig. 7-2). Supporting the leakage theory are the following findings: the incidence and severity of headache were found to be proportionate to the size of the needle, and the CSF pressure was found absent or negligible when lumbar puncture was performed following PLPC.[85]

Cerebral Vasodilation

Cerebral vasodilation is an auxiliary factor in producing PLPC.[54] As a result of leakage of CSF and diminution of the CSF volume, there is compensatory vasodilatation of the cerebral blood vessels. This leads to increased weight of the brain

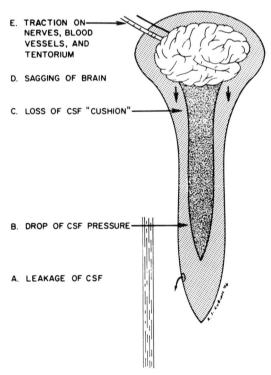

E. TRACTION ON NERVES, BLOOD VESSELS, AND TENTORIUM

D. SAGGING OF BRAIN

C. LOSS OF CSF "CUSHION"

B. DROP OF CSF PRESSURE

A. LEAKAGE OF CSF

Fig. 7-2. Mechanism of post-lumbar-puncture cephalgia.

which causes its further "sagging" with the patient's erect position. It also causes "vascular headaches" due to the distention of the blood vessels and perivascular edema. In a susceptible patient with prolonged PLPC, vascular changes such as perivascular edema and fibrosis, muscle spasm, tension, and anxiety play an important role in perpetuating the headache that once has been initiated by leakage of CSF. Therefore, in PLPC, as in any painful condition, the earlier the treatment the better the ultimate result.

PREDISPOSING FACTORS TO POST-LUMBAR-PUNCTURE CEPHALGIA

Not every case of lumbar puncture is followed by cephalgia. The following factors affect the incidence of PLPC:

Parturition

Parturition, as well as the size of the needle used, and the number of dural punctures are the most important factors. During pregnancy, the gravid uterus partially obstructs the inferior vena cava. Accordingly, the blood has to be shunted through the vertebral venous plexus to the azygos veins to reach the heart. This leads to dilation of the vertebral veins and, subsequently, diminution in the CSF volume. With delivery and loss of abdominal compression, the vena caval obstruction disappears and the vertebral veins are no longer engorged. Moreover, there is diuresis on the second or third postpartum day. Therefore, the leakage of CSF, the diuresis, and the end of the vertebral vasodilation lead to a lax dura with a decrease in the subarachnoid pressure and sagging of the brain, especially when the patient assumes the erect posture.

Method of Delivery

Vaginal delivery is associated with the highest incidence of PLPC,[53,85] being 6 times higher than in surgical operations, and twice as high as in cesarean section. The reasons behind the lower incidence of PLPC in cesarean section compared to vaginal delivery are the better attention to hydration, the more liberal use of narcotics, and the distracting effect of the abdominal incision in cesarean section.

Sex

The incidence of PLPC is 14 per cent in females compared to 7 per cent in males.[85] If the obstetric cases are excluded, the incidence of PLPC in females remains higher (12%).

Age

The incidence of headache at the age of 20 is 4 times higher than at the age of 60.[85] This is due to the decreased elasticity of the blood vessels and the tentoria making them less stretchable, the decreased number of sensory nerves, and the increased pain threshold in the geriatric patient.

Dehydration

Dehydrated patients have a higher incidence of PLPC. Proper hydration is an important prophylactic and curative measure of PLPC.[46]

Needle Size and Shape

The larger the gauge of the needle, the wider the dural rent becomes, leading to more CSF leakage and to higher possibility and severity of PLPC. The relation of headache to the size of the needle is in support of the leakage theory as being the cause of PLPC (Table 7-2).[12,14,37,45,59,66,68, 76,80,85]

The use of tapered needles for subarachnoid block has been recommended.[57] The alleged advantages are that the terminal bevel and shaft that puncture the dura are of a smaller gauge than the proximal portion of the shaft. Thus it diminishes the incidence of PLPC, reduces the problem of bending, and gives greater maneu-

Table 7.2. The Relation of the Size of the Lumbar-Puncture Needle to the Incidence of Headache

		Internal Diameter (mm.)		
Gauge	External Diameter (mm.)	Regular-wall	Thin-wall	Incidence of Headache
17	1.49	1.04	1.16	75
22	0.71	0.40	0.46	12
24	0.56	0.30	0.36	6
25*	0.51	0.25	0.30	4
26*	0.46	0.25	0.30	2
32	0.23	0.10	0.13	1.5

*Note that although the internal diameters of the 25- and 26-gauge needles are the same, the external diameter of the 26-gauge needle is smaller. Therefore, although the flow rate of C.S.F. or injected solution is the same with both needles, the dural rent, and subsequently the incidence of headache, is less with the 26-gauge needle.

verability than a regular spinal needle of a uniform gauge throughout its length. However, when a 25-gauge tapered needle was compared to a 25-gauge regular needle, the incidence and severity of headache with the former type was significantly higher than with the latter.[1] The reason for this is that the length of the 25-gauge portion of the tapered needle is only 4.76 mm. and the diameter of the subarachnoid space in the lumbar region is 10 to 15 mm. Therefore, the tapered needle could be so advanced that the dura is punctured by the larger and thicker part of the shaft, producing a larger dural rent and, subsequently, a higher incidence of cephalgia (Fig. 7-3).

Number of Dural Punctures

If there are multiple dural punctures, the volume of CSF leakage is higher than if one puncture is produced using the same size needle.

Experience of the Operator

The incidence of headache is lower with experienced operators than those with limited experience. With the same operator, the incidence of PLPC decreases as more experience in the technique of lumbar puncture is gained.

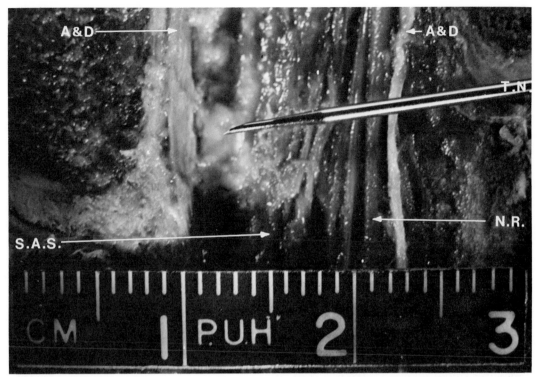

Fig. 7-3.   Photomicrograph showing thick part of tapered needle (T.N.) piercing dura. A and D = arachnoid and dura; N.R. = nerve root; S.A.S. = subarachnoid space. (Abouleish, E., Yamaoka, H. and Hingson, R. A.: Evaluation of a tapered spinal needle. Anesth. Analg., 53:258, 1974)

Direction of the Bevel of the Spinal Needle

When the bevel of the lumbar-puncture needle is parallel to the dural fibers, the latter are separated and then come together after the needle is withdrawn. When the needle bevel is perpendicular to the dural fibers, the latter are cut and it becomes difficult for the dural rent to close after the removal of the needle. Therefore, when inserting a lumbar-puncture needle, the bevel should be directed toward one side of the patient rather than cephalad or caudad because the dural fibers run longitudinally. Considering this factor, some needles have a pencil-like tip in order to separate rather than cut the dural fibers. It has also been noticed that if the needle is inserted obliquely instead of at a right angle, the holes in the dura and arachnoid are not opposite each other. Thus leakage of CSF is said to be prevented when the needle is withdrawn and the meninges return in contact.[66] However, when using a fine needle such as a 25- or 26-gauge, factors such as the direction of the bevel and the angle of insertion are of minor importance.[85]

The Patient's Expectation

If a person expects headache to follow a lumbar puncture, she already has put herself into a group that has a higher incidence of PLPC.

Previous Incidence of Headache or Migraine

Patients who have frequent headaches or migraines have a low threshold for PLPC and, therefore, are poor candidates for spinal anesthesia. The development of severe PLPC following a nontraumatic lumbar puncture with a fine needle is a contraindication to subsequent spinal anesthesia because the incidence of PLPC is higher in such patients.[19]

High Altitudes

There is a higher incidence and severity of PLPC at high altitudes.[75,83] This may be due to the higher than normal CSF pressure, thus increasing the leakage following lumbar puncture.[75]

SIGNS AND SYMPTOMS OF POST-LUMBAR-PUNCTURE CEPHALGIA

Time of Onset

PLPC usually occurs within a week following lumbar puncture. The severer the headache, the earlier its onset. In a study of 107 patients who had a severe headache following spinal analgesia, 98 per cent of PLPC occurred within 3 days, and none after the fourth day (Table 7-3). When the dura is inadvertently punctured by a 17-gauge needle during an epidural attempt, headache may occur immediately, especially if the patient is sitting up; in all cases, PLPC appears within 3 days from the time of dural puncture.

Relationship to Posture

PLPC is characteristically related to posture, i.e., it appears or is accentuated by assuming the erect position, and is relieved or eliminated by lying down.

Severity

PLPC is classified into three groups according to its duration and its effect on the patient's activity:

1. *Mild headache*: if it lasts less than 24 hours.

2. *Moderate headache*: if it lasts more than 24 hours and less than 5 days provided it is not incapacitating (i.e., not interfering with the patient's activity and her ability to take care of herself and/or her baby).

3. *Severe headache*: if it lasts 5 days or more, is incapacitating, or both. In 90 per cent of these cases the headache is associated with other symptoms.

Sites of PLPC

PLPC is usually bilateral, either frontal, occipital, or both (Table 7-4). the patient commonly describes a severe headache as starting behind the eyes, extending to the occiput, and reaching down the neck and shoulders.

Associated Symptoms of PLPC

1. Neckache and stiffness of the neck are the most common associated symptoms with PLPC (Table 7-5). The cause of these complications is traction on the structures at the base of the skull and upper cervical nerves. When the condition is severe, the headache and neckache extend down the shoulders.

Table 7-3. Time of Onset of Headache Following Dural Puncture

Number of Cases With Severe PLPC		Time of Onset of Headache
Spinal (24–26 gauge)	Epidural (17–gauge)	
0	2	Immediate
19	3	12 hours
29	3	12–24 hours
44	2	24–48 hours
13	1	48–72 hours
2	0	72–96 hours (3–4 days)
0	0	96–129 hours (4–5 days)
0	0	5 days
Totals: 107	11	

Table 7-4. Sites of Severe Headache

Site	Percentage of Cases
Occipital	25
Frontal	22
Both frontal and occipital	25
Entire head	22
Temporo-occipital	4
Vertex	2

Table 7-5. Associated Symptoms of PLPC

Symptom	Percentage of Cases
Neckache and/or stiffness of neck	57
Pain extending down to shoulders	9
Backache	35
Nausea	22
Blurred vision	10
Tinnitus	5
Vomiting	2
Total:	140

2. Backache is the second most common associated symptom.

3. Nausea and vomiting may also occur when the patient stands. This can be due to the headache itself or to dysfunction of the labyrinth.

4. "Plugging" of the ears, tinnitus, and vertigo are frequent complaints.[85] These symptoms are due to dysfunction of the internal ear. There is a correlation between CSF pressure and cochlear function, and communication between the two has been proven.[49] Experimentally, a decrease in CSF pressure is associated with a fall in the intralabyrinthine pressure and followed by a functional disability of the ear to transmit high tones.[49] Clinically, normal audiograms are restituted following elevation of CSF pressure in patients who have complained of headaches and decreased hearing after spinal anesthesia.[85] Therefore, a drop in CSF pressure following lumbar puncture leads to these auditory and vestibular dysfunctions.

5. Blurring of vision, occurring in 10 per cent of cases with severe PLPC, can be due to traction on the ophthalmic nerves. If this traction is prolonged or severe, cranial nerve palsy can occur.[30,58] The palsy is usually unilateral and the most common time of onset is usually the second week. The cranial nerves most commonly involved are in this order: abducent, trochlear, and oculomotor nerves.[57] The blurring of vision becomes associated with squint, diplopia, and the other characteristics of the specific nerve palsy. The prog-

nosis is good and the patient usually recovers in 6 to 8 weeks.[85]

A patient with severe PLPC may develop more than one associated symptom (Table 7-5).

Duration of PLPC

In 72 per cent of cases, even without treatment, PLPC usually terminates within 1 week from onset: 24 per cent within 2 days; 29 per cent within 2 to 4 days; and 19 per cent within 5 to 7 days.[4] However, it may last for weeks, months, and even a year.[30]

DIFFERENTIAL DIAGNOSIS OF PLPC

Postanesthesia headache can follow spinal as well as general anesthesia. The incidence of headache following general anesthesia varies from 2.7 per cent to 35 per cent.[33,35,59] There are many causes of headaches other than anesthesia. Fever, hypertension, postpartum toxemia, severe anemia, and sinusitis are but a few causes of headache. Chemical and bacterial meningitis, which are associated with increased CSF pressure and characterized by headache that is worse when lying down, should be of historic nature. Using aseptic techniques, removing the excess of the degerming solution from the needles used, and utilizing the new local anesthetic drugs are preventive measures against bacterial and chemical meningitis. PLPC is differentiated from other causes of cephalgia by the headache worsening or only appearing on standing up, and being relieved or ameliorated by lying down.

TREATMENT OF PLPC

The facts that PLPC, in the majority of cases, is spontaneously relieved and that its signs and symptoms are only subjective, make it difficult to evaluate the numerous available lines of treatment (see list of treatment of PLPC, below, and Fig. 7-4). The choice of a certain line or lines of

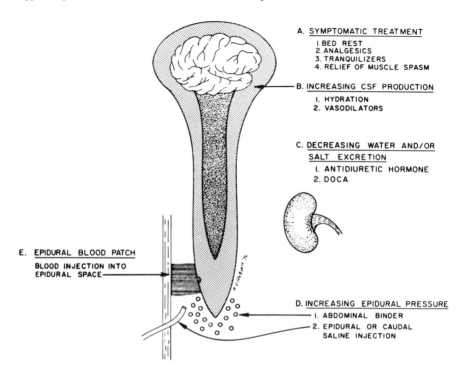

Fig. 7-4.   Treatment of post-lumbar-puncture cephalgia.

treatment depends on the severity of the headache and the anesthesiologist's preference. On the whole, the following methods are used:

Treatment of PLPC

In 72% even without treatment→ cured

H →Hydration
E → Epidural saline (flap-valve)
A →Abdominal binder
D →Drugs: Vasodilator→ Thorazine
　　　　Muscle relaxant→ diazepam
　　　　Antihistamine→ Phenergan
A →Analgesics
C →Clot (epidural blood patch)
H →Head lowered
E → Electrolyte retention = desoxycorti-
　　costerone acetate, DOCA
　　　Linguets or
　　　I.M. injection, 5 mg. t.i.d.

Symptomatic Treatment

Bed Rest

Staying flat in bed to prevent PLPC is of no value;[51,56,85] it only postpones its occur-rence and may suggest to the patient the feeling of headache.[10] Early ambulation, as soon as the effects of spinal block wear off, results in better acceptance of spinal anes-thesia by the patient.[51] Prolonged rest in bed does not enhance healing of the dural rent; it may even cause problems such as vasomotor instability,[16] and may predis-pose to venous thrombosis. Therefore stay-ing in bed is left to the patient's discretion, and other aggressive methods to terminate the cephalgia should be used in intracta-ble or severe cases.

Analgesics

Various analgesics, from salicylates to codeine, are used to relieve the headache. However, the use of narcotics is not advis-able because PLPC may be sufficiently pro-longed to make addiction a real hazard.

Tranquilizers

Benadryl and Dramamine are some-times recommended.[57] Probably their mechanism of action on headache is to relieve the "tension," thus breaking the vicious circle of pain, tension, more pain, etc., and subsequently curing the headache.

Relief of Muscle Spasm

As mentioned previously, neckache and stiffness of the neck are commonly associated with headache. In such cases, the author usually prescribes 5 mg. diazepam tablets to be taken 3 times daily to relieve the muscle spasm and the nervous tension. Diazepam as well as many tranquilizers are transmitted through lactation to the neonate. Therefore, they should not be used in cases of breast feeding.

INCREASING CSF PRODUCTION

Hydration

Hydration not only prevents but also relieves spinal headache. However, if the patient is not dehydrated, overhydration in a patient with normal renal function does not cure the headache unless combined with measures to prevent water and salt excretion. Intravenous fluid therapy is not required as long as the patient can drink.

Vasodilators

Nicotinic acid and Priscoline have been used to produce vasodilatation of the choroid plexus, thus promoting the secretion of CSF.[34,53] At present, such a method is rarely used because cerebral vasodilatation increases the weight of the brain, thus augmenting the traction on the sensitive intracranial structures. This is why the results of the use of vasodilator drugs as well as stellate ganglion blockade have been disappointing.[57] Carbon dioxide has potent vasodilating and antidiuretic effects.[78] It is claimed to increase the CSF production and hasten the recovery from PLPC. It is administered by inhaling 5.6 per cent CO_2 in oxygen for 10 minutes. The procedure is repeated once every 24 hours for 3 days. The author does not recommend this

treatment due to the need to induce sleep by intravenous thiopental prior to each administration.

DECREASING WATER AND SALT EXCRETION

Vasopressin

The antidiuretic component of the posterior pituitary extract (ADH, vasopressin, Pitressin) has been used to treat PLPC.[46,79] Its intramuscular injection causes a rise of CSF pressure whereas its intrathecal injection is ineffective. The increase in CSF pressure is independent of the rise in blood pressure because intramuscular epinephrine does not cause much change in CSF pressure.[79] However, recently it has been found that the prophylactic use of vasopressin does not differ from that of sodium chloride when used as a placebo; both are followed by almost the same incidence of PLPC.[6] The side effects in the form of diarrhea, abdominal cramps, and sweating are 27 per cent with vasopressin, compared to 4 per cent with the placebo. Vasopressin has a direct vasoconstrictor effect, and the coronary arteries are not spared from this action. Some patients with coronary insufficiency experience anginal pain even with minute quantities of vasopressin.[41] Vasopressin-induced myocardial ischemia has led to severe reactions, and has even caused death. Consequently, its use to relieve headache is not recommended.

Mineralocorticoids

Mineralocorticoids, such as desoxycorticosterone acetate (DOCA), act on the renal tubules to retain Na^+, and subsequently Cl^- and water. This leads to expansion of the extracellular compartment including the CSF. Asbell[5] claimed success in 92 per cent of cases following the intramuscular injection of DOCA. Pfeffer[67] claimed excellent results in 35 patients following its oral administration. Wolfson, Siker, and Gray[88] found it valuable in relieving the headache following pneumoencephalograph in eight out of 12 patients. DOCA is usually administered either as a 5-mg. linguet or an intramuscular injection every 8 hours.

INCREASING EPIDURAL PRESSURE

Abdominal Binder

An abdominal binder has been utilized to prevent as well as treat PLPC. It assists the re-establishment of maternal CSF dynamics that existed prior to delivery. By its compressing action on the uterus, the binder reproduces the predelivery vena caval obstruction, thus shunting blood into the vertebral veins. This causes splinting of the dura and prevents the sagging of the brain as well as the traction on the sensitive intracranial structures. It also relieves headache by raising the epidural pressure which reduces or prevents leakage of CSF, thus allowing the fibrin deposition to seal the dural rent and permit its repair.[38]

The abdominal binder was introduced in 1951 by Hanahan and Redding.[48] Leighton and Hershenson[55] found PLPC to occur in 3.4 per cent of cases following use of an abdominal binder compared to 26 per cent in controls. Ainslie[4] claimed a 100 per cent relief of PLPC following the use of an abdominal binder. Beck[9] studied two consecutive groups of 100 patients each. The only difference in management was the use in one group of an abdominal binder from the delivery to the date of discharge. Without a binder the incidence of headache was 18 per cent, 14 per cent being mild and 4 per cent being severe. With the binder there was only a 4 per cent incidence of mild headache. However, following inadvertent dural puncture with a 16-gauge needle during epidural analgesia, the incidence of PLPC was 76.5 per cent,[19] a figure which is not significantly different from that observed when no abdominal binder has been used.[24] Therefore, although an abdominal binder is recommended, the results of its prophylactic use when the dura is punctured dur-

ing epidural analgesia are not as satisfactory as with subarachnoid block.

For treating PLPC, prior to the application of the abdominal binder, a test as to its efficiency is performed. The patient is asked to stand. The operator, with one hand against the patient's back as a brace, presses with his fist gently but firmly in the epigastric area just below the xiphoid process. The pressure of the fist is increased slowly but steadily until the patient spontaneously notes a reduction or relief of the headache.[4] Such a pressure on the abdomen is capable of raising the epidural pressure and, subsequently, the CSF pressure to 200 or more mm. H_2O.[38]

For the abdominal binder to be effective, it is important to be properly applied. Whether it is used for prophylaxis or treatment, the abdominal binder should be tight, short of discomfort. It can be loosened before meals and on retiring to bed.

Therefore, use of the abdominal binder in obstetric patients is recommended in every case. It not only reduces the incidence of PLPC but also gives support to the patient's back.

Epidural or Caudal Saline Injection

Epidural or caudal saline injection has been used for prophylaxis as well as treatment of PLPC.[19,20,21,72] As a prophylactic measure following inadvertent dural puncture during epidural analgesia, the epidural injection of 60 ml. of saline, which is repeated once the following day, reduces the incidence of headache from 76.5 per cent to 12.5 per cent.[19] Following inadvertent dural puncture during epidural analgesia, Crawford[20] used an epidural infusion of 1 to 1.5 liters of Hartmann's solution at a rate of about 15 to 20 drops per minute for 24 hours after delivery. The incidence of headache in the control group was 77.5 per cent; yet in the treated group only 31 per cent developed mild headache. However, this continuous epidural infusion over 24 hours with the confinement to bed is distressing in patients who have had a vaginal delivery. Also, while the drip was in progress, 25 per cent of the patients experienced severe interscapular pain of unknown origin. Occasionally this pain was so severe as to require the administration of a narcotic.[21]

As a curative measure, the epidural injection of 30 ml. of saline usually causes an immediate relief of the headache. This is due to the increase in the epidural pressure[82] which not only prevents the leakage of CSF but also causes "lifting up" of the brain. In 50 per cent of cases the relief of headache is permanent although the injected saline is absorbed within a few hours.[72] The reason for such a permanent cure is that the increased epidural pressure produced by the saline injection causes inversion of a flap valve through which CSF was leaking.[24] Injection of saline by way of the caudal route causes insignificant increase of pressure in the epidural space in the lumbar region.[82] This is probably due to the escape of a large proportion of the injected fluid through the wide sacral openings into the pelvis. The fibrous bands anchoring the dural cul de sac to the sacral promontory promote the escape of saline toward the pelvis instead of it spreading cephalad toward the epidural space. Therefore for the treatment of PLPC, if saline injection is chosen, the lumbar route is more rational than the caudal one.

EPIDURAL BLOOD PATCH

History

There have been various attempts to close dural rents and thus prevent the escape of CSF. Nelson in 1930 placed pieces of catgut in the epidural space. However, such insertion was difficult and caused serious neurologic complications, such as cauda equina lesions. Nelson also suggested the possible importance of blood plugging the hole in the dura caused by the spinal needle. Such a technique, later called epidural blood patch (EBP), was started in 1960 by James B. Gormley. He believed that the incidence of headache was not as high as anticipated when a bloody tap was produced because of a higher incidence of repair of the dural rent. He reasoned that if a patch or a sealing material could be placed adjacent to the arachnoid puncture then, theoretically, a permanent closure could be accomplished. Therefore, blood was injected epidurally in 7 patients, including himself, who had suffered from PLPC, and this was followed by prompt and complete relief. Since then EBP has been used successfully for treatment of severe intractable PLPC.[2,7,11,16,28,29,32,39,43,65,86]

Indications

EBP is indicated for the treatment of severe PLPC, i.e., when the headache is prolonged for more than 5 days or is incapacitating. The prophylactic use of EBP is not recommended because it has not been more successful than the epidural injection of saline in preventing PLPC, especially if injected through an epidural catheter. Moreover, not every patient who has lumbar puncture develops severe PLPC. Thus, it is unfair to expose the patient to an unnecessary procedure.

Contraindications

Anticoagulant Therapy or Blood Dyscrasias. Dural, epidural, or caudal puncture is contraindicated when the patient has a bleeding tendency. This is because of the danger of injuring a blood vessel in the vertebral canal and the formation of a hematoma with subsequent cord compression and paraplegia.[25]

Fever. A bacteremic state may be present in a patient who has a fever. Thus, the injection of blood from a feverish patient into the epidural space is not advisable, especially in the presence of a fistula between the epidural and subarachnoid spaces.

Infection of the Back. Even a sweat rash or acne of the back is a contraindication to

EBP because of the possibility of introducing infection into the epidural space.

Bleeding During the Procedure From an Injured Epidural Blood Vessel. No further blood should be injected before reevaluating the patient's condition in 24 hours.[27,77] The introduction of additional blood may, concomitant with epidural bleeding, cause significant increase in the volume of the epidural clot and result in increased morbidity.[15]

Patient's Refusal. The procedure, the success rate, the alternatives, and the usual complications should be explained to the patient. She must accept the procedure and sign the consent form. If EBP is really indicated, the patient usually welcomes it.

Procedure

1. Positioning the Patient. EBP is usually performed in the patient's bed to allow her to rest for 1 hour following the procedure. The operator helps the patient to lie in the left lateral position with the shoulders and pelvis parallel and both perpendicular to the edge of the bed.

2. Preparing the Instruments. EBP should be performed under complete aseptic technique. The sterile epidural tray is opened by the operator who, as well as all the attendants in the room, is wearing a mask and cap. A sterile saline ampule or vial is added to the tray for lubricating the syringes. A 5-ml. syringe is filled with about 2 ml. of 1 per cent lidocaine for local infiltration of the skin prior to the epidural procedure. It goes without saying that the operator has washed his hands and is wearing sterile gloves before touching any of the contents of the tray.

3. Preparing the Patient's Back. The patient's back is cleansed twice with 1 per cent Betadine solution. The excess of the antiseptic solution is removed and the area for epidural puncture is isolated with towels.

4. Performing the Epidural Puncture. When PLPC occurs following one lumbar puncture, the same interspace is used for EBP; if lumbar puncture was attempted in more than one interspace, the lowermost one is chosen because it is easier for epidurally injected fluids to spread cephalad than caudal.[13] The skin is infiltrated with 1 per cent lidocaine. The epidural needle is introduced and the epidural space is identified by the technique with which the operator is most familiar. The author utilizes the technique of loss of resistance using air (for details see Chap. 14, Epidural Analgesia).

5. Aspirating Blood. After adequately sterilizing the skin of the forearm with 1 per cent Betadine followed by 70 per cent alcohol, the assistant using a sterile syringe and needle aspirates 10 ml. of blood. A large vein is preferable to allow free flow of blood. The filled syringe is handed over to the operator.

6. Injecting Blood. Blood is injected slowly, at the rate of 1 ml. per 2 seconds, through the epidural needle. If blood is rapidly injected, the patient feels marked back and neck pain during the process of injection.

7. Placing of Antibiotic or Germicidal Ointment. An ointment such as Betadine or Bacitracin is placed on the site of epidural puncture, covered by 4 × 4 gauze, taped, and the patient is turned on her back.

8. Resting for 1 Hour. The patient is asked to stay in the supine position for 1 hour following the procedure.

9. Evaluating the Treatment. Following this period of bed rest the patient is asked to stand up and move her head from one side to the other. The patient is usually at first suspicious, and then happily surprised by the absence of headache and the associated symptoms. The dramatic relief of these symptoms following a successful EBP is very impressive.

Success Rate (Table 7-6)

Since the technique of EBP was started in 1960, 642 cases have been reported by the end of 1975 with an average success

Table 7-6. The Success Rates of Epidural Blood Patch

Reference	Year	Number of Cases	Number of Successes	Percentage of Success
Gormley	1960	7	7	100
DiGiovanni and Dunbar	1970	45	41	91
Glass and DuPont	1972	43	40	93
Glass and Kennedy	1972	50	47	94
DuPont and Shire	1972	41	40	97.5
DiGiovanni *et al.*	1972	63	61	97
Vondrell and Bernards	1973	60	58	96.5
Blok	1973	22	20	91
Cass and Edlist	1974	1	1	100
Balagot	1974	7	7	100
Ostheimer *et al.*	1974	185	182	98.5
Abouleish *et al.*	1975	118	115	97.5
	Totals:	642	619	*Average:* 96.5

rate of 96.5 per cent. Following the first EBP there is about 8 per cent recurrence of headache which is relieved by a second patch.[2] The headache can recur within 36 hours. Therefore, if EBP is done as an outpatient procedure, the patient should be warned and asked to report to the treating physician at the end of 48 hours or if headache recurs.

Failure Rate

There is an ultimate 3 to 5 per cent failure rate which is mainly due to:

1. *Improper Diagnosis.* As explained before, postanesthetic headache can be due to many factors. Therefore, before doing an EBP, the anesthesiologist should be sure of the diagnosis.

2. *Improper Placement of the Blood.* If the blood is injected outside the epidural or subarachnoid space, or in the epidural space far away from the dural rent (e.g. through an epidural catheter), headache will not be relieved.

Complications

During the Procedure

Neckache and Backache. These are usually due to rapid injection. They can also be due to blood injection into the ligaments of the back. The incidence of neckache is 0.9 per cent, and of backache is 1.8 per cent.[2]

Usually such a problem can be avoided by slow injection. However, if it occurs, the patient should be reassured with or without the supplementation of 5 mg. of diazepam.

Dural Puncture. The epidural space should be carefully identified to avoid accidental dural puncture with the 17-gauge epidural needle. DuPont and Shire[32] encountered such a complication in five out of 41 cases, DiGiovanni and Dunbar[28] in one out of 45 cases, Vondrell and Bernards[86] in several out of 60 cases, and Abouleish and coworkers in one out of 118 patients. If such a complication occurs, the needle should be withdrawn until its tip lies in the epidural space, and then the blood is injected very slowly. The success rate of EBP after accidental dural puncture varies. In DiGiovanni and Dunbar's and Abouleish's series, the headache recurred worse than before EBP. In DuPont and Shire's report the headache was cured, while in Vondrell and Bernards' series the results were mixed. Failure of EBP or recurrence of headache under these circumstances does not preclude another attempt in 24 hours.

Paresthesia. The incidence of paresthesia during injection is 0.9 per cent.[2] This is only a temporary complication because long-term follow-up did not reveal any problem.[2,27]

Cramps in the Lower Abdomen. This occurred in one out of 185 cases.[65]

During 48 Hours Following EBP

Backache. This is the commonest complication, occurring in about one-third of the patients and lasting for 24 to 48 hours.

Transient Elevation of Body Temperature. Within 12 hours of EBP, 5 per cent of the patients developed a 1°C. rise in body temperature, lasting for 12 to 24 hours.[2] None of these patients developed any problem in the long-term follow-up. This benign rise in body temperature is probably due to the absorption of the blood. Parenteral injection of autologous blood (autohemotherapy), frequently used for treatment of many illnesses including uveitis and allergic diseases, was also accompanied by a rise in body temperature.[31] This line of treatment, introduced in 1913, was in vogue especially in France and Germany before the cortisone era.

Complications Lasting More than 2 Days. In a series of 118 patients who were followed for up to 2 years, there were no major complications that could be attributed to epidural blood patch.[2] The problems encountered were:

Backache. Nineteen per cent had residual backache for a variable period of time lasting from between 3 to 100 days (mean, 27.7 days). This backache did not interfere with the activities of the patients, who were all ambulatory. However, there were 2 cases of reported severe back pain radiating to the lower limbs with limitation of leg movement shortly after epidural blood injection. This pain lasted for a period extending from a few hours to 2 days and gradually disappeared in about a week without any residual symptoms.[15,17] The cause of such a complication is not clear.

Limited Back Flexion. This occurred in 1 per cent of the cases.[2]

Difficult Back Extension. This was present in 2 per cent of the patients.[2]

Occasional Radiating Pains Down Both Legs. This occurred in two out of 98 patients who were examined about one year following EBP. However, one of them, who was under psychiatric treatment, complained of pain in other parts of the body. Neither patient showed signs of radicular sensory or motor loss.

Cranial Nerve Palsies. In two out of 118 patients, cranial nerve palsies occurred.[2] One patient developed right facial nerve palsy 5 days after EBP, while the other developed ataxia and vertigo 10 days after EBP. These problems were, most probably, a coincidence. However, cranial nerve palsy can follow spinal, intravenous, or inhalation anesthesia.[18,60,63] After lumbar puncture, the nerve most commonly involved is the abducent, followed by the oculomotor, and then the trochlear.[57] The cause of cranial nerve lesions after lumbar puncture, as explained previously, is mainly the drop in CSF pressure, with subsequent traction on cranial nerves. If cranial nerve palsies were secondary to EBP, the mechanism, and therefore the nerves involved, would be different than in lumbar puncture. The sudden changes in CSF dynamics as a result of leakage, possible increased production, and abrupt cessation of leakage, might be responsible. Since there is a correlation between CSF pressure and cochlear function, and the communication between the two has been proven,[49] the functional disturbance of the episodes of vertigo, tinnitus, and imbalance in one patient can be explained. The facial nerve palsy in the other patient is more difficult to describe on the basis of changes in CSF dynamics. But both cranial nerves VII and VIII enter the same bone, the petrous portion of the temporal bone, through the same orifice, the internal acoustic meatus, and the facial nerve runs between the cochlea and semicircular canals.[44] Therefore, although cranial nerve palsy has not been proven to be secondary to EBP, long-term follow-up of more cases performed under this relatively new procedure is required.

Sequelae

Danger of Cauda Equina Lesions. One of the theoretical objections to EBP is the danger of cord compression leading to cauda equina lesions. Such problems do occur when hematomas are associated with trauma, blood coagulopathy, and anticoagulants with or without epidural catheters.[25,73] In these cases, trauma to, or hemorrhage into, the spinal cord or other parts of the nervous system cannot be excluded as important contributing factors to a large space-occupying lesion. With EBP, 10 ml. of blood injected therapeutically, in the absence of anticoagulants or infection, either local or systematic, and under controlled condition, is a different situation.

Danger of Adhesions Between the Dura and Ligamentum Flavum.[26] This can possibly lead to inadvertent dural puncture if subsequent epidural block is attempted, and may limit or prevent the spread of the local anesthetic in the epidural space. However, such a theoretical objection has been ruled out.[3] At Magee-Womens Hospital, eight cases of epidural analgesia were performed 6 months to 2 years following EBP. The "snap" of ligamentum flavum was distinctly felt, the epidural space was easily identified, and there was no undue resistance to injection of the local anesthetics or to the advancement of the epidural catheters. The extent of the blocks as well as the onset and duration of action of the drugs were in accordance with what is expected under normal circumstances. Moreover, injection of a radiopaque dye (meglumine iothalamate) into the epidural space 1 to 2 years after EBP showed normal spread, both longitudinally into the space and laterally through the intervertebral foramina (unpublished data).

In conclusion, EBP does not prevent either normal physical or chemical spread of solutions into the epidural spread. Also, caudal and spinal analgesia were used successfully following EBP.[3] During lumbar puncture, the ligamentum flavum was distinctly felt from the dura. Therefore, previous administration of EBP should not obviate the use of vertebral blocks.

RECOMMENDED LINES OF TREATMENT OF PLPC

Prophylaxis

It is important to bear in mind that the best way to treat PLPC is to avoid its occurrence in the first place. The use of fine needles such as 26-gauge, avoidance of multiple punctures, attention to hydration, and the use of an abdominal binder are important points to follow in order to prevent PLPC.

Curative Measures

If PLPC occurs, abdominal binder, DOCA in the form of 5-mg. linguets 3 times daily, plenty of oral fluids, and 5-mg. diazepam tablets 3 times a day are recommended. If in spite of this treatment the headache, which is usually associated with other manifestations, does not improve and is incapacitating, EBP is used.

REFERENCES

1. Abouleish, E., Amortegui, A. J., and Taylor, F. H.: Are bacterial filters needed in continuous epidural analgesia for obstetrics? Anesthesiology, *46*:351, 1977.
1a. Abouleish, E., Yamaoka, H., and Hingson, R. A.: Evaluation of a tapered spinal needle. Anesth. Analg., *53*:258, 1974.
2. Abouleish, E., *et al.*: Long-term follow-up of epidural blood patch. Anesth. Analg., *54*:459, 1975.
3. ———: Regional analgesia following epidural blood patch. Anesth. Analg., *54*:634, 1975.
4. Ainslie, W. H.: Simple relief of post-spinal headache. J. Med. Soc. N.J., *65*:546, 1968.
5. Asbell, N.: Post-spinal headache; treatment with desoxycorticosterone acetate. J. Med. Soc. N.J., *46*:433, 1949.
6. Aziz, H., Pearce, J., and Miller, E.: Vasopressin in prevention of lumbar puncture headache. Br. Med. J., *4*:677, 1968.
7. Balagot, R. C., *et al.*: The prophylactic epidural blood patch. [Letter] J.A.M.A., *228*:1369, 1974.
8. Ball, C. G., *et al.*: Case history number 86: an unusual complication of lumbar puncture: a CSF cutaneous fistula. Anesth. Analg., *54*:691, 1975.

9. Beck, W. W., Jr.: Prevention of the postpartum spinal headache. Am. J. Obstet. Gynecol., *115*:354, 1973.

10. Blau, A.: Reactions following spinal puncture. Urol. Cutan. Rev., *45*:239, 1941.

11. Blok, R. J.: Headache following spinal anesthesia: treatment by epidural blood patch. J. Am. Osteopath. Assoc., *73*:128, 1973.

12. Boman, K.: Spinal anesthesia and hypotension headache. Acta Chir. Scand., *102*:110, 1951.

13. Burn, J. M., Guyer, P. B., and Langdon, L.: The spread of solutions injected into the epidural space: a study of using epidurograms in patients with the lumbosciatic syndrome. Br. J. Anaesth., *45*:338, 1973.

14. Cann, J. E., and Wycoff, C. C.: Incidence of headache with use of 27-gauge spinal needle. Anesthesiology, *11*:294, 1950.

15. Case history: complications following epidural "blood patch" for post-lumbar-puncture headache. Anesth. Analg., *52*:67, 1973.

16. Cass, W., and Edlist, G.: Postspinal headache. Successful use of epidural blood patch 11 weeks after onset. J.A.M.A., *227*:786, 1974.

17. Cornwall, R. D., and Dolan, W. M.: Radicular back pain following lumbar epidural blood patch. Anesthesiology, *43*:692, 1975.

18. Courville, C. B.: Untoward Effects of Nitrous Oxide Anesthesia. Mountain View, Cal., Pacific Press Publishing Association, 1939.

19. Craft, J. B., Epstein, B. S., and Coakley, C. S.: Prophylaxis of dural-puncture headache with epidural saline. Anesth. Analg., *52*:228, 1973.

20. Crawford, J. S.: The prevention of headache consequent upon dural puncture. Br. J. Anaesth., *44*:598, 1972.

21. ———: Epidural drip and post-spinal headache. [Letter] Br. J. Anaesth., *45*:1177, 1973.

22. ———: Pathology in the extradural space. Br. J. Anaesth., *47*:412, 1975.

23. Cutler, R. W., Murray, J. E., and Moody, R. A.: Overproduction of cerebrospinal fluid in communicating hydrocephalus. A case report. Neurology, *23*:1, 1973.

24. Dawkins, C. J.: An analysis of the complications of epidural and caudal block. Anaesthesia, *24*:554, 1969.

25. DeAngelis, J.: Hazards of subdural and epidural anesthesia during anticoagulant therapy: a case report and review. Anesth. Analg., *51*:676, 1972.

26. DeKrey, J. A.: Epidural injection of autologous blood for post-lumbar-puncture headache. [To the editor] Anesth. Analg., *52*:218, 1973.

27. DiGiovanni, A. J.: Discussion. Case history: Complications following epidural "blood patch" for post-lumbar-puncture headache. Anesth. Analg., *52*:67, 1973.

28. DiGiovanni, A. J., and Dunbar, B. S.: Epidural injections of autologous blood for postlumbar-puncture headache. Anesth. Analg., *49*:268, 1970.

29. DiGiovanni, A. J., Galbert, M. W., and Whale, W. M.: Epidural injection of autologous blood for postlumbar-puncture headache. II. Additional clinical experiences and laboratory investigation. Anesth. Analg., *51*:226, 1972.

30. Dripps, R. D., and Vandam, L. D.: Long-term follow-up of patients who received 10,098 spinal anesthetics; failure to discover major neurological sequelae. J.A.M.A., *156*:1486, 1954.

31. Duke-Elder, S.: System of Ophthalmology. St. Louis, C. V. Mosby, 1962.

32. DuPont, F. S., and Shire, R. D.: Epidural blood patch. An unusual approach to the problem of post-spinal anesthetic headache. Mich. Med., *71*:105, 1972.

33. Edmons-Seal, J., and Eve, N. H.: Minot sequelae of anaesthesia: a pilot study. Br. J. Anaesth., *34*:44, 1962.

34. Elam, J. O.: Catheter subarachnoid block for labor and delivery: a differential segmental technic employing hyperbaric lidocaine. Anesth. Analg, *49*:1007, 1970.

35. Fahy, A., Watson, B. G., and Marchall, M.: Post-anaesthetic follow-up by questionnaire: a research tool. Br. J. Anaesth., *41*:439, 1969.

36. Forestner, J. E., and Raj, P. P.: Inadvertent epidural injection of thiopental: a case report. Anesth. Analg., *54*:406, 1975.

37. Furmin, M. J.: Spinal anesthesia using a 32-gauge needle. Anesthesiology, *30*:599, 1969.

38. Gilland, O.: How to take the headache out of spinal taps. Headache, *8*:154, 1969.

39. Glass, P. M., and Kennedy, W. F., Jr.: Headache following subarachnoid puncture. Treatment with epidural blood patch. J.A.M.A., *219*:203, 1972.

40. Goldberg, N. B., Sawinski, V. J., and Goldberg, A. F.: Human cerebrospinal fluid osmolality at 37-degree C. Anesthesiology, *26*:829, 1965.

41. Goodman, L. S., and Gilman, A. (eds.): The Pharmacological Basis of Therapeutics. Ed. 5, p. 854. New York, Macmillan, 1975.

42. Goonewardene, T. W., *et al.*: Accidental subarachnoid injection of gallamine. Br. J. Anaesth., *47*:889, 1975.

43. Gormley, J. B.: Treatment of postspinal headache. Anesthesiology, *21*:565, 1960.

44. Gray, H.: Anatomy of the Human Body. Ed. 28. Philadelphia, Lee & Febiger, 1967.

45. Greene, B. A.: A 26-gauge lumbar puncture needle: its value in the prophylaxis of headache following spinal analgesia for vaginal delivery. Anesthesiology, *11*:464, 1950.

46. Greene, B. A., Goldsmith, M., and Lichtig, S.: Prevention of headache after spinal analgesia for vaginal delivery by use of hydration and a 24-gauge needle. Am. J. Obstet. Gynecol., *58*:709, 1949.

47. Guyton, A. C.: Textbook of Medical Physiology. Ed. 4. Philadelphia, W. B. Saunders, 1971.

48. Hanahan, P. W., and Redding, T.: Study of post-spinal anesthesia headaches. Am. J. Obstet. Gynecol., *61*:173, 1951.

49. Hughson, W.: A note on the relationship of cerebrospinal and intralabyrinthine pressures. Am. J. Physiol., *101*:396, 1932.

50. Hurst, E. W.: Adhesive arachnoiditis and vascular blockage casued by detergents and other chemical irritants: experimental study. J. Path. Bact., *70*:167, 1955.

51. Jones, R. J.: The role of recumbency in the pre-

vention and treatment of postspinal headache. Anesth. Analg., *53*:788, 1974.

52. Kim, Y., Mazza, W. M., and Marx, G. F.: Massive spinal block with hemicranial palsy after a "test dose" for extra dural analgesia. Anesthesiology, *43*:370, 1975.

53. Krueger, J. E.: Etiology and treatment of post-spinal headaches. Anesth. Analg., *32*:190, 1953.

54. Kunkle, E. C., Ray, B. S., and Wolff, H. G.: Experimental studies on headache: analysis of the headache associated with changes in intracranial pressure. Arch. Neurol. Psychiat., *49*:323, 1943.

55. Leighton, H. T., and Hershenson, B. B.: "Spinal" headache; clinical study. Obstet. Gynecol., *1*:426, 1953.

56. Levin, M. J.: Lumbar puncture headaches. Bull. U.S. Army Med. Dept. No. 82, pp. 107–110, 1944.

57. Lund, P. C.: Principles and Practice of Spinal Anesthesia. Springfield, Ill. Charles C Thomas, 1971.

58. Lund, P. C., and Cwik, J. C.: Modern trends in spinal anaesthesia. Can. Anaesth. Soc. J., *15*:118, 1968.

59. McDowell, S. A., Dundee, J. W., and Pandit, S. K.: Para-anaesthetic headache in female patients. Anaesthesia, *24*:334, 1970.

60. Moore, D. C.: Complications of Regional Anesthesia. Springfield, Ill., Charles C Thomas, 1955.

61. Nicholson, M. J.: Comment. Case history: complications following epidural "blood patch" for postlumbar-puncture headache. Anesth. Analg., *52*:67, 1973.

62. Nicholson, M. J., and Eversole, M. H.: Neurologic complications of spinal anesthesia. J.A.M.A., *132*:679, 1946.

63. Norman, J. E.: Nerve palsy following general anaesthesia. Anaesthesia, *10*:87, 1955.

64. Oppelt, W. W., et al.: Effects of acid-base alterations on cerebrospinal fluid production. Proc. Soc. Exp. Biol. Med., *114*:86, 1963.

65. Ostheimer, G. W., Palahniuk, R. J., and Shnider, S. M.: Epidural blood patch for postlumbar-puncture headache. [Letter] Anesthesiology, *41*:307, 1974.

66. Owen, C. K., et al.: Twenty-six gauge spinal needles for prevention of spinal headache. Am. J. Surg., *85*:98, 1955.

67. Pfeffer, R. I.: Treatment of postspinal headache with buccal tablets of desoxycorticosterone acetate. Am. J. Obstet. Gynecol., *65*:21, 1953.

68. Phillips, O. C., et al.: Neurologic complications following spinal anesthesia with lidocaine: a prospective review of 10,440 cases. Anesthesiology, *30*:284, 1969.

69. The physician and the Law. Anesth. Analg., *51*:48, 1972.

70. Plum, F., and Siesjo, B. K.: Recent advances in CSF physiology. Anesthesiology, *42*:708, 1975.

71. Reisner, L. S.: Epidural test solution or spinal fluid? Anesthesiology, *44*:451, 1976.

72. Rice, G. G., and Dabbs, H. C.: The use of peridural and subarachnoid injection of saline solution in the treatment of severe postspinal headaches. Anesthesiology, *11*:17, 1950.

73. Russman, B. S., and Kazi, K. H.: Spinal epidural hematoma and the Brown-Seguard Syndrome. Neurology, *21*:1066, 1971.

74. Saady, A.: Epidural abscess complicating thoracic epidural analgesia. Anesthesiology, *44*:244, 1976.

75. Safar, P., and Tenicela, R.: High altitude physiology in relation to anesthesia and inhalation therapy. Anesthesiology, *25*:515, 1964.

76. Sergent, W. F., et al.: Twenty-six gauge spinal needles for the prevention of spinal headache. Am. J. Surg., *85*:98, 1955.

77. Shantha, T. R., McWhirter, W. R., and Dunbar, R. W.: Discussion. Case history: complications following epidural "blood patch" for postlumbar-puncture headache. Anesth. Analg., *52*:67, 1973.

78. Sikh, S. S., and Agarwal, G.: Post-spinal headache. A preliminary report on the effect of inhaled carbon dioxide. Anaesthesia, *29*:297, 1974.

79. Solomon, H. C.: Raising cerebrospinal fluid pressure with special regard to the effect on lumbar puncture headache. J.A.M.A., *82*:297, 1924.

80. Tourtellotte, W. E., et al.: Postlumbar Puncture Headaches. Springfield, Ill., Charles C Thomas, 1964.

81. Usubiaga, J. E.: Neurological complications following epidural anesthesia. Int. Anesthesiol. Clin., *13*(2):3, 1975.

82. Usubiaga, J. E., et al.: Effect of saline injections on epidural and subarachnoid space pressures and relation to postspinal anesthesia headache. Anesth. Analg., *46*:293, 1967.

83. Vacanti, J. J.: Post-spinal headache and air travel. Anesthesiology, *37*:358, 1972.

84. Vandam, L. D., and Dripps, R. D.: Long-term follow-up of patients who received 10,098 spinal anesthetics: incidence and analysis of minor sensory neurological defects. Surgery, *38*:463, 1955.

85. ———: Long-term follow-up of patients who received 10,098 spinal anesthetics: syndrome of decreased intracranial pressure (headache and ocular and auditory difficulties). J.A.M.A., *161*:586, 1956.

86. Vondrell, J. J., and Bernards, W. C.: Epidural "blood patch" for the treatment of postspinal puncture headaches. Wis. Med. J., *72*:132, 1973.

87. Winkelman, N. W.: Neurologic symptoms following accidental intraspinal detergent injection. Neurology, *2*:284, 1952.

88. Wolfson, B., Siker, E. S., and Gray, G. H.: Post-pneumoencephalography headache. A study of incidence and an attempt at therapy. Anaesthesia, *25*:328, 1970.

89. Wolman, I. J., Evans, B., and Lasker, S.: The specific gravity of cerebrospinal fluid. Am. J. Clin. Pathol., *16*:33, 1946.

8

Vomiting, Regurgitation, and Aspiration in Obstetrics

Ezzat Abouleish, M. D.

Aspiration of vomitus into the lungs during obstetric anesthesia was first reported by Hall in 1940 and clarified by Mendelson in 1946. Since then, anesthesiologists have become more and more aware of its danger. Many articles and reviews have been published dealing with this potentially lethal complication. With present advances in the management of cardiac, toxemic, and hemorrhagic patients during pregnancy and labor, aspiration stands out as a prominent cause of maternal mortality and morbidity.[10] It is universally accepted as the most frequent, single cause of obstetric death due to anesthesia. Merrill and Hingson,[61] on the basis of a review of two and a half million deliveries, estimated that the number of maternal deaths due to aspiration in the United States is about 100 every year. Phillips and coworkers[69] estimated that in a community of one million American people, there was one death every year from this cause.

In England, Edwards and Hingson[27] reviewed one thousand deaths associated with anesthesia and reported more than 50 per cent of all obstetric anesthetic mishaps were due to aspiration of vomitus. A subsequent report from England and Wales[85] showed a 40 per cent reduction in deaths due to anesthesia with, however, aspiration responsible for 60 per cent of the maternal anesthetic deaths. In 1966, a follow-up survey showed that of the fourteen avoidable obstetric deaths under anesthesia, twelve were due to aspiration.[59]

ANATOMY AND PHYSIOLOGY OF VOMITING AND REGURGITATION

While vomiting is an active process and requires motor activity, regurgitation is a passive process enhanced by motor paralysis. Both processes, however, may lead to aspiration of gastric contents with the same ultimate result.

Vomiting

Vomiting is defined as the forceful expulsion of gastric and intestinal contents through the mouth. It requires adequate stimulation of the vomiting center in the medulla which, by the way of the efferent pathways, sends impulses to the target structures involved in the act of vomiting. Interruption of this reflex arc in any part of the pathway can prevent vomiting.

The stimulus to the vomiting center could arise from: the gastrointestinal tract (e.g., stimulation of the back of the tongue or throat, overdistention of the stomach, or intestinal obstruction); other viscera, such as severe uterine contractions or injury of the uterus; painful conditions, in-

138

cluding pain of labor; vestibular stimulation (e.g., motion sickness); drugs (e.g., morphine), which act by stimulating both the vestibular and the chemoreceptor trigger nuclei;[32] and psychological conditions, such as anxiety and apprehension.

The vomiting center (Fig. 8-1) lies deep in the medulla in relation to its connections: the nuclei of the vagus, from which it receives impulses and through which it sends messages; the nucleus of tractus solitarius, which controls salivation; the vestibular nucleus, which sends impulses to it; the respiratory center; and the vasomotor center. These are all involved in the act of vomiting.

The chemoreceptor trigger zone (Fig. 8-1) is situated dorsal to the vomiting center, in the floor of the fourth ventricle. Chemical stimulation, as by digitalis, and chemical inhibition, as by chlorpromazine, act primarily on this center, from which impulses are sent to the vomiting center. On the other hand, nervous stimuli (except motion sickness) act directly on the vomiting center. Destruction of the chemoreceptor trigger zone prevents vomiting caused by drugs acting centrally but does not prevent vomiting resulting from gastrointestinal tract irritation.[36]

The efferent pathways of vomiting include the phrenic nerves (C3 to C5), the intercostal nerves (T1 to T12 inclusive), and the cranial nerves—mainly the vagus, glossopharyngeal, and accessory nerves. Immediately preceding vomiting, there is a sensation of nausea, with increased salivation, dilatation of the pupils, tachypnea, slow or irregular pulse, hypotension, pallor, and sweating.

The act of vomiting itself involves many pathways, including voluntary and involuntary muscles. To understand these pathways, the mechanism should first be considered. Following a deep breath, the glottis and nasopharynx are closed to prevent vomitus from entering the trachea and the nose. The cricopharyngeal muscle (considered the upper sphincter of the esophagus) is relaxed to allow passage of the vomitus into the pharynx and mouth for expulsion. There is simultaneous descent of the diaphragm, forced expiration, and contraction of the abdominal muscles.

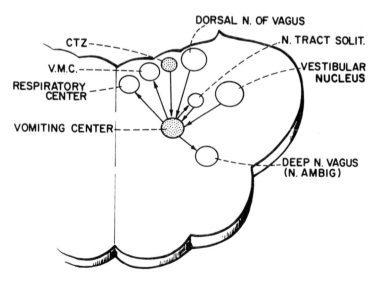

Fig. 8-1.   Cross section of the medulla oblongata showing vomiting center and its connections. (Abouleish, E., and Grenvik, A.: Vomiting, regurgitation, and aspiration in obstetrics. Pa. Med., 77:45, 1974)

CTZ = CHEMORECEPTOR TRIGGER ZONE
V.M.C. = VASOMOTOR CENTER
N. AMBIG = NUCLEUS AMBIGUUS

This increases the intra-abdominal and intrathoracic pressures. The muscles of the stomach and esophagus relax, and the raised intra-abdominal pressure is directly transmitted to the stomach, forcing its contents into the esophagus, which evacuates its contents into the pharynx and mouth. Emptying of both stomach and esophagus is promoted by peristaltic waves opposite the usual direction. During the act of vomiting, no inspiration takes place because the larynx is closed, but a deep breath follows; and if the oropharyngeal airway is not clear at that time, vomitus will be aspirated deep into the bronchi.

Regurgitation

During anesthesia, regurgitation is a more frequent and more serious complication than vomiting. This is because regurgitation is a passive process which may not show obvious signs until aspiration results,

and it can occur at any time, whether or not a muscle relaxant is used. Vomiting, on the other hand, requires motor activity and may occur only at certain stages during induction or recovery from anesthesia. The normal intragastric pressure is 10 to 12 cm. H_2O,[71] and all that is required for regurgitation to occur is a pressure gradient high enough to overcome the sphincter mechanisms at the lower and upper ends of the esophagus.[16]

The Gastroesophageal Junction

Normally, the intra-abdominal pressure is higher than the intrathoracic pressure. If there were no mechanism to occlude the esophagus, the stomach contents would readily pass into the esophagus when favored by gravity. This closure mechanism (see Fig. 8-2) can possibly be due to a sphincter at the gastroesophageal junction. The so-called *cardiac sphincter* is not an

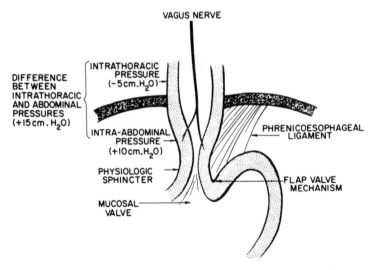

FLAP VALVE MECHANISM: THE ACUTE ANGLE BETWEEN THE STOMACH AND ESOPHAGUS.

MUCOSAL VALVE: FOLDS OF GASTRIC MUCOSA HELP IN CLOSING THE GASTROESOPHAGEAL JUNCTION.

PHYSIOLOGIC SPHINCTER: STIMULATION OF VAGUS NERVE RELAXES THE SPHINCTER. ATROPINE ADMINISTRATION INCREASES ITS TONE.

DIFFERENCE IN PRESSURE ON THE TERMINAL PORTION OF ESOPHAGUS: THIS AMOUNTS TO 15cm. H_2O

PHRENICOESOPHAGEAL LIGAMENT: KEEPS THE TERMINAL PORTION OF THE ESOPHAGUS INTRA-ABDOMINALLY AND MAINTAINS THE ACUTE GASTROESOPHAGEAL ANGLE.

Fig. 8-2. Protective mechanisms against gastroesophageal regurgitation. (Abouleish, E., and Grenvik, A.: Vomiting, regurgitation, and aspiration in obstetrics. Pa. Med., 77:45, 1974)

anatomical structure although it often acts in a physiologic manner as a sphincter. It maintains a higher pressure than either the adjacent parts of the stomach or the esophagus. Stimulation of the vagus nerve relaxes the sphincter while stimulation of the sympathetic innervation constricts it. Drugs that affect the autonomic nervous system exert a similar action on the gastroesophageal junction. Thus, atropine increases the tone of the cardiac sphincter and neostigmine relaxes it.

The gastroesophageal angle is usually acute so that the mucosal folds act as a flap valve.[33,55,75] Clinically and experimentally, it has been found that factors which modify this angle change the tendency for reflux. Increasing the gastroesophageal angle, such as in "short esophagus" associated with hiatus hernia, enhances the tendency to regurgitate. A rise in intragastric pressure during stomach distention also increases the angle and predisposes to regurgitation. On the other hand, a simple rise in intra-abdominal pressure should act against reflux by potentiating the flap valve closure.

The crura of the diaphragm (mainly the right crus) have been considered to play an important role in preventing regurgitation through contraction.[88] However, destruction or displacement of the crura alone does not cause reflux.[14] Therefore the current view is that the diaphragm does not play a direct role in preventing regurgitation.

Folds of gastric mucosa may help in closing the gastroesophageal junction. They are responsible for watertight closure. Insertion of a gastric tube renders closure by these mucosal folds inefficient. Overdistention of the stomach or the lower end of the esophagus stretches and separates these folds and increases the tendency to regurgitate.

The terminal portion of the esophagus, about 2 or 3 cm., lies below the diaphragm. Normally this portion is subjected to an outside pressure of $+10$ cm. H_2O, which represents normal intra-abdominal pressure. The thoracic portion of the esophagus is exposed to a pressure of -5 cm. H_2O (i.e., normal intrathoracic pressure). This creates a pressure difference of 15 cm. H_2O against the two portions of the esophagus which keeps its terminal part closed, opening only to allow forward flow when the pressure gradient is overcome. Any increase in abdominal pressure will promote regurgitation by increasing the intragastric pressure, but at the same time, the increase in intra-abdominal pressure keeps the terminal portion of the esophagus closed. This is a protective mechanism against reflux in persons with a normal gastroesophageal junction. In patients with an abnormal gastroesophageal junction or with overdistended stomach, straining can cause reflux.[56] Further, an independent rise in intragastric pressure above the intra-abdominal pressure would overcome this valve mechanism.[21]

The phrenicoesophageal "ligament," extending from the diaphragm to the terminal part of the esophagus, holds this portion of the esophagus in the abdomen and prevents its rise into the thorax.[16] Absence, atrophy, or attenuation of this ligament (e.g., by hiatus herniation) will allow the esophagus to lie totally intrathoracic. Thus, the previous mechanical factor, which depends on the difference in pressure to which the terminal portion of the esophagus is exposed, would not exist. A slight increase in intra-gastric pressure could then cause regurgitation.

Upper Esophageal Sphincter

The cricopharyngeal muscle is a striated muscle and acts as the sphincter at the upper end of the esophagus. It forms the lower part of the inferior constrictor muscle and is innervated, through the vagus, by the cranial part of the accessory nerve. Normally, the esophagus can hold large volumes of fluid (up to 500 ml.) without spilling over into the pharynx.[68,75] Paralysis of the cricopharyngeal muscle by muscle relaxants or deep general anesthesia, or stretching this muscle by insertion of a laryngoscope, can lead to a sudden gush of large quantities of fluid contained in the esophagus.

FACTORS PREDISPOSING TO VOMITING AND REGURGITATION DURING PARTURITION

Many factors and conditions predispose to vomiting and regurgitation in parturient women. For instance, labor may start immediately after a meal. Even fluid intake during labor is not as safe as once thought, because hypertonic fluids can remain in the stomach for long periods.[64] Once labor starts, the only safe way of administering fluids is intravenously.

Normal evacuation time for the stomach is 3 to 4 hours. Pregnancy itself has little or no effect on this evacuation time,[50] but labor pain can prolong the time by several hours. Apprehension, exhaustion, hypotension, and certain drugs may also prolong evacuation time. Narcotics such as meperidine (Demerol) act by increasing the tone of the antral portion of the stomach and the first part of the duodenum.[32] Atropine and scopolamine can prolong evacuation time by inhibiting motor activity of the stomach.[32] Further, there may be dryness of the mouth due to inadequate hydration and administration of scopolamine, tranquilizers, and/or analgesics. This may lead to swallowing of air with gastric distention.

The gravid uterus increases intra-abdominal pressure and, subsequently, the intragastric pressure. The lithotomy position increases intragastric pressure more than the supine position.[92] Direct pressure is usually applied to the abdomen in an effort to aid expulsion of the fetus. Unfortunately, this pressure is not always limited to the fundus of the uterus and may thus increase intragastric pressure.

Acid gastric secretions by the pregnant patient at term do not differ specifically from those of the nonpregnant adult.[42a] The volume of gastric contents during pregnancy normally varies from a few to over 300 ml.[81] In cases of prolonged labor, pylorospasm may occur due to pain, anxiety, and narcotics; in such cases, although food material may be absent, the stomach may still be full of acid secretions, and aspiration of these secretions could lead to disaster. In a case reported by Adams and coworkers,[4] the estimated volume of gastric contents was 2500 ml. in a patient who was in labor for more than 26 hours and had received 900 mg. of meperidine.

Anesthetic factors can predispose to vomiting and regurgitation by (1) airway obstruction which enhances regurgitation.[26,68,79] This can be due to the rise of intragastric pressure by forceful contractions of the diaphragm. (2) Positive-pressure ventilation before intubation may cause air to enter the esophagus and distend the stomach. This becomes particularly serious in cases of respiratory obstruction where gases are administered by excessive pressure in an attempt to overcome the obstruction. (3) Succinylcholine fasciculations can increase intragastric pressure not by direct action on the gastric musculature but rather by increasing intra-abdominal pressure. (4) Stormy induction can lead to bucking and coughing, which also increase intragastric pressure. (5) Each time direct intubation is attempted, the cricopharyngeal sphincter is stretched and made incompetent. During prolonged intubation attempts, anesthesia may lighten enough or paralysis may fade so that vomiting occurs. (6) Esophageal intubation not only renders the cricopharyngeal sphincter incompetent, but also allows gases to be delivered directly into the stomach.[72] These dangers are not much less serious in awake intubation. Therefore, the keystone for management of full stomach, whether the patient is awake or under general anesthesia, is skillful intubation.

PATHOLOGY FOLLOWING ASPIRATION

The results of aspiration of gastric content will vary according to (1) aspirated gastric content being solid or liquid; (2) pH of the aspirated material; and (3) superimposed bacterial infection. Consequently, three classic types of the aspiration syndrome have been described. The first is due to mechanical obstruction, the second to acute chemical inflammation, and the third to bacterial endotoxins; but any combinations of these may also occur.

Mechanical Obstruction of the Airway

Mechanical obstruction of the air passage above the carina by food can cause immediate death. Distal to the carina, lobar or segmental collapse occurs, the extent of which depends on the site of bronchial obstruction. Single or multiple areas of collapse may result. If the patient is supine, as is usually the case at the time of aspiration, the most common site of atelectasis is the apical segment of the right lower lobe. Atelectasis is due to mechanical obstruction by the aspirated material as well as to secretions which are produced in response to stimulation of the bronchial mucosa by this material. Depression of ciliary activity and the cough reflex by anesthesia delays removal of the obstructing material. Bacterial growth distal to obstruction may supervene, leading to pneumonitis, lung abscess, bronchiectasis, and empyema.

Acute Chemical Pneumonitis

Acute chemical pneumonitis was first described by Mendelson.[60] He showed experimentally in rabbits that acid vomitus caused irritation of the lungs, with resulting bronchospasm and patchy areas of hemorrhage and edema. He injected either 0.1 N hydrochloric acid or unneutralized liquid human gastric content into the trachea of different rabbits. At autopsy, both experiments showed congestion and edema throughout the lungs, peribronchial hemorrhage, and exudate with areas of secondary emphysema. The bronchial mucous membrane showed sloughing in scattered areas. When normal saline, distilled water, or neutralized liquid gastric contents was injected into the trachea of a rabbit, a brief phase of obstructive respiration ensued, but breathing quickly returned to normal. These lungs only showed scattered areas of atelectasis.

In 1961, Bannister, Sattilaro, and Otis,[11] also using rabbits, confirmed the occurrence of aspiration pneumonitis following instillation of hydrochloric acid. They extended the experiment in two ways: (1) by instilling separately in different rabbits the following solutions in the same volume (4 ml./kg. of body weight): (a) hydrochloric acid, 0.1 N; (b) sodium bicarbonate, 0.46 N; (c) sodium bicarbonate, 0.23 N; (d) sodium lactate, 0.1 N; (e) sodium hydroxide, 0.1 N; (f) sodium chloride, 0.16 N (normal saline); and (g) calcium gluconate. Both 0.1 N sodium hydroxide and 0.1 N hydrochloric acid produced equally severe lesions. All other solutions produced either no damage or only slight damage. (2) In another group of rabbits, they instilled hydrochloric acid first, followed by one of the six fluids listed above (b–g). It was found that the lesions were aggravated in all cases, including those receiving normal saline. Bannister, Sattilaro, and Otis[11] explained this on the basis that the large volume of fluid served to push the hydrochloric acid deeper into the lungs; also, that mixing of the acid and treatment solution was impossible because of the minute size of the interface; and that hydrochloric acid probably causes damage within a very short time. Mucklow and Larard[66] added that, even if normal saline and hydrochloric acid were completely mixed, the damage would still worsen. This is due to the fact that if equal volumes of hydrochloric acid (e.g., of pH 1.6) and normal saline are added together, the pH only increases to 1.8, but the resultant fluid mixture is twice in volume; since Teabeaut[84] found that all solutions with a pH less than 2.5 produced lesions of aspiration pneumonitis, the extent of damage would be more widely spread with little change in severity.

Alexander,[5] also using rabbits, instilled either 0.1 N hydrochloric acid, water, or normal saline (4 ml./kg.). The animals were sacrificed 30 minutes later and the lungs were studied macroscopically and microscopically, by light and electron microscopy. He found that the initial lesion from hydrochloric acid, water, or normal saline was similar. There was damage to the alveolar-capillary membrane leading to an exudate separating the basement membrane from the capillary endothelium (Fig. 8-3). This separation leads to interference with gaseous exchange across the alveolar-capillary membrane. It explains the early respiratory distress that happens before the appearance of physical signs such as crepitations and frank pulmonary edema. With acid aspiration the subsequent lesion affected 80 per cent of the lung tissue, whereas with water or normal saline this figure was only 30 per cent. Further, the degree of damage was more severe with acid aspiration, i.e., there was more congestion, plasma exudate, infiltration by inflammatory cells, necrosis of alveolar epithelial cells, and pulmonary edema.

Thus, aspiration of water or normal saline is not completely innocuous. These findings may further explain the results of Bannister, Sattilaro, and Otis[11] who found exaggeration of the lesions when instillation of hydrochloric acid was followed by an equal volume of saline. Therefore, these facts should be borne in mind when deciding whether or not to irrigate the tracheobronchial tree. In our opinion, irrigation should be used only in the obstructive type of aspiration to loosen food particles, thick mucus, or blood. Irrigation is not recommended in pure chemical pneumonitis. Further, when indicated, only small quantities (5 ml.) of physiologic saline solution, ideally buffered to normal pH, should be used at a time.

Pneumonitis With Acute Endotoxin Shock

Pneumonitis with acute endotoxin shock occurs when aspirated material from the gastrointestinal tract has a high pH and is bacterially contaminated,[4] such as in long-standing ileus. Although not as common as the two previously described aspiration syndromes, this one leads to severe bacterial pneumonia and the mortality is even higher than in Mendelson's syndrome.

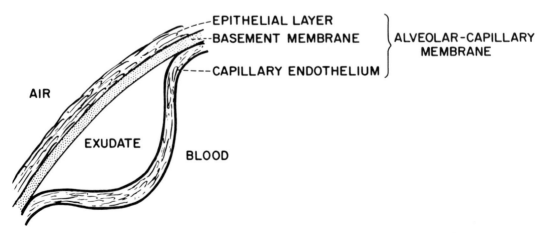

Fig. 8-3.   Initial damage in aspiration syndrome. (Abouleish, E., and Grenvik, A.: Vomiting, regurgitation, and aspiration in obstetrics. Pa. Med., 77:45, 1974)

CLINICAL PICTURE OF ASPIRATION

The clinical picture of aspiration could be that of respiratory obstruction, acute chemical irritation, shock, or a mixture of these in varying degrees. The initial effect of any aspirated material is laryngospasm (if the vocal cords are not paralyzed) which, if not relieved, may result in death from hypoxia and cardiac arrest.

In the obstruction type of aspiration, if the obstruction is distal to the carina or only partial, the clinical picture is that of hypoxia with partial airway obstruction. In the unparalyzed patient, at first there is moderate hyperpnea followed by great respiratory difficulty, particularly during the expiratory phase. This may lead to exhaustion with hypercapnia, and finally apnea may occur. There may also be cyanosis, bronchospasm, and increased resistance to ventilation. During the initial stage, sympathetic activity is increased. Thus, there is tachycardia and a rise in arterial pressure which later falls. X-ray of the chest reveals a rather uniform density of the affected area with mediastinal shift. The heart ultimately fails, the ventricles dilate and may finally fibrillate, leading to death. If the patient survives, secondary infection usually supervenes, with signs of consolidation which may progress into lung abscess, bronchiectasis, or empyema.

In the chemical pneumonitis type of aspiration (Mendelson's syndrome), although the pathologic lesion occurs immediately, the clinical picture may not be noticed for a few hours.[66] This could depend on the quantity of aspirated fluid and its pH, the response of the patient, and the alertness of the anesthesiologist. A "golden rule" to follow is: aspiration should be suspected, until proven otherwise, in any emergency case having or having had general anesthesia, with development of cyanosis, tachypnea, tachycardia, and bronchospasm. In Mendelson's syndrome, no signs of mediastinal shift are seen, but chest x-ray films usually show irregular mottled densities. Progressive cardiac embarrassment and pulmonary edema may supervene. An important differential diagnosis is acute left ventricular failure. If vomiting or regurgitation precedes the clinical picture, or food material is found in the respiratory passages, the diagnosis is easy. In silent aspiration, the differential diagnosis of left ventricular failure and Mendelson's syndrome could be very difficult because both conditions may lead to the same clinical picture since Mendelson's syndrome ultimately also results in pulmonary edema and heart failure. History of previous cardiac disease, apparent cause for acute left ventricular failure, and progress of the condition can aid in the differentiation. The triphasic sequence of immediate respiratory distress with bronchospasm and cyanosis, followed by partial recovery, and a final phase of gradual return of respiratory dysfunction, is characteristic of Mendelson's syndrome.

Pneumonitis with endotoxic shock following aspiration is more common in surgical than in obstetric patients because it is usually associated with intestinal obstruction. The patient vomits or regurgitates alkaline gastrointestinal fluid containing large amounts of bacteria. Shock may supervene rapidly. Bronchial as well as blood cultures show gram-negative organisms similar to those of the intestinal flora.

Pulmonary edema following aspiration results mainly from injury to the alveolar-capillary membrane. Other contributing factors of pulmonary edema are: (1) mechanical factors: obstruction of the bronchioles and loss of surfactant decrease pulmonary compliance and lead to increased respiratory work which creates greater negative pressure within the alveoli; (2) pulmonary hypertension from hypoxia and acidosis raises intravascular pressure within the pulmonary capillaries; and (3) hypoxia, increased vascular resistance, and acidosis, which is both respiratory and metabolic, cause acute heart failure.

PROPHYLAXIS OF ASPIRATION

In obstetrics, every possible precaution should be taken to avoid the occurrence of vomiting and regurgitation. No treatment for aspiration is as effective as proplylactic measures taken to prevent it, since neglecting one single precaution can make the difference between life and death for a previously healthy woman. *The following principles are of extreme importance.*

1. Every delivery patient should be considered as having a full stomach and should be treated accordingly.

2. The possibility of regurgitation and aspiration in vaginal delivery is greater than in cesarean section delivery because the lithotomy position and the application of extra-abdominal pressure to aid fetal delivery increase the intra-abdominal pressure. Therefore, vaginal delivery under general anesthesia should be performed with greatest care. "Give the patient a whiff!" may be the password to a dangerous and potentially fatal complication.

3. General anesthesia for emergency obstetrics should be administered by the most competent person available who is aware of the problems, takes all the necessary precautions, and is capable of performing a rapid, atraumatic intubation.

The author favors *maternity centers* in large communities rather than the practice of having obstetric patients dispersed over too many hospitals in the same area. By centralization, obstetric complications, including aspiration, would be minimized because the following could be provided:

1. Twenty-four-hour coverage by experienced obstetric anesthesiologists and nurse anesthetists[12,22,23]

2. Better equipment and facilities to prevent complications and to deal with them if they occur

3. Better obstetric team, including other physicians and nursing staff, whose management and cooperation will be reflected on the anesthetic mortality and morbidity in obstetrics.

The following precautions should always be considered: (1) The patient, her relatives, and all nursing staff should be instructed that *no food or drinks* be given to the mother once labor begins. Fluid and energy sources must be supplied intravenously. (2) General anesthesia should be avoided if possible. Regional analgesia, when properly administered, gives complete relief of pain without loss of protective reflexes. If no hypotension or hypoxia is allowed with regional anesthesia, the incidence of nausea and vomiting is less than with general anesthesia or narcotics. General anesthesia should be used rarely for vaginal delivery because of the great risk of aspiration. However, a patient under high subarachnoid block can also regurgitate and aspirate while unable to cough because of the associated paralysis of the abdominal muscles. Therefore, the anesthesiologist should be aware of this possibility.

The need for general anesthesia in obstetrics is quite limited. It is only indicated if there is a contraindication to regional analgesia or uterine relaxation is required; even the latter indication can be waived owing to the development of specific uterine-relaxing drugs (see Chap. 10 Oxytocic and Tocolytic Agents). The limited use of general anesthesia and the proper administration of regional analgesia are responsible for the absence of maternal mortality due to anesthesia and the high success rate of pain relief in obstetrics.[1]

PRECAUTIONS WITH GENERAL ANESTHESIA

Certain precautions should be taken if the need for general anesthesia arises. Skill, attention to details, and proper judgment are important points that can prevent complications.

Separating the Gastrointestinal Tract From the Respiratory System

If there is no connection between the gastrointestinal tract and the respiratory system, aspiration cannot occur. This can be achieved by sealing one or the other system and connecting it to the outside. (1) The gastrointestinal tract can be sealed by using a cuffed esophageal tube. Although the concept of preventing regurgitation by inflating a cuff at the esophagus has appealed to many,[29,35,45,54] its safety is doubtful. The esophagus is a distensible organ. Therefore, it is difficult to maintain a reasonable seal with a cuffed tube.[43,79] Moreover if vomiting occurs, the increase in pressure distal to the cuff may distend the esophagus, making a previously satisfactory seal useless, or it may dislodge the esophageal tube altogether.[79] (2) The respiratory tract can be sealed by using a cuffed endotracheal tube. There is no doubt that sealing the respiratory tract from the gastrointestinal tract by the use of a cuffed endotracheal tube provides the best protection against aspiration. Therefore, adequate consideration should be given to the possible ways of preventing aspiration during the two critical periods when a cuffed endotracheal tube is not in place. *The first critical period* is from the start of induction to the inflation of the endotracheal tube cuff. Vomiting and regurgitation during induction of anesthesia have been long recognized as the most important causes of mortality and morbidity in parturients submitted to general anesthesia. Although there is general agreement to the dangers involved, the preferred method of induction varies. None of the three methods available (awake intubation, inhalation induction, intravenous "crash" induction) is foolproof and none is suitable for an inexperienced or unskilled physician or nurse anesthetist. *The second critical period* is from the time of the removal of the endotracheal tube until the recovery of all the protective reflexes. The endotracheal tube should be left with the cuff inflated in the trachea as long as it is tolerated and under no circumstances removed before return of the protective reflexes.

Awake Intubation. With experience, gentleness, and proper explanation, the passage of a tube in an awake patient can be made tolerable. Intravenous diazepam, 5 mg., may help to relax and sedate the patient. Diazepam in such a dose is safe to use in obstetric anesthesia.[30] The patient is carefully positioned with the neck flexed and the head extended at the atlanto-occipital joint. The patient is asked to open her mouth at which time the tongue, pharynx, and palate are sprayed with 4 per cent lidocaine. The patient is told that a light will be used in her throat to position a tube, and the laryngoscope is slowly advanced. Additional lidocaine may be used to spray the valleculae and the anterior surface of the epiglottis, but not the larynx. The patient is asked to relax and breathe deeply. The tube is inserted when the cords are widely open. Once the tube is in place, the cuff is inflated and an oropharyngeal airway is inserted in order to avoid the patient biting on the tube when the laryngoscope is removed. Anesthesia is induced rapidly by the intravenous route if the patient's condition permits. In case of difficulty, nasopharyngeal spray is used, followed by blind nasal intubation. In experienced hands, blind nasal intubation has a high rate of success with very little discomfort to the patient. The administration of carbon dioxide or intravenous doxapram (1 mg./kg.) before nasal intubation increases the success rate since the vocal cords open widely during hyperventilation. In experienced hands, the use of the fiberoptic laryngoscope has proven advantageous in difficult cases.[80,83]

Theoretically, awake intubation would be the safest method of induction of anesthesia because with this method the respiratory tract is sealed from the gastrointestinal tract before loss of consciousness. Moreover, the patient is spontaneously breathing, and therefore, adequate time is available. However, awake intubation has several disadvantages. It does not always eliminate the danger of regurgitation and aspiration. Fluid may have accumulated in the esophagus, and stretching of the cricopharyngeal muscle by the laryngoscope will make that sphincter incompetent so that a sudden gush of gastric fluid may enter the trachea. This can be provoked by inadequate topical anesthesia of the oropharynx, at which time the insertion of the laryngoscope may stimulate the vomiting reflex. Local anesthetic so liberally applied as to include the larynx is also dangerous, because if regurgitation occurs, no protective reflex is present to prevent aspiration. Further, the experience can be unpleasant for the patient, especially if technical difficulty is encountered. The technique is easy in edentulous and frail patients, but in young healthy individuals with a full set of teeth, as in the majority of obstetric patients, the technique is relatively difficult and requires much skill since muscular relaxation is usually inadequate.

Inhalation Induction. After the usual check of the anesthesia machine and other equipment, including the suction apparatus, anesthesia is induced while the patient lies horizontally supine. A high flow of gases is used to help the rapid elimination of nitrogen. The carbon dioxide absorber may be turned off at the start and 5 per cent carbon dioxide added to inhaled gases to prevent breath-holding, an essential preliminary to active vomiting.[43]

Hyperventilation as well as the acceptance of rapidly increasing concentrations of potent inhalation anesthetics will speed the induction period.[38] Slow induction can initiate vomiting because the patient may remain in the excitement stage too long, and central stimulation of vomiting may occur. With the original technique, either ether or cyclopropane was used.[13,43] Later on, other anesthetics were employed, including methoxyflurane.[44] In lambs, Motoyama and co-workers[65] found that hypercapnia had no adverse effect on the fetus. Ivankovic, Elam, and Huffman[44] confirmed this finding in humans. They also found that umbilical vein oxygen tension and Apgar scores were higher and the time to sustain respiration was shorter in the hypercapnic group, than in the normocapnic group. This was attributed to the possibility of stimulation of the respiratory centers of the neonates by hypercapnia.

The main advantage of this technique is that apnea resulting from the use of relaxants is avoided. Therefore, there is adequate time for intubation in difficult cases. Also, the use of blind nasal intubation is accompanied by a higher success rate as a result of hypercapnia and presence of muscle tone of the pharynx. Further, the presence of spontaneous respiration eliminates the need for positive-pressure ventilation prior to intubation, thus preventing the rise of intragastric pressure from pushing gases into the stomach. If vomiting or regurgitation does occur, the protective reflexes are still active.

With the described technique, the induction period is shortened during inhalation induction, but it is still much longer than with the intravenous method. The longer the period of unconsciousness before intubation, the higher the risk of vomiting and regurgitation. Moreover, the longer the period of administration of general anesthesia prior to delivery the more depressed the baby will be.[58] Also, the relaxation is not as ideal as with the use of muscle relaxants, and premature attempts at intubation before an adequate level of anesthesia is reached can lead to disaster. Inadequate relaxation makes laryngoscopy difficult and prolonged, the anesthesia level becomes lighter, and the vomiting reflex is stimulated by the laryngoscope.

Intravenous "Crash" Induction. This is our method of choice because induction is rapid (the period between loss of consciousness and sealing of the trachea is very short), fetal depression is minimal, and the technique is pleasant for the mother. However, the mother is paralyzed, and oxygenation depends on preliminary breathing of oxygen. Thus, the time allowed for intubation is limited. Further, if attempt at intubation is prolonged, the patient may recover partially from the state of paralysis and active vomiting may occur. Therefore, if an intubation problem is anticipated, such as in a patient with a markedly receding jaw, it is best to resort to other methods of induction or to avoid general anesthesia altogether.

The usual time for injection of succinylcholine is immediately after sleep induction by thiopental. To further shorten the induction period, injection of mixtures of thiopental and succinylcholine has been advocated.[46] Yet there is no guarantee that all patients will become unconscious before the action of succinylcholine takes place; some will still be conscious and frightened by the inability to breathe.[6]

Reducing Intragastric Pressure

For those patients in whom a full stomach is suspected, it has been assumed that the danger of aspiration could be avoided by emptying the stomach prior to induction. However, complete emptying of the stomach is usually impossible. The aim is to evacuate as much as possible in order to reduce intragastric pressure far *below the critical pressure at which reflux occurs.* This critical level varies between 15 and 70 cm. H_2O, with an average of 30 cm. H_2O.[18,33] Lowering of intragastric pressure prior to anesthesia can be achieved by inducing vomiting or introducing a stomach tube.

Induction of vomiting can be evoked by stimulating the back of the tongue or the pharyngeal wall. Some patients are able to do this themselves or it can be done with a catheter. Certain drugs stimulate the vomiting center by way of the chemoreceptor trigger zone. The most common emetic drug is apomorphine.[20,41,42,89] However, this drug is not always effective, and complete emptying of the stomach is not guaranteed. Drug-induced vomiting is also

unpleasant to the patient, and such drugs may produce cardiovascular collapse.

Insertion of a gastric tube is the most common method for evacuation of the stomach.[12,27,72,73] Again, complete evacuation should not be expected. Even a wide-bore stomach tube is not necessarily able to remove all large food particles, but at least the intragastric pressure is lowered and can be reduced further by suction just prior to induction. Moreover, by leaving the distal end of the tube open, it can act as a safety valve for any increase in the intragastric pressure during induction. Therefore, the method of choice for evacuating the stomach is to use a nasogastric tube. The question is whether it should be inserted prior to anesthesia in every obstetric patient. Although this is more ideal, it is difficult to practice for several reasons; for example, to a patient in labor, the need for anesthesia may be so urgent that no time can be spared for emptying of the stomach.

Although we consider all mothers in labor as having full stomachs and being potential candidates for vomiting or regurgitation, we divide them into two groups in regard to the need for a stomach tube. (1) The stomach is *certain* to contain food when labor has started within 6 hours of food intake. In this group, if time allows, the widest possible stomach tube is inserted prior to anesthesia. To make the patient relatively comfortable and to minimize trauma, 4 per cent lidocaine is administered as nasal drops a few minutes before insertion of the tube. The tube is then well lubricated with lidocaine gel. Positive evidence that the tube is in the stomach is confirmed by aspiration of gastric fluid or by injection of air into the tube while auscultating the left hypochondriac region.[43] Do not inject fluid into the stomach tube to comfirm its position because in a moribund patient the tube could be in the tracheobronchial tree.[43] Apply gentle suction since excessive suction can cause occlusion of the tube. (2) The stomach is *likely* to contain food when labor has started more than 6 hours after food intake. In this group, no stomach tube is inserted before induction, but all other precautions for "crash" induction are adhered to.

When the patient is under anesthesia, insertion of a nasogastric tube may be more difficult. Therefore, the author always prefers to insert it before induction. If insertion of a nasogastric tube is required in an anesthetized, intubated patient, gently lifting of the larynx can allow the tube to pass easily through the upper part of the esophagus.[78] In case there is difficulty in introducing the nasogastric tube in the anesthetized or comatose patient, one method is to insert it through the nose, and pull the distal end through the mouth for a distance of about 45 cm. A noncuffed Magill endotracheal tube with a side slit is inserted through the mouth into the esophagus. When the Magill tube is in the esophagus, the nasogastric tube is passed down through it into the stomach. The slit Magill tube is then removed from the nasogastric tube. When the nasogastric tube is in the stomach, it is fixed to the nose and side of the face in such a way that it does not cause pressure on the external nares.

Use of Antacids

Gastric aspirate pH is an important factor in determining the severity of the chemical irritation. In a study of 18 patients with aspiration pneumonitis, by Lewis, Burgess, and Hampson,[52] all patients with a gastric aspirate of pH less than 1.75 died, whereas only one, probably unrelated death occurred when the aspirate pH was greater than 2.4. Therefore, administration of antacids is considered an important prophylactic measure.[70] Taylor and Pryse-Davies[81] introduced prophylactic ingestion of magnesium trisilicate mixture (BPC) in order to maintain acidity of the gastric contents above pH 2.5 during labor. Williams and Crawford[91] recommended the administration of 15 ml. of magnesium trisilicate mixture orally every

2 hours to maintain the gastric contents pH above 3.0. Thus, presumably if such contents are aspirated, the Mendelson syndrome will not develop. The composition of the recommended mixture is as follows: magnesium carbonate, 5.0 g.; magnesium trisilicate, 5.0 g.; sodium bicarbonade, 5.0 g.; and peppermint water to 100 ml. Repeated administration of this mixture can increase the blood level of magnesium in the mother, but such an increase is highly unlikely to be detrimental to either mother or infant.[8] Unfortunately, it seems that preoperative alkali therapy gives a false sense of security and cannot be relied upon to prevent development of pneumonitis should aspiration occur, since Adams and coworkers[4] reported a case of massive severe pneumonitis in a patient who received magnesium trisilicate mixture before induction of anesthesia.

The administration of antacid usually raises the pH of the stomach contents, but this is not guaranteed. If no antacid is used, 50 per cent of the patients have gastric contents of a pH lower than 3. If antacids are given regularly every 2 hours, the percentage drops to 20.

It is a dilemma to decide which antacid to use in obstetrics and what regimen to follow. Some recommend the administration of antacid every 2 hours to all parturients.[19] However, a single-dose antacid is a more practical method and does not add to the burden of the nursing staff. Using the pH of 3 as the critical level of the acidity of gastric contents, White, Clark, and Stanley-Jones[90] found no significant difference in the protective efficacy of the 2-hourly regimen of magnesium trisilicate mixture and that of a single-dose 0.3 M sodium citrate[49] administered a few minutes prior to anesthesia. Sodium citrate 0.3 M, is a clear solution devoid of the particulate matter present in many of the commercial antacids which may cause pulmonary lesion if aspirated.[48] The addition of 20 per cent of syrup makes it palatable without significantly changing its pH. This mixture has been found be practical and inexpensive, does not require refrigeration, and is stable for at least two months (pH about 8.5)[2]

In conclusion, the author recommends the use of 15 ml. of 0.3 M sodium citrate as a single dose prior to general anesthesia. He is, until proven otherwise, against the routine use of antacids to all parturients.

Prevention of Succinylcholine Fasciculations

Succinylcholine fasciculations raise intragastric pressure.[7,62,71,77] This rise in pressure is more significant in adults than in children.[73] The fasciculations can raise the pressure to as high as 50 cm. H_2O and overcome the sphincter mechanism at the gastroesophageal junction. However, these fasciculations can be prevented by prior administration of a small dose of a nondepolarizing muscle relaxant, e.g., 3 mg. of d-tubocurarine. To obtain adequate relaxation, the dose of succinlycholine must be increased from 1 mg./kg. to 1.5 mg./kg. when a dose of nondepolarizing muscle relaxant has been used.[24]

The use of a nondepolarizing muscle relaxant prior to succinylcholine administration is the classic method. However, the increased intragastric pressure following succinylcholine is due to the increased intra-abdominal pressure. Thus, there is also an associated increased pressure on the outer wall of the abdominal esophagus. If the stomach is not overdistended, the increased pressure on the esophageal wall can balance the increased intragastric pressure and succinylcholine will not cause regurgitation. Moreover, curare even in such a small dose sometimes causes blurring of vision which in unpremedicated patients causes much distress and anxiety. In conclusion, the administration of a nondepolarizing muscle relaxant before succinylcholine has to be reevaluated.

Position During Induction

In patients who are fasting and submitted to routine anesthesia and surgery, intragastric pressure is most often below 10 cm. H_2O, although pressures of 15 to 16 cm. H_2O are not infrequent.[56,68,71] In patients with abdominal distention, such as with a gravid uterus, O'Mullane[68] measured pressures of 15 to 18 cm. H_2O. Placing a patient in a *40-degree head-up tilt* will raise the larynx 19 cm. above the gastroesophageal junction.[76] In this position it is assumed that gastric contents will not reach the laryngeal level, even if forced into the esophagus;[40,76] but this is not always the case. Regurgitation may still occur in this position.[13,78] The results of regurgitation become very serious in an anesthetized, paralyzed patient since aspiration becomes inevitable; even fatal aspiration has been recorded in the head-up position.[66] Postural hypotension during induction is also likely to occur, especially in hypovolemic patients. To avoid this postural hypotension, Stept and Safar[78] recommend the V-position with the trunk elevated 30 degrees and the feet raised.

The use of thiopental-muscle-relaxant induction with *head-down tilt* was recommended by Mucklow and Larard[66] on the assumption that if regurgitation does occur, gravity will prevent aspiration. It also avoids cardiovascular collapse that can occur in the head-up position. However, the best way to avoid aspiration is to prevent regurgitation in the first place. This position definitely favors such a complication.

Another method is to place the patient in the *lateral position with a slight head-down tilt,* and induce anesthesia by inhalation anesthetics. Hyperventilation, with CO_2 admixture, may be used to speed up induction and depress the vomiting mechanism. But the disadvantages of this technique are that regurgitation can still take place, particularly if respiratory obstruction occurs, and conditions for intubation are not optimal.

Head-up, head-down, and lateral positions, although each offering some benefit, all have disadvantages which outweigh the advantages. Therefore, we recommend *the horizontal supine position* with which the anesthesiologist is most familiar. If other precautions are taken and rapid induction with skillful intubation is performed, the risk of aspiration should be very small. A pillow under the head facilitates intubation, since it places the head and neck in optimal position to visualize the larynx. Neglect of this often leads to problems and no chances should be taken in a patient with a full stomach.

Cricoid Pressure

The use of cricoid pressure to prevent regurgitation in the unconscious and paralyzed patient was first recommended by Sellick.[74] In the Sellick maneuver, the cricoid cartilage is pressed against the body of the sixth cervical vertebra, thus occluding the esophagus. It also facilitates intubation by bringing the larynx into view. Postmortem studies were done to determine quantitatively the efficiency of cricoid pressure in preventing regurgitation of gastric contents.[28,73] Cricoid compression was found to provide protection against regurgitation until intraesophageal pressure reaches 50 to 100 cm. H_2O. The presence of a nasogastric tube was thought to diminish the effectiveness of this method in occluding the esophageal lumen.[43,87] But Salem[73] found, in children, that the nasogastric tube does not interfere with the efficiency of cricoid pressure in preventing regurgitation. A patent nasogastric tube is a safety valve against excessive rise in intragastric pressure and subsequent regurgitation. Thus, the presence of the nasogastric tube and cricoid pressure are synergistic rather than antagonistic. The disadvantages of the Sellick maneuver are the theoretically possible rupture of the esophagus if vomiting occurs while cricoid pressure is maintained,[74] and possible trauma to the larynx if the pressure applied is too excessive. Therefore, only a trained assistant who is aware of these dangers should be allowed to apply cricoid pressure. The patient's cricoid could be outlined with surface marking before induction.[20]

TECHNIQUE OF INTRAVENOUS "CRASH" INDUCTION

This technique is used for vaginal delivery or cesarean section when general anesthesia is indicated. If possible, intravenous infusion should be started outside the operating room using a plastic cannula that is well fixed to the skin to ensure against its dislodgement at the critical moment. Sometimes this complication occurs, and before another vein is cannulated the patient vomits. A blood pressure cuff and a stethoscope are applied. If there is indication to insert a nasogastric tube, do not hesitate to do so. If a nasogastric tube is present, let it remain *in situ* after making certain that it is well fixed and patent. Make sure at least three cuffed oral tubes of different sizes and one nasal tube are available. Check the cuffs and connect a syringe for air injection to the cuff of the most suitable tube. The tubes should be well lubricated and have a straight connector attached. If a stylet is used, it should be well lubricated and easy to remove and reinsert. Test the laryngoscope and have an extra one available in case the light fails. Use the type of laryngoscope with which you are familiar. Have an airway or a bite block ready. There should be extra full cylinders of oxygen and nitrous oxide on the machine in addition to those in use. Do not be misled by the attached label. Check the cylinders yourself. There should be a powerful suction available. Have a tonsil suction tip attached and several rubber or plastic sterile suction tubes available. Check the suction for leakage. Check the drugs you may need for anesthesia and for resuscitation if aspiration should occur.

The delivery or operating table is kept horizontal but should allow tilting if vomiting occurs. Put a pillow under the patient's head for comfort and proper positioning during laryngoscopy. Allow the patient to breathe 100 per cent oxygen at a high flow rate with a well-fitting mask. The patient should breathe oxygen spontaneously until paralysis is complete. Do not use positive-pressure ventilation. Inject intravenously 0.4 to 0.6 mg. of atropine. The patient might feel some palpitation following the injection. Curare, 3 mg., may be intravenously injected. During the next 3 minutes: apply electrocardiograph electrodes and a precordial stethoscope; continue oxygen administration and apply gentle suction to the stomach tube, if present, to reduce intragastric pressure. Attach a plastic bag to the nasogastric tube and allow the end to hang down below the stomach level. Gravity will facilitate drainage and prevent the building up of excessive pressure. After the 3-minute interval, start induction by intravenous injection of a predetermined dose of thiobarbiturate directly into the vein or the intravenous tubing as close to the vein as possible. The usual dose is 4 mg./kg.[47] which is reduced in a patient who is hypovolemic or critically ill. Ketamine may be administered in such cases.[17,63] Tilt the head gently backward and ask the assistant to apply and maintain firm cricoid pressure until the cuff of the endotracheal tube is inflated. When the eyelash reflex disappears (indicating loss of consciousness) inject succinylcholine in one dose. The dose is 1.5 mg./kg. injected directly into the patient's vein or into the intravenous tubing as close to the patient's vein as possible. Continue oxygen administration. When respiration ceases, remove the mask quickly and perform intubation. Quick, gentle intubation is the key to success. Never try to intubate a partially paralyzed patient. Inflate the cuff, connect the tube to the anesthesia machine, squeeze the bag to make sure there is no leakage around the cuff, then ask the assistant to release the cricoid pressure.

In cases of vaginal delivery, lithotomy position is instituted after intubation. Maintain anesthesia with a 4:2 mixture of nitrous oxide and oxygen, and succinylcholine drip of 0.1 per cent concentration. To avoid bacterial contamination, a small bottle of 250 ml. of succinylcholine mixture, which is disposed of at the end of the procedure, is preferred to a larger bottle

used for more than one patient. The rate of succinylcholine drip is regulated by the aid of a peripheral nerve stimulator or by allowing slight respiratory movements. If complete muscular paralysis is maintained throughout the procedure, resumption of adequate ventilation after the end of operation may be unduly delayed. Following clamping of the umbilical cord, inject intravenously 0.2 mg./kg. morphine and 0.1 mg./kg. diazepam to a maximum of 15 mg. and 7.5 mg. respectively.[3] Continue the $N_2O:O_2$ (4:2) mixture and controlled ventilation until the end of the procedure.

TREATMENT OF ASPIRATION

Treatment of aspiration is divided into (1) immediate treatment until the situation is under control; and (2) subsequent treatment which deals with continued support of the vital systems and the follow-up of the patient.

Immediate Treatment

If the patient vomits or regurgitates, the table or bed is rapidly tilted to a 30 to 40 degree head-down position to have the larynx at a higher level than the pharynx and to allow gastric material to drain to the outside. The patient is also rapidly rolled to her side to confine any aspiration to the dependent lung and to facilitate drainage of vomitus from the mouth.

The mouth and pharynx should be suctioned as rapidly as possible. If solid material is found, it is scooped out e.g., using a finger wrapped in gauze. If the patient is not paralyzed, insert a bite block or the finger might be injured. If it is difficult to open the patient's mouth, try to open the clenched jaws by using the crossed finger maneuver. If possible, avoid muscle relaxants because of the danger of combined loss of protective laryngeal reflex and paralysis of the cricopharyngeal sphincter. However, do not waste too much time in trying to open the mouth if respiratory obstruction is evident. In such cases, aspirate the pharynx with a large catheter and administer 100 per cent oxygen while an assistant injects succinylcholine intravenously and applies pressure on the cricoid. Once relaxation occurs, open the mouth quickly, remove rapidly any foreign material or mucus to get a clear view of the larynx, intubate, and inflate the cuff. Following this, the assistant can release the cricoid pressure.

In all cases of suspected aspiration, laryngoscopy and intubation are performed. This is to assure a patent airway, allow suction of aspirated material, facilitate assisted or controlled respiration, and prevent further aspiration. If the condition of the patient allows, suck through the endotracheal tube before administering 100 per cent oxygen by positive-pressure ventilation. This is to prevent pushing aspirated material beyond your reach. As a rule, suction should be brief (less than 15 seconds) to avoid cardiac arrest from hypoxia, give 100 per cent oxygen both before and after suctioning. Observe chest expansion, adventitious sounds, and change in the patient's color. Continue 100 per cent oxygen administration until the patient has improved, e.g., as demonstrated by arterial blood gas analysis.

Bronchial irrigation is indicated only in the obstructive type of aspiration. Five ml. of normal saline is instilled into the tracheobronchial tree, followed immediately by suction. This is preceded and followed by oxygenation. The sequence is repeated until the aspirated fluid is clear. Further, 200 mg. of hydrocortisone or its equivalent should be given intravenously.

To evacuate the stomach, a nasogastric tube should be inserted. The evacuated material should be sent for pH determination. Some workers have suggested that in patients with aspiration pneumonitis, the pH of the pharyngeal or tracheal aspirate reflects the original pH of the aspirated fluid. But Awe, Fletcher, and Jacob[9] found that the pH of tracheobronchial secretions rose rapidly in dogs following aspiration as large quantities of blood-tinged fluid, rich in protein, poured into the lumen. On the other hand, analysis of gastric juice within 4 hours of aspiration closely resembles that of the aspirate.[52] The pH of the gastric contents is of importance for treatment and prognosis of the patient. Tracheobronchial aspirate is collected in a special sterile container for culture and sensitivity determination. Give a broad-spectrum antibiotic as an immediate emergency measure, such as 0.5 g. of tetracycline, by intravenous drip. This antibiotic should be continued until the culture and sensitivity results are reported and the most suitable antibiotic can be selected.

If the patient has bronchospasm, give aminophylline, 250 mg. slowly intravenously, followed by 250 mg. in 250 ml. of fluid as a drip. Rapid intravenous administration of aminophylline can cause hypotension.[32] Isoproterenol inhalation (0.5 mg. in 3 ml. of normal saline) can be given with a nebulizer. In patients with pronounced cardiac arrhythmia, we prefer a beta-2-agent, such as isoetharine (Bronkosol), 0.5 ml. in 3 to 5 ml. of normal saline.

Subsequent Treatment

If aspiration occurs during induction of anesthesia for elective surgery, the operation should be postponed until the patient has recovered completely. Unfortunately, this cannot be applied to obstetric emergencies. In these situations, the delivery or operation must be expedited.

Once the initial danger of asphyxia is overcome and the patient is well oxygenated, *bronchoscopy* may be undertaken to ensure that the segmental bronchi are patent. This could be an immediate lifesaving procedure when solid food particles are causing obstruction. On the other hand, bronchoscopy is not an easy procedure in this situation. It can be quite traumatic and can exaggerate hypoxia if not done properly. Bonchoscopy should not be performed in every case of vomiting or regurgitation, but when necessary it should be performed by an experienced person. The history, physical examination, x-ray of the chest, and nature of the gastric contents help in deciding the indication and urgency for bronchoscopy.

In some cases of vomiting, it is apparent that there is no soiling of the respiratory tract, and all that is required is *observation*. In other cases, after the initial phase of cyanosis and bronchospasm, there may be an apparent improvement followed by respiratory dysfunction. Therefore, all cases with vomiting or regurgitation should be meticulously observed for at least 48 hours for signs of respiratory insufficiency and treatment initiated accordingly.

Mechanical ventilation through an endotracheal tube is required if the patient shows the following signs and symptoms:[12] dyspnea; cyanosis; tachypnea; tachycardia; tracheal tug; retraction; flaring; the use of accessory muscles of respiration; PaO_2 less than 200 mm. Hg on 100 per cent oxygen; $paCO_2$ higher than 50 mm. Hg; arterial pH less than 7.2; increased dead space (V_D/V_T more than 60 per cent); vital capacity less than 15 ml./kg.; effective compliance less than 15 ml./cm. H_2O. In such cases, intubation and institution of intermittent positive-pressure ventilation may be of great value.[53,67] *The advantages of intermittent positive-pressure ventilation in these cases are:* (1) it relieves the patient's exhaustion and dyspnea; (2) it improves alveolar ventilation ($PaCO_2$ decreases) and reduces right-to-left shunting (PaO_2 increases); (3) it is beneficial in preventing and treating acute pulmonary edema by reducing transmural pulmonary arterial pressure;[34] and (4) it allows removal of secretions by suction.

Chemical pneumonitis can lower pulmonary compliance due to exudate, bronchospasm, and loss of surfactants. In such cases, ventilation with a slow rate and large tidal volume may be required. Large doses of narcotics may be needed to sedate the patient and to allow control of ventilation. One must bear in mind that hypoxia is an important reason for the patient to fight the ventilator. For control of respiration, increase in oxygen concentration, initial hyperventilation, and narcotics are preferred to the administration of a muscle relaxant. *Tracheostomy* may be required later in the course of the disease.

Inspired oxygen concentration should be high enough to relieve hypoxemia which may cause acidosis, myocardial depression, and pulmonary edema. Therefore, inspired oxygen concentration is temporarily raised (even to 100 per cent) to obtain a nearly normal PaO_2 of at least 70 mm. Hg. Sometimes such a level of PaO_2 cannot be achieved in spite of 100 per cent oxygen in the inspired mixture. In such cases, positive-end expiratory pressure (PEEP) is utilized. If $PaCO_2$ is low, dead-space tubing should be added or $FICO_2$ control instituted.[15] There is the possibility of oxygen toxicity when a patient is exposed to high oxygen pressure for a long time, but the dangers of hypoxia outweigh the dangers of oxygen toxicity and 100 per cent oxygen must be given when required. On the other hand, inspired oxygen concentration should not be kept higher than required to maintain a near normal PaO_2.[12]

Humidification of inspired gases is important since dry gases inhibit ciliary action, decrease pulmonary compliance, and cause sticky secretions that are difficult to remove. Aseptic techniques and gentleness are essential for intermittent suction through endotracheal or tracheostomy tubes. Superimposed infection can lead to deterioration in the pulmonary condition of these patients. Trauma from the suction catheter and infection can also be important causes of tracheal stenosis.[4]

In patients who need prolonged respiratory support and have desiccated secretion, instilling a few milliliters of normal saline solution is often required before suctioning, in order to loosen secretions and prevent atelectasis. Administration of aminophylline, corticosteroids, isoproterenol inhalation, and removal of secretions and foreign materials help to relieve associated bronchospasm. Repeated determinations of arterial Po_2, Pco_2, pH, and other pulmonary function tests are required to guide treatment and follow-up of these cases.

The cardiovascular condition of patients with aspiration pneumonitis should be closely monitored. Hypovolemia is suggested by tachycardia, falling blood pressure, rising hematocrit, low central venous pressure, and decreased measured blood volumes. Hypovolemia plays an important role in the hypotension seen in these cases.[9] The deficit should be replaced by moderate volumes of fluids, mainly colloids. Larger volumes of electrolyte solutions restore circulation, but often at the expense of increasing alveolar-arterial oxygen tension difference, decreasing PaO_2, and increasing interstitial edema of the lungs.

If tachycardia and hypotension are associated with high central venous pressure, and the latter rises more by rapid administration of 200 ml. of fluid, then heart failure may complicate the picture and rapid digitalization is required. After full digitalization, hypovolemia may become more evident and need correction. Also, if pulmonary edema develops at any time during the course of the disease, rapid digitalization is indicated together with other lines of treatment, intermittent positive-pressure ventilation with high inspired oxygen concentration, isoproterenol, narcotics, diuretics, intravenous fluid restriction, and so on.

Antibiotics are required to combat infection of the respiratory system, especially if corticosteroids are administered. Because organisms in the respiratory system may change during the course of prolonged respiratory support, repeated cultures and sensitivity tests should be performed (e.g., 2 to 3 times a week).

Administration of corticosteroids is still controversial. On the whole, they have been accepted in the treatment of the aspiration syndrome.[10] Corticosteroids inhibit the inflammatory reaction of the pulmonary tissue and bronchial tree to the chemical irritation by aspirated acidic fluid and products of cell injury.[11,25,39,57] They may improve the diffusing capacity of the lung in advanced cases that require prolonged intermittent positive-pressure ventilation.[4] Direct instillation of hydrocortisone into the tracheobronchial tree was considered to be effective in inhibiting the inflammatory reaction;[51,86] but more recently Taylor and Pryse-Davies,[82] in similar experiments, found that endotracheal hydrocortisone or fluocinolone did not affect the course of pulmonary pathology produced by hydrochloric acid solutions of low pH. They also found that steroids produce lesions of their own. Therefore, it is not recommended to give steroids by endotracheal instillation. The route of choice is parenterally, either intravenously or intramuscularly. After initial intravenous injection of 200 mg. of hydrocortisone, 100 mg. every 6 hours is required. In certain cases, as in a patient with toxemia of pregnancy when sodium retention is to be avoided, dexamethasone may be used instead in equivalent doses (100 mg. of hydrocortisone equals 3.75 mg. of dexamethasone). The duration of the treatment with corticosteroids depends on the progress of the case. Toward the end of a prolonged course, either gradual diminution of the dose and/or administration of ACTH may be required.

PROGNOSIS FOLLOWING ASPIRATION

In the obstructive type of aspiration, the prognosis will depend on the degree of obstruction and subsequent atelectasis, the onset of bacterial infection, the efficiency of treatment, and the resistance of the patient. The course may be quite protracted.

In Mendelson's syndrome, with proper treatment the patient usually recovers completely within 24 to 36 hours if the pH of the aspirated material is not too low and bacterial infection does not supervene. Nearly all 40 cases of Mendelson's original series recovered after an afebrile illness, and only four developed pneumonia with one developing a lung abscess. Rarely does the patient rapidly develop acute pulmonary edema and heart failure, subsequently leading to death; but respiratory insufficiency may follow the initial period of respiratory distress and prolong the recovery period. The main factors leading to poor prognosis are (1) low pH of gastric aspirate, (2) advanced age, (3) prolonged hypoxia, (4) pulmonary infection, and (5) previous pulmonary or cardiovascular disease.

The septic pneumonitis type of aspiration has the highest mortality rate and the prognosis depends largely on the underlying disease causing intestinal obstruction.

CONCLUSION

In obstetric anesthesia, aspiration of gastric contents has been one of the leading causes of mortality and morbidity. However, during the 11-year period from July 1966 through June 1977 at Magee-Womens Hospital in Pittsburgh, Pennsylvania, 64,008 obstetric anesthetics were given without a single death caused by aspiration. This is essentially due to avoidance of general anesthesia whenever possible. Intravertebral blocks were utilized in 78 per cent of the cases while general anesthesia was administered in only 9 per cent. When general anesthesia is used, the patient is considered to have a full stomach, and meticulous attention is paid to all details to avoid vomiting and regurgitation since prophylaxis, as always, is the best way to avoid the serious consequence of aspiration. Should aspiration still occur, early diagnosis, adequate treatment, and follow-up are mandatory for recovery. Complete understanding of the basic pathophysiology is essential for applying prophylactic measures, early diagnosis of aspiration, adequate therapy, and proper follow-up.

REFERENCES

1. Abouleish, E., and Grenvik, A.: Vomiting, regurgitation, and aspiration in obstetrics. Pa. Med., 77:45, 1974.
2. Abouleish, E., and Schenle, I. A.: Efficiency of antacid therapy. Br. J. Anaesth., 49:394, 1977.
3. Abouleish, E., and Taylor, F. H.: Effect of morphine-diazepam on signs of anesthesia and dreams of patients under N_2O for cesarean section. Anesth. Analg., 55:702, 1976.
4. Adams, A. P., *et al.*: A case of massive aspiration of gastric contents during obstetric anesthesia; treatment by tracheostomy and prolonged intermittent positive pressure ventilation. Br. J. Anaesth., 41:176, 1969.
5. Alexander, I. G. S.: The ultrastructure of the pulmonary alveolar vessels in Mendelson's syndrome (acid pulmonary aspiration). Br. J. Anaesth., 40:408, 1968.
6. Alexander, J.: Thiopentone-suxamethonium mixture. [Correspondence] Br. J. Anaesth., 43:591, 1971.
7. Anderson, N.: Changes in intragastric pressure following administration of suxamethonium. Br. J. Anaesth., 34:363, 1962.
8. Aviet, T. A., and Crawford, J. S.: Serum magnesium levels and magnesium trisilicate therapy in labour. Br. J. Anaesth., 43:183, 1971.
9. Awe, C. W., Fletcher, W. S., and Jacob, S. W.: The pathophysiology of aspiration pneumonitis. Surgery, 60:232, 1966.
10. Baggish, M. S., and Hooper, S.; Aspiration as a cause of maternal death. Obstet. Gynecol., 43:327, 1974.
11. Bannister, W. K., Sattilaro, A. J., and Otis, R. D.: Therapeutic aspects of aspiration pneumonitis in experimental animals. Anesthesiology, 22:440, 1961.
11a. Bendixen, H. H., et al.: Respiratory Care. C. V. Mosby, St. Louis, 1965.
12. Bonica, J. J.: Principles and Practice of Obstetric Analgesia and Anesthesia. Philadelphia, F. A. Davis, 1967.
13. Bourne, J. G.: Anesthesia and the vomiting hazard. A safe method for obstetric and other emergencies. Anesthesia, 17:379, 1962.
14. Braasch, J. W., and Ellis, F. H.: The gastroesophageal sphincter mechanism. Surgery, 39:901, 1956.
15. Breivik, H., *et al.*: Normalizing low arterial CO_2 tension during mechanical ventilation. Chest, 63:525, 1973.
16. Brown, H. G.: The applied anatomy of vomiting. Br. J. Anaesth., 35:136, 1963.
17. Chodoff, P., and Stella, J.: Use of C1-581, a phencyclidine derivative for obstetric anesthesia. Anesth. Analg. 45:527, 1966.
18. Clark, G. G., and Riddoch, M. E.: Observations on the human cardia at operation. Br. Anaesth., 34:875, 1962.
19. Crawford, J. S.: The anaesthetist's contribution to maternal mortality. Br. J. Anaesth., 42:70, 1079.
20. ———: Anaesthesia for obstetric emergencies. Br. J. Anaesth., 43:864, 1971.

21. Creamer, B., Harrison, G. K., and Pierce, J. W.: Further observations on the gastroesophageal junction. Thorax, *14*:132, 1959.

22. Cull, W. A.: Twenty-four-hour obstetric anesthesia coverage. J.A.M.A., *172*:416, 1960.

23. Cull, W. A., and Hingson, R. A.: Dedication, education and organization in the round-the-clock-staffing of a modern obstetrical analgesia and anesthesia service. Bull, Mat. Welf., *4*:17, 1957.

24. Cullen, D.: The effect of pretreatment with nondepolarizing muscle relaxants on the neuromuscular blocking action of succinylcholine. Anesthesiology, *35*:572, 1971.

25. Dines, D. E., Baker, W. G., and Scantland, W. A.: Aspiration pneumonitis—Mendelson's syndrome. J.A.M.A., *176*:229, 1961.

26. Dornhurst, A. C., Harrison, K., and Pierce, J. W.: Observations on the normal esophagus and cardia. Lancet, *1*:695, 1954.

27. Edwards, G., and Hingson, R. A.: Deaths associated with anesthesia, A report on 1000 cases. Anesthesia, *2*:194, 1956.

28. Fanning, G. L.: The efficiency of cricoid pressure in regurgitation of gastric contents. Anesthesiology, *32*:535, 1970.

29. Fisher, C. W.: Prevention of aspiration of gastric contents. Anesthesiology, *14*:506, 1953.

30. Flowers, C. S., Rudolph, A. J., and Desmond, M. M.: Diazepam (Valium) as an adjunct in obstetric analgesia. Obstet. Gynecol., *34*:68, 1969.

31. Ghoneim, M. M., and Long, J. P.: Interaction between magnesium and other neuromuscular blocking agents. Anesthesiology, *32*:23, 1970.

32. Goodman, L., and Gilman, A.: The Pharmacological Basis of Therapeutics. Ed. 4. New York, Macmillan, 1970.

33. Greenan, J.: The cardio-esophageal junction. Br. J. Anaesth., *33*:432, 1961.

34. Grenvik, A.: Respiratory, circulatory and metabolic effects of respirator treatment. A clinical study in postoperative thoracic surgical patients. Acta Anesthesiol. Scand.[Suppl.]*19*, 1, 1966.

35. Guiffrida, J. G., and Bizzari, D.: Intubation of the esophagus. Am. J. Surg., *93*:329, 1957.

36. Guyton, A. C.: Textbook of Medical Physiology, Ed. 3. Philadelphia, W. B. Saunders, 1967.

37. Hall, C. C.: Aspiration pneumonitis, an obstetric hazard. J.A.M.A., *114*:728, 1940.

38. Hamelberg, W., and Bosomworth, P. P.: Aspiration pneumonitis: experimental studies and clinical observations. Anesth. Analg., *43*:669, 1964.

39. Hausmann, W., and Lunt, R. L.: Problem of treatment of peptic aspiration pneumonia following obstetric anesthesia (Mendelson's syndrome). J. Obstet. Gynaecol. Br. Emp., *62*:509, 1955.

40. Hodges, R. J. H., *et al.*: General anesthesia for operative obstetrics with special reference to the use of thiopentone and suxamethonium. Br. J. Anesth., *31*:152, 1959.

41. Holdsworth, J. D., Furness, R. M. B., and Roulston, R. G.: A comparison of apomorphine and stomach tubes for emptying the stomach before general anesthesia in obstetrics. Br. J. Anaesth., *46*:526, 1974.

42. Holmes, J. M.: Prevention of inhaled vomit during obstetric anesthesia. J. Obstet. Gynaecol. Br., Emp., *63*:239, 1956.

42a. Hunt, J. N., and Murray, F. A.: Gastric function in pregnancy. J. Obstet. Gynec. Brit. Commonw. *65*:78, 1958.

43. Inkster, J. S.: The induction of anesthesia in patients likely to vomit with special reference to intestinal obstructpon. Br. J. Anaesth., *35*:160, 1963.

44. Ivankovic, A. D., Elam, J. O., and Huffman, J.: Effect of maternal hypercapnia on newborn infants. Am. J. Obstet. Gynecol., *107*:939, 1970.

45. Kausch, W.: Zur Narkose beim Ileus. Klin. Wochenschr., *40*:753, 1903.

46. Khawaja, A. A.: Thiopentone-suxamethonium mixture: a method for reducing the aspiration hazard during induction of anesthesia. Br. J. Anaesth., *43*:100, 1971.

47. Kosaka, Y., Takahashi, T., and Mark, L. C.: Intravenous thiobarbiturate anesthesia for cesarean section. Anesthesiology, *31*:489, 1969.

48. Kuchling, A., Joyce, T. A., and Cook, S.: The pulmonary lesion of antacid aspiration. American Society of Anesthesiologists. Annual Meeting, Pp. 281–282. 1975. Abstracts of Scientific Papers.

49. Lahiri, S. K., Thomas, T. A., and Hodgson, R. M. H.: Single-dose antacid therapy for the prevention of Mendelson's Syndrome. Br. J. Anaesth., *45*:1143, 1973.

50. LaSalvia, L. A., and Steffen, E. A.: Delayed gastric emptying time in labor. Am. J. Obstet. Gynecol., *59*:1075, 1950.

51. Lewinski, A.: Evaluation of methods employed in the treatment of the chemical pneumonitis of aspiration. Anesthesiology, *26*:37, 1965.

52. Lewis, R. T., Burgess, J. H., and Hampson, L. G.: Cardiorespiratory studies in critical illness. Changes in aspiration pneumonitis. Arch. Surg., *103*:336, 1971.

53. McCormick, P. W.: The severe pulmonary aspiration syndrome in obstetrics. Proc. R. Soc. Med., *59*:66, 1966.

54. Macintosh, R. R.: A cuffed stomach tube. Br. Med. J., *2*:545, 1951.

55. Marchand, P.: The gastro-esophageal "sphincter" and the mechanism of regurgitation. Br. J. Surg., *42*:504, 1954.

56. ———: A study of the forces productive of gastro-oesophageal regurgitation and herniation through the diaphragmatic hiatus. Thorax, *12*:189, 1957.

57. Marshall, B. M., and Gordon, R. A.: Vomiting regurgitation and aspiration in anesthesia. 1. Can. Anaesth. Soc. J., *5*:274, 1958.

58. Marx, G. F., Joshi, C. W., and Orkin, L. R.: Placenta transmission of nitrous oxide. Anesthesiology, *32*:429, 1970.

59. Maternal deaths. [Editorial] Br. Med. J.,*2*(1):319, 1966.

60. Mendelson, C. L.: Aspiration of stomach contents into lungs during obstetric anesthesia. Am. J. Obstet. Gynecol., *52*:191, 1946.

61. Merrill, R. B., and Hingson, R. A.: Study of incidence of maternal mortality from aspiration of

vomitus during anesthesia occurring in major obstetric hospitals in the United States. Anesth. Analg., *30*:121, 1951.

62. Miller, R. D.: Inhibition of succinylocholine induced increased intragastric pressure by nondepolarizing muscle relaxants. American Society of Anesthesiologists, Abstract of Scientific Paper, 1969.

63. Moore, J., McNabb, I. G., and Dundee, J. W.: Preliminary report of ketamine in obstetrics. Br. J. Anesth., *43*:779, 1971.

64. Morton, H., and Wylie, W.: Anesthesic deaths due to regurgitation or vomiting. Anesthesia, *6*:190, 1951.

65. Motoyama, E. K., *et al.*: The effect of changes in maternal pH and PCO_2 of fetal lambs. Anesthesiology, *28*:891, 1967.

66. Mucklow, R. G., and Larard D. G.: The effect of the inhalation of vomitus on the lungs: clinical considerations. Br. J. Anaesth., *35*:153, 1963.

67. Nicholl, R. M., Holland, E. L., and Brown, S. S.: Mendelson's syndrome: its treatment by tracheostomy and hydrocortisone. Br. Med. J., *2*:745, 1967.

68. O'Mullane, E. J.: Vomiting and regurgitation during anesthesia. Lancet, *1*:1209, 1954.

69. Phillips, O. C., *et al*: The role of anesthesia in obstetric mortality. Anesth. Analg., *40*:557, 1961.

70. Roberts, R. B., and Shirley, M. A.: The obstetrician's role in reducing the risk of aspiration pneumonitis, with particular reference to the use of oral antacids. Am. J. Obstet., Gynecol., *124*:611, 1976.

71. Roe, R. B.: The effect of suxamethonium on intragastric pressures. Anesthesia, *17*:179, 1962.

72. Salem, R.: Anesthetic management of patient with a "full stomach." A critical review. Anesth., Analg., *49*:47, 1970.

73. ———: Prevention of aspiration in pediatric anesthesia. Audio Digest, *13*:23, 1971.

74. Sellick, B. A.: Cricoid pressure to control regurgitation of stomach contents during induction of anaesthesia. Lancet, *2*:404, 1961.

75. Sinclair, R. N.: Oesophageal cardiac and regurgitation. Br. J. Anesth., *31*:15, 1959.

76. Snow, R. G., and Nunn, J. F.: Induction of anesthesia in the foot down position with a full stomach. Br. J. Anaesth., *31*:493, 1959.

77. Spence, A. A., Moir, D. D. and Finlay, W. E. I.: Observations on intragastric pressure. Anaesthesia, *22*:249, 1967.

78. Stept, W. J., and Safar, P.: Rapid induction/intubation for prevention of gastric-content aspiration. Anesth., Analg., *49*:633, 1970.

79. Stevens, J. H.: Anaesthetic problems of intestinal obstruction in adults. Br. J. Anaesth. *36*:438, 1964.

80. Stiles, C. M., Stiles, O. R., and Denson, J. S.: A flexible fiber optic laryngoscope. J.A.M.A., *221*(11):1246, 1972.

81. Taylor, G., and Pryse-Davies, J.: Prophylactic use of antacids in the prevention of the acid-pulmonary-aspiration-syndrome (Mendelson's Syndrome). Lancet, *1*:228, 1966.

82. ———: Evaluation of endotracheal steroid therapy in acid pulmonary aspiration syndrome (Mendelson's syndrome). Anesthesiology, *29*:17, 1968.

83. Taylor, P. A., and Towey, R. M.: The bronchofiberscope as an aid to endotracheal intubation. Br. J. Anaesth., *44*:611, 1972.

84. Teabeaut, J. R.: Aspiration of gastric contents, experimental study. Am. J. Pathol. *28*:51, 1952.

85. Walker, A. L., *et al.*: Report on Confidential Inquiries into Maternal Deaths in England and Wales, 1955–57. London, Her Majesty's Stationery Office, 1960.

86. Wamberg, K., and Zeskov, B.: Experimental studies of the course and treatment of aspiration pneumonia. Preliminary report. Anesth., Analg., *45*:230, 1966.

87. Weaver, D. C.: Preventing aspiration deaths during anesthesia. J.A.M.A., *188*:971, 1964.

88. Whillis, J.: Some observations on the anatomy and physiology of the lower oesophagus. Thesis for M. D. (Duneim), 1930.

89. White, R. T.: Apomorphine as emetic prior to obstetric anesthesia. Prevention of inhaled vomitus. Obstet. Gynecol., *14*:111, 1959.

90. White, W. D., Clark, J. M., and Stanley-Jones, G. H. M. [Correspondence] The efficiency of antacid therapy. Br. J. Anaesth., *48*:1117, 1976.

91. Williams, M., and Crawford, J. S.: Titration of secretion. Br. J. Anaesth., *4*:783, 1971.

92. Wylie, W. D.: The use of muscle relaxants at induction of anesthesia of patients with a full stomach. Br. J. Anaesth., *35*:168, 1963.

9

Amniotic Fluid Embolism and Disseminated Intravascular Coagulopathy

Ezzat Abouleish, M.D.

DEFINITION

Amniotic fluid embolism is the syndrome resulting from the infusion of amniotic fluid into the maternal circulation, causing acute cardiorespiratory failure which may be followed by a coagulation disorder. The coagulation disorder will be referred to in this chapter as disseminated intravascular coagulopathy (DIC); other synonyms used in the literature are consumption coagulopathy, intravascular coagulation, and the defibrination syndrome.

The anesthesiologist is commonly present when amniotic fluid embolism occurs and usually plays a major role in its treatment. Therefore, he should thoroughly understand the syndrome including the coagulation disorder.

HISTORY

Amniotic fluid embolism was first described by Richard Meyer in 1926. At postmortem, he noticed the presence of fetal debris in the pulmonary blood vessels of a young woman who had died suddenly in labor. The following year amniotic fluid embolism was induced experimentally in

animals by Warden.[15] However, it was not until 1941 that the syndrome was clearly described by Stainer and Lushbaugh.[60a] They presented the first eight documented cases of amniotic fluid embolism. Furthermore, they intravenously administered meconium and amniotic fluid to animals, thus producing anaphylactic shock, pulmonary edema, and death. Microscopic examination of the small arteries, arterioles, and capillaries of the pulmonary vascular bed of the animals revealed the same embolic material as that seen in their first eight patients. Hence, the syndrome became a distinct clinical entity which should be suspected in any case of sudden cardiorespiratory collapse during labor, delivery, or immediately thereafter.[59]

INCIDENCE

The incidence of fatal amniotic fluid embolism varies between 1:10,000 to 1:25,000 deliveries.[1,15,22,59] However, there are many cases of minor amniotic fluid emboli that pass unnoticed or cause few problems, thus being difficult to document.

As the overall maternal death rate has decreased in recent decades, amniotic fluid

160

embolism as a cause of death has increased in relative incidence and importance. Indeed, in some obstetrical medical centers, it is the leading cause of death.[1,59] Fifty per cent of patients who survive the amniotic fluid embolism develop disseminated intravascular coagulopathy, and 50 per cent of these bleed to death. Therefore it is essential to understand the physiology of blood coagulation and lysis, as well as disseminated intravascular coagulopathy.

PHYSIOLOGY AND PHYSIOPATHOLOGY RELATED TO AMNIOTIC FLUID EMBOLISM AND DISSEMINATED INTRAVASCULAR COAGULOPATHY

BLOOD COAGULATION

The platelets are the first components of the blood to react to injury of a blood vessel. Initially, platelets aggregate due to exposure to collagen of the injured blood vessel. The platelets release adenosine diphosphate (ADP) which causes additional platelets to aggregate and adhere to each other to form the hemostatic plug. Serotonin is also released and causes vasoconstriction (Figure 9-1).

The platelet aggregation and the vasoconstriction stop the bleeding temporarily; but fibrin, the end product of a complex interaction of the multiple clotting factors, is necessary for complete cessation of bleeding. This coagulation process is accompanied by another process, fibrinolysis, to prevent excessive deposition of fibrin and to keep the blood clot localized to the site of injury.

The various factors that interact to cause blood coagulation are listed below. They have been assigned numbers, not according to their order in the process of blood coagulation, but according to the order of their discovery. Three elements for blood coagulation are considered "labile," that is, easily destroyed by storage or common blood bank techniques. These elements are the platelets, factor V, and factor VIII. The platelets take part in every stage of the clotting mechanism. They accelerate the clotting steps and take part in activating factors V, IX, and X. They are also essential for clot retraction. Platelet function and survival are markedly compromised if stored at refrigerator temperatures. In platelet-concentrate bags, their survival and function are preserved for 72 hours if

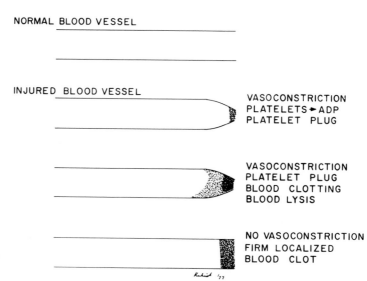

Fig. 9-1. Hemostasis after blood vessel injury.

kept at 22° C. Fresh-frozen plasma preserves factors V and VIII as well as the stable plasma factors which include factors II, VII, IX, X, XI, XII, and XIII. Factor XIII is responsible for clot stabilization and, when deficient, causes late (postoperative) bleeding. There is no factor presently designated VI. Ca$^+$ is called factor IV. Factor III is the thromboplastin released from injured tissues, and factor I is fibrinogen.[56] Plasma deficiencies of the vitamin-K-dependent factors (II, VII, IX, X) can be treated with liquid or fresh-frozen plasma; intravenous vitamin K can be used but is slow and does not even begin to work until 4 hours after its administration.[56] Plasminogen and all blood coagulation factors except platelets and factor VIII are probably made in the liver.[4]

Figure 9-2 shows the elements in the order of their activation during blood

International Nomenclature for Blood Coagulation Factors

Factor I,	fibrinogen
Factor II,	prothrombin
Factor III,	tissue factor (tissue thromboplastin)
Factor IV,	calcium
Factor V,	proaccelerin
Factor VI,	*Obsolete*
Factor VII,	proconvertin
Factor VIII,	antihemophilic factor (AHF)
Factor IX,	plasma thromboplastin component (PTC; also called Christmas factor)
Factor X,	Stuart-Prower factor
Factor XI,	plasma thromboplastin antecedent (PTA)
Factor XII,	Hageman factor
Factor XIII,	fibrin stabilizing factor (FSF)

coagulation. *The first step* is the formation of prothrombin activator through a series of cascade reactions initiated by a tissue factor.[20] *The second step* is the formation of thrombin by the action of prothrombin activator on prothrombin. *The third step* is the

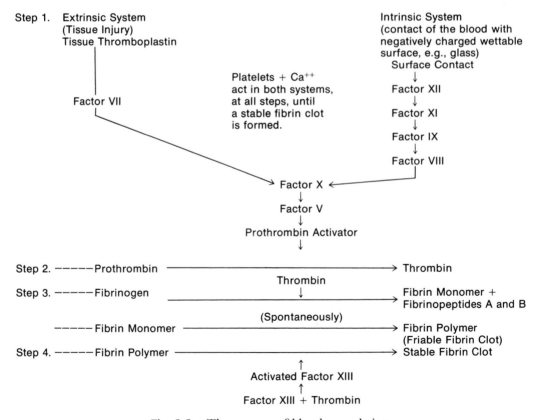

Fig. 9-2. The process of blood coagulation.

formation of the fibrin clot. Thrombin acts on fibrinogen to form fibrin monomer and fibrinopeptides A and B which are produced as by-products and have heparinlike activity. Normally these peptides A and B, which help to prevent excessive coagulation, are removed easily from the circulation and have no systemic effect. They are also small in size and produce no immunologic reaction. The fibrin monomer then spontaneously changes its configuration into fibrin polymer which is still friable. *The fourth step* is the formation of a stable firm blood clot. Factor XIII, which is activated by thrombin, acts on the fibrin threads to make them interlace and form a strong fibrin clot. It is interesting that factor XIII is also important for the activation of fibroblasts, and its deficiency not only affects blood clotting but also the scartissue formation. *Thrombin has multiple actions.* Its main action, as mentioned before, is to convert fibrinogen into fibrin. It also activates factor XIII, acts on the platelets to cause further release of ADP and serotonin, and activates another system, the fibrinolysis or blood lysis system, which normally prevents excessive coagulation.

FIBRINOLYSIS

In the plasma there is an inactive globulin fraction called plasminogen. It becomes activated into a proteolytic enzyme called plasmin by many factors, e.g., thrombin, activated factor XII, tissue factors including placental extracts, urokinase, and amniotic fluid (Fig. 9-3). Normally plasmin action is localized to prevent excessive fibrin deposition. Plasmin is neutralized by an albumin fraction called antiplasmin, and thus it is not normally detected in the systemic circulation. Normally the coagulation and fibrinolytic mechanisms are in a state of dynamic equilibrium which keeps the vascular compartment intact and patent: the coagulation system lays down fibrin to seal any gaps in the vascular endothelium, and the fibrinolytic mechanism prevents excessive coagulation and removes the deposits of fibrin after they have served their hemostatic function.

In pathologic conditions plasmin is formed in excessive quantities. Thus, the antiplasmin is no longer sufficient to inhibit its effect and the plasmin attacks not only fibrin but also other blood coagulation constituents, namely fibrinogen and factors V and VIII. The result of lysis of fibrin and fibrinogen is the formation of fibrin and fibrinogen split products, which are also called fibrin and fibrinogen degradation products. They are designated as X, Y, D, and E fragments.[21,38] The molecular weight of fibrinogen is 350,000 while that of the fibrin and fibrinogen split

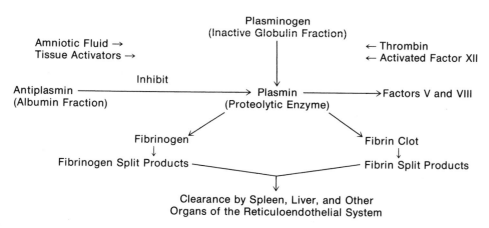

Fig. 9-3.   Fibrinolysis.

products ranges between 30,000 and 50,000. Early in the process of fibrinolysis these split products are phagocytosed by the reticuloendothelial system, and thus are not easily detected in the circulation. When their production becomes excessive, they circulate and prevent blood coagulation by having an antithrombin action as well as by preventing the aggregation of platelets and the polymerization of fibrin.[25]

DISSEMINATED INTRAVASCULAR COAGULOPATHY

Under certain pathologic conditions there is hypercoagulability of the blood leading to excessive and widespread coagulation. As a compensatory mechanism, in order to remove the excessive deposition of fibrin from the circulatory bed and to restore the perfusion of tissues, the fibrinolytic system is activated into a process called secondary fibrinolysis. However, the associated excessive plasmin liberation leads to destruction of certain blood coagulation factors and to the circulation of excessive amounts of fibrin and fibrinogen split products. *Therefore, with disseminated intravascular coagulopathy there is excessive bleeding due to:* (1) consumption of the coagulation factors as a result of the hypercoagulatory state of the blood (there may also be an associated decreased production of these factors[58]); (2) the circulation of heparinlike substances such as fibrin and fibrinogen split products and fibrinopeptides A and B preventing blood coagulation; and (3) the breakdown of the blood clots by plasmin.

Disseminated intravascular coagulopathy can occur as a result of many conditions. Shock itself can cause DIC or accentuate it through the stagnation of blood, acidosis, and hypoxia.[27] Hemolyzed blood such as with mismatched blood transfusion, overheated blood, or snake venom can cause DIC.[40] Generalized sepsis, whether bacterial, viral, or rickettsial, causes damage to capillary endothelium and activation of blood

coagulation by the toxins. Neoplasms cause DIC by the chronic release of low-grade thromboplastic materials from the tumors. DIC can also occur secondary to malignant hyperpyrexia, extensive burns, drug reactions, or cardiopulmonary bypass.[29,55]

If the causative factor for DIC is removed, the fibrin and fibrinogen split products will be cleared by the reticuloendothelial system within 2 to 19 hours. The coagulation factors will return to near-normal levels in 12 hours provided the liver is normal and its perfusion is adequate. A rise in the platelet count to normal value may take as long as a week[58] but generally rises quickly with effective therapy.

Primary fibrinolysis refers to activation of the fibrinolytic system without concomitant disseminated coagulation.[39] This condition is very rare and is associated with primary hepatoma and hepatic cavernous hemangioma, and with metastatic carcinoma of the prostate. It can be difficult to differentiate primary fibrinolysis from DIC with secondary fibrinolysis. However, primary fibrinolysis is accompanied by a normal platelet count because of the absence of extensive coagulation in the system, and negative ethanol and protamine gel tests (see later).

EFFECTS OF PREGNANCY, PARTURITION, AND PUERPERIUM ON BLOOD COAGULATION

Effects of Pregnancy on Blood Coagulation

During pregnancy the platelet count does not show significant changes from the normal levels of between 200,000 to 300,000 per mm.[3] of blood. However, the platelet levels are sometimes elevated in healthy pregnant women at term;[41] therefore, a "low normal" value should be regarded with suspicion. On the other hand, fibrinogen and the other blood coagulation factors increase progressively throughout pregnancy;[46] e.g., the normal nonpregnant level of fibrinogen is 250 to 300 mg. per cent; during pregnancy it increases to between 400 and 500 mg. per cent, and increases even more with toxemias of pregnancy. Fibrinogen levels at or below 300 mg. per cent at term should be considered abnormally low. Considering the increase in the blood volume and the hemodilution, there is a total increase of about 40 per cent of the blood coagulation factors during pregnancy as compared with the non-pregnant state. This increase in the coagulation factors is associated with a decrease in the fibrinolytic system.[8]

BLOOD COAGULATION CHANGES WITH PARTURITION

Parturition presents a serious challenge to the integrity of the vascular component. As the placenta separates, the large and numerous maternal blood vessels at the placental site must close, or otherwise fatal hemorrhage can occur. The contraction of the myometrium—"the living ligatures" of the uterus—plays an important role in controlling blood loss at delivery, helped by an efficient coagulation mechanism. This heavy demand on the coagulation factors is provided by their raised levels during pregnancy.

The clotting time of blood obtained from uterine veins is significantly shortened compared to the clotting time obtained from a peripheral vessel or from the same uterine vein prior to placental separation. There is also a decrease in fibrinogen level in blood obtained from uterine as well as systemic veins due to the increased usage of fibrinogen and the deposition of fibrin at the placental sites. There is also increased fibrinolytic activity during the third stage of labor. This is reflected in a fall in plasminogen level as well as a rise in fibrin and fibrinogen split products in blood of both the systemic and the uterine veins.[8,9] In the hemorrhagic complications of pregnancy, particularly abruptio placentae, much more striking changes in blood coagulation occur both in the uterine and systemic veins.[7]

BLOOD COAGULATION DURING THE PUERPERIUM

During the two weeks after delivery, levels of the coagulation factors, including fibrinogen, platelets, and factor VIII, progressively increase. For example, the highest level of plasma fibrinogen is found 10 to 14 days following parturition, with a mean level of 536 mg. per cent in the peripheral blood.[9] The plasminogen level which decreased during the placental separation reaches normal value in a few hours and remains virtually unchanged during the postpartum period. These changes are important predisposing factors for postpartum thromboembolic complications which are 3 to 4 times higher than during pregnancy. The usual increase in the fibrin and fibrinogen split products, which is maximum at the sixth to the ninth postpartum day, may reflect increased lysis of the intravascular fibrin deposits.

AMNIOTIC FLUID

FUNCTIONS

During fetal development, the amniotic fluid serves both as a mechanical cushion against external trauma to the fetus and as a medium for its free mobility.[19] The fluid also acts as a thermal insulator against extremes of temperatures as well as a reservoir for fetal wastes. Nutritive elements such as lipids, carbohydrates, and proteins, as well as electrolytes could be incorporated into the fetus from the amniotic fluid through swallowing and intestinal absorption.

VOLUME

The amniotic fluid gradually increases during pregnancy to reach a maximum of 1,000 ml. At 38 weeks of gestation, the total exchange of amniotic fluid is about 500 ml./hour.[45]

COMPOSITION

Early in pregnancy amniotic fluid is a dialysate of the maternal serum. Near term it is hypotonic due to dilution by the very hypotonic fetal urine. It has a low concentration of dextrose (10 to 60 mg.%) which increases with diabetes mellitus (20 to 140 mg.%). It has a very low Po_2, a high Pco_2, and a low pH (from 6.9 to 7.15). The blood gases of amniotic fluid do not correlate with the fetal condition. It has no fibrinogen. The total lipids are 50 to 60 mg. per cent, with 50 per cent in the form of fatty acids. Amniotic fluid contains prostaglandins, a group of vasoactive hormones, some of which are capable of producing peripheral vasodilatation and pulmonary vasoconstriction.[34] The cells in the amniotic fluid are derived either from the fetus or the amnion. At term the fetal squamous cells constitute 50 per cent of all the cell population. Amniotic fluid usually contains meconium in the presence of acute or chronic fetal hypoxia; this is the result of the hypoxic relaxation of the fetal anal sphincter or due to vagal gastrointestinal stimulation.[52] Amniotic fluid may contain mucin which is also derived from the fetal intestinal tract and essentially represents contamination of amniotic fluid by meconium. Fetal hair (lanugo hair) and fat from vernix caseosa can be detected in the amniotic fluid. The presence of the fetal squames, meconium, mucin and/or lanugo hair in the maternal circulation is diagnostic of amniotic fluid embolism. However, these materials of fetal origin require special stains and may be missed if regular staining techniques are used.[15,47]

PATHOGENESIS OF AMNIOTIC FLUID EMBOLISM

For amniotic fluid embolism to occur, amniotic fluid has to gain access to the maternal circulation. Therefore, *the membranes must be ruptured at some point.* In those cases in which it has been stated that the membranes were intact, it is likely that they had been torn at the placental margin.[14] The force of expulsion causes the membranes to tear at the junction of the part fixed to the placenta and the mobile or bulging portion.

There should be a breach in the maternal circulation in a vicinity close to the site of ruptured membranes through which amniotic fluid enters. The usual described site is a laceration of an endocervical vein produced by the rapid dilatation of the cervix.[54] In abruptio placentae, placenta previa, as well as in complete or partial tear of the uterine wall, maternal blood may gain access to amniotic fluid and vice versa.[14]

Once a communication is established between the amniotic fluid and the maternal circulation, force is required to push amniotic fluid into the circulation. This is usually achieved by the uterine contractions raising the intrauterine pressure. Therefore, it is classically stated that amniotic fluid embolism is associated with exceptionally strong uterine contractions whether spontaneous or induced. Blunt trauma to the abdomen (e.g., automobile accident) was once reported to initiate the incident.[44] *When amniotic fluid enters the maternal circulation it produces three things:* first, pulmonary embolism; second, disseminated intravascular coagulopathy; and third, uterine atony.

PULMONARY EMBOLISM

As amniotic fluid reaches the pulmonary vascular bed, it causes mechanical obstruction of the lumen and chemical irritation of the endothelium (Fig. 9-4). The chemical irritation causes (1) endothelial swelling which adds to the mechanical obstruction, (2) reflex pulmonary arteriolar spasm of the affected blood vessels as well as the unaffected ones, (3) bronchospasm, and (4) attraction of platelets which aggregate and initiate a coagulation process, increase the mechanical obstruction, and augment the chemical irritation. The net result is acute pulmonary hypertension, leading to reflex

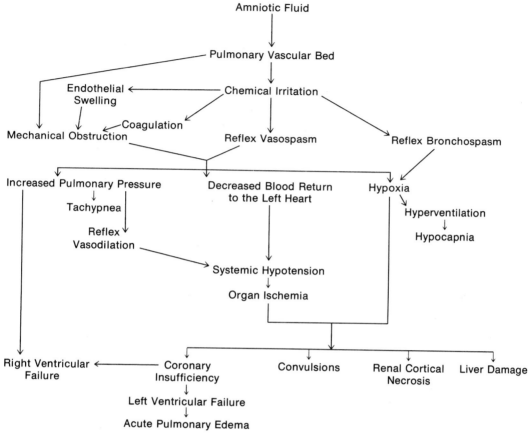

Fig. 9-4. Pathogenesis of the cardiopulmonary effects of amniotic fluid embolism.

tachypnea, peripheral vasodilation, and systemic hypotension.[54] Due to increased pulmonary resistance there is an added right ventricular strain which may lead to acute heart failure. Owing to the block in the pulmonary circulation there is decreased blood return to the left side of the heart, leading to diminished cardiac output, hypotension, and ischemia of visceral organs, particularly the heart and brain, which may lead to acute left ventricular failure and convulsions. As a result of the diminished and uneven perfusion of the alveoli and the associated bronchospasm, there is a deranged ventilation to perfusion ratio (V/Q) with subsequent low Pao$_2$ and tissue hypoxia.[59] As a result of hypoxia, hyperventilation occurs, leading to hypocapnia. Acute pulmonary edema

may ultimately result from acute heart failure and the augmenting effect of hypoxia on the capillary leakage.

DISSEMINATED INTRAVASCULAR COAGULOPATHY

As amniotic fluid enters the maternal circulation it initiates blood coagulation and fibrinolysis, thus producing DIC. Both *in vivo* and *in vitro* studies have shown that amniotic fluid has a strong blood coagulant effect.[15,16,63] It activates factor X, an effect similar to that of Russell's venom.[16,49] It also can activate the lysis system.[60] Therefore, amniotic fluid causes liberation of plasmin indirectly through excessive formation of thrombin and directly by acting on plasminogen (Fig. 9-5). The first vessels

Actions of Amniotic Fluid Embolism		Drugs That Can Be Used
A. Hypercoagulation	Amniotic fluid ↓ Prothrombin activator ↓ Prothrombin → Thrombin ↓ Fibrinogen → Fibrin	*Heparin:* inhibits blood coagulation at all stages (requires antithrombin III)
B. Fibrinolysis	Amniotic fluid + Thrombin ↓ Plasminogen → Plasmin	*Epsilon aminocaproic acid* (Amicar): antiplasminogen *Apritonin* (Trasylol): antiplasmin

Fig. 9-5.   Actions of amniotic fluid on blood coagulation, and the drugs used for disseminated intravascular coagulopathy.

exposed to amniotic fluid are the uterine veins. DIC in them leads to uterine bleeding owing to lysis of the blood clots at the placental site and increased venous pressure.

UTERINE ATONY

The association of hypotension and increased pressure in the uterine veins leads to decreased uterine perfusion, and subsequently uterine atony with further postpartum bleeding. Uterine atony can also be due to a direct depressant effect of amniotic fluid on the uterine muscles.[14]

THE CAUSATIVE CONSTITUENTS IN AMNIOTIC FLUID RESPONSIBLE FOR THE PRODUCTION OF THE AMNIOTIC FLUID EMBOLISM SYNDROME

THE PARTICULATE MATTERS IN AMNIOTIC FLUID

The particulate matters in amniotic fluid are the squames, meconium, mucin, and lanugo hair. There is evidence that they cause both mechanical obstruction and chemical irritation, and are always present in the pulmonary circulation in fatal cases. However, amniotic fluid embolism can be experimentally produced before or after removal of these particulate matters.[3] Moreover, there are few squames in the amniotic fluid before the 32nd week of

pregnancy,[33] and despite of this, amniotic fluid embolism has been described in a patient whose gestation was only 18 weeks.[63]

THE FAT CONTENT IN AMNIOTIC FLUID

As described before, amniotic fluid contains 50 to 60 mg. per cent of lipids, and half of them are in the form of fatty acids. It is not known whether or not the syndrome of pulmonary embolism is due to these lipids or how much is their contribution.

PROSTAGLANDINS IN AMNIOTIC FLUID

As mentioned before, amniotic fluid contains prostaglandins. The role of these vasoactive substances in the syndrome of amniotic fluid embolism has yet to be explored.

PLACENTAL TISSUES

Both the placenta and decidua are known to have high concentrations of thromboplastinlike materials.[11] These substances have been considered to play an essential role in producing postpartum hemostasis following the separation of the placenta.[9] At the same time, entry of these thromboplastinlike materials in large quantities into the maternal circulation may be implicated as the mechanism responsible for DIC in obstetrics. In the rhesus monkey, the intravenous injection of a cell-free homogenate of placental tissue causes cardiovascular collapse, apnea, and extensive blood clotting in the vascular tree.[42] The effect is dose-related. The prior administration of a small dose of placental extract or heparin protects the animal from the adverse effect of subsequent large doses of placental extract by preventing blood coagulation. It could be that tissues from damaged, degenerated, or necrotic placenta reach the maternal circulation and initiate intravascular coagulopathy in some cases of abruptio placentae, intrauterine salt infusion, or fetal death.[42]

Experimental Amniotic Fluid Embolism

Animal studies of amniotic fluid infusion are conflicting and inconclusive, perhaps because of species differences. Intravenous injection of human amniotic fluid into dogs produced systemic hypotension and pulmonary hypertension.[3] However, a less pronounced effect occurred when dogs were injected with autogenous amniotic fluid.

In ewes, the syndrome of cardiopulmonary collapse followed intravenous administration of autogenous amniotic fluid, whether or not amniotic fluid was filtered.[54] On the other hand, no changes were observed in cardiovascular and respiratory systems following intravenous infusion of autogenous amniotic fluid in the rhesus monkey.[2]

PATHOLOGY

The Lungs

The postmortem examination of the lungs of patients who die as a result of amniotic fluid embolism shows acute pulmonary edema in 70 per cent of the cases.[47] Focal atelectasis with areas of acute emphysema occurs in 40 per cent of cases. There is also infiltration with polymorphonuclear leukocytes. Utilizing special stains, amniotic fluid debris is readily identifiable in pulmonary arterioles and small arteries (Fig. 9-6). Mucin is found in all cases and fetal squames can be identified in 80 per cent of cases. No correlation has been found between the degree of embolization and the severity of the acute episode or the subsequent clinical course.

The Uterus

There may be signs of uterine laceration or rupture. Amniotic fluid debris in the uterine veins and venules can be detected in 50 per cent of cases (Fig. 9-7).

The Heart

There is marked dilatation of the right ventricle. Amniotic fluid debris may be found in the right side of the heart.

Other Organs

Other organs usually show signs of hypoxia. Very rarely amniotic fluid debris can be identified in these organs.

PREDISPOSING FACTORS TO AMNIOTIC FLUID EMBOLISM AND DISSEMINATED INTRAVASCULAR COAGULOPATHY

Patient's Age

The age ranges from 20 to 42 years, with an average age of 32 years.[47] Sixty per cent of the cases of amniotic fluid embolism occur in patients who are over 30 years of age. With increasing age, the placenta can be diseased, thus becoming rich in thromboplastins. However, amniotic fluid embolism can occur in any age.

Parity

Amniotic fluid embolism is more common in multipara; only 10 per cent of cases are nulliparous.

Gestation Age

Classically, the patient is full-term and in active labor. However, amniotic fluid em-

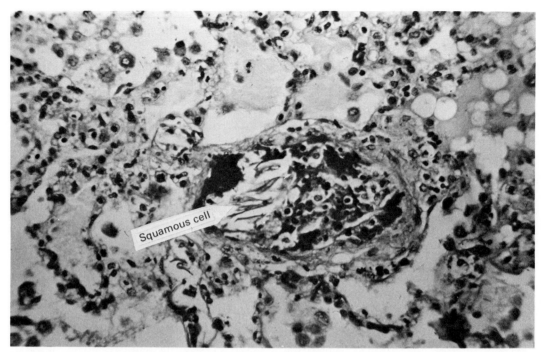

Fig. 9-6.   In the lung: squamous cells in a pulmonary vessel and pulmonary edema. (Abouleish, E.: Amniotic fluid embolism: report of a fatal case. Anesth. Analg., *53*:549, 1974)

bolism can occur in a patient who is not in labor,[47] and even at midtrimester.[63]

Course of Labor

The labor is usually described as "hard," "tumultuous," or "rapid," i.e., associated with either spontaneous or induced strong uterine contractions. Such a rapid course produces favorable conditions for embolism by causing tearing of the endocervical veins, rupturing the membranes, and pumping amniotic fluid into the maternal circulation. However, amniotic fluid embolism has been described in patients with a normal course of labor.[15]

Size of the Fetus

In early literature amniotic fluid embolism was described to be associated with a large fetus. However, the size of the fetus in most cases is within the normal range.[47]

Abruptio Placentae

Amniotic fluid embolism is associated with abruptio placentae in 45 per cent of the cases. The mechanisms are the consumption of the blood coagulation factors due to the separation of the placenta and accumulation of a large blood clot,[48] the breach in the maternal circulation through which amniotic fluid can gain access, and the hypertonic uterus. Abruptio placentae is usually associated with toxemia which is another important predisposing factor.

Toxemias of Pregnancy

Preeclampsia and eclampsia create favorable conditions for amniotic fluid embolism and DIC. The blood coagulation factors are elevated, the placenta may separate, the uterus may become hyperirritable, and the fetus may be dead. In fact DIC is sometimes considered the pathogenesis of severe toxemia.[4]

Meconium Staining

In 35 per cent of the patients who died of amniotic fluid embolism, meconium

Fig. 9-7. Squamous cells in a uterine vein. (Abouleish, E.: Amniotic fluid embolism: report of a fatal case. Anesth. Analg., *53*:549, 1974)

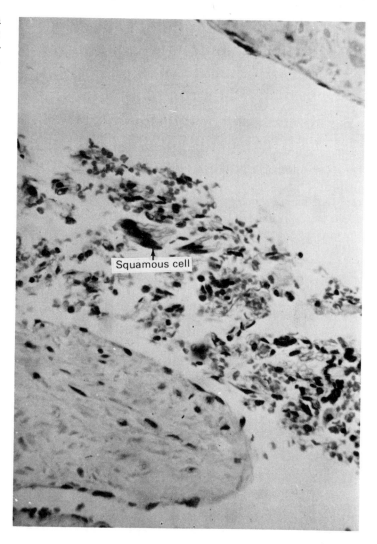

Squamous cell

staining of the amniotic fluid prior to embolization was described.

Dead Fetus

Antepartum coagulation defect occurs in approximately 25 per cent of cases of prolonged retention of a dead fetus *in utero*.[15] A dead fetus is present in 40 per cent of fatal cases of amniotic fluid embolism: 75 per cent of which show evidence of fetal death prior to embolization, and 25 per cent die during the course of the disease.

If a dead fetus is retained for more than 3 to 4 weeks there is a gradual decline of the maternal fibrinogen level which may lead to severe bleeding at delivery.[53] Moreover, there is a threefold increase in diffusion through the amniotic membranes of a dead fetus when compared with those of a normal fetus. The former membranes are also friable, and their strength and elasticity are markedly reduced.[17] As a result of these changes there is increased formation of thromboplastins from the dead fetus and placenta, and enhanced diffusion through the membranes which also tear easily allowing the escape of amniotic fluid.

Intra-amniotic Infusion of Hypertonic Saline to Terminate Pregnancy During the Second Trimester

The use of this method to terminate pregnancy can lead to DIC.[6,10,13] Most of these patients exhibit laboratory evidence suggestive of activation of the blood coagulation with a mild secondary fibrinolysis. One out of every 1500 cases develops severe coagulopathy requiring blood transfusion. The peak of coagulation abnormalities usually occurs within 24 hours after the saline infusion and returns to normal level by 48 hours.

The causes of coagulopathy in these cases are:

1. Death of the fetus which occurs within 1 hour following saline instillation

2. Injury to the placenta by the needle, especially if repeated attempts have been performed

3. Creation of a channel by the needle between the amniotic sac and the maternal blood vessels in the uterine wall

4. Swelling of the placenta very shortly after the saline injection which can lead to its tearing and the allowance of amniotic fluid to enter the maternal circulation.

Hysterotomy

The use of this surgical procedure for the termination of pregnancy during the second trimester, especially in elderly gravidas, can lead to DIC.[57] Fortunately, such a coagulation problem does not occur with cesarean section. During the years from 1968 through 1970, at Magee-Womens Hospital, 49 hysterotomies were performed with a 6.1 per cent incidence of DIC. During the same period, 1,270 cesarean sections were done with no coagulopathy complications. The cause of DIC in association with hysterotomy is not yet clear.

Use of Excessive Force in the Insertion of Uterine Catheters

The use of excessive force to insert an intra-amniotic catheter for recording the uterine activity may force amniotic fluid into the placental sinusoids or into an endocervical vein.[12]

Severe Abdominal Trauma

Severe abdominal trauma such as may occur in an automobile accident can force amniotic fluid into the maternal circulation, even in the absence of an occult uterine rupture.[44]

SIGNS AND SYMPTOMS
PRESENTING SYMPTOMS

In many cases amniotic fluid infusion passes unnoticed. For example, one of the reasons for shivering during parturition can be due to the introduction of a foreign protein into the maternal circulation associated with a minor amniotic fluid embolization.[50]

Massive amniotic fluid embolism strikes with sudden onset. The presenting symptoms are: (1) dyspnea and cyanosis in 50 per cent of cases; (2) sudden profound shock, out of proportion to the amount of bleeding, in 30 per cent of cases; and (3) convulsions, which may be preceded by hyperreflexia, apprehension or irrational behavior, in 20 per cent of cases.[47]

The clinical sequence of events, on the whole, can be divided into:

1. An initial stage of cardiopulmonary collapse with hypoxia of the brain

2. A following stage of coagulopathy manifested mainly as severe uterine bleeding.

RESPIRATORY MANIFESTATIONS

The respiratory manifestations of the initial stage of amniotic fluid embolism are dyspnea, tachypnea, hyperpnea, cyanosis, and bronchospasm. Later on, signs of acute pulmonary edema such as frothy sanguineous sputum and widespread rales and crepitation may occur.

CARDIOVASCULAR SIGNS AND SYMPTOMS

The cardiovascular signs and symptoms are hypotension, tachycardia, arrhythmia, and cardiac arrest in severe cases.

CENTRAL NERVOUS SYSTEM MANIFESTATIONS

Owing to hypoxia and hypotension, effects on the central nervous system, e.g. convulsions, are among the earliest manifestations of the syndrome. Ultimately, the patient may lapse into a coma, develop respiratory failure and die.

RENAL MANIFESTATIONS

If the patient survives the cardiorespiratory collapse, effects on the kidneys may present as renal cortical necrosis if hypotension is prolonged or DIC occurs.

DISSEMINATED INTRAVASCULAR COAGULOPATHY

DIC usually occurs postpartum within 90 minutes after the onset of embolization, but may be delayed up to 4 hours. It usually presents as uterine atony and bleeding which are resistant to treatment.

CHANGES IN ELECTROCARDIOGRAM

The ECG usually shows nonspecific changes. It may show tachycardia, arrhythmias, and right ventricular strain.

CHANGES SHOWN ON X-RAY

In massive pulmonary embolism, signs of increased right heart work load may be noted, including prominence of the proximal pulmonary artery plus right atrial and ventricular enlargement.[31]

LUNG SCAN

With amniotic fluid embolism, lung scan may show reduced radioactivity in some areas of the lung field up to 6 days after the accident.[12]

CHANGES IN CENTRAL VENOUS PRESSURE

With the onset of pulmonary hypertension and right ventricular strain there is increase in central nervous pressure. However, with the occurrence of bleeding the central venous pressure falls. If the catheter reaches the right side of the heart, aspirated blood may contain fetal squames or other debris.

LABORATORY TESTS

The blood coagulation factors are raised in pregnancy, and what are considered normal values for nonpregnant women are considered low with pregnancy. Moreover, the changes in the blood coagulation factors are more important than the absolute values. Therefore, when amniotic fluid embolism first strikes, the blood laboratory should be called immediately to obtain blood samples in order to have a baseline. Also, the blood bank should be alerted to crossmatch packed red cells and make available fresh-frozen plasma, platelet concentrates, and so on, and to be ready in case of bleeding.

For the diagnosis of amniotic fluid embolism, the clinical picture is the most important tool. The laboratory tests are used to confirm the diagnosis, guide the treatment, and help in the follow-up.

Quick Tests

In every case of suspected amniotic fluid embolism or DIC the following tests provide, with a reasonsble degree of confidence, a quick confirmation of the diagnosis of DIC. The results are usually obtained within 15 to 30 minutes:

Exposure of Blood to Thrombin. The patient's blood is added to a test tube containing thrombin to bypass all defects in coagulation before the fibrinogen transformation to fibrin. If the blood clots, the fibrinogen level is above 60 mg. per cent.

Blood Smear. As the *red blood cells* pass through the microcirculation, partially occluded by fibrin deposition, they become fragmented or abnormal in shape. The presence of fragmented red blood corpuscles, called helmet cells or schistocytes, is suggestive of DIC (Fig. 9-8). However, in early cases of DIC, these abnormal red cells are removed from the circulation by the spleen, and only when they are excessive do they appear in the peripheral circulation. If the patient has had a splenectomy, fragmented red blood corpuscles can be detected quite early in DIC. If the number of *platelets* in the blood field is much reduced and large platelets appear, DIC should be suspected. The appearance of these premature, large platelets indicates a greater platelet consumption with release of younger, larger platelets.

Platelet Count. The findings in the blood smear are confirmed by a platelet count. The critical level below which bleeding occurs is 50,000/mm.[3]

The Blood Clot. The clotting of 5 ml. of the patient's blood in a test tube is observed. If the blood clot is friable and small or the blood does not clot at all, DIC should be suspected.[43]

Coagulation Screen Profile

In any case of presumed DIC a coagulation screen profile is performed as early as possible, and always before heparin administration.

Early in DIC. Owing to the hyper-

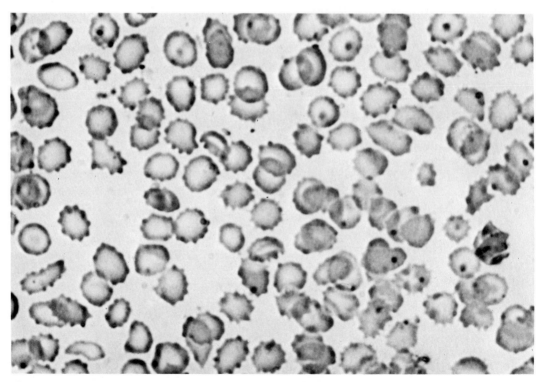

Fig. 9-8. A peripheral blood smear in disseminated intravascular coagulopathy showing deformed red blood corpuscles (schistocytes or helmet cells). Notice the film attached to the periphery of the red cells giving them a gearlike appearance.

coagulability stage of the blood, the prothrombin time and the partial thromboplastin time are faster than normal; the fibrinogen level and the platelet count may be still within normal ranges.

With Progress of DIC. The prothrombin time and the partial thromboplastin time become normal, then prolonged. The platelet count and the fibrinogen level progressively decrease owing to their consumption and the destructive effect of plasmin on fibrinogen. Therefore, the two most important blood tests in DIC are serial platelet count and fibrinogen level. They are not only important for diagnosis

but also for the follow-up. Fibrin and fibrinogen split products indicate the activation of the lysis system and the degree of its severity.

Special Tests

The blood coagulation tests are shown in Table 9-1. It usually takes from 45 minutes to 1 hour to obtain their results. Some of these tests will be explained in detail in order to understand their significance.

Tests for Fibrin and Fibrinogen Split Products. These split products, although smaller than fibrin or fibrinogen, are still

Table 9-1. Blood Coagulation Factors and Laboratory Tests for DIC

Laboratory Tests	*Normal Test Results*	*Test Results in Conditions in Which Gross Bleeding Occurs*	*Change With DIC*
Fibrinogen: Nonpregnant state	250 to 300 mg. %	<100 mg.%	
Pregnant state	400 to 500 mg.%	<150 mg. %	
Platelet count	200,000 to 300,000/mm.³	<50,000/mm.³	Lowered levels
Factor V	70 to 120%		
Factor VII	70 to 120%		
Factor VIII	70 to 120%		
Plasma Hb			Increased level
Prothrombin time	<12 sec.	>100 sec.	
Partial thromboplastin time	35 to 50 sec.	>100 sec.	
Thrombin time	15 to 20 sec.	>100 sec.	Prolonged times*
Bleeding time	1 to 7 min.	> 15 min.	
Coagulation time (Lee-White)	At 37°C.—6 to 12 min. At room temp.—10 to 18 minutes	> 20 min.	
Euglobulin lysis time		<1 hour (primary fibrinolysis) < 2 hours (secondary fibrinolysis)	Shortened time
Fibrinogen and fibrin split products			
Counter electrophoretic test (MISFI)	Negative	Positive	
Hemagglutination inhibition test	<16 μg./ml.	>200 μg./ml.	Positive tests
Staph clumping test	1:4 dilution	Positive at more dilutions	
Ethanol and protamine gel tests	Negative	Positive (secondary fibrinolysis) Negative (primary fibrinolysis)	

*In early DIC these times are shortened due to the hypercoagulation state.

big enough to be antigenic, which is important for their identification.

Counter Electrophoretic Test. The test most commonly used is called MISFI (Molecules Immunologically Similar to Fibrinogen). This test does not differentiate between fibrinogen and the split products. Therefore one has to get rid of fibrinogen from the blood sample before conducting the test. This is achieved by collecting blood in a special test tube, called the "fast" serum tube, containing thrombin and epsilon amniocaproic acid (EACA). The presence of thrombin will eliminate fibrinogen by changing it into a fibrin clot. Normally, the thrombin liberated will activate plasminogen in the clot to form plasmin which acts on fibrin and liberates split products, thus giving a false positive test. That is why EACA is added to inhibit plasminogen and prevent such a reaction. Therefore, normally the split products are not detected using this test which, if positive, is indicative of a pathologic condition.

Hemagglutination Inhibition Test. In contrast to the previous qualitative test, this test is quantitative and the fibrin and fibrinogen split products are estimated in μg./ml. In the normal nonpregnant state the level of these split products is 4 μg./ml. In normal pregnancy, the level increases up to 16 μg./ml. and remains at a slightly higher level for up to 6 weeks after delivery. In eclampsia it is high, up to 180 μg./ml. Bleeding occurs if the level exceeds 200 μg./ml.

Staph Clumping Test. Normally split products are detected with a dilution of less than 1:4. If this test is positive with more dilution, it is indicative of a pathologic condition. The degree of dilution serves as a quantitative test.

Ethanol and Protamine Gel Tests. In DIC a fibrin split product molecule combines with a fibrin monomer to form a complex. This combination breaks up in the presence of ethanol or protamine, and the liberated fibrin monomers join together to form a gel. Thus, if this test is positive, it not only shows the presence of fibrin split products, but also fibrin monomer molecules, indicating both hypercoagulation and fibrinolysis.

Euglobulin Lysis Time. If this time is short it signifies the presence of plasmin causing the lysis. If the time is less than 1 hour, primary fibrinolysis is suspected. If the time is less than 2 hours, it is indicative of DIC.

Plasma Hb. Owing to hemolysis of the trapped red blood corpuscles in the microthrombi of the small blood vessels, Hb is liberated and the free plasma Hb increases. After centrifugation of a blood sample, the serum may have a reddish shade rather than the characteristic straw color.

It is optimum to be able at any time to have a coagulation profile and consult a hematologist. However, such an ideal situation is not always present. Therefore, the previously described quick tests can confirm the clinical diagnosis. For performing the coagulation profile, blood samples are collected in a special series of test tubes under certain regulations from the specific blood laboratory. Blood is then centrifuged, decanted, and the serum or plasma is frozen until the hematologist is available.

THROMBOELASTOGRAPH

The thromboelastograph is a mechanical-optical system in which the blood sample is placed into a cup.[18,56] A steel cylinder attached to a torsion wire is lowered into the metal cup which is slowly oscillating. As the clot forms, the cylinder becomes attached to the oscillating cup by way of the fibrin strands. The oscillations of the cylinder are then transmitted to a mirror attached to the torsion wire. The mirror reflects a fixed light source into 2 scales, one a direct visual read-out and the other a reel of photographic film (Fig. 9-9). Therefore, the oscillations can be visually seen and

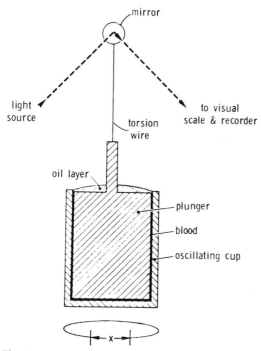

Fig. 9-9. Thromboelastograph. (Ryan, G. M., Boyan, C. P., and Howland, W. S.: Clotting problems during surgery. Surg. Clin. North Am., *49*:233, 1969)

recorded on the film. A rapid read-out graph can also be obtained using a special electronic attachment.[35] The thromboelastogram gives a picture of the blood coagulation as a whole (Fig. 9-10). If there is a

plasma coagulation factor deficiency or the patient is under anticoagulant therapy, the time necessary for initiation of the clot formation will be prolonged. On the other hand, if the blood is hypercoagulable, the onset of oscillations is shortened. The width of the bullet-shaped tracing depends on the elasticity and firmness of the blood clot. If there is platelet deficiency and/or decreased coagulation factors the degree of oscillations is limited. If there is lysis the oscillations will fade away quickly as a result of destruction of the fibrin threads (Fig. 9-11). The use of the thromboelastograph has been established in surgery;[28,30,56] its usefulness in obstetrics is yet to be determined.

DIFFERENTIAL DIAGNOSIS

Amniotic fluid embolism should be suspected in any obstetric patient who suddenly develops dyspnea, cyanosis, shock, and/or convulsions. However, amniotic fluid embolism does not always cause a generalized reaction. Thus, it should be considered in any case of postpartum uterine atony or bleeding diathesis, especially if associated with a dead fetus. Among the many conditions that can be mistaken for amniotic fluid embolism are:

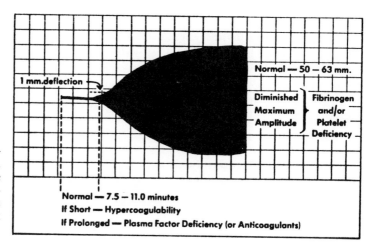

Fig. 9-10. A normal thromboelastogram. (Howland, W. S.: Use of halothane [Fluothane] in radical abdominal surgery. Clinical aspects of anesthesiology. Ayerst Laboratories, 1972)

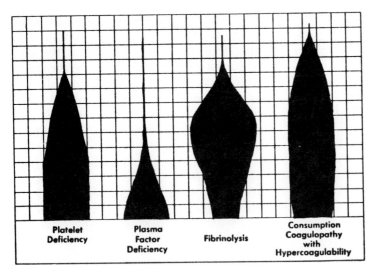

Fig. 9-11 Abnormal thromboelastogram. (Howland, W. S.: Use of halothane [Fluothane] in radical abdominal surgery. Clinical aspects of anesthesiology. Ayerst Laboratories, 1972)

Aspiration Pneumonitis

Aspiration pneumonitis causes cyanosis, tachypnea, tachycardia, hypotension, and acute pulmonary edema. However, it usually occurs in a patient who is unconscious or unable to cough, and there is some evidence of regurgitation or vomiting.

Local Anesthetic Drug Toxicity

Drug toxicity can cause apprehension followed by sudden onset of convulsions. However, the close temporal relationship between the drug administration and the onset of symptoms indicates the real cause of the syndrome.

Eclampsia

Eclampsia causes hyperreflexia, excitability, and convulsions. However, with eclampsia the blood pressure is elevated rather than lowered, there is usually a history of toxemia, and edema of the lower limbs or generalized edema may be present.

Cerebrovascular Accident Such as Subarachnoid Hemmorrhage

A cerebrovascular accident causes sudden onset of unconsciousness. However, the absence of central cyanosis and hypotension, the presence of lateralization, and the examination of the cerebrospinal fluid should help to reach the correct diagnosis.

Pulmonary Embolism Due to Other Causes

A thrombus can be dislodged from one of the lower limbs or the pelvic veins and cause pulmonary embolism. However, such a complication usually occurs later in the postpartum period and there may be evidence of venous thrombosis. Cardiac vulvular diseases may predispose to embolization, either into the systemic or pulmonary circulation. However, the history of cardiac disease and the examination of the patient should give a clue to the source of the problem. Air embolism can occur during labor, but is very rare. The circumstances surrounding the incident (e.g., vaginal douching or following the administration of blood under pressure) and the auscultation of a typical water-wheel murmur over the precordium help to differentiate the condition.[59]

Acute Heart Failure Secondary to Heart Disease

Heart failure may cause acute pulmonary edema, cyanosis, and hypotension.

However, the history and physical examination should distinguish the cause.

Hemorrhagic Conditions in Obstetrics

Conditions such as placenta previa, abruptio placentae, ruptured uterus, lacerated cervix, and retained placental tissues may be mistaken for amniotic fluid embolism. However, careful history and physical examination should direct the physician to the right diagnosis. The presence of central cyanosis rules out bleeding *per se* as the cause of the problem.[1] Moreover, central venous pressure is abnormally low with bleeding whereas it is usually high in amniotic fluid embolism.

In any case of postpartum uterine atony, especially if resistant to treatment, amniotic fluid embolism should be considered and blood coagulation studies should be done.

PROPHYLAXIS

Intravenous Infusion

Every parturient should have an *intravenous infusion using a cannula*. This not only permits supplying her with fluids and nutrients, but also allows the administration of drugs and blood if required. Once amniotic fluid embolism develops, it becomes difficult to start an intravenous infusion because of the profound peripheral vascular collapse, and valuable time will be lost if a cutdown is necessary.

Uterine Contractions

The uterus should not be stimulated at a frequency greater than 1 contraction every 3 minutes and the baseline should not be higher than 10 torr. Excessively strong or frequent contractions should be a matter of concern.

Prolonged Fetal Death

The use of oxytocic drugs should be carefully used in such cases.

Ruptured Membranes

Once the cervix is fully dilated, the membranes should be ruptured. Otherwise the strong expulsive movements can cause them to tear proximal to the presenting part near the placental margin. This would allow amniotic fluid to be pumped into the maternal circulation rather than being expelled.

Stripping of the Membranes From the Cervix

The use of this procedure to induce labor is inadvisable because it exposes the endocervical veins to amniotic fluid.

Amniocentesis

Amniocentesis should be carefully performed especially in cases of hydramnios. The placenta should be well localized by sonography prior to amniocentesis. Excessive aspiration of amniotic fluid should not be allowed; otherwise premature separation of the placenta may occur or a maternal blood vessel may tear.

Instrumentation

The insertion of instruments into the uterus such as intrauterine catheters should be gently performed.

Precautions in Predisposing Conditions

In cases of toxemia, abruptio placentae, intrauterine fetal death, and other predisposing conditions, the patient should be carefully watched and a blood sample withdrawn to establish a baseline of the coagulation factors.

TREATMENT

The treatment of amniotic fluid embolism falls under two categories: first, treatment of the initial cardiorespiratory collapse, and second, treatment of bleeding diathesis.

CARDIOPULMONARY RESUSCITATION

The patient should be well monitored, including monitoring of the ECG and blood gases.

1. *Oxygen* should be administered, preferably by an endotracheal tube, in order to alleviate hypoxia and relieve the pulmonary vasoconstriction.

2. *Positive-pressure ventilation* helps to prevent or overcome pulmonary edema.

3. *Two intravenous cannulas* are inserted to be ready if DIC should occur.

4. *Intravenous fluids are administered with caution* because of the right ventricular strain.

5. *Central venous pressure monitoring* helps to establish the diagnosis by aspirating blood containing amniotic fluid debris from the right side of the heart, and is also important for the follow-up and the regulation of fluid administration. On the one hand it prevents overloading the right ventricle, and on the other hand it allows adequate fluid replacement to prevent vasoconstriction and sludging, a process that may accentuate DIC. The aim is to keep central venous pressure within normal range (5 to 15 cm. H_2O); however, the changes in the pressure with fluid administration are more important than the absolute reading.

6. *Isoproterenol,* a strong beta stimulant agent, improves the cardiac function and relieves the pulmonary vasoconstriction.[24] However, it should be administered cautiously because it can cause peripheral vasodilation and a further drop in blood pressure. It also increases pulmonary ventilation and reverses bronchospasm in experimental amniotic fluid embolism.[26] One mg. of isoproterenol is added to 500 ml. of diluent and the drug is injected slowly, either by an intravenous drip or a Harvard pump. The pulse, blood pressure, and central venous pressure are watched during the drug administration. The pulse rate is kept below 110; otherwise arrhythmias oc-

cur. If the heart rate reaches above 110 without improvement in the central venous pressure or blood pressure, then digitalization should be considered. Other vasopressors such as epinephrine or mephentermine may be used as an alternative to isoproterenol to maintain an adequate blood pressure. Aminophylline is also recommended to produce bronchodilatation and cardiac stimulation.

Dopamine, a new cardiac stimulant, may offer some advantages over isoproterenol. For example, infusion rates of the two drugs that increase the cardiac output to the same extent in dogs are associated with a fall in blood pressure in case of isoproterenol in contrast to a rise in blood pressure with dopamine.[36] Also, the infusion rates of isoproterenol which raise cardiac output are usually associated with a fall in superior mesenteric and renal flow, the converse being true with dopamine. The usual dopamine therapy in cardiogenic shock is begun with an initial infusion rate of 2 to 5 μg./kg./min. and adjusted to produce, if possible, a blood pressure of 100 mm. Hg systolic or more, and a satisfactory urinary output.[61] Doses in excess of 10 μg./kg./min. are not advisable. The use of dopamine in amniotic fluid embolism has to be explored.

7. *Intravenous digitalization* is required in the face of a rising central venous pressure and deteriorating cardiovascular condition, especially if the patient is not responding to isoproterenol. Cedilanid, 0.8 to 1.6 mg., is administered intravenously over a period of 5 to 10 minutes.

8. *Cortisone* helps to reduce pulmonary edema, decreases the endothelial swelling and the chemical reaction, reduces the pulmonary pressure, and increases the cardiac response to catecholamines. The recommended dose is 2 g. of hydrocortisone by an intravenous push followed by 1 g. administered by intravenous infusion drip every 6 hours for 24 hours.

9. *A urinary catheter* should be inserted which helps to regulate the fluid balance.

Adequate urine output, as an indication of sufficient renal perfusion, is aimed at to avoid renal cortical necrosis.

10. *Addition of CO₂* to the inspired mixture or increasing the dead space is required to correct the hypocapnia resulting from the hyperventilation. Serial blood gases are required for follow-up.

11. *A Swan-Ganz catheter* may be used. In special centers, the insertion of such a catheter to measure the pulmonary capillary wedge pressure is helpful for regulating the fluid intake and guiding the therapy.

TREATMENT OF THE BLEEDING DIATHESIS

To prevent, abort, or terminate dangerous DIC associated with amniotic fluid embolism, the cause should be removed as early as possible. Therefore the fetus should be delivered and the placenta removed by the most expeditious method.[22] *If bleeding occurs, the coagulation factors should be replaced and the blood volume should be maintained.* Therefore, there are three lines of treatment: correcting the blood coagulation, replacing the blood loss, and treating the uterine atony.

CORRECTING THE BLOOD COAGULATION

Replacement Therapy

Fibrinogen. Each gram of infused fibrinogen raises the plasma level by 40 mg. per cent. At the present time commercial fibrinogen is rarely administered because it carries with it a high risk of hepatitis. Fibrinogen, however, can be supplied with fresh-frozen plasma. Each 100 ml. of fresh-frozen plasma contains about 300 mg. of fibrinogen. Therefore, the administration of 1 liter of fresh-frozen plasma provides the patient with about 3 g. of fibrinogen, thus raising the fibrinogen level by about 120 mg. per cent and bringing it close to the critical level of 150 mg. per cent. This may be sufficient to correct the hypofibrinogenemia. Another good source for fibrinogen is cryoprecipitate.[32] Cryoprecipitate contains about 200 mg. of fibrinogen per cryoprecipitate bag in a volume of 20 to 25 ml. The administration of fresh-frozen plasma and/or cryoprecipitate carries a much lower risk of hepatitis than commercial fibrinogen.

Other Coagulation Elements. Fresh-frozen plasma contains all coagulation factors except the platelets. However, fresh-frozen plasma should be type-specific, although group AB fresh-frozen plasma contains no anti-A or anti-B and can be considered universal donor plasma. It must be stored frozen and thawed before use for 15 to 30 minutes at 37°C. This temperature should not be raised to shorten the required time. Fresh-frozen plasma is not only administered to treat a bleeding diathesis, but also to prevent it in a patient receiving massive blood transfusion. After every 10 units of transfused bank blood, 500 ml. of fresh-frozen plasma must be given. The platelet count rarely falls below 50,000 after massive transfusion and, therefore, the prophylactic use of platelet concentrates is generally not required.[56]

Platelets. The indications for platelet transfusion are a platelet count below 50,000/mm.[3], poor clot retraction, and poor platelet function as seen in the thromboelastogram.[56] It is usually supplied in single random donor concentrates. Each unit of platelet concentrate increases the platelet count by 7,000 to 9,000/mm.[3] in a 70-kg. person.

Calcium administration is not required in DIC or following massive transfusion. So long as the parathyroids are active, Ca^{++} can be mobilized easily from the huge Ca^{++} stores in the body, namely the bones. Moreover, in a patient who is digitalized and/or on isoproterenol, serious arrhythmias may follow Ca^{++} administration. Therefore, it is only when the patient has parathyroidectomy that serum Ca^{++}

should be watched carefully and administered if necessary.

Drug Administration

Heparin. Heparin inhibits blood coagulation in all stages, e.g., it prevents thromboplastin formation, the prothrombin transformation into thrombin, and thrombin action on fibrinogen. For heparin to act, it requires the presence of a naturally occurring substance, antithrombin III.[23] The rationale for using heparin in DIC is to prevent the hypercoagulation, thus preserving the coagulation products and stopping the activation of plasminogen by the liberated thrombin. Meanwhile the reticuloendothelial system takes care of the fibrin and fibrinogen split products, and hence bleeding stops. The dose recommended is just enough to prevent the hypercoagulation; therefore, it is about one-third the full heparinization dose used with cardiopulmonary bypass. The dose recommended for DIC with amniotic fluid embolism is 0.5 mg./kg. intravenously every 4 to 6 hours for 48 hours.[12] The use of heparin in the obstetric patient with DIC is still controversial because of the absence of adequate data for its proper evaluation.[12,25,32,37,40,44,51,57,62] The use of heparin in chronic cases where the triggering mechanism is still present, such as the release of thromboplastin from a tumor, has been proven to be successful. However, its role in acute cases is uncertain[25] and may be followed by serious or fatal hemorrhage.[25,57] The use of heparin in patients with fibrinogen levels less than 50 mg. per cent can produce fatal bleeding. The major therapy in obstetric cases is to remove the cause by emptying the uterus.

Antiproteolytic Drugs. To stop fibrinolysis, there are two drugs which can be used, namely, epsilon aminocaproic acid (Amicar) and aprotinin (Trasylol).[58] The former drug is an antiplasminogen and the latter is an antiplasmin. The rationale for using them is to stop bleeding if there is fibrinolysis. However, in DIC the primary cause is usually hypercoagulation

of the blood and not fibrinolysis. Therefore, if epsilon aminocaproic acid (EACA) is administered in these cases, extensive fibrin thrombi will develop and produce even more tissue ischemia. On the other hand, if fibrinolysis is the primary cause, which is very rare, EACA will correct the coagulopathy. Hence the indications for EACA are:

1. Primary fibrinolysis
2. Local irrigation in a patient with bleeding following prostatic surgery[58]
3. Secondary fibrinolysis, provided intravenous heparin is administered half an hour before its administration, and heparin therapy is continued thereafter

The recommended dose of EACA is 1 g. by intravenous push followed by 1 g. every 4 hours in the form of an intravenous drip. In advanced cases of DIC much of plasminogen has been transformed into plasmin. Thus EACA will not be quite effective, and aprotinin is the drug of choice (Fig. 9-5).

In obstetric patients with DIC, neither EACA nor aprotinin is required since they both carry a high risk of thrombosis and pulmonary embolism. EACA also crosses the blood-placental barrier and causes hyaline membrane disease of the newborn.[5]

REPLACING THE BLOOD LOSS

Sometime during pregnancy every woman should be typed and screened to determine her ABO and Rh_0 blood group and to exclude irregular antibodies.

It is always preferable to give blood of the same ABO group and Rh type. In sudden massive bleeding in a previously typed and screened patient with a negative antibody screen, uncrossmatched ABO and $Rh_0(D)$ type-specific whole blood or packed red blood cells may be given with less than a one in 10,000 chance of a hemolytic transfusion. If ABO group-specific blood is not available, then one must switch to the next appropriate ABO blood group and must use packed red blood cells instead of whole blood to minimize the amount of anti-A and/or anti-B infused into the patient. For example, if the patient is group AB, then, after group AB, group A is the next most appropriate, followed by group B and then group O, which is the worst ABO type to give to a group AB patient. If the patient is group A, then only A and O can be given. If the patient is group B, then only B and O can be given. And if the patient is group O, only group O can be used. If there is difficulty in determining the $Rh_0(D)$ status of the *woman* then $Rh_0(D)$-negative blood should be used if possible. Fresh blood, i.e., blood less than 24 hours old, is generally not available in many blood banks because of the time necessary to completely process the blood (ABO, Rh, serology, antibody screening and hepatitis testing). Therefore, when required, one relies on packed red cells and fresh-frozen plasma as a substitute. The use of blood warmers and microaggregate blood filters is important especially in amniotic fluid embolism.

The central venous pressure, pulse, blood pressure, and urinary output are monitored to regulate the rate and volume of blood transfusion. Hypovolemia is dangerous in DIC because the coagulopathy state deteriorates and the kidneys may be seriously damaged. Therefore, the golden rule is to try maintain the blood volume as normal as possible despite the excessive bleeding.

Treating the Uterine Atony

Massage of the uterus, oxytocics, and uterine pack can be used to improve the uterine tone. Improving the circulatory status helps to terminate such a resistant and serious complication.[15]

PROGNOSIS

Maternal Prognosis

Amniotic fluid embolism has a very high mortality rate.[47] Fifty per cent of the patients who develop it die within 1 hour of the incident. Fifty per cent of those who survive develop DIC. Fifty per cent of those who acquire DIC die because of uncontrolled bleeding and/or renal cortical necrosis.

Fetal Prognosis

Because amniotic fluid embolism occurs before delivery, fetal hypoxia occurs and the fetus usually dies if not delivered promptly. Rarely, if the mother is dead and the fetus is still alive, postmortem cesarean section can be performed to save the baby. This situation has been reported in 5 cases and resulted in delivering 4 live babies.[47]

REFERENCES

1. Abouleish, E.: Amnioctic fluid embolism: report of a fatal case. Anesth. Analg., *53*:549, 1974.
2. Adamsons, K., Mueller-Heubach, E., and Myers, R. E.: The innocuousness of amniotic fluid infusion in the pregnant rhesus monkey. Am. J. Obstet. Gynecol., *109*:977, 1971.
3. Attwood, H. D., and Downing, E. S.: Experimental amniotic fluid and meconium embolism. Surg. Gynecol. Obstet., *120*:255, 1965.
4. Beecham, J. B., Watson, W. J., and Clapp, J. F., III: Eclampsia, preeclampsia and disseminated intravascular coagulation. Obstet. Gynecol., *43*:576, 1974.
5. Beller, F. K.: Treatment of coagulation disorders in pregnancy. Clin. Obstet. Gynecol., 7:372, 1964.
6. Beller, F. K., *et al.*: Consumptive coagulopathy associated with intra-amniotic infusion of hypertonic salt. Am. J. Obstet. Gynecol., *112*:534, 1972.
7. Bonnar, J., McNicol, G. P., and Douglas, A. S.: Fibrinolytic enzyme system and pregnancy. Br. Med. J., *3*:387, 1969.
8. ———: Coagulation and fibrinolytic mechanisms during and after normal childbirth. Br. Med. J., 2:200, 1970.
9. Bonnar, J., *et al.*: Haemostatic mechanism in the uterine circulation during placental separation. Br. Med. J., 2:564, 1970.
10. Brown, F. D., Davidson, E. C., Jr., and Phillips, L. L.: Coagulation changes after hypertonic saline infusion for late abortions. Obstet. Gynecol., *39*:538, 1972.
11. Chargaff, E.: The isolation of preparations of thromboplastic protein from human organs. J. Biol. Chem., *161*:389, 1945.
12. Chung, A. F., and Merkatz, I. R.: Survival following amniotic fluid embolism with early heparinization. Obstet. Gynecol., *42*:809, 1973.
13. Cohen, E., and Ballard, C. A.: Consumption coagulopathy associated with intra-amniotic saline instillation and the effect of intravenous oxytocin. Obstet. Gynecol., *43*:300, 1974.

14. Courtney, L. D.: Amniotic fluid embolism. Br. Med. J., *1*:545, 1970.
15. ———:Amniotic fluid embolism. Obstet. Gynecol. Surv., *29*:169, 1974.
16. Courtney, L. D., and Allington, M.: Effect of amniotic fluid on blood coagulation. Br. J. Haematol., *22*:353, 1972.
17. Courtney, L. D., Boxall, R. R., and Child, P.: Permeability of membranes of dead fetus. Br. Med. J., *1*:492, 1972.
18. Czemba, G. F.: Blood coagulation measurement. Med. Electron. Data, vol. 1, pp. 112–113, Sept.–Oct., 1970.
19. DeVoe, S. J., and Schwartz, R. H.: Determination of maturity and well-being using maternal and amniotic fluids. *In* Gruenwald, P.: The Placenta and Its Maternal Supply Line. Ed. 2, p. 261, Baltimore, University Park Press, 1975.
20. Deykin, D.: Thrombogenesis. N. Engl. J. Med., *276*:622, 1967.
21. ———: The clinical challenge of disseminated intravascular coagulation. N. Engl. J. Med.,*283*:36, 1971.
22. Ebner, H.: The obstetric anesthesiologist: his role in coagulation disorders in the parturient. Anesth. Analg., *50*:131, 1971.
23. Gilcher, R. O.: Thrombolytic agents and prophylactic heparinization. Abstract, The 10th Annual Postgraduate Symposium on Critical Care Medicine, University of Pittsburgh, May 7, 1976.
24. Goodman, L. S., and Gilman, A.: The Pharmacological Basis of Therapeutics. Ed. 5. New York, Macmillan, 1975.
25. Green, D., *et al.*: The role of heparin in the management of consumption coagulopathy. Med. Clin. North Am., *56*:193, 1972.
26. Halmagyi, D. F. J., Starzecki, B., and Shearman, R. P.: Experimental amniotic fluid embolism: mechanism and treatment. Am. J. Obstet. Gynecol., *84*:251, 1962.
27. Hardaway, R. M.: Syndromes of Disseminated Intravascular Coagulation. With special reference to Shock and Hemorrhage. Springfield, Ill., Charles C Thomas, 1966.
28. Howland, W. S.: Use of halothane (Fluothane) in radical abdominal surgery. Clinical Aspects of Anesthesiology. Ayerst Laboratories, 1972.
29. Howland, W. S., Schweizer, O., and Gould, P. A.: Comparison of intraoperative measurements of coagulation. Anesth. Analg., *53*:657, 1974.
30. Howland, W. S., *et al.*: Coagulation abnormalities associated with liver transplantation. Surgery, *68*:591, 1970.
31. James, F. M.: When amniotic fluid embolism strikes. Immediate oxygen, vasoactive drugs, urged to stave off total collapse. Clin. Trends Anesth., *2*:1, 1972.
32. Jewett, J. F.: Committee on maternal welfare. Amniotic-fluid infusion. N. Engl. J. Med., *292*:973, 1975.
33. Josey, W. E.: Hypofibrinogenemia complicating uterine rupture: relationship to amniotic fluid embolism. Am. J. Obstet. Gynecol., *94*:29, 1966.
34. Karim, S. M. M., The Prostaglandins, Progress in Research. New York, Wiley-Interscience, 1972.

35. Leeming, M. N., Ryan, G. M., and Howland, W. S.: Rapid read out device for thromboelastography. J. Lab. Clin. Med., *73*:163, 1969.
36. MacCannell, K. L.: Pharmacological role of dopamine in catecholamine therapy. Abstracts and Proceedings of a Symposium, Dopamine in Clinical Use. P. 7. Institute of Cardiology of Montreal, Quebec, Canada, March 29, 1976. Excerpta Medica, Amsterdam.
37. Maki, M., *et al.*: Heparin treatment of amniotic fluid embolism. Tohoku J. Exp. Med., *97*:155, 1969.
38. Marder, V. J., Matchett, M. O., and Sherry, S.: Detection of serum fibrinogen and fibrin degradation products: comparison of six techniques using purified products and application in clinical studies. Am. J. Med., *51*:71, 1971.
39. Miller, R. D.: Complications of massive blood transfusion. Anesthesiology, *39*:82, 1973.
40. ———: Theoretical, practical evidence is lacking; corticosteroids use held unjustified in treating intravascular hemolysis. Clin. Trends Anesth., *5*:89, 1975.
41. Mor, A., *et al.*: Platelet counts in pregnancy and labor: a comparative study. Obstet. Gynecol., *16*:338, 1960.
42. Mueller-Heubach, E.: Production of disseminated intravascular coagulation in monkeys by injection of cell-free extracts of placenta. Mt. Sinai J. Med. N.Y., *42*:415, 1975.
43. Nossel, H. L., Marcus, A., and Merskey, C.: Understanding coagulation: clinical applications vols 3 and 5. The Surgical Team, Sept.–Oct., 1974.
44. Olcott, C., IV, *et al.*: Amniotic fluid embolism and disseminated intravascular coagulation after blunt abdominal trauma. Obstet. Gynecol. Surv., *29*:208, 1973.
45. Ostergard, D. R.: The physiology and clinical importance of amniotic fluid. A review. Obstet. Gynecol. Surv., *25*:297, 1970.
46. Pechet, L., and Alexander, B.: Increased clotting factors in pregnancy. N. Engl. J. Med.,*265*:1093, 1961.
47. Peterson, E. P., and Taylor, H. B.: Amniotic fluid embolism: an analysis of 40 cases. Obstet. Gynecol., *35*:787, 1970.
48. Phillips, J. M., and Evans, J. A.: Acute anesthetic and obstetric management of patients with severe abruptio placentae. Anesth. Analg., *49*:998, 1970.
49. Phillips, L. L., and Davidson, E. C., Jr.: Procoagulant properties of amniotic fluid. Am. J. Obstet. Gynecol., *113*:911, 1972.
50. Phillips, O. C.: Guest discussion. *In* Ebner, H.: The obstetric anesthesiologist: his role in coagulation disorders in the parturient. Anesth. Analg., *50*:138, 1971.
51. Prichard, J. A.: Heparin in disseminated intravascular coagulation. Am. J. Obstet. Gynecol., *115*:871, 1973.
52. Quilligan, E. J.: Changes in the status of the fetus. *In* Romney, S. L. *et al.* (eds.): Gynecology and Obstetrics, the Health Care of Women, pp. 280. New York, McGraw-Hill, 1975.

53. Reid, D. E., *et al*.: Intravascular clotting and afibrinogenemia, presumptive lethal factors in syndrome of amniotic fluid embolism. Am. J. Obstet. Gynecol., *66*:465, 1953.

54. Reis, R. L., Pierce, W. S., and Behrendt, D. M.: Hemodynamic effects of amniotic fluid embolism. Surg. Gynecol. Obstet., *129*:45, 1969.

55. Ryan, G.: Management of consumption coagulopathy. Low-dose heparin, EACA, and platelet transfusion advised for hemorrhage. Clin. Trends Anesth., *3*:197, 1973.

56. Ryan, G. M., Boyan, C. P., and Howland, W. S.: Clotting problems during surgery. Surg. Clin. North. Am., *49*:233, 1969.

57. Sabbagha, R. E., and Hayashi, T. T.: Disseminated intravascular coagulation complicating hysterotomy in elderly gravidas. Obstet. Gynecol. *38*:844, 1971.

58. Sherman, L. A., Wessler, S., and Avioli, V.: Therapeutic problems of disseminated intravascular coagulation. Arch. Intern. Med., *132*:446, 1973.

59. Shnider, S. M., and Moya, F.: Amniotic fluid embolism. Review article. Anesthesiology, *22*:108, 1961.

60. Stefanini, M., and Turpini, R. A.: Fibrinogenopenic accident of pregnancy and delivery: syndrome with multiple etiological mechanisms. Ann. N.Y. Acad. Sci., *75*:601, 1959.

60a.Steiner, P. E., and Lushbaugh, C. C.: Maternal pulmonary embolism by amniotic fluid as cause of obstetrical shock and unexpected deaths in obstetrics. JAMA, *117*:1245, and 1340, 1941.

61. Teesdale, S. J.: Dopamine in clinical practice. Abstracts and Proceedings of a Symposium, Dopamine in Clinical Use. Institute of Cardiology of Montreal, Quebec, Canada, March 29, 1976. Pp. 11, Excerpta Medica, Amsterdam.

62. Waxman, B., and Grambrill, R.: Use of heparin in disseminated intravascular coagulation. Am. J. Obstet. Gynecol., *112*:434, 1972.

63. Weiner, A. E., and Reid, D. E.: The pathogenesis of amniotic fluid embolism. III. Coagulant activity of amniotic fluid. New Engl. J. Med., *243*:597, 1950.

64. Woodfield, D. G., Galloway, R. K., and Smart, G. E.: Coagulation effect associated with presumed amniotic fluid embolism in the mid-trimester of pregnancy. J. Obstet. Gynaecol. Br. Commonw., *78*:423, 1971.

10

Oxytocic and Tocolytic Agents

Ezzat Abouleish, M.D.

Oxytocic and tocolytic agents have significant actions on the mother and/or the fetus. They are frequently used in obstetrics and the anesthesiologist should be aware of their effects.

OXYTOCIC DRUGS

Oxytocic drugs include oxytocin, ergot alkaloids, and prostaglandins.

OXYTOCIN
HISTORY

The posterior pituitary gland secretes a hormone called Pituitrin. In 1938, two derivatives of it were separated, one with mainly an oxytocic action called, oxytocin, Pitocin, and the other with vasopressor and antidiuretic effects, called vasopressin, Pitressin, or antidiuretic hormone (ADH). Pituitrin, owing to its vasopressin component, is capable of producing severe and persistent hypertension. Following its use, cases of cerebral hemorrhage have been reported, particularly when combined with vasopressors. Severe hypotension, arrhythmias, and shock were also noticed and attributed to coronary vasospasm and severe myocardial ischemia. Therefore, the name "Pituitrin shock" was adopted. These severe reactions occurred in anesthetized as well as in awake patients. Owing

to its serious cardiovascular complications, the use of Pituitrin has been abandoned.

The natural oxytocin, although considered to act only as an oxytocic drug, caused hypertension, hypotension, and even cardiac arrest, mainly due to its contamination with vasopressin. Being of animal origin, its protein content could have also caused anaphylactic reaction. However, in 1955, oxytocin was synthesized and universally used as an oxytocic agent.

STRUCTURE

The structure of oxytocin is similar to that of the antidiuretic hormone. Each is composed of a ring of nine aminoacids, seven of which are identical in both compounds.

PHARMACOLOGIC ACTIONS
Oxytocic Effect

Both oxytocin and ergot preparations stimulate uterine contractions. With advance in gestation the uterus, which is estrogen-dependent, becomes especially sensitive to their effects.[16] With increasing dosage of the oxytocic drug, the frequency and strength of uterine contractions increase, the baseline tonus is elevated, and eventually tetanic contractions result. Oxytocin has the advantage over ergot al-

186

kaloids in that its action can be easily regulated to obtain rhythmic uterine contractions. Therefore, oxytocin has been used for induction and augmentation of labor whereas ergot has been used for control of postpartum hemorrhage. In the parturient, the fetal heart rate and uterine contractions should be monitored during the administration of oxytocin. Too frequent uterine contractions can interfere with the uteroplacental circulation, resulting in fetal asphyxia. The combination of oxytocin and epidural analgesia calls for more attention. The hypotensive effect of the latter plus the oxytocic action of the former can cause marked fetal bradycardia.[38]

For the termination of pregnancy in the second trimester, oxytocin is used to augment uterine contractions following the intra-amniotic injection of hypertonic saline. In the third trimester when intrauterine fetal death is diagnosed, labor is induced using oxytocin infusion. The use of oxytocin in association with a dead fetus requires extra caution irrespective of the stage of gestation. Under these circumstances, there is always a danger of amniotic fluid embolism and the development of disseminated intravascular coagulopathy (see Chap. 9).

Side Effects

The main side effect of the use of oxytocin is its actions on the cardiovascular system. The anesthesiologist should be aware of these actions, which can be quite dangerous. Oxytocin causes vasodilation of both alpha- and beta-adrenoreceptive blood vessels.[22] The action occurs in less than 30 seconds after administration of oxytocin and is maintained for 3 to 5 minutes.[17] The vasodilating effect of oxytocin causes transient hypotension; the degree and duration of which are proportionate to the dose of the drug and the rate of injection. The average drop in blood pressure after oxytocin injection (0.1 unit/kg.) in the form of an intravenous

bolus is 45 per cent.[40] Hypotension due to oxytocin is minimized by the lithotomy position.[22] However, such hypotension becomes especially dangerous in a hypovolemic patient in whom vasoconstriction is an important factor in maintaining the blood pressure.

Tachycardia occurs 5 to 10 seconds after the onset of hypotension, with an average increase in heart rate of 20 beats/min.[40] The tachycardia, which is reflex in origin and secondary to the hypotension, is associated with S-T segment depression and T wave inversion, denoting myocardial ischemia. This is due to coronary insufficiency as a result of hypotension, combined with increased oxygen demand secondary to the tachycardia.[5,22,31] There is also mild myocardial depression manifested by the antiarrhythmic properties of oxytocin.[29] Such mild myocardial depression becomes significant in a patient with cardiac disease.

Therefore, if oxytocin is required, it can be injected either intramuscularly or by intravenous pump or drip; it should not be administered by intravenous bolus in a dose exceeding 2 units.

When administered in a large dose over a prolonged period of time, even synthetic oxytocin has antidiuretic action.[16] Therefore, caution should be taken in administering the drug, and fluids should be restricted in patients with toxemia, renal disease, or cardiac problems.

ERGOT ALKALOIDS

History

The fungus product ergot has been employed in obstetrics for the past four centuries.[37] Its uterotonic action was initially documented by Adam Lonicer in 1582. European midwives utilized the substance throughout the seventeenth and eighteenth centuries.[11] The toxicity of ergot, however, tended to limit its usage. Its propensity for producing "Saint Anthony's fire" became well known. This descriptive term referred to the red face associated with a burning feeling in the affected limbs which occurred as a result of ergot-induced vasospasm. When the spasm persisted, dry gangrene of the limbs developed. The use of ergot in modern history was revived in 1932 by Moir. Thereafter, many ergot derivatives have been introduced, and it is claimed that they produce less vasoconstriction, thus, less toxic reactions.

STRUCTURE

Ergot is obtained from the fungus *Claviceps purpurea* that grows over rye and other grains. Ergot has many alkaloids which are divided mainly into two groups. The first group is the amine group which on hydrolysis yields lysergic acid and an amine, and the second group is the amino group which has a higher molecular weight and on hydrolysis yields lysergic acid and an amino group. An example of the first group is ergonovine (ergometrine), and an example of the second group is ergotamine.

The addition of a methyl group, e.g., methylergonovine (Methergine), is supposed to cause less vasoconstriction and less endothelial damage. Dihydrogenation of the alkaloids leads to less vasoconstriction, less oxytocic action, and increased adrenergic blocking effect.

PHARMACOLOGIC ACTIONS

The main actions of ergot alkaloids are oxytocic, vasoconstrictive, adrenergic blocking, and mixed excitatory and depressive effects on the central nervous system. An example of the central nervous system excitatory action of ergot is vomiting due to stimulation of the chemoreceptor trigger zone. An example of the central nervous system depressive action of ergot is respiratory depression and the failure of the vasomotor center to respond to impulses from the carotid sinus. The main

therapeutic action of ergot is its oxytocic effect, and the important side effect is the vasoconstriction.

Ergot preparations, in contrast to oxytocin, are known to cause vasoconstriction.[16] The vasoconstrictive action of ergonovine is less than that of other ergot alkaloids, and methylation further reduces its vasoconstrictive effects. A pressor effect has been seen in about 48 per cent of patients following ergonovine administration and in 22 per cent of patients following methylergonovine administration.[37] The incidence of severe hypertension (systolic elevation of greater than 25 torr and diastolic elevation of greater than 20 torr) was reported in 2 per cent of cases following intravenous injection of methylergonovine and in 4.6 per cent with concomitant administration of vasopressor.

Hypertension also can follow the intramuscular injection of ergot alkaloids.[9] Vasoconstriction, through a direct stimulation of blood vessels both at the arterial and venous sides,[6] leads to increased peripheral resistance and a rise in both arterial blood pressure and central venous pressure. Ergot also has a depressant effect on the vasomotor center, preventing compensatory vasodilation secondary to afferent impulses from the baroreceptors. The increased venous return to the heart following relief of the inferior vena caval compression after delivery and the diminution of the vascular bed following tetanic contraction of the uterus potentiate the postpartum rise in blood pressure. The vasoconstrictive effect of ergot becomes manifest in 3 minutes and lasts for several hours.[22]

Blood pressure elevation following ergot preparations is particularly pronounced in toxemias of pregnancy, hypertension, presence of hypoxia, administration of vasopressors,[9] or marked apprehension.[3] Since the incidence of a dangerous rise in blood pressure after the administration of ergot alkaloids is rare and hypertension would otherwise be attributed to postpartum toxemia, some physicians continue to give ergot intravenously. However, this is particularly dangerous in patients with cardiovascular disease, hypertension, respiratory disease, renal disease, or chronic anemia. Sudden hypertension produced by ergot causes a strain on the heart and may be associated with coronary vasoconstriction, leading to myocardial ischemia, acute heart failure, and acute pulmonary edema. It may also lead to cerebral edema or even to cerebral hemorrhage.[9] Retinal detachment following intravenous injection of 0.2 mg. of methylergonovine and 5 units of oxytocin has also been described.[15] The mechanism causing the detachment was thought to be spasm of the choroidal vessels, producing an increase in choroidal hydrostatic pressure and transudation of fluid into the subretinal space.

If ergot is administered during general anesthesia under such potent drugs as halothane, or during regional analgesia, its vasoconstrictive action may be counteracted by the vasodilative effect of these techniques. Thus, the hypertensive effect of ergot may be masked and the lungs and brain may be temporarily protected from edema or hemorrhage until the vasodilation wears off.[1]

To treat the hypertensive episode produced by ergot, slow intravenous injection of 12.5 to 15 mg. of chlorpromazine is recommended. Hydralazine infusion has also been effective, since it causes generalized vasodilation, particularly of the renal vessels.[7]

Although pharmaceutic literature[35] suggests that methylergonovine maleate might be slowly injected intravenously over a period of no less than 60 seconds while monitoring the blood pressure, this is not safe enough in view of the delay (3 minutes) of the hypertensive response.[22] Therefore, if ergot is to be used, it should be administered by the intramuscular route for a life-threatening uterine atony resistant to oxytocin.

Since the vasoconstrictive effect of ergot is opposite to the vasodilative action of oxytocin, this may lead to the erroneous assumption that, by simultaneous intravenous administration of both drugs, the effect of one will nullify that of the other. However, because onset and duration of action of the two drugs are so different, the patient would be exposed to the harmful effects of both (Fig. 10-1).

PROSTAGLANDINS

HISTORY

In 1930 prostaglandin was first obtained from the vesicular and prostatic glands, hence the name prostaglandin. It was first thought that prostaglandin was one substance, but now it is identified to be a large group of substances. Prostaglandins were synthesized, more or less simultaneously, in 1964 and 1965 in the Netherlands and the United States.[30]

STRUCTURE

Prostaglandins are 20-carbon fatty acids. There are primary six prostaglandins: E_1 E_2, E_3, $F_{1\alpha}$, $F_{2\alpha}$, and $F_{3\alpha}$. In obstetrics, the commonly used ones are E_1, E_2, and $F_{2\alpha}$.

DISTRIBUTION

Prostaglandins have been found in tissues of various species ranging from man to coral. Human semen has the highest concentration, containing 13 to 14 naturally occurring prostaglandins.

METABOLISM

After intravenous injection, prostaglandins are rapidly cleared from the circulation due to uptake by tissues, especially the lungs and liver, and hydrolysis by an enzyme called prostaglandin dehydrogenase.

MECHANISM OF ACTION

The mechanism of action of prostaglandins is still not clearly defined. They act

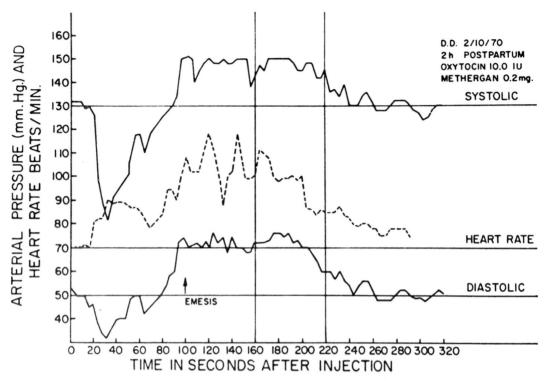

Fig. 10-1.   Combination of oxytocin and methylergonovine. In a postpartum patient, the simultaneous administration of oxytocin, 10 I.U., and methylergonovine, 0.2 mg., shows the cardiovascular effects of both drugs. The initial sharp reduction in systolic and diastolic pressure plus an increase in heart rate was followed by a rapid rise in blood pressure and continued rise in heart rate. All parameters had returned to near the preinjection levels within 6 minutes after the injection. (Hendricks, C. H., and Brenner, W. E.: Cardiovascular effects of oxytocic drugs used post partum. Am. J. Obstet. Gynecol., *108*:751, 1970)

mainly at a local level, probably on the cell membrane, and cause the release of bound Ca++. They also stimulate adenyl cyclase, resulting in an increase in tissue levels of cyclic AMP.

PHARMACOLOGIC ACTIONS

Prostaglandins affect almost all the systems of the body.

Effects on the Reproductive System

Several prostaglandins can be absorbed from the vagina in amounts sufficient to produce physiologically active concentrations in the plasma. This probably helps to regulate the motility of the female reproductive system to produce fertilization of

the ovum and its transfer to the uterus.[19] Therefore, diminished prostaglandins in the semen may be responsible for infertility in some cases.

Prostaglandins play an important role in initiating menstruation, probably by causing lysis of the corpus luteum. They can stimulate or inhibit uterine contractions depending on the type of the drug, the species involved, the endocrine state of the animal, and whether it is an *in vivo* or *in vitro* study. The pregnant uterus of all studied animals responds to prostaglandins, whether E or F, with contraction. The action is not blocked by atropine, antihistamines, or ganglionic blockers.

Effects on the Gastrointestinal Tract

Prostaglandins play an important role in regulating the gastrointestinal tract motility. Therapeutic doses of the drug may cause gastrointestinal stimulation evidenced by marked diarrhea and vomiting.[25]

Effects on the Cardiovascular System

In man as well as in experimental animals, intravenous injection of prostaglandin A lowers the blood pressure, decreases peripheral resistance, and reflexly increases the cardiac output.[20] This effect is mainly due to a direct vasodilating effect; atropine, ganglionic blockers, or beta-adrenergic blockers cannot counteract it. The vascular effects of prostaglandin A may be beneficial in the treatment of hypertension. Prostaglandin A also improves the renal blood flow and enhances water and salt excretion. The use of prostaglandins in preeclampsia has to be examined.

In humans, the prostaglandins commonly used for inducing abortion, namely E_2 and $F_{2\alpha}$, have minimal effects on the cardiovascular system.

Effects on the Respiratory System

The lung contains large quantities of prostaglandins and is important for their removal from the circulation. The effect of prostaglandins on the smooth muscles of the tracheobronchial tree varies with the type of hormone and the species studied. On the whole prostaglandin F constricts and prostaglandin E relaxes the bronchial smooth muscle. In asthmatic patients, the infusion of prostaglandin $F_{2\alpha}$ for induction of abortion can initiate bronchospasm.[30] Thus, it is postulated that normally a balance exists in the respiratory system between these two types of prostaglandins. If prostaglandin F outweighs prostaglandin E, asthma occurs.[39] The administration of prostaglandin E or drugs to antagonize prostaglandin F is a new approach to the management of bronchial asthma.

CONCLUSION

The use of prostaglandins in obstetrics is growing. However, the side effects such as nausea, vomiting, diarrhea, and headache may set limitations to their widespread use.

TOCOLYTIC AGENTS

There are many drugs which can inhibit the uterine contractions and relax the myometrium. These drugs are used for two purposes: to allow intrauterine manipulations during delivery, and to stop premature labor.

DRUGS THAT ALLOW INTRAUTERINE MANIPULATIONS DURING DELIVERY

It is frequently necessary to administer anesthesia to cause uterine relaxation in order to permit intrauterine manipulation (e.g., breech delivery, manual removal of the placenta, or delivery of the second twin). Since chloroform is too toxic and ether is explosive, the commonly used anesthetic drug for this purpose is halothane. Under these circumstances, the patient is managed in the same way as for general anesthesia, i.e., antacid administration, "crash" induction, and endotracheal intubation. Anesthesia is deepened using 1.5 to 2.5 per cent halothane in oxygen. Since halothane is a cardiovascular depressant especially in these high concentrations, hydration and adequate replacement of any blood loss should precede and accompany the anesthesia. The patient should receive atropine as a premedicant to avoid halothane bradycardia. The ECG should be monitored and the blood pressure should be closely followed. Vigorous hyperventilation should be avoided to prevent overdosage; it is preferable, once the effects of succinylcholine wear off, to keep the patient spontaneously breathing with assisted ventilation every second breath. The halothane administration should be terminated as soon as the intrauterine manipulation ends, otherwise uterine atony may lead to post-partum bleeding. If required, anesthesia can thereafter be maintained with nitrous oxide and oxygen.

DRUGS USED TO STOP PREMATURE LABOR

Since prematurity is a leading cause of perinatal death, various attempts have been made in cases of premature labor to prolong pregnancy by pharmacologic means.

The indication for the use of drugs to stop premature labor is fetal prematurity as evidenced by an estimated fetal weight more than 500 g. and less than 2,500 g. and/or gestation age of less than 36 weeks.

The contraindications for the use of these drugs are when it is safer for the infant to be outside than inside the uterus, as, for instance, with abruptio placentae, pre-eclampsia, hypertensive heart disease and other conditions leading to intrauterine growth retardation. Other contraindications are ruptured membranes with intrauterine infection, and advanced labor, e.g., cervical dilatation more than 4 cm. and/or cervical effacement of more than 50 per cent. Of course, a dead or grossly deformed fetus is a contraindication for attempting to prolong pregnancy.

Many drugs have been used for the treatment of premature labor, mainly ethanol, magnesium sulfate, prostaglandin inhibitors, β_2-adrenergic receptor stimulators, and others.

ETHANOL

History

Alcohol has long been used for obstetric analgesia, and it was noted that when given too early in labor, the contractions stopped.[4,10]

Mechanism of Action

There are two ways to control uterine contractions. One way is to prevent the myometrium from responding to internal and external stimuli, e.g., beta-adrenergic compounds; the other way is to decrease the stimuli reaching the uterus. Alcohol constitutes the latter approach. Ethyl alcohol is known to inhibit the release of the antidiuretic hormone as well as the release of oxytocin during parturition and lactation in rabbits, and during lactation in humans.[13]

Administration

Ethanol is administered in the form of an intravenous infusion. One hundred ml. of 95 per cent ethanol is added to 900 ml. of 5 per cent dextrose in water, making a total of 1,000 ml. of 9.5 per cent (V/V) ethanol in dextrose solution.[14] The loading dose is 7.5 ml./kg./hour for 2 hours (e.g., for a 70-kg. female, the 1,000 ml. is initially administered). The maintenance dose is 1.5 ml./kg./hour. This scheme gives an alcohol blood level of 0.10 to 0.16 per cent.

Undesirable Maternal Side Effects

The inhibitory action of ethanol on the uterine contractions is dose-related. Thus, its use is limited by the side effects seen at higher doses, such as nausea, vomiting, stupor, and respiratory depression.

The administration of alcohol to the mother causes mild metabolic changes, namely lactacidemia.[30a]

Effect on the Fetus and Neonate

Alcohol is of small molecular size, poorly ionizable, and fat-soluble. Therefore, it is rapidly diffusible across cellular membranes including the placenta.

In ewes, after intravenous infusion to the mother, alcohol, as expected, is rapidly transmitted to the fetus. There is a significant correlation between the maternal and fetal blood levels of alcohol, and the peak concentration is similar in both.[30]

After discontinuation of the alcohol infusion, both fetal and maternal blood levels remain high for several hours, with fetal blood levels sometimes exceeding the maternal levels.

In an experimental study on anesthetized monkeys, fetal tachycardia, hypotension, and acidosis have been reported after ethanol infusion in rates 2 to 4 times higher than those used in women.[18] Similar effects were not observed by others.[12]

Clinically, no untoward effects have been observed on most of the fetuses or neonates. However, if alcohol fails to stop premature labor, the delivered baby may have hypotonia and mild acidosis which is a mixture of lactacidemia and respiratory acidosis as a result of respiratory depression. If these complications are added to prematurity, the neonate can be in trouble and the perinatologists should be aware of these possibilities and ready to treat them.

Success Rate

Alcohol has been successfully used to stop premature labor.[1,14] However, alcohol administration is not successful in stopping labor in one-third of the cases with intact membranes and in all of the cases with ruptured membranes.[14] Recently, immunoassay studies have shown that oxytocin is not elevated in maternal blood prior to or during labor. This may account for the inability of ethanol to significantly inhibit human labor in some cases.

Role in Obstetrics

At present, there is a tendency to use ethanol in combination with other tocolytic agents.[42]

MAGNESIUM SULFATE

Mechanism of Action

The mechanism by which magnesium sulfate ($MgSO_4$) inhibits the uterine contractions is not yet settled, but it probably involves competing with Ca^{++} at the cell level.

Administration

The initial dose of magnesium sulfate is 2 g. administered by intravenous bolus. The maintenance dose is about 2 g./hour by continuous infusion. The patient should be closely followed lest $MgSO_4$ toxicity arise in the form of hypotonia, areflexia, stupor, and respiratory and cardiovascular depression. The aim is to have a $MgSO_4$ blood level of 6 to 8 mEq./liter, and below the toxic level of 12 to 14 mEq./liter. The urine output should be monitored because overdosage easily arises with oliguria. To treat magnesium sulfate overdosage, calcium gluconate, 10 ml. of a 10 per cent solution, is intravenously injected.

Effect on the Neonate

The effect on the neonate, if delivered while the mother is under $MgSO_4$ therapy, is generalized central nervous system depression and hypotonia (see also Chap. 3, The Placenta and Placental Transfer of Drugs at Term).

PROSTAGLANDIN INHIBITORS

Prostaglandins play an important role in the mechanism of onset of labor. They have also been used to induce labor and abortion. Drugs that inhibit endogenous prostaglandins have a promising future in the control of premature labor. Aspirin inhibits prostaglandin biosynthesis. In experimental animals, aspirin can prevent abortion by inhibiting premature contractions.[29] Similarly, indomethacin, which is 23 times more potent than aspirin, prolongs gestation in both the rat and rhesus monkey.[29,34]

BETA$_2$-ADRENERGIC RECEPTOR STIMULATORS

Beta receptors have different geographical distributions and pharmacologic responses. β_1 receptors are predominantly present in the heart and the gastroinestinal tract, whereas β_2 receptors are mostly present in the uterus, bronchial tree, and blood vessels. The myometrial cells are activated through changes in extra- and intracellular ionic equilibrium leading to changes in action potential. After reaching a critical level, propagation of the impulse leads to a uterine contraction. Adrenergic neurotransmitters influence these cellular mechanisms, activating uterine contractility through α-adrenergic receptor stimulation and inhibiting it through β-adrenergic receptor stimulation. For example, epinephrine inhibits whereas norepinephrine enhances uterine contractions. Administration of isoproterenol, although it can inhibit uterine activity, has undesirable side effects on the cardiovascular system, such as tachycardia and arrhythmias. Beta stimulants, used to correct hypotension with regional analgesia, cause temporary suppression of uterine contractions.

Several drugs are currently being evaluated for potential use in the treatment of premature labor. These agents are selected for study on the basis of their relative predominance of uterine-inhibiting activity relative to the undesirable cardiovascular responses of tachycardia and hypotension. Among these agents are isoxsuprine, mesuprine, ritodrine, and terbutaline. Only after thorough experimental and human studies will the drug of choice emerge. A brief resumé of some of these drugs follows.

Terbutaline

This drug inhibits uterine activity at term *in vitro*[2] and *in vivo*, both in ewes[32] and in humans[21] It also antagonizes the uterine effect of injected oxytocin.[32]

Administration. Terbutaline can be administered in the form of a continuous infusion to treat premature labor. The loading dose is 10 to 25 μg./min. for 1 hour. Then, at intervals of 30 minutes, the dose is gradually decreased by 5 μg. until the lowest maintenance dose is reached. The infusion is stopped after 8 hours, provided uterine activity has completely ceased. This is followed by intramuscular injections every 4 hours for 24 hours, then oral administration until the time considered safe to deliver the baby.

Effect on the Mother. The effect on the mother is mainly in the form of maternal tachycardia. Hypotension may occur if the patient has been dehydrated. Therefore, hypovolemia should be corrected before the drug is administered.

Effect on the Fetus. In the rhesus monkey, terbutaline dose not significantly change the maternal or fetal acid-base state.[8] In ewes, the uterine blood flow is not adversely changed, and the fetal blood pressure is not altered.[8]

Ritodrine

Ritodrine is another β_2-adrenergic receptor stimulator which has been used to treat premature labor. It is related to isoxsuprine, but is 5 times more effective on the human myometrium, has less cardiovascular side effects, and is effective both orally and intravenously.[42] Following prolonged administration of the drug, no fetal abnormalities have been found. Moreover, there is experimental evidence that fetal weight is increased compared to the control animals, probably due to increase in uterine blood flow.[42] During intravenous infusion, a rise in the fetal heart rate of less than 20 beats/min. has been observed, while the Po_2 and acid-base state remain normal.

OTHER DRUGS

Progesterone

Exogenous progesterone is ineffective as a treatment for premature labor.[42]

Diazoxide

Diazoxide is a strong tocolytic agent. It is probably not a β stimulant since most of its effects are not blocked by beta blockers. Its mechanism of action is unknown. However, it has a relaxant action on the smooth muscles of the blood vessels and has been used clinically as an antihypertensive agent. If administered very slowly, the hypotensive effect is minimal, yet the uterine inhibition persists. In the baboon, in a dose of 0.06 mg./kg./hour it does not adversely affect the maternal or fetal acid-base state.[8] In ewes, it does not significantly alter the uterine blood flow.[8] It is a strong uterine inhibitor, but, because of hypotension, the safety margin of the drug is very narrow, requiring maternal and fetal surveillance.

CONCLUSION

To allow intrauterine manipulation, halothane anesthesia is still the method of choice. However, there is a possibility that in the future other tocolytic agents, e.g., β_2-adrenergic receptor stimulators, may be used instead. The latter drugs offer the advantage of specificity while the patient's consciousness is retained, and thus, the danger of aspiration is eliminated.

To treat premature labor, ethanol is still used in many institutions. β_2 stimulants have now been introduced as well and are safer and more successful than ethanol. Terbutaline has minimal side effects and a safe therapeutic index. If it fails, diazoxide should be used instead, or a combination of terbutaline and ethanol tried. The prostaglandin inhibitors may be the future drugs for uterine inhibition. Since the anesthesiologist may be asked to administer anesthesia to a mother who is under the effect of one or more of these tocolytic agents, and the infant may be delivered with some of these drugs in its bloodstream, he should be aware of their pharmacologic effects on both the mother and fetus.

REFERENCES

1. Abouleish, E.: Postpartum hypertension and convulsion after oxytocic drugs. Anesth., Analg., *55*:813, 1976.
2. Andersson, K. E., Ingemarsson, I., and Persson, C. G. A.: Effect of terbutaline on human uterine motility at term. Acta Obstet. Gynecol. Scand., *54*:165, 1975.
3. Baillie, T. W.: Vasopressor activity of ergometrine maleate in anesthetized parturient women. Br. Med. J., *1*:585, 1963.
4. Belinkoff, S., and Hall, J.: Intravenous alcohol during labor. Am. J. Obstet. Gynecol., *59*:429, 1950.
5. Bergquist, J. R., and Kaiser, I. H.: Cardiovascular effects of intravenous syntocinen. Obstet. Gynecol., *13*:360, 1959.
6. Brooke, O. G., and Robinson, B. F.: Effect of ergotamine and ergometrine on forearm venous compliance in man. Br. Med. J., *1*:139, 1970.
7. Browning, D. J.: Serious side effects of ergometrine and its use in routine obstetric practice. Med. J. Aust., *1*:957, 1974.
8. Caritis, S.: Unpublished data, 1976.
9. Casady, G. M., Moore, D. C., and Bridenbaugh, D. L.: Postpartum hypertension after use of vasoconstrictor and oxytocic drugs. J.A.M.A., *172*:101, 1960.
10. Chapman, E. R., and Williams, J. T., Jr.: Intravenous alcohol as obstetrical analgesia. Am. J. Obstet. Gynecol., *61*:676, 1951.
11. Condie, D. F.: Churchill's Theory and Practice of Midwifery, New American Edition. P. 262. Philadelphia, Henry C. Lea, 1866.
12. Dilts, P. V., Jr.: Effect of ethanol on maternal and fetal acid-base balance. Am. J. Obstet. Gynecol., *107*:1018, 1970.
13. Fuchs, A. R.: The inhibitory effect of ethanol on the release of oxytocin during parturition in the rabbit. J. Endocrinol., *35*:125, 1966.
14. Fuchs, F., *et al.*: Effect of alcohol on threatened premature labor. Am. J. Obstet. Gynecol., *99*:627, 1967.
15. Gombos, G. M., Howitt, D., and Chem, S.: Bilateral retinal detachment occurring in the immediate postpartum period after methylergonovine and oxytocin administration. Eye Ear Nose Throat Mon., *48*:680, 1969.
16. Goodman, L. S., and Gilman, A.: The Pharmacological Basis of Therapeutics. Ed. 5. New York, Macmillan, 1975.
17. Hendricks, C. H., and Brenner, W. E.: Cardiovascular effects of oxytocic drugs used postpartum. Am. J. Obstet. Gynecol., *108*:751, 1970
18. Horiguchi, T., *et al.*: Effect of ethanol upon uterine activity and fetal acid-base state of the rhesus monkey. Am. J. Obstet. Gynecol., *109*:910, 1971.
19. Horton, E. W.: Hypothesis on physiological roles of prostaglandins. Physiol., Rev., *49*:122, 1969.
20. ———: Cardiovascular system. *In* Horton, E. W. (ed.): *Prostaglandins.* Pp. 150–153. New York, Springer-Verlag, 1972.
21. Ingermarsson, I.: Effect of terbutaline on premature labor. Am. J. Obstet. Gynecol., *125*:520, 1976.
22. Johnstone, M.: The cardiovascular effects of oxytocic drugs. Br. J. Anaesth., *44*:826, 1972.
23. Karim, S. M. M.: Response of pregnant human

uterus to prostaglandin-$F_{2\alpha}$-induction of labour. Br. Med. J., *4*:621, 1968.

24. ———: Once-a-month vaginal administration of prostaglandins E_2 and $F_{2\alpha}$ for fertility control. Contraception, *3*:173, 1971.

25. ———: Prostaglandins and human reproduction: physiological roles and clinical uses of prostaglandins in relation to human reproduction. *In* Karim, S. M. M. (ed.): Prostaglandins: Progress in Research. Pp. 71–164, New York, Wiley-Interscience, 1972.

26. Karim, S. M. M., and Filshie, G. M.: Use of prostaglandin E_2 for therapeutic abortion. Br. Med. J., *3*:198, 1970.

27. Karim, S. M. M., and Sharma, S. D.: Termination of second trimester pregnancy with 15-methylanalogues of prostaglandins E_2 and $F_{2\alpha}$. J. Obstet. Gynecol. Br. Commonw., *79*:737, 1972.

28. Karim, S. M. M., *et al.*: Induction of labour with prostaglandin E_2. J. Obstet Gynecol. Br. Commonw., *77*:200, 1970.

29. Katz, R. L.: Antiarrhythmic and cardiovascular effects of synthetic oxytocin. Anesthesiology, *25*:653, 1964.

30. Katz, R. L., and Katz, G. J.: Prostaglandins—basic and clinical consideration. Anesthesiology, *40*:471, 1974.

30a.Mann, L. I. *et al.*: Placental transport of alcohol and its effect on maternal and fetal acid-base balance. Am. J. Obstet. Gynecol., *122*:837, 1975.

31. Mayes, B. Y., and Shearman, R. P.: Experience with synthetic oxytocin—the effects on cardiovascular system and its use for the induction of labour and control of the third stage. J. Obstet. Gynecol. Br. Commonw, *63*:812, 1956.

32. Milliez, J. M., *et al.*: Effect of terbutaline on oxytocic-induced labor in sheep. Abstracts of the Society of Obstetrical Anesthesia and Perinatology, 1976.

33. Moir, C., and Dale, H.: Action of ergot preparations on puerperal uterus. Clinical investigation with special reference to active constituent of ergot as yet unidentified. Br. Med. J. *1*:1119, 1932.

34. Novy, M., Cook, M., and Manaugh, L.: Indomethacin block of normal onset of parturition in primates. Am. J. Obstet. Gynecol., *118*:412, 1974.

35. Physicians' Desk Reference. Ed. 30. p. 1348. Oradell, N.J. Medical Economics Company, 1976.

36. Population Report: Prostaglandins. Series G, No 1. Department of Medical and Public Affairs, The George Washington University Medical Center, Washington, D.C., April, 1973.

37. Ringrose, C. A. D.: The obstetrical use of ergot: a violation of the doctrine "Primum non nocere." Can. Med. Assoc. J. *87*:712, 1962.

38. Schifrin, B. S.: Fetal heart rate patterns following epidural anaesthesia and oxytocin infusion during labour. J. Obstet. Gynecol. Br. Commonw., *79*:332, 1972.

39. Sweatman, W. J. F., and Collier, H. O. J.: Effects of prostaglandins on human bronchial muscle. Nature [Lond.], *217*:69, 1968.

40. Weis, F. R., and Peak, J.: Effects of oxytocin on blood pressure during anesthesia. Anesthesiology, *40*:189, 1974.

41. Woodbury, R. A., *et al.*: Cardiac and blood pressure effects of Pitocin (oxytocin) in man. J. Pharmacol. Exp. Ther., *81*:95, 1944.

42. Zuspan, F. P.: Premature labor: its management and therapy. J. Reprod. Med., *9* (3):93, 1972.

11

Antenatal Evaluation of the Fetus

Steve N. Caritis, M.D. and Eberhard Mueller-Heubach, M.D.

An estimated 55,000 fetal deaths occur annually in the United States.[44] Although a disproportionately large percentage of these fetal deaths occur in a small group of women with some obstetric or medical complication, a significant number occur in otherwise "uncomplicated" pregnancies.[43] Periodic antenatal maternal and fetal assessment is therefore essential in all pregnant patients, but more extensive surveillance is required for those patients at high risk.

Until recently the antenatal assessment of fetal well-being was limited to periodic auscultation of the fetal heart rate; fetal growth was assessed by measurement of the fundal height; and estimates of fetal maturity were based on such imprecise means as patient estimation of last menstrual period, fetal radiography, and measurement of amniotic fluid bilirubin and creatinine. Techniques have now been developed which enable the clinician to accurately assess placental function and fetal growth, maturity, and well-being. Contemporary management of the obstetric patient requires a thorough knowledge of these techniques and their limitations.

The methods used to assess the fetal state antenatally may be divided into tests that evaluate fetal growth and maturity and tests that assess placental function and fetal well-being. Listed below are a few of these methods.

Methods Used to Assess the Fetal State

I. *Fetal growth*
  1. Serial ultrasonic fetal measurements
    a. Biparietal diameter
    b. Other
  2. Serial fundal height measurement
II. *Fetal maturity*
  1. Lecithin-sphingomyelin ratio
  2. Foam stability (shake) test
  3. Ultrasonographic fetal measurement
  4. Amniotic fluid creatinine
  5. Fetal radiography
III. *Placental function and fetal well-being*
  1. Oxytocin challenge test
  2. Serial urinary estriol determinations
  3. Amniotic fluid assessment
    a. Meconium detection
    b. Bilirubin (optical density at 450 mμ)
  4. *In utero* fetal respiratory movements
  5. Systolic time intervals

ASSESSMENT OF FETAL GROWTH

The realization that infants of similar gestational age may vary in birth weight has led to a redefinition of fetal growth and maturity according to both gestational age and birth weight rather than either parameter alone. Previously, maturity had been defined by birth weight alone.[70] An infant weighing less than 2500 g. was deemed premature while infants weighing 2500 g. or more were considered to be at term. It is now apparent that birth weight alone is not an accurate indicator of gestational age and that both birth weight and gestational age must be utilized in order to assess fetal maturity and growth. At any given gestational age, the distribution of birth weights in any given population approximates a bell-shaped curve.[6,35] By definition of the standard curve, 95 per cent of the sample population lies within two standard deviations of the mean. This population of infants is termed appropriate for gestational age, i.e., their birth weight is within two standard deviations of the mean for their gestational peers. Infants whose weight is more than two standard deviations above the mean at a given gestational age are termed large for gestational age, and infants whose weight is more than two standard deviations below the mean are termed small for gestational age.

Fetal and neonatal outcome is strongly affected by the pattern of intrauterine growth.[5] The infant who is large for gestational age (e.g., the infant of a diabetic mother) is more prone to the consequences of fetopelvic disproportion such as trauma from shoulder dystocia, difficult forceps delivery, and an increased risk of delivery by cesarean section. The newborn who is small for gestational age is frequently the product of a pregnancy complicated by severe hypertension, preeclampsia, or malnutrition. These small-for-gestational-age babies are at increased risk throughout the entire perinatal period. Antepartum fetal death, intrapartum asphyxia, meconium aspiration, neonatal hypoglycemia, hypocalcemia, and intraventricular hemorrhage are some of the problems that are commonly seen in these infants.[3,5,67] In addition, animal studies have indicated that growth retardation may be accompanied by a reduction in brain cell number and size.[71,73] Similar findings in humans have been reported,[26] but evidence is still inconclusive. The afore-mentioned problems encountered by the small-for-gestational-age infant emphasize the importance of antenatal assessment of fetal growth. Early detection of intrauterine fetal growth retardation enables the physician to minimize the potential hazards commonly encountered by these fetuses. Weekly oxytocin challenge testing, electronic and biochemical monitoring during labor, and, in severe cases, preterm delivery will increase the possibility for a good outcome.

Serial Ultrasonic Fetal Measurements

Biparietal Diameter. In obstetrics, ultrasound waves are commonly used to outline the fetus and placenta.[17] The measurement of the fetal biparietal diameter has become a routine method of assessing gestational age and fetal growth. A single biparietal measurement is very reproducible (error, less than 1 mm).[18] The accuracy of ultrasound in the measurement of the fetal biparietal diameter has been substantiated by caliper measurements of the biparietal diameter of newborns delivered by cesarean section shortly after ultrasonographic measurement.[16] The measurement of the biparietal diameter in a large population of fetuses at various gestational ages has led to a statistical definition of fetal growth which may be used to predict gestational age by a single measurement of the fetal biparietal diameter (Fig. 11-1).[19] Measurements at 20 to 25 weeks' gestation are fairly accurate in predicting gestational age since the standard deviation in the biparietal diameter among fetuses of similar gestational age is small at this time (± 11 days). Later in gestation a single reading is less precise in assessing gestational age because of large differences in biparietal diameter among fetuses of the same gestational age. Ultrasonography is of great value in those instances in which gestational age is uncertain early in pregnancy. An ultrasonographic determination at 20 weeks gestation can in many instances resolve this dilemma.

Intrauterine growth retardation can be detected by means of serial biparietal diameter measurements. Weekly increments of fetal growth have been determined and deviations from the norm may indicate a growth disorder.[19] A lack of growth in the

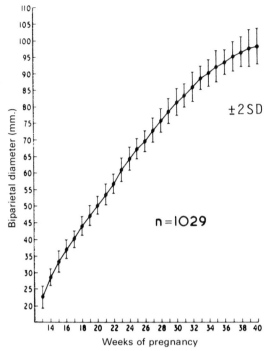

Fig. 11-1. Mean biparietal diameter at various gestational ages. (Campbell, S.: Ultrasonic and radiological examination. *In* Gruenwald, P. (ed.): The Placenta and Its Maternal Supply Line. Pp. 281–306. Baltimore, University Park Press, 1975)

fetal biparietal diameter over a 3- to 4-week period of time is highly suggestive of intrauterine fetal growth retardation.

Other. In addition to the measurement of the fetal biparietal diameter, fetal gestational age and growth may be assessed by a multitude of other fetal measurements. Measurement of fetal thoracic and abdominal size provides dimensions which have been correlated with intrauterine fetal growth.[4,8,36] Campbell and coworkers have calculated daily fetal urine production rates by measurement of the fetal bladder capacity. Gestational age as well as fetal growth can be evaluated with this technique.[20,72]

Serial Fundal Height Measurements

A single fundal height measurement does not provide an accurate assessment of fetal growth; however, serial fundal height measurements performed by the same examiner may be helpful in this regard. This method can detect severe cases of intrauterine fetal growth retardation. When ultrasonography is not available, the only simple method of assessing fetal growth available to the clinician is serial fundal height measurements. Although this technique of assessing fetal growth is ignored by many physicians, the performance of the measurement is justified because it draws the clinician's attention to the growing fetus.

ASSESSMENT OF FETAL MATURITY

Preterm delivery should not be performed unless some estimate of fetal maturity has been obtained, except in cases of extreme emergency. Each test of fetal maturity provides an estimate of the maturity of a single or group of fetal organ systems. Since the major cause of death in the preterm infant is hyaline membrane disease, knowledge of the state of pulmonary maturity is more important than knowing the state of maturity of other organ systems. For instance, the presence of renal or skeletal maturity does not preclude the possibility of the neonate developing hyaline membrane disease.

In the pregnancy complicated by obstetric or medical disease, preterm delivery for fetal or maternal reasons may be necessary. Termination of pregnancy prior to the 36th week may be required in the rhesus-sensitized, diabetic, or hypertensive patient. Fortunately, the development of fetal pulmonary maturity is variable, and in some instances lung maturity occurs as early as 30 weeks gestation.[61] If pulmonary maturity exists, a stressed preterm fetus may be delivered irrespective of gestational age.

The following tests are of value in the determination of fetal maturity:

Lecithin-Sphingomyelin Ratio

The lecithin-sphingomyelin ratio is used to estimate fetal pulmonary maturity.

Lecithin is a surface-active phospholipid that appears to be responsible for the stability of the alveolus. Surface tension in the alveolus is decreased by lecithin, preventing alveolar collapse. Lecithin is produced by the type-2 alveolar cell, and low levels of it may be detected as early as 20 weeks gestation. A sudden rise in the concentration of lecithin in amniotic fluid occurs at approximately 34 to 35 weeks gestation, while the concentration of sphingomyelin, another pulmonary phospholipid with surface-active properties, decreases at this time (Fig. 11-2). Sphingomyelin is included in the determination to correct for differences in amniotic fluid volume. A lecithin-sphingomyelin ratio greater than 2.0 in the amniotic fluid indicates that the fetus is at very low risk for developing or dying from hyaline membrane disease. A lecithin-sphingomyelin ratio less than 2.0 is associated with an increased risk of death from hyaline membrane disease.[30] In infants of diabetic mothers, respiratory distress can occur even with lecithin-sphingomyelin ratios greater than 2.0.[51] In such cases elective delivery should be postponed until the lecithin-sphingomyelin ratio is greater than 2.5 and, when possible, the gestation exceeds 37 weeks. Several studies have reported an acceleration of fetal pulmonary maturation in cases of chronic fetal stress such as severe diabetes with vascular complications, intrauterine fetal growth retardation, and third trimester bleeding.[31,38] Other studies have failed to substantiate this pulmonary accelerative effect of fetal stress.[33,51]

Determination of the lecithin-sphingomyelin ratio requires a minimum of 5 ml. of amniotic fluid, and approximately 4 hours are necessary to perform the test. The lecithin-sphingomyelin ratio is a highly reproducible and very accurate means of assessing the risks for neonatal hyaline membrane disease. However, the results of the lecithin-sphingomyelin ratio determination can be altered by the presence of meconium or blood in the amniotic fluid.[42,45]

Foam Stability (Shake) Test

The foam stability (shake) test first described by Clements[26] is also based on the fact that lecithin possesses surface-active properties. Aliquots of amniotic fluid are

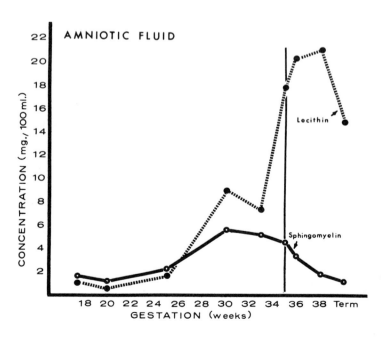

Fig. 11-2. Mean concentrations in amniotic fluid of sphingomyelin and lecithin during gestation. (Gluck, L., *et al.*: Diagnosis of the respiratory distress syndrome by amniocentesis. Am. J. Obstet. Gynecol., *109*:440, 1971)

mixed with increasing amounts of 95 per cent ethanol and physiologic saline in small test tubes. The tubes are gently agitated and the presence or absence of stable bubbles at the air-liquid interface is noted. Amniotic fluid with sufficient surface-active material will foam, resulting in a complete circle of bubbles at the top of the liquid. Various dilutions of the amniotic fluid allow for a semiquantitative assessment of surface-active material. This test is simple to perform, requires a minimum of equipment, and can be done with only 3 ml. of amniotic fluid. The result is obtained in 5 minutes. Contaminants such as meconium and blood invalidate the test.[26] Many studies suggest that a positive shake test at a dilution of 1:2 is frequently associated with a mature lecithin-sphingomyelin ratio and a low incidence of hyaline membrane disease. A negative test, however, does not accurately predict the occurrence of hyaline membrane disease.[21,63]

Fetal Ultrasonographic Measurement

See above, Assessment of Fetal Growth.

Amniotic Fluid Creatinine Concentration

The concentration of creatinine in amniotic fluid may be utilized to estimate fetal gestational age.[56] Amniotic fluid creatinine increases progressively during pregnancy, and after 37 weeks the concentration exceeds values of 2.0 mg. per cent in the majority of cases. The quantity of creatinine in amniotic fluid relates to renal function of the fetus and is influenced by maternal and fetal conditions.[22] Since the occurrence of hyaline membrane disease is related to gestational age, any test that estimates gestational age will indirectly provide a statistical measure of the possibility for the development of hyaline membrane disease. Amniotic fluid creatinine determinations are of value whenever the lecithin-sphingomyelin ratio or shake test cannot be performed or the results obtained are questionable, for example, in cases of blood or meconium staining of the amniotic fluid.[37]

Fetal Radiography

Prior to the development of the above-mentioned tests, radiographic study of the fetal skeleton was commonly used to assess gestational age.[9] The hazards of irradiation do not make this an ideal test. The distal femoral epiphyses and proximal tibial epiphyses are most often evaluated for ossification. Other radiographic studies of the fetal skeleton have been utilized to estimate gestational age but have not added to the accuracy of predicting fetal maturity.[9,23]

ASSESSMENT OF PLACENTAL FUNCTION AND FETAL WELL-BEING

Until recently, the state of fetal well-being could not be accurately assessed. Periodic auscultation of the fetal heart rate during each prenatal visit provided evidence of fetal life, but fetal condition could not be determined. The absence of fetal movement and fetal cardiac activity shortly after a recent "normal" prenatal examination was not a rare occurrence, emphasizing the limitations of these examinations. Recently, however, the ability to evaluate the intrauterine patient has improved considerably and fetal health may be predicted with great accuracy.

Monitoring the fetal condition throughout pregnancy is essential, particularly in pregnancies complicated by maternal or fetal disease since the incidence of antepartum fetal death is greater in these conditions. Periodic assurances of fetal stability will decrease the number of stillbirths and will also decrease the number of unnecessary preterm deliveries performed because of suspected fetal distress.

Oxytocin Challenge Test

The oxytocin challenge test is based on the experience that a compromised fetus will display alterations of the fetal heart rate during periods of additional stress such as those produced by uterine contractions. A characteristic slowing of the fetal heart rate can be produced whenever fetal arterial oxygen tension is transiently decreased to approximately 18 torr.[15,53] Since the slowing of the fetal heart rate occurs late in the uterine contraction phase, it is termed a late deceleration. The precise cause of this type of deceleration has not been clearly defined but fetal arterial hypoxia may play a major role.[15] During a uterine contraction, blood flow to the uterus and intervillous space is reduced, resulting in a transient reduction of oxygen delivery to the fetus.[1,54] In the uncompromised, well-oxygenated fetus, the partial pressure of oxygen in arterial blood ranges between 30 and 40 torr with a saturation of hemoglobin of approximately 60 to 80 per cent.[27,49] During a uterine contraction fetal oxygen levels decrease, but in a well-oxygenated fetus the reduction in oxygen tension does not exceed the critical levels required to produce a deceleration of the fetal heart rate. However, in the case of a compromised fetus in whom the levels of oxygenation may already be reduced, any further diminution of oxygen delivery can result in fetal arterial hypoxia of a sufficient degree to result in the characteristic late deceleration. Recurrent late decelerations of the fetal heart rate most often indicate fetal compromise. The oxytocin challenge test is based on the recognition of this fact and provides an excellent means of assessing the state of fetal well-being.

To perform the oxytocin challenge test the patient is placed in a semi-Fowler's position to avoid supine hypotension, and a fetal monitor is applied. This instrument is used to obtain a continuous recording of fetal heart rate and uterine activity (Fig. 11-3A). The fetal heart rate may be obtained by the use of phonocardiography, Doppler cardiography, or the fetal electrocardiogram which may be obtained from electrodes placed on the maternal abdomen. An indication of uterine activity is obtained with a tokodynamometer which is placed on the maternal abdomen; however, this device does not provide a quantitative measure of uterine pressure. During a uterine contraction, the contour of the maternal abdomen is altered and these changes are detected by the tokodynamometer. Uterine activity and fetal heart rate are monitored for 15 minutes in order to establish a baseline. If uterine contractions are already present, further augmentation of labor is unnecessary. A minimum of 3 contractions must occur over a 10-minute period. If these criteria are not met, dilute oxytocin is infused by means of a pump into a maternal vein. The infusion is begun at 0.5 mU./min. and is increased every 15 minutes until the desired uterine activity occurs (i.e., 3 contractions over a 10-minute period). The infusion is then discontinued.

The oxytocin challenge test is interpreted as positive, suspicious, unsatisfactory, hyperstimulation, or negative. A *positive* test consists of recurrent late decelerations of the fetal heart rate (Fig. 11-3B). Nonrecurrent late decelerations do not constitute a positive test. Such a test is termed *suspicious* and is repeated in 24 hours. Even with judicious use of oxytocin, *hyperstimulation* of the uterine musculature can occur. This may temporarily compromise uteroplacental blood flow and lead to late decelerations of the fetal heart rate. Such iatrogenic causes of late deceleration do not allow for the valid assessment of fetal well-being, and therefore the test must be repeated at some other time. Hyperstimulation exists whenever uterine contractions occur more frequently than every 2 minutes or whenever any contraction exceeds 90 seconds in duration.[58] The presence of hyperstimulation in an otherwise adequate test does not prevent the test from being interpreted as negative if no decelerations occur. This indicates that fetal oxygenation is such that even with exceptional duress fetal hypoxia does not occur. An *unsatisfactory* test is one in which

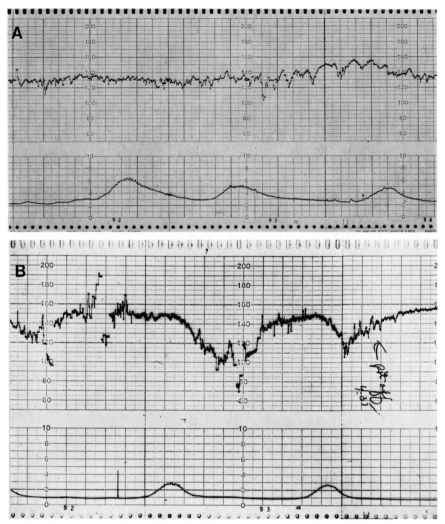

Fig. 11-3. Continuous recording of the fetal heart rate and uterine activity. Paper speed 3 cm./ min. *A*. Negative oxytocin challenge test. *B*. Positive oxytocin challenge test demonstrating late decelerations of the fetal heart rate.

definite fetal evaluation is not possible. Causes for an unsatisfactory test are multiple, but the most common are the inability to elicit 3 contractions in the specified 10-minute period, and the inability to obtain a technically adequate fetal heart rate recording. In these instances the test should be repeated within 24 hours. If there are no late decelerations of the fetal heart rate, the test may be called *negative* and in such instances is repeated weekly.

The oxytocin challenge test has proven to be exceptionally accurate in predicting the absence of fetal compromise. A negative test is more than 99 per cent accurate in predicting that the fetus will not die over the ensuing seven days.[32,58] Fetal death resulting from acute accidents such as abruptio placentae or cord complications cannot be considered as test failures. In patients with diabetes mellitus, chronic hypertension, or preeclampsia, the incidence of fetal compromise increases as pregnancy proceeds. The physician must balance the risk of intrauterine fetal death against the risk of neonatal morbidity and mortality as a result of preterm delivery. The weekly oxytocin challenge test enables the pregnancy to continue until the fetus is capable of survival in an extrauterine environment.

The accuracy of a positive oxytocin challenge test in predicting fetal compromise is less than that of the negative oxytocin challenge test in predicting fetal well-being. In about 20 per cent of cases a positive oxytocin challenge test is not associated with fetal compromise and these fetuses may be delivered vaginally without evidence of acidosis, late decelerations, or low Apgar scores. An additional 60 per cent of fetuses with a positive oxytocin challenge test will survive 7 days after the test but will subsequently demonstrate growth retardation or evidence of fetal distress during labor. The remaining 20 per cent of fetuses with a positive oxytocin challenge test will succumb within 7 days after the test.[34,60,64] The percentage of false positive tests varies among reports and may reflect differences in the criteria which are used to label an oxytocin challenge test as positive.

There are several possible causes for a false positive oxytocin challenge test. Cord compression or other reflex mechanisms in the fetus which are not hypoxic in nature may cause decelerations that may be mistaken for late decelerations. In addition, late decelerations may occur which are not due to chronic fetal distress. Excessive oxytocin administration and maternal hypotension and/or dehydration may be associated with a transient reduction in uteroplacental perfusion and late decelerations of the fetal heart rate. In such cases, even a previously well-oxygenated fetus may appear to be compromised. Failure to recognize these conditions may account for a substantial number of false positive tests.

If delivery is indicated because of a positive oxytocin challenge test, the membranes should be ruptured and the fetus evaluated by direct biophysical and biochemical means. Obtaining the fetal heart rate directly from the fetal electrocardiogram and assessing uterine activity with the use of an intrauterine pressure catheter will provide more accurate information about fetal well-being. Late or otherwise suspicious decelerations detected by external means may prove to be entirely benign when assessed by internal methods, obviating the need for cesarean section. When possible, biochemical analysis of fetal capillary blood should also be performed, especially if some question exists relative to the interpretation of the fetal heart rate pattern.

The performance of the oxytocin challenge test requires well-trained personnel with expertise in biophysical fetal monitoring techniques. The availability of several means for obtaining the fetal heart rate facilitates the acquisition of data. The average time required to perform the test is approximately 90 minutes. Interpretation of the test requires a thorough knowledge of fetal cardiovascular physiology as well as some understanding of the technical aspects of fetal heart rate monitoring. In most institutions the oxytocin challenge test has replaced the determination of 24-hour urinary estriol excretion as the primary method of evaluating fetal well-being.

Serial Urinary Estriol Determinations

The 24-hour urinary excretion of estriol has been regarded by some as a valid means of assessing the fetoplacental unit in late pregnancy.[7,41,62] Others feel the test is inaccurate and expensive.[13,46] The metabolic pathways leading to the production of estriol are complicated and will not be discussed here. The interested reader is referred to several recent reviews.[29,68] The production of estriol is dependent on a functioning fetoplacental unit since both fetal and placental enzymes are necessary for estriol synthesis. The maternal organism also contributes to the total estriol production. The 24-hour urinary excretion of estriol increases with advancing gestational age. Absolute values vary widely from patient to patient, but in a given patient the urinary estriol production is more constant although large daily variations may be seen. The completeness of 24-hour urine collections is assured by the determination of urinary creatinine (a value greater than 1.0 gm./24-hour specimen is suggestive of an adequate urinary collection). A single 24-hour urinary estriol determination is not helpful unless the value is extremely low. Levels less than 4 mg./24 hours after the 36th week of pregnancy are frequently associated with impending or preexisting fetal death. Serial 24-hour urinary estriol determinations minimize the error due to normal daily variation and allow for the continuous assessment of placental function using the patient as her own control. Absolute values are not as important as trends. A decrease of 40 per cent or greater from previous values in the quantity of estriol excreted over a 24-hour period indicates fetal jeopardy. In such cases, additional diagnostic procedures such as the oxytocin challenge test may be performed to substantiate the estriol results. In instances in which the oxytocin challenge test is negative but estriol excretion has decreased more than 40 per cent, most physicians would rely more heavily on the former test.[32]

Goebelsman and coworkers have indicated that daily estriol determinations are necessary, with urine collections performed in the hospital, if the results are to be reliable.[39] In many centers, urine collections are performed on an out-patient basis and then only 2 to 3 times weekly. Such infrequent and potentially incomplete collections could account for the apparent inaccuracy of urinary estriol assays in the detection of fetal distress. Supporters believe that estriol assays are helpful in the management of diabetes, chronic hypertension, preeclampsia, prolonged gestation, and intrauterine fetal growth retardation. The test is not of value in the rhesus-sensitized pregnancy. Since the pregnant diabetic is frequently hospitalized several weeks prior to her anticipated delivery date, the daily collection of urine is easily performed and may provide valuable adjunctive information. The high risk of antepartum fetal death in the diabetic patient justifies the use of all possible parameters to assess fetal and placental function. Therefore, in the diabetic patient both the oxytocin challenge test and daily estriol determinations should be performed. Patients with chronic hypertension and/or intrauterine fetal growth retardation may excrete chronically low levels of urinary estrogens, making the interpretation of changes in daily excretion very difficult.

Urinary estriol excretion is altered by certain drugs (e.g., Mandelamine, ampicillin, and corticosteroids). In addition, glucose in the urine may interfere with assay techniques. The test requires approximately 6 to 8 hours for its performance. Because of the cost, reproducibility, and need for repetitive analysis, the assay of urinary estriol has been supplanted by the oxytocin challenge test in many centers.

Amniotic Fluid Assessment

Meconium Detection. The presence of meconium in amniotic fluid may be an indication of fetal jeopardy. Meconium staining of the amniotic fluid prior to the onset of labor is accompanied by fetal acidosis in as many as 9 per cent of cases, and in addition, up to 31 per cent of such cases may be associated with fetal acidosis during the intrapartum period.[12,48] Neonatal mortality rates may be increased 20-fold in the presence of meconium-stained amniotic fluid.[66] Meconium in the amniotic fluid is also associated with increased neonatal morbidity due to aspiration penumonitis. Acute or chronic hypoxia may result in fetal gasping, with resulting aspiration of amniotic fluid into the tracheobronchial tree. The highly irritant properties of meconium will cause severe respiratory compromise in the neonate.

Although in many instances the presence of meconium does not result in a poor fetal outcome, early detection of stained fluid will decrease perinatal mortality rates.[59] Saling reported a decrease in perinatal mortality from 2.5 per cent to 0.9 per cent in cases of suspected postdatism and from 8.3 per cent to 1.7 per cent in cases of toxemia by the use of amnioscopy to detect meconium prior to labor. The technique of amnioscopy has been described by Saling and others.[50,59] An endoscope is placed through the partially dilated cervix and a characteristic greenish tinge is noted whenever meconium is present. In approximately 5 per cent of cases, amniotic fluid which appears clear on amnioscopy will contain meconium; however, in only 1 to 2 per cent of cases will meconium which is noted to be present on amnioscopy not be confirmed at amniotomy.[50] Amnioscopy provides useful adjunctive information to other methods of fetal surveillance. It is particularly helpful in instances of questionable prolonged gestation. It also provides a means by which intra-amniotic fetal hemorrhage may be detected.

Change in Optical Density at 450 mμ. In the Rh-sensitized pregnancy the severity of fetal disease can only be assessed by the spectrophotometric measurement of bilirubinoid products in the amniotic fluid. The state of fetal well-being cannot be assessed adequately by analysis of urinary estriol excretion or by the oxytocin challenge test. Severe fetal anemia may be associated with normal estriol excretion values and a negative oxytocin challenge test. The anlaysis of amniotic fluid in the management of the rhesus-sensitized patient is discussed in several texts dealing with rhesus disease.[24,57]

Fetal Respiration

Barcroft observed movements of the fetal thorax during his pioneering studies in fetal lambs.[2] Dawes and coworkers evaluated the respiratory movements of chronically instrumented fetal lambs and demonstrated the presence of intrauterine fetal respirations.[28] During any 24-hour period, these respiratory movements occurred up to 40 per cent of the time in healthy fetuses. Subsequently, Boddy demonstrated the presence of respiratory movements in human fetuses using ultrasound techniques.[11]

The mechanisms responsible for the initiation and maintenance of fetal respiratory movements have not been defined. However, sufficient data have accumulated indicating that the assessment of fetal respiratory movement is a promising method of evaluating fetal well-being.[10,11,28,47] Boddy has reported that the human fetus spends approximately 80 per cent of the time engaged in some form of respiratory activity. Animal studies have demonstrated that fetal hypoxia will abolish rhythmic respiratory movements, whereas fetal hypercapnia increases these movements. The combination of fetal hypoxia and hypercapnia results in fetal gasping which is associated with intrathoracic pressures as high as -40 torr. A marked decrease in fetal respiratory activity has been noted prior to intrauterine fetal death or in association with fetal compromise. Boddy has successfully predicted the occurrence of intrauterine fetal death in a group of high-risk patients.[10]

At present fetal respiratory activity in the human is most often detected by the use of ultrasound. A great deal of technical expertise is necessary in order to obtain valid data. The advantage of this technique over currently available methods of assessing fetal well-being has not been fully evaluated.

Systolic Time Intervals

In adults, myocardial function has been assessed by the study of several intervals in the cardiac cycle. The preejection period defines the time interval from the electrical activation of the myocardium to the opening of the aortic valve (Fig. 11-4).[69] In the fetus, the preejection period is obtained by the use of a fetal scalp electrode and an ultrasonic transducer which is placed on the maternal abdomen to obtain fetal aortic valvular opening.[40] Since the Q wave of the fetal electrocardiogram is poorly defined, with a scalp electrode the interval between the fetal R wave and aortic valvular opening is utilized to determine the preejection period. This period has been demonstrated to be independent of heart rate.[65] The interval increases with increasing gestational age.[52] In a normal fetus of 38 to 40 weeks gestation, the average interval is approximately 70 milliseconds. In experimental studies, compression of the umbilical cord results in prolongation of the preejection period. Acidosis also results in prolongation of the preejection period. However, the effects of hypoxia are not certain. Organ noted a decrease in this interval in hypoxic fetal lambs, whereas Murata noted a prolongation of this period in hypoxic fetal monkeys.[52,55]

The clinical value of measuring the preejection period has not been determined. The close correlation between fetal acidosis and the length of the preejection period is promising. However, the technical problems associated with this method of fetal monitoring currently make it less desirable than the methods now at hand.

REFERENCES

1. Assali, N. S., *et al.*: Measurement of uterine blood flow and uterine metabolism. J. Physiol. [Lond.], *195*:614, 1958.
2. Barcroft, J., and Barron, D. H.: The genesis of respiratory movements in the foetus of the sheep. J. Physiol,. [Lond.] *88*:56, 1937.

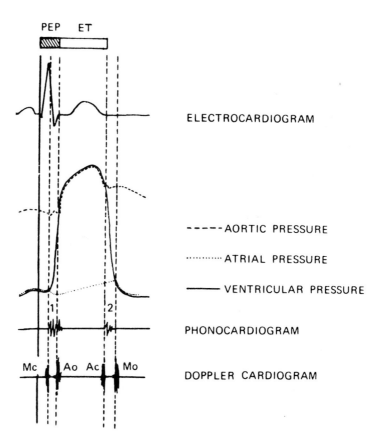

Fig. 11-4. Schematic presentation of the systolic time intervals of the cardiac cycle. PEP = preejection period; ET = ventricular ejection time; 1 = first heart sound; 2 = second heart sound; MC = mitral closure; AO = aortic opening; AC = aortic closure; MO = mitral opening. (Hon, E. H., *et al.*: Continuous microfilm display of the electromechanical intervals of the cardiac cycle. Obstet. Gynecol., *43*:722, 1974)

3. Bard, H.: Intrauterine growth retardation, Clin. Obstet. Gynecol., *13*:511, 1970.
4. Bartolucci, L.: Biparietal diameter of the skull and fetal weight in the second trimester: An allometric relationship. Am. J. Obstet. Gynecol., *122*:439, 1975.
5. Battaglia, F. C.: Intrauterine growth retardation. Am. J. Obstet. Gynecol., *106*:1103, 1970.
6. Battaglia, F. C., Frazier, T. M., and Hellegers, A. E.: Birth weight, gestational age and pregnancy outcome with special reference to high birth weight-low gestational age infant. Pediatrics, *37*:417, 1966.
7. Beischer, N. A., *et al.*: The incidence and significance of low estriol excretion in an obstetric population. J. Obstet. Gynecol., Br. Commonw., *75*:1024, 1968.
8. Berger, G. S., Edelman, D. A., and Kerenyi, T. D.: Fetal crown, rump length and biparietal diameter in the second trimester of pregnancy. Am. J. Obstet. Gynecol., *122*:9, 1975.
9. Bluth, I.: The antenatal study of the fetus. Clin. Obstet. Gynecol., *9*:22, 1966.
10. Boddy, K., and Dawes, G. S.: Fetal breathing. Obstet. Gynecol. Sur., *30*:589, 1975.
11. Boddy, K., and Robinson, J. S.: External method for detection of fetal breathing in utero. Lancet, *2*:1231, 1971.
12. Bollinger, J., *et al.*: Hat die Amnioskopie heute noch ihre Berechtigung? Eine Analyse von 4000 Amnioskopien. Fortschr. Med., *90*:937, 1972.
13. Booth, R. T., *et al.*: Urinary hormone excretion in abnormal pregnancy. J. Obstet. Gynecol., Br. Commonw., *72*:229, 1965.
14. Brandfass, R. T., and Howland, H. J.: Determination of fetal weight by long bone measurements. Obstet. Gynecol., *29*:230, 1970.
15. Caldeyro-Barcia, R., *et al.*: Correlation of intrapartum changes in fetal heart rate with fetal blood oxygen and acid-base state. *In* Adamsons, K. (ed.): Diagnosis and Treatment of Fetal Disorders. Pp. 205–225. New York, Springer-Verlag, 1968.
16. Campbell, S.: An improved method of fetal cephalometry by ultrasound. J. Obstet. Gynecol. Br. Commonw., *75*:568, 1968.
17. ———Ultrasound in obstetrics. Br. J. Hosp. Med., *8*:541, 1972.
18. ———Ultrasonic and radiologic examination. *In* Gruenwald, P. (ed.): The Placenta and the Maternal Supply. Pp. 281–306, Baltimore, University Park Press, 1975.
19. Campbell, S., and Newman, G. B.: Growth of the fetal biparietal diameter during normal pregnancy. J. Obstet. Gynecol. Br. Commonw., *78*:513, 1971.
20. Campbell, S., Wladimiroff, J. W., and Dewhurst, C. J.: The antenatal measurement of fetal urine production. J. Obstet. Gynecol. Br. Commonw., *80*:680, 1973.
21. Caspi, E., Schreyer, P., and Tamier, I.: The amniotic fluid foam test, L/S ratio, and total phospholipids in the evaluation of fetal lung maturity. Am. J. Obstet. Gynecol., *122*:323, 1975.
22. Cassady, G.: Amniocentesis. Clin. Perinatol., *1*:87, 1974.
23. Chang, L. W. M., *et al.*: Device to estimate fetal age. Obstet. Gynecol., *38*:154, 1971.
24. Charles, A. G., and Friedman, E. A.: (eds.): Rh Isoimmunication and Erythroblastosis Fetalis. New York, Appleton-Century-Crofts, 1969.
25. Chase, H. P., *et al.*:Alterations in human brain biochemistry following intrauterine growth retardation. Pediatrics, *50*:403, 1972.
26. Clements, J. A., *et al.*: Assessment of the risk of the respiratory distress syndrome by a rapid test for surfactant in amniotic fluid. N. Engl. J. Med., *286*:1077, 1972.
27. Comline, R. S., and Silver, M.: Daily changes in fetal and maternal blood of conscious and pregnant ewes with catheters in umbilical and uterine vessels. J. Physiol. [Lond.], *209*:567, 1970.
28. Dawes, G. S., *et al.*: Respiratory movements and rapid eye movement in the fetal lamb. J. Physiol. [Lond.], *220*:119, 1972.
29. Diczfalusy, E.: Endocrine functions of the human fetus. Am. J. Obstet. Gynecol., *119*:419, 1974.
30. Donald, I. R., *et al.*: Clinical experience with the amniotic fluid lecithin sphingomyelin ratio. Am. J. Obstet. Gynecol., *115*:547, 1973.
31. Dyson, D., Blake, M., and Cassady, G.: Amniotic fluid lecithin sphingomyelin ratio in complicated pregnancies. Am. J. Obstet. Gynecol., *112*:772, 1975.
32. Freeman, R. K.: The use of the oxytocin challenge test for antepartum clinical evaluation of uteroplacental respiratory function. Am. J. Obstet. Gynecol., *121*:481, 1975.
33. Freeman, R. K., *et al.*: Clinical experience with the amniotic fluid lecithin sphingomyelin ratio. Am. J. Obstet. Gynecol., *119*:239, 1974.
34. ———An evaluation of the significance of a positive oxytocin challenge test. Obstet. Gynecol., *47*:8, 1976.
35. Fujikura, T., and Neiman, W. H.: Birth weight, gestational age and type of delivery in rhesus monkeys. Am. J. Obstet. Gynecol., *97*:76, 1967.
36. Garrett, W. J., and Robinson, D. E.: Assessment of fetal size and growth rate by ultrasonic echoscopy. Obstet. Gynecol., *38*:525, 1971.
37. Gibbons, J. M., Huntley, T. E., and Corral, A. G.: Effect of maternal blood contamination on amniotic fluid analysis. Obstet. Gynecol., *44*:657, 1974.
38. Gluck, L., Kulovich, M. V., and Gould, J. B.: The effects of maternal disease on maturation of human fetal lung. Soc. Pediatr. Res., *6*:409, 1972.
39. Goebelsmann, U., *et al.*: Estriol and pregnancy; daily urinary estriol assays in the management of the pregnant diabetic woman. Am. J. Obstet. Gynecol., *15*:795, 1973.
40. Goodlin, R. C., Girard, J., and Hollmen, A.: Systolic time intervals in the fetus and neonate. Obstet. Gynecol., *39*:295, 1972.
41. Greene, J. W., Jr., and Touchstone, J. C.: Urinary estriol as an index of placental function. Am. J. Obstet. Gynecol., *85*:1, 1963.
42. Harding, P., *et al.*: Amniotic fluid phospholipids

and fetal maturity. Am. J. Obstet. Gynecol., *115*:298, 1973.

43. Hobel, C. J., *et al.*: Prenatal and intrapartum high-risk screening. Am. J. Obstet. Gynecol., *117*:1, 1973.

44. Hoffman, H. J., *et al.*: Analysis of birth weight, gestational age and fetal viability, U.S. births, 1968. Obstet. Gynecol. Surv., *29*:651, 1974.

45. Kulkarni, B. D., *et al.*: Determination of lecithin sphingomyelin ratios in amniotic fluid. Obstet. Gynecol., *40*:173, 1972.

46. MacLeod, S. C., *et al.*: The value of urinary estriol mesaurements during pregnancy. Aust. N.Z. J. Obstet. Gynecol., 7:25, 1967.

47. Martin, C. B., *et al.*: Respiratory movements in fetal rhesus monkeys. Am. J. Obstet. Gynecol., *119*:939, 1974.

48. Mathews, C. D. and Martin, M. R.: Early detection of meconium stained liquor during labor; a contribution of fetal care. Am. J. Obstet. Gynecol., *120*:808, 1974.

49. Meschia, G., *et al.*: The hemoglobin, oxygen, carbon dioxide, and hydrogen ion concentrations in the umbilical bloods of sheep and goats as sampled via indwelling plastic catheters. Q. J. Exp. Physiol., *50*: 185, 1965.

50. Mueller-Heubach, E.: Amnioscopy. Clin. Perinatol., *1*:81, 1974.

51. Mueller-Heubach, E., Caritis, S. N., and Edelstone, D. I.: Management of pregnant diabetics using L/S ratios, urinary estrogens and oxytocin challenge test. Abstract no. 170, 4th European Congress of Perinatal Medicine, Uppsala, 1976.

52. Murata, Y., and Martin, C. B.: Systolic time intervals of the fetal cardiac cycle. Obstet. Gynecol., *44*:224, 1974.

53. Myers, R. E., Mueller-Heubach, E., and Adamsons, K.: Predictability of the state of fetal oxygenation from a quantitative analysis of the components of late deceleration. Am. J. Obstet. Gynecol., *115*:1083, 1973.

54. Novy, M. J., Thomas, C. L., and Lees, M. H.: Uterine contractility and regional blood flow responses to oxytocin and prostaglandin E_2 in pregnant rhesus monkeys. Am. J. Obstet. Gynecol., *122*:419, 1975.

55. Organ, L. W., *et al.*: The pre-ejection period of the fetal heart: response to stress in the term fetal lamb. Am. J. Obstet. Gynecol., *115*:377, 1973.

56. Pitkin, R. M., and Zwirek, S. J.: Amniotic fluid creatinine. Am. J. Obstet. Gynecol., *98*:1135, 1967.

57. Queenan, J. T. (ed.): Modern Management of the Rh Problem. New York, Harper & Row, 1967.

58. Ray, M., *et al.*: Clinical experience with the oxytocin challenge test. Am. J. Obstet. Gynecol., *114*:1, 1972.

59. Saling, E., Amnioscopy. Clin. Obstet. Gynecol., *9*:472, 1966.

60. Schiffrin, B., *et al.*: Contraction stress tests for antepartum fetal evaluation. Obstet. Gynecol., *45*:433, 1975.

61. Schulman, J. D., *et al.*: Lecithin sphingomyelin ratios in amniotic fluid. Obstet. Gynecol., *40*:697, 1972.

62. Schwarz, R. H., and Fields, G. A.: The management of the pregnant diabetic. Obstet. Gynecol., Surg., *26*:277, 1971.

63. Shephard, B., Buhi, W., and Spellacy, W.: Critical analysis of the amniotic fluid shake test. Obstet. Gynecol., *43*:558, 1974.

64. Spurrett, B.: Stressed cardiotocography in late pregnancy. Obstet. Gynecol. Br. Commonw., *78*:894, 1971.

65. Talley, R. C., Meyer, J. F., and McNay, N. L.: Evaluation of the pre-ejection period as an estimate of myocardial contractility in dogs. Am. J. Cardiol., *27*:384, 1971.

66. Ting, P., and Brady, J. P.: Tracheal suction in meconium aspiration. Am. J. Obstet. Gynecol., *122*:767, 1975.

67. Usher, R.: Clinical and therapeutic aspects of fetal malnutrition. Pediatr. Clin. North Am., *17*:169, 1970.

68. Villee, D. B.: Development of endocrine function in the human placenta and fetus. N. Engl. J. Med., *281*:473, 1969.

69. Weissler, A. M., Harris, W. S., and Schoenfeld, C. D.: Systolic time intervals in heart failure in man. Circulation, *37*:149, 1968.

70. W.H.O., Expert Group on Prematurity: Final Report. W.H.O. Technical Report Series No. 27, Geneva, 1950.

71. Winick, M.: Nutrition and nerve cell growth. Proceedings of the 53rd Annual Meeting of the Federation of American Societies for Experimental Biology, Atlantic City, N. J., April, 1969.

72. Wladimiroff, J. W., and Campbell, S.: Fetal urine production rates in normal and complicated pregnancy. Lancet, *1*:151, 1974.

73. Zanenhof, S., Marthens, E., and Margolis, F. L.: DNA (cell number) and protein in neonatal brain; alteration by maternal dietary protein restriction. Science, *160*:322, 1968.

12

Evaluation of Fetal Condition During Labor and Delivery

Eberhard Mueller-Heubach, M. D. and Steve N. Caritis, M.D.

During labor and delivery, the human fetus is subjected to transient alterations in its oxygen supply which are well tolerated by the vast majority of fetuses. However, in a small percentage of fetuses the degree of oxygen deprivation may be sufficient to interfere with the energy transformation in vital organs of the fetus to an extent that permanent damage is incurred. The organ which is most sensitive to oxygen deprivation is the fetal brain. Varying degrees of brain damage may result from lack of oxygen supply to the fetus during labor and delivery, ranging from minimal brain damage to severe cerebral palsy.

With the development of the Apgar scoring system[3] physicians started to take a closer look at the newborn immediately after delivery, and it was recognized that difficult labors and deliveries resulted in neonates with lower Apgar scores. Data from a collaborative project indicated that in newborns of a given birth weight with Apgar scores of 3 or less at 5 minutes of age there was an incidence of neurologic deficit at 1 year of age 3 times higher than in neonates of similar birth weight with 5-minute Apgar scores of 7 or more.[14] Assessment of the Apgar score of the newborn and the pH of umbilical cord blood has demonstrated that Apgar scores are lower whenever the cord blood is aci-

dotic.[25] Generally, acidosis of fetal blood reflects oxygen deprivation of tissues and conversion to anaerobic glycolysis for energy transformation. Extensive experimental work with models of fetal asphyxia in the subhuman primate has elucidated the mechanisms of perinatal brain damage.[34]

With the increasing clinical and experimental evidence relating neonatal outcome to events occurring during labor and delivery, obstetricians became eager to find new methods of ascertaining the state of fetal oxygenation and searched for ways of detecting changes in fetal oxygen supply before these changes endangered the integrity of the fetal nervous system. The crude method of intermittent auscultation of the fetal heart rate was found to be an unreliable indicator of fetal condition.

UTERINE BLOOD FLOW AND FETAL OXYGENATION DURING LABOR

The principles of placental blood flow have been elucidated by the cineradiographic studies of Ramsey and coworkers[39] in the rhesus monkey. (Details of these principles can be found in Chap. 3, The Placenta and Placental Transfer of Drugs at Term.) Uterine vascular resistance is at a minimum at any given stage in gestation, and autoregulatory mechanisms to increase uterine blood flow by decreasing uterine vascular resistance do not exist.[17] Uterine blood flow is directly dependent on perfusion pressure of the uterine vasculature[29] and no preferential circulatory adjustments to maintain uterine perfusion occur when systemic changes in the maternal circulation take place.

The branches of the uterine vessels which traverse the myometrium to and from the intervillous space are compressed during uterine contractions, resulting in an interruption of blood flow to and from the intervillous space.[39] As the myometrial fibers start to contract, the pressure exerted on the vessels traversing the myometrium reaches and exceeds the pressure within the veins, thus preventing venous outflow from the intervillous space. As the myometrial fibers continue to contract, the pressure within the arterial vessels leading to the intervillous space is exceeded and arterial inflow to the intervillous space is interrupted. When the myometrium starts to relax during the second half of a uterine contraction this sequence of hemodynamic events is reversed. Therefore, fetal oxygen supply is intermittently interrupted during labor. Adequate fetal oxygenation requires periodic uterine relaxation during which sufficient amounts of oxygen are delivered to fetal tissues to meet fetal metabolic requirements. During a uterine contraction the fetus is dependent upon the oxygen stored in the intervillous space and the umbilical circulation. The periodic reduction in fetal oxygen delivery results in a limited degree of fetal metabolic acidosis which is present even in normal labors. However, this does not affect the integrity of fetal tissues.

FACTORS ADVERSELY AFFECTING FETAL OXYGENATION

Any decrease in the oxygen content of the maternal blood perfusing the placenta will impair the oxygen supply to the fetus.

Maternal respiratory or cardiac disorders may endanger the fetus if these conditions result in a decrease in the oxygen content of maternal blood. Since most oxygen is bound to hemoglobin, the oxygen-carrying capacity of maternal blood is reduced when the mother is anemic. Thus, fetuses of anemic mothers are more likely to become distressed during labor and delivery. The greater affinity of hemoglobin for carbon monoxide and the higher concentrations of carbon monoxide in the blood of smokers may decrease the oxygen content of maternal blood if the mother smokes.

Factors which may decrease uterine perfusion will reduce oxygen transport to the fetus. Hypotension, whether due to regional anesthesia or the supine position, or maternal dehydration are important causes of impaired placental blood flow which may result in fetal hypoxia.[31] Many alpha-sympathomimetic agents act by vasoconstriction of certain regional vascular beds including the uterine vasculature. Although systemic blood pressure may be restored by these agents, perfusion of the uterus and placental gas exchange can be markedly reduced.[46] These important considerations will be presented elsewhere in this book in more detail.

Inadequate pain control as well as anxiety and fear in the pregnant patient during labor and delivery may produce increased release of catecholamines from the adrenal medulla. Studies in subhuman primates have demonstrated that prolonged infusions of catecholamines produce impairment of fetal oxygenation.[1] This impairment is the result of a direct constrictive effect of catecholamines on the uterine vasculature, although in some instances increased uterine activity contributed to the decrease in fetal oxygen supply. Electrical stimulation of lumbar sympathetic nerves in pregnant ewes has been shown to decrease uterine blood flow.[18] These findings point to the importance of adequate pain control in the obstetric patient.

It has been recognized that the supine position which laboring women traditionally assume in most countries may reduce the blood flow to the uterus.[18] In some instances the pregnant uterus may compress the inferior vena cava, reducing venous return to the maternal heart and producing the syndrome of supine hypotension. Laboring patients should be encouraged to lie on their side which prevents compression of the inferior vena cava and possibly even the abdominal aorta by the pregnant uterus. It is of interest to note that women of some primitive tribes do not labor in a supine but in a squatting position which never exposes their fetuses to the risk of hypoxia as a result of supine hypotension.

Maternal conditions which may be accompanied by vasoconstriction of the uterine vasculature such as preeclampsia or chronic hypertension reduce placental blood flow and jeopardize the fetus. Lowering of maternal blood pressure in these situations may decrease the perfusion pressure of the uterine vascular bed and endanger the fetus even more. Therefore, antihypertensive therapy should probably be initiated only when maternal blood pressure has reached levels which endanger the mother.

On the fetal side the most frequent factors which interfere acutely with fetal oxygenation are problems with the umbilical cord. Fetal anemia together with edema of the placental villi as found in erythroblastosis may lead to fetal death probably as a result of high-output heart failure in response to the decreased oxygen-carrying capacity of fetal blood.

MONITORING OF FETAL CONDITION DURING LABOR AND DELIVERY

As knowledge of fetal physiology has expanded, techniques have been developed which allow a better assessment of fetal well-being during labor and delivery than was possible with the traditional auscultation of fetal heart rate every few minutes. Biophysical and biochemical techniques of fetal assessment have been developed. These techniques have become almost universally accepted and are practiced at many major obstetrical services.

BIOPHYSICAL MONITORING OF THE FETUS

Continuous electronic monitoring of fetal heart rate and uterine activity was pioneered by Hon,[21] Hammacher,[19] and Caldeyro-Barcia.[12] The high metabolic requirements of the fetal myocardium are responsible for the sensitivity of the fetal heart to decreases in oxygenation. Specific changes in fetal heart rate have been recognized as indicators of fetal oxygen deprivation, hemodynamic changes in the umbilical circulation, or compression of the fetal head.

Technique of Biophysical Monitoring

Two approaches can be taken to obtain a continuous electronic recording of fetal heart rate and uterine activity. The *indirect external approach* can be utilized prior to cervical dilatation and rupture of membranes. An external tokodynamometer fastened to a belt is placed on the maternal abdomen over the uterus for recording of uterine activity. In the center of this tokodynamometer is a pin which is depressed whenever the uterus changes its contour during a uterine contraction. This method of recording uterine activity gives an indication of when a uterine contraction occurs; however, uterine activity cannot be adequately quantitated in this fashion. The input signal for the cardiotachometer which records fetal heart rate can be obtained externally in several ways. Most frequently an ultrasound transducer which emits and receives high-frequency sound is placed on the maternal abdomen. The sound waves are reflected by the moving interfaces of the fetal heart and are received by the transducer, providing an input for the cardiotachometer. The fetal heart rate signal can also be obtained by means of phonocardiography from the maternal abdomen. However, this approach is prone to artifacts as a result of a poor signal to noise ratio. Finally, electrodes placed on the maternal abdomen can be used to record electrical activity of the fetal heart, with the R wave of the fetal electrocardiogram providing the input signal for the cardiotachometer. Due to the much greater amplitude of the maternal ECG complexes the recording of the fetal electrocardiogram from the maternal abdomen is not always successful.

Direct or internal biophysical monitoring requires rupture of the membranes as well as a limited degree of cervical dilatation. Uterine activity is recorded by means of a fluid-filled plastic catheter which is introduced into the uterine cavity and connected to a strain gauge. This allows accurate measurement of the intrauterine pressure which is created during a uterine contraction. The fetal electrocardiogram is obtained by means of a spiral electrode which is attached superficially to the presenting part of the fetus. The R wave is used as input for the cardiotachometer. The recording of fetal heart rate obtained in this manner is generally far superior to any externally obtained input signal for fetal heart rate monitoring.

With limited experience technically adequate tracings of fetal heart rate and uterine activity can be obtained. Postpartum infection has not been a problem with the direct, invasive method of fetal monitoring.[47] Rare cases of uterine perforations during introduction of the intrauterine catheter are the result of forceful manipulations and can be avoided.

Interpretation of Fetal Heart Rate Tracings

Baseline fetal heart rate is generally a poor indicator of fetal condition.[7] The normal range of fetal heart rate is 120 to 155 beats per minute. Tachycardia is

thought to be related to mild hypoxia, and is frequently seen with maternal fever. Fetal bradycardia below 100 beats per minute present for a long period of time may indicate a defect in electrical conduction of the fetal heart. In experimental studies in the rhesus monkey, baseline fetal heart rate did not change significantly during prolonged and severe fetal hypoxia and acidosis.[32]

Decelerative Patterns of Fetal Heart Rate. Three distinct patterns of transient deceleration of fetal heart rate have been recognized. These decelerations have a temporal relationship to uterine contractions and are labeled accordingly as early, variable, and late decelerations.

In *early decelerations* of fetal heart rate the deceleration coincides with the occurrence of the uterine contraction and is usually of limited amplitude. They are thought to represent a vagal reflex resulting from fetal head compression and can be abolished by the administration of atropine. The presence of early decelerations is not an indication of fetal jeopardy.

Variable decelerations are characterized by a variable temporal relationship to uterine contractions. The amplitude of the variable deceleration is usually greater than that of other types of decelerations with rapid decrease and recovery of fetal heart rate (Fig. 12-1). Variable decelerations are the result of umbilical cord compression and can frequently be relieved by a change in maternal position when the umbilical cord is compressed between a fetal part and the uterine wall. This decelerative pattern is the most frequently observed one. If variable decelerations of fetal heart rate are severe and repetitive over a prolonged time period, they have the potential to interfere with fetal oxygenation.[28] Less severe variable decelerations during a limited period of time usually do not jeopardize the fetus. Assessment of fetal condition by other techniques is indicated whenever persistent variable decelerations of the fetal heart rate are seen during the

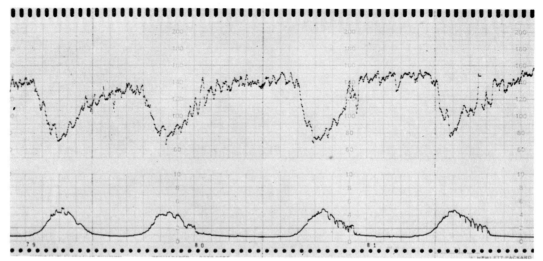

Fig. 12-1.   Variable decelerations of fetal heart rate. The upper tracing represents fetal heart rate and the lower tracing represents intrauterine pressure.

course of labor to ascertain whether these episodes of umbilical cord compression compromise oxygen supply to the fetus.

The most ominous decelerative pattern of fetal heart rate in terms of fetal well-being is that of *late decelerations* (Fig. 12-2). The onset of a late deceleration follows the onset of a uterine contraction with a latency period of 10 to 40 seconds. Late decelerations are an indication of fetal oxygen deprivation. Experimental work in the rhesus monkey has clearly shown that the latency period between onset of uterine contraction and onset of late deceleration correlates well with the degree of oxygenation of fetal arterial blood prior to the uterine contraction.[35] A similar relation-

ship was also demonstrated between fetal oxygenation and the rate of decrease in fetal heart rate during a late deceleration. Figure 12-3 illustrates that the absolute decrease in fetal heart rate during a late deceleration depends upon the degree of fetal oxygenation prior to the uterine contraction. A certain oxygen content of fetal arterial blood is necessary to sustain fetal myocardial performance. If fetal oxygenation is compromised, further reduction in oxygen transfer to the fetus as a result of a uterine contraction will produce late decelerations of fetal heart rate since the high metabolic requirements of the fetal myocardium cannot be met. Experimental work in rhesus monkeys indicates that dur-

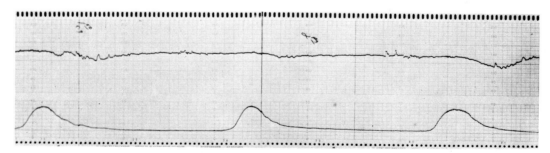

Fig. 12-2.   Late decelerations of fetal heart rate. The upper tracing represents fetal heart rate and the lower tracing represents uterine activity.

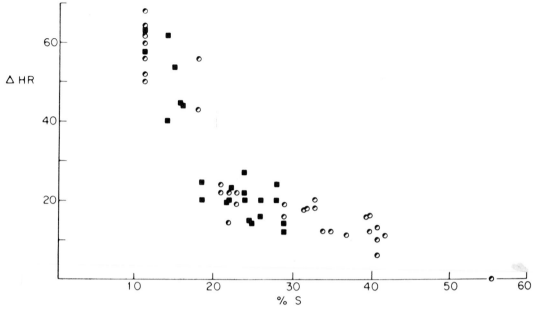

Fig. 12-3.   Decrease in fetal heart rate (beats per minute) of two rhesus monkey fetuses during late decelerations as a function of hemoglobin saturation with oxygen (%) of fetal arterial blood before onset of the uterine contractions. (Myers, R. E., Mueller-Heubach, E., and Adamsons, K.: Predictability of the state of fetal oxygenation from a quantitative analysis of the components of late deceleration. Am. J. Obstet. Gynecol., *115*:1083, 1973)

ing fetal asphyxia there is a decrease in the cardiac output of the fetus, with preferential distribution to the brain, myocardium, and adrenals.[6] This probably accounts for the significant degree of desaturation of fetal arterial blood which is present whenever late decelerations are observed.

Beat-to-Beat Variability of Fetal Heart Rate. Since the time intervals between R waves of the fetal ECG complex are not exactly the same, an irregularity of the baseline fetal heart rate is observed which has been labeled "beat-to-beat variability." It is being increasingly recognized that beat-to-beat variability of fetal heart rate reflects fetal well-being. In order to appreciate this beat-to-beat variability, fetal heart rate recordings have to be obtained by means of instantaneous cardiotachometers which do not average several incoming electrical signals but print out every single electrical input signal coming from the fetal heart. More severe degrees

of fetal acidosis have been found in the presence of late decelerations of fetal heart rate whenever beat-to-beat variability was decreased compared to late decelerations with normal fetal heart rate variability.[38] Efforts are being made to quantitate variability of fetal heart rate electronically.[49] It is thought that normal beat-to-beat variability reflects the integrity of the fetal autonomic nervous system with its interplay of sympathetic and parasympathetic discharges. Figure 12-4 illustrates simultaneous recording of fetal heart rate externally by means of an ultrasound transducer and internally by means of a spiral electrode. The technical quality of an externally obtained input signal of fetal heart rate is inadequate to allow accurate evaluation of beat-to-beat variability because of artifacts. In the illustration, beat-to-beat variability appears normal when judged by the externally obtained recording whereas in reality variability is decreased as indi-

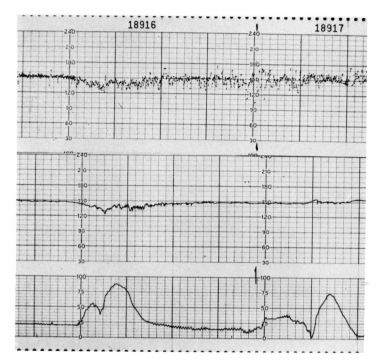

Fig. 12-4. Beat-to-beat variability of fetal heart rate recorded externally (upper tracing) versus internally (middle tracing). The lower tracing represents intra-uterine pressure. (See text for details.)

cated by the direct recording of fetal heart rate from the presenting part of the fetus.

Most pharmacologic agents used for pain control or sedation in the pregnant patient during labor are transferred rapidly across the placenta and decrease normal beat-to-beat variability of fetal heart rate.[10,45] This fact is essential in the interpretation of fetal heart rate variability in order to prevent a false diagnosis of fetal compromise when beat-to-beat variability is depressed as a result of drug administration to the mother. Loss of variability due to drugs can be corrected by administration of physostigmine to the mother.[16]

BIOCHEMICAL EVALUATION OF THE FETUS DURING LABOR

Glucose is the main metabolic fuel of the fetus. In the presence of adequate fetal oxygenation energy transformation in fetal tissues occurs by means of the aerobic pathway of glycolysis, and hydrogen ions generated in this process are oxidized to water. This biologic oxidation cannot take place during hypoxia and, as a result, energy is created through anaerobic glycolysis and the generated hydrogen ions accumulate in the tissues. Therefore, hydrogen ion concentration or its negative logarithm (pH) is an indicator of fetal oxygen availability. During episodes of fetal asphyxia, oxygen tension (P_{O_2}) and hemoglobin saturation with oxygen (S) decrease rapidly while carbon dioxide tension (P_{CO_2}) increases rapidly. The pH value decreases more gradually and the base deficit increases at a similar rate. Following restoration of normal placental gas exchange, these parameters return to normal at their respective rates of change. Thus, at the onset of an episode of fetal oxygen deprivation pH and base deficit may still be near normal while P_{O_2}, P_{CO_2} and S have already markedly decreased. Conversely, following termination of an episode of oxygen deprivation P_{O_2}, P_{CO_2} and S may have already returned to normal while pH and base deficit are still abnormal. It is for these reasons that an indicator with a slower rate of change, such as pH or base deficit, is more suitable whenever fetal well-being is assessed only intermittently.

Technique of Fetal Blood Sampling

The biochemical assessment of fetal well-being has been pioneered by Saling.[43] He developed a microtechnique of sampling fetal blood from the presenting part of the fetus which has become widely practiced. Disposable sets containing the equipment necessary to obtain fetal capillary blood samples are available. (Fig. 12-5). The mother is either placed in a supine position with her hips elevated or in a Sims position with her knees flexed. A conical endoscope is introduced into the vagina and the cervix and held against the presenting part of the fetus. This requires ruptured membranes and a cervical dilatation of at least 1 cm. A light source is at-

tached to the distal end of the endoscope. The illuminated presenting part is dried with cotton swabs and some silicone is applied to aid the formation of blood drops. A 2-mm. blade on a rod is then used to incise the presenting part superficially. The blood drops forming at the site of incision are collected in long heparinized capillary tubes. The blood in the tubes is mixed by means of an internal mixing rod which is moved by an external magnet. The pH, Po_2, Pco_2, and base deficit can be determined from 0.2 to 0.3 ml. of blood; for pH determination alone 0.05 ml. of blood is sufficient. A variety of instruments are currently available to perform these determinations.

Indications for Fetal Blood Sampling

Since sampling of fetal blood can be done only intermittently, certain indications have to be established for when to

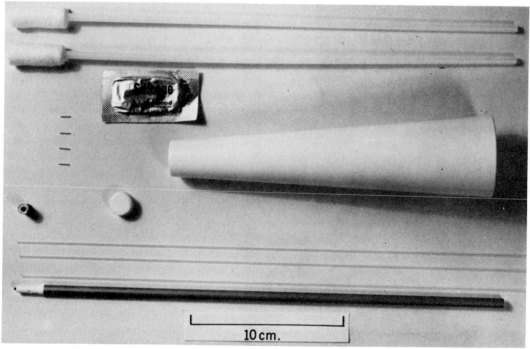

Fig. 12-5. Equipment for fetal blood sampling (see text for details of technique). Conical endoscope *(center right)*; cotton swabs and silicone *(top)*; rod with 2-mm. blade and heparinized capillary tubes *(bottom)*; clay to seal capillary tubes, external magnet and internal mixing rods *(center left)*.

perform this procedure. We recommend fetal blood sampling whenever clinical signs of fetal distress are present or suspected (with the exception of placenta previa or prolapsed cord). For example, conditions which make the fetus more prone to asphyxia such as toxemia, chronic hypertension, or maternal cardiac disease are indications for fetal blood sampling. The presence of meconium in the amniotic fluid is an indication for sampling of fetal blood. Whenever a fetus is biophysically monitored and abnormal or equivocal patterns of fetal heart rate are observed, the condition of the fetus should also be assessed biochemically. Before operative intervention for presumed fetal distress is considered, a fetal blood sample should be obtained first.

Interpretation of Results From Fetal Blood Sampling

The normal values of pH, P_{O_2}, P_{CO_2}, and base deficit of human fetal blood prior to the onset of labor are unknown. Experimental studies in various species have been performed, giving some indication of normal values of these parameters although the experimental procedure itself has the potential of changing these values. The intermittent measurements of oxygen and carbon dioxide tension in fetal blood do not optimally indicate fetal condition.[20,48] The rapid rate of change in these parameters is one of the major reasons for this, as has been outlined above. Furthermore, since the P_{O_2} and P_{CO_2} of fetal blood are markedly different from ambient air, it is difficult to avoid changes in oxygen and carbon dioxide tension by exposure to air. The pH and base deficit have been recognized as the most suitable indicators of fetal condition as assessed from fetal blood. The pH of fetal arterial blood is lower than the pH of maternal blood and probably ranges around 7.35 before labor. Based on clinical experience, pH values of fetal blood above 7.25 are considered normal.[44] During the normal course of labor and delivery there is a decrease in the pH of fetal blood as labor advances, but fetal blood pH usually remains above 7.25.[26] According to Saling, pH values of fetal blood between 7.20 and 7.25 are considered "preacidotic" whereas those below 7.20 are considered "acidotic."[44] Whenever a pH value in the "preacidotic" range is obtained, the fetal blood sample should be repeated within 20 minutes to ascertain whether the fetus is deteriorating or recovering.

After Saling reported his technique of fetal blood sampling in 1961[43] it was doubted at first that blood obtained from the presenting part of the fetus is representative of blood in its systemic circulation since various degrees of caput succedaneum resulting from venous stasis are usually seen during labor and delivery. Experimental studies in rhesus monkeys with simultaneous sampling of blood from the carotid artery, jugular vein and scalp of the fetus *in utero* during labor revealed an excellent correlation between the pH values of fetal blood obtained from these various sites.[2]

Since the effect of labor and delivery on the fetus is usually assessed by the Apgar score during the immediate neonatal period, it was soon recognized that there were occasional discrepancies between the pH values of fetal blood shortly before delivery and the expected condition of the newborn immediately after birth.[11] In approximately 10 per cent of fetuses pH values in the normal range are found during fetal blood sampling before delivery and the Apgar score is below 7 at 1 minute of age. It is important to note that in most of these cases neonatal depression is not the result of fetal oxygen deprivation, but usually reflects drug depression of the neonate as a result of placental transfer of narcotics and/or sedatives administered to the mother before delivery. Conversely, in about 8 per cent of fetuses acidosis is diagnosed by means of fetal blood sampling before delivery but vigorous neonates with high Apgar scores are delivered. During prolonged labors maternal acidosis may occur as a result of the muscular efforts of the mother. Although the permeability of the placenta to hydrogen ion is limited, maternal acidosis of some duration may eventually be reflected in fetal acidosis. This acidosis then is not a result of fetal oxygen deprivation. To avoid this difficulty in interpretation of results of fetal blood sampling, Beard[5] has suggested obtaining a simultaneous maternal blood sample when a fetal blood sample indicates fetal acidosis to determine the difference in base deficit between maternal and fetal blood. The value for the difference in base deficit should be less than 3 mEq./l. when placental perfusion is normal.

Complications

Complications of fetal blood sampling are rare. Exsanguination of the fetus has not occurred since the blades used to incise the presenting part of the fetus have been limited in size. Bleeding complications of fetal blood sampling are generally the first indication of a hemorrhagic disorder of the fetus.[4,24] Breakage of the blade is an extremely rare occurrence[41] and is usually related to inexperience of the person performing the procedure. Abscesses at the site of blood sampling have been occasionally reported.[4,27] These are generally small and rarely lead to septicemia. The risks of fetal blood sampling are extremely small compared to the benefits.

COMPARISON OF BIOPHYSICAL AND BIOCHEMICAL METHODS OF FETAL EVALUATION

Continuous monitoring of fetal heart rate and fetal blood sampling are methods which complement each other, and the use of one technique does not make the other unnecessary. In many instances abnormal patterns of fetal heart rate cannot be clearly related to fetal compromise. For example, a decrease in beat-to-beat varia-

bility of fetal heart rate during labor may indicate fetal jeopardy or reflect the effect of drugs previously administered to the mother. The presence of variable decelerations may possibly lead to fetal asphyxia, but this does not occur unless this type of deceleration is severe and persists for a prolonged period. Fetal blood sampling can provide information about the condition of the fetus in these cases. As a result of these considerations, many major obstetrical services use fetal heart rate monitoring as a method to screen their obstetric population at risk, and use fetal blood sampling to verify abnormalities of fetal heart rate. Clinical data have indicated that the intrapartum fetal death rate in a monitored high-risk population is lower than in a nonmonitored low-risk population.[37] This strongly suggests routine monitoring of all obstetric patients. Although the rate of primary cesarean sections has increased during the last years in most obstetrical departments, it has been shown that in those obstetrical services which possess considerable experience with fetal monitoring the number of cesarean sections performed because of fetal distress has either remained the same[40] or even decreased.[13]

CURRENT DEVELOPMENTS

A variety of new concepts are presently under investigation to assess fetal condition during labor and delivery. The use of computers in the evaluation of fetal heart rate tracings is being investigated at various institutions. Fetal electroencephalography has been used in sheep[30] and in humans[42] to assess changes in fetal brain potentials in response to fetal oxygen deprivation. Evaluation of these recordings is difficult even with the use of computers.[13] The preejection phase of the fetal heart is another parameter which is currently being investigated as an indicator of fetal well-being.[33,36]

The recognition of rhythmic fetal

breathing movements has aroused interest in the relationship between fetal breathing and fetal well-being.[9]

One of the most promising developments is that of a transcutaneous P_{O_2} electrode which allows recording of fetal oxygen tension from the presenting fetal part.[22] A good correlation has been found between oxygen tension measured with this electrode and oxygen tension of arterial blood obtained by means of an arterial catheter.[23] With this technique of continuous recording of fetal oxygen tension, alterations in oxygen availability to fetal tissues could be identified most rapidly.

REFERENCES

1. Adamsons, K., Mueller-Heubach, E., and Myers, R. E.: Production of fetal asphyxia in the rhesus monkey by administration of catecholamines to the mother. Am. J. Obstet. Gynecol., *109*:248, 1971.
2. Adamsons, K., *et al.*: The validity of capillary blood in the assessment of the acid-base state of the fetus. *In* Adamsons, K. (ed.): Diagnosis and Treatment of Fetal Disorders. Pp. 175–177. New York, Springer-Verlag. 1968.
3. Apgar, V., *et al.*: Evaluation of the newborn infant. second report. J.A.M.A., *168*:1985, 1958.
4. Balfour, H. H., *et al.*: Complications of fetal blood sampling. Am. J. Obstet. Gynecol., *107*:288, 1970.
5. Beard, R. W.: Maternal-fetal acid-base relationships. *In* Adamsons, K. (ed.): Diagnosis and Treatment of Fetal Disorders. Pp. 151–162. New York, Springer-Verlag, 1968.
6. Behrman, R. E., *et al.*: Distribution of the circulation in the normal and asphyxiated fetal primate. Am. J. Obstet. Gynecol., *108*:956, 1970.
7. Benson, R. C., *et al.*: Fetal heart rate as a predictor of fetal distress. Obstet. Gynecol., *32*:259, 1968.
8. Bieniarz, J., *et al.*: Aortocaval compression by the uterus in late human pregnancy. Am. J. Obstet. Gynecol., *100*:203, 1968.
9. Boddy, K., and Robinson, J. S.: External method for detection of fetal breathing in utero. Lancet, *2*:1231, 1971.
10. Boehm, F., and Growden, J.: The effect of scopolamine on fetal heart rate baseline variability. Am. J. Obstet. Gynecol., *120*:1099, 1974.
11. Bowe, E. T., *et al.*: Reliability of fetal blood sampling. Am. J. Obstet. Gynecol., *107*:279, 1970
12. Caldeyro-Barcia, *et al.*: Significado de los cambios registrados en la frecuencia cardiaca fetal durante el parto. V. Congreso Medico del Uruguay, *4*:1741, 1962.
13. Chik, L., *et al.*: Computer interpreted fetal elec-

14. Drage, J. S., and Berendes, H.: Apgar scores and outcome of the newborn. Pediat., Clin. North Am., *13*:635, 1966.
15. Edington, P. T., Sibanda, J., and Beard, R. W.: Influence on clinical practice of routine intrapartum fetal monitoring. Br. Med. J., *3*:341, 1975.
16. Eglimez, A., Boehm, F. H., and Smith, B. E.: Placental transfer and transplacental fetal pharmacology of physostigmine. World Congress on Anesthesiology, Abstract 253, 1976.
17. Greiss, F. C.: A clinical concept of uterine blood flow during pregnancy. Obstet. Gynecol., *30*:595, 1967.
18. Greiss, F. C., and Gobble, F. L.: Effect of sympathetic nerve stimulation on the uterine vascular bed. Am. J. Obstet. Gynecol., *97*:962, 1967.
19. Hammacher, K., *et al.*: Foetal heart frequency and perinatal condition of the fetus and newborn. Gynaecologia, *166*:410, 1968.
20. Haworth, S. G., Milic, A. B., and Adamsons, K.: Biochemical indices of fetal condition. Clin. Obstet. Gynecol., *11*:1182, 1968.
21. Hon, E. H.: The electronic evaluation of fetal heart rate. Preliminary report. Am. J. Obstet. Gynecol., *75*:215, 1958.
22. Huch, A., *et al.*: Erste Erfahrungen mit kontinuierlicher transcutaner PO_2-Registrierung bei Mutter und Kind sub partu. Geburtsh. Frauenheilk., *33*:856, 1973.
23. Huch, R., Lübbers, D. W., and Huch, A.: Quantitative continuous measurement of partial oxygen pressure on the skin of adults and new-born babies. Pfluegers Arch., *337*:185, 1972.
24. Hull, M. G. R., and Wilson, J. A.: Massive scalp hemorrhage after fetal blood sampling due to hemorrhagic disease. Br. Med. J., *4*:321, 1972.
25. James, L. S., *et al.*: The acid-base status of human infants in relation to birth asphyxia and the onset of respiration. J. Pediat., *52*:379, 1958.
26. Kubli, F.: Influence of labor on fetal acid-base balance. Clin. Obstet. Gynecol., *11*:168, 1968.
27. Kubli, F., *et al.*: Microanalysis of fetal blood. A critical study of the method. German Med. Monthly, *12*:315, 1967.
28. ———: Observations on heart rate and pH in the human fetus during labor. Am. J. Obstet. Gynecol., *104*:1190, 1969.
29. Ladner, C. N., *et al.*: Dynamics of uterine circulation in pregnant and nonpregnant sheep. Am. J. Physiol., *218*:257, 1970.
30. Mann, L. I., Prichard, J. W., and Symmes, D.: EEG, EKG, and acid-base observations during acute fetal hypoxia. Am. J. Obstet. Gynecol., *106*:39, 1970.
31. Mueller-Heubach, E., Myers, R. E., and Adamsons, K.: Maternal factors affecting fetal condition during labor and delivery. Obstet. Gynecol. Digest, *16*(10):11, 1974.
32. ———: Heart rate and blood pressure as indicators of fetal oxygenation during prolonged partial asphyxia in the rhesus monkey. 4th Euro-

pean Congress on Perinatal Medicine, Abstract IV-5/1, 1974.

33. Murata, Y., and Martin, C. B.: Systolic time intervals of the fetal cardiac cycle. Obstet. Gynecol., *44*:224, 1974.

34. Myers, R. E.: Two patterns of perinatal brain damage and their conditions of occurrence. Am. J. Obstet. Gynecol., *112*:246, 1972.

35. Myers, R. E., Mueller-Heubach, E., and Adamsons, K.: Predictability of the state of fetal oxygenation from a quantitative analysis of the components of late deceleration. Am. J. Obstet. Gynecol., *115*:1083, 1973.

36. Organ, L. W., *et al.*: The pre-ejection period of the fetal heart: detection during labor with Doppler ultrasound. Am. J. Obstet. Gynecol., *115*:369, 1973.

37. Paul, R. H.: Clinical fetal monitoring. Experience on a large clinical service. Am. J. Obstet. Gynecol., *113*:573, 1972.

38. Paul, R. H., *et al.*: Clinical fetal monitoring. VII. The evaluation and significance of intrapartum base-line FHR variability. Am. J. Obstet. Gynecol., *123*:206, 1975.

39. Ramsey, E. M., Corner, G. W., and Donner, M. W.: Serial and cineradiographic visualization of maternal circulation in the primate (hemochorial) placenta. Am. J. Obstet. Gynecol., *86*:213, 1963.

40. Rey, H.: Personal communication.

41. Roberts, H. R. N.: and Whitehouse, W. L.: Broken blade in foetal blood sampling. Br. Med. J., *2*:510, 1969.

42. Rosen, M. G., Scibetta, J. J., and Hochberg, C. J.: Human fetal electroencephalogram. III. Pattern changes in presence of fetal heart rate alterations and after use of maternal medications. Obstet. Gynecol., *36*:132, 1970.

43. Saling, E.: Neues Vorgehen zur Untersuchung des Kindes unter der Geburt. Einführung, Technik und Grundlagen. Arch. Gynaekol., *196*:108, 1962.

44. Saling, E., and Schneider, D.: Biochemical supervision of the fetus during labour. J. Obstet. Gynaecol. Br. Commonw., *74*:799, 1967.

45. Scher, J., Hailey, D. M., and Beard, R. W.: The effects of diazepam on the fetus. J. Obstet. Gynaecol. Br. Commonw., *79*:635, 1972.

46. Schnider, S. M., *et al.*: Vasopressors in obstetrics. Am. J. Obstet. Gynecol., *106*:680, 1970.

47. Wiechetek, W. J., Horiguchi, T., and Dillon, T. F.: Puerperal morbidity and internal fetal monitoring. Am. J. Obstet. Gynecol., *119*:230, 1974.

48. Wood, C., Lumley, J., and Renou, P.: A clinical assessment of foetal diagnostic methods. J. Obstet. Gynaecol. Br. Commonw., *74*:823, 1967.

49. Yeh, S. Y., Forsythe, A., and Hon, E. H.: Quantification of fetal heart beat-to-beat interval differences. Obstet. Gynecol., *41*:355, 1973.

Part Two

Techniques of Obstetric Anesthesia and Analgesia

13

Caudal Analgesia

Ezzat Abouleish, M.D.

DEFINITION

Caudal analgesia is one form of epidural block in which the local anesthetic drugs are injected into the epidural space by way of the sacral hiatus. Caudal epidural block, sacral epidural block, caudal peridural block, caudal epidural analgesia, and caudal anesthesia are all synonyms.

HISTORY

Caudal analgesia was first described separately by Cathelin[23] and Sicard[85] in 1901, and was introduced for obstetrics in 1909 by Stoeckel.[88] In 1942, Hingson and Edwards[47] published an account of their experience with continuous caudal analgesia. Thereafter Hingson, through his enthusiasm, dedication, publications, and teaching, popularized the technique.[45,46,48]

ANATOMY AND PHYSIOLOGY RELATIVE TO CAUDAL ANALGESIA

SITES OF ACTION OF LOCAL ANESTHETIC DRUGS FOLLOWING EPIDURAL OR CAUDAL ANALGESIA

The nerve roots in the epidural space are covered by the pia, the arachnoid, and the thick dura, which is relatively impermeable to local anesthetics. Therefore, the site of action of local anesthetics is not at the epidural space, but somewhere else. The main site of action of local anesthetics injected into the epidural space is in the subarachnoid space through the arachnoid villi, followed by neuraxial spread, then paravertebral block. The least important site is the diffusion through the dura to reach the posterior root ganglion cells. The possible sites are discussed below.

The Paravertebral Spaces

Epidurally injected fluids (e.g., methylene blue) were found to spread outside the vertebral column into the paravertebral space. There the dura no longer exists since it becomes continuous with the perineural sheath which can be readily penetrated by the local anesthetic. Hence, epidural analgesia can be considered as diffuse bilateral paravertebral block.[86] Although the paravertebral spaces were the first to be considered as the site of action, during pregnancy and old age paravertebral spread of injected fluid is limited, yet epidural analgesia can be quite extensive.[55] These findings are against the paravertebral spaces being the site of action.

The Posterior Root Ganglia

Since the dura covering the posterior root ganglia is thin, it was thought that local anesthetics can readily penetrate it to reach the ganglia and affect the nerve cells.[16] This explained the phenomenon of having extensive sensory blockade with minimal motor paralysis since the anterior nerve roots are covered with thicker dura. However, following epidural injection of a radiolabeled local anesthetic, very small amounts of the drug were found in the posterior root ganglia;[25] moreover, some new local anesthetics, such as etidocaine, produce more motor block than sensory loss.

The Central Nervous System

Local anesthetics injected into the epidural space spread toward the central nervous system along the perivascular spaces to cause blockage at the spinal cord. This theory of neuraxial spread is supported by:

1. Retrieval of C^{14} from the spinal cord following injection of labeled local anesthetics into the epidural space[26]

2. Change of the analgesia level pattern on the body surface with time.[95] During the induction of epidural analgesia, the level of analgesia is slanting, suggesting a dermatomal pattern. During the regression of the block, the analgesia level becomes transverse, suggesting spinal cord involvement.

3. Increase of the knee jerk and the development of a positive Babinski sign following the injection of local anesthetics into the thoracic epidural space to produce a segmental block above the l2 segment. This suggests involvement of the long pathways in the spinal cord.[16] Moreover, by acting on various spinal cord laminae different local anesthetics have preferential blocks. This explains the finding that etidocaine has an intense, prolonged motor effect whereas its sensory effect is weak compared to bupivacaine.[19a]

The Subarachnoid Space

It has been known for years that the local anesthetic drugs injected into the epidural space can gain access to the subarachnoid space where the nerve roots are covered only by the thin pia and are more susceptible to blockade. The way the drugs reach the subarachnoid space was not settled until Shantha and Evans[83] found that this can be accomplished through the spinal arachnoid villi which are similar to the brain villi. Thus, the epidural space becomes separated from the subarachnoid space only by the thin layers of the arachnoid villi made of actively permeable cells which allow transmission of local anesthetics. These villi are mainly present close to the nerve roots where most of the local anesthetic is taken up, leaving a small amount free to diffuse into the main subarachnoid space (Fig. 13-1).

Distal to the intervertebral foramina, the meninges are extended along the nerve roots in the form of perineurons and epineurons. Although the subarachnoid space anatomically ends at the junction of the anterior and posterior nerve roots at the intervertebral foramina, it extends along nerve roots as a potential, and, in some individuals as an actual extension of the subarachnoid space for a variable distance. Therefore, local anesthetics injected for peripheral nerve block can spread centrally to the subarachnoid space. This explains the occasional total spinal anesthesia following such blocks as paravertebral, celiac, or interscalene.

FACTORS CONTROLLING THE SPREAD OF LOCAL ANESTHETICS INJECTED INTO THE EPIDURAL SPACE

The term "spread" here refers to dermatomal spread evidenced by the level of analgesia, and not to physical spread determined by radiopaque dye. The two are related but not synonyms. The physical spread in the epidural space could be limited, while the dermatomal spread could be quite extensive owing to the action of local anesthetics on nerve tissues beyond the epidural space. As an example, injection of 8 ml. of 0.25 per cent bupivacaine with radiopaque dye in the lumbar

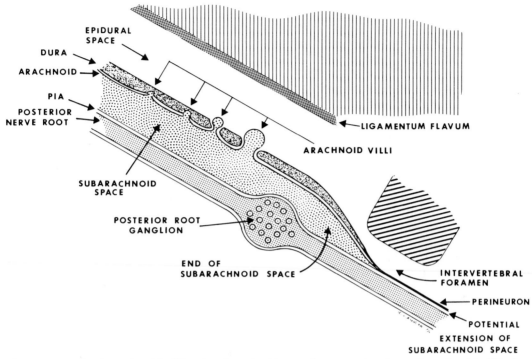

Fig. 13-1. Spinal arachnoid villi. The dura is thin or absent at the sites of arachnoid villi, thus reducing the barrier between the epidural and subarachnoid spaces.

epidural space showed only spread of the solution from T8 to L3, as evidenced by x-ray, while perineal analgesia was excellent.[20]

Whether the local anesthetic is injected into the lumbar or the sacral regions of the epidural space, its spread is affected by the following factors:

Volume of the Local Anesthetic

The larger the volume of a drug injected into the epidural space, the wider it spreads. In adults the volume of local anesthetic injected into the epidural space is usually 1.5 ml. per segment. However, with limited blocks there is a tendency to use larger volumes of drug to ensure adequate analgesia and decrease the interval between refills.[30] For example, during the first stage of labor, to produce a block of 4 segments extending from T10 to L1, 6 to 8 ml. of the local anesthetic is injected into the lumbar epidural space. If the pa-

tient is ready for delivery, the block should include all the 14 segments extending from T10 to the coccygeal nerve. The volume of the local anesthetic in this case is usually 15 to 20 ml.

Concentration of the Local Anesthetic

The higher the concentration, the more is the spread of the local anesthetic,[17,55] which is probably due to more diffusion of the drug. With bupivacaine the volume plays a more important role in controlling the extent of analgesia, while the concentration is more important for producing muscular relaxation, intensity of analgesia, onset of action, and duration of effect.

Specific Gravity of the Local Anesthetic

The epidural space has no fluid and the pressure is relatively subatmospheric.[59] The spread of a local anesthetic injected into the epidural space can be controlled by gravity. For example, if a sacral block is desired, the patient is kept in the sitting position when the drug is injected in the lumbar epidural space. However, it should be remembered that the local anesthetics are usually hypobaric compared to cerebrospinal fluid, and accidental injection of these drugs into the subarachnoid space with the patient sitting up can cause massive spinal, and even cranial, block.[51]

Height of the Patient

The volume of local anesthetic, whether for epidural or caudal analgesia, varies according to the height of the patient. For example, for cesarean section under lumbar epidural analgesia, the volume of 0.75 per cent bupivacaine is 15 ml. for a patient 150 cm. (5 feet) tall, with a change of 1 ml. for each 2.5-cm. (inch) deviation. However, personal variations should be expected, because the height of a patient does not always correlate with the length of the vertebral column.

Site of Injection of the Local Anesthetic

The Site in Relation to the Thoracic Region. The negative epidural pressure is most pronounced in the thoracic region.[59] This explains the more cephalad spread of the local anesthetic injected into the lumbar region.[20] Moreover, the dura is anchored to the lumbosacral angle by fibrous tissue which varies in density in different individuals. If this fibrous tissue is thick, it may interfere with the spread of the local anesthetic. This explains the occasional failure to achieve an adequate upper level of analgesia when a local anesthetic is injected into the lower sacral region, as well as the occasional inadequacy of perineal analgesia when a local anesthetic is injected into the lumbar region. The third anatomical factor that affects mainly the cephalad spread of local anesthetic is the sacral foramina. In order to achieve a certain thoracic segmental level, the volume injected through the lower caudal canal has to be increased to make up for the loss of solution through these foramina.

The Site in Relation to the Nerve Segments to Be Blocked. The nearer the site of injection or the tip of the catheter to the nerves to be blocked, the more reliable is the effect and the smaller is the dose of local anesthetic required. Therefore, for abdominal analgesia the epidural catheter can be inserted in the thoracic region. However, it is customary to insert the catheter in the lumbar region and advance it cephalad. The lumbar region is preferred because the vertical direction of the spinous processes of the thoracic vertebrae makes epidural technique more difficult. Moreover, although the spinal cord in the thoracic region is separated from the epidural space by the dura, arachnoid, and cerebrospinal fluid, the lumbar region is preferred to avoid any chance of injury to the spinal cord.

Escape of the Epidurally Injected Local Anesthetic Through the Intervertebral Foramina

The less the escape of local anesthetic through the intervertebral foramina, the wider is the spread. In late pregnancy the dilated vertebral veins passing through the intervertebral foramina reduce this escape area. In old age, there is increased condensation of fibrous tissue that tends to occlude these foramina.[16,83,86] Therefore, the dose of local anesthetic in the parturient or the aged should be reduced by one-third compared to the nonpregnant or young patient.[17]

The Space Available in the Epidural Canal Through Which a Certain Volume of the Local Anesthetic Spreads

Owing to compression of the inferior vena cava by the gravid uterus, the vertebral venous plexus is distended, thus diminishing the space available in the epidural canal for the local anesthetic which spreads more longitudinally. This factor has also been demonstrated experimentally in dogs by the wider spread of contrast media injected into the epidural space following inflation of balloons placed in the inferior vena cava.[44]

Age of Patient

Bromage has shown that the dose of local anesthetic is reduced proportionately to age above 18½ years, e.g., at the age of 60 it is reduced by one-third.[19a] In addition to the previously mentioned sclerosis of the intervertebral foramina limiting the escape of the local anesthetic in old age, this reduction in requirement can be due to decreased number of myelinated fibers,[26] greater neuraxial spread,[18] and more diffusion through the spinal arachnoid villi.[83]

Direction of the Opening of the Tuohy Needle or the Epidural Catheter

Local anesthetics spread more in the same direction as that of the opening of the Tuohy needle or tip of the epidural catheter. This is why in some centers when lumbar epidural analgesia is used for vaginal delivery, the catheter is directed caudad in order to achieve good perineal analgesia.

Rate of Injection

The more rapid the injection is, the more extensive and thinner the spread of the local anesthetic. This can lead to a marked sympathetic blockade associated with a short duration of analgesia. The usual rate of injection is 1 ml. per second.

Coughing or Straining

Coughing or straining will increase the spread of the local anesthetic by causing congestion of the vertebral veins and diminishing the available epidural space.

Gross Obesity or Marked Abdominal Distention

Gross obesity or marked distention of the abdomen will extend the dispersion of the local anesthetic drug in the epidural space, probably by increasing the extradural venous pressure.[17]

ANATOMY RELATIVE TO CAUDAL ANALGESIA

The Sacrum

The sacral bone is triangular in shape with its base cephalad where it articulates with the 5th lumbar vertebra (Fig. 13-2). Its apex is caudad where it is attached to the coccyx by the sacrococcygeal ligaments.[37] Laterally it articulates with the iliac bones through the two sacroiliac joints. The sacrum is composed of 5 fused vertebrae. It has a smooth, concave anterior surface which forms part of the posterior wall of the pelvis. Anterior to it lie the pelvic organs (e.g., the rectum). Its anterior surface has 4 openings, called the anterior sacral foramina, for the anterior primary rami of the sacral nerves and blood vessels. The posterior surface of the sacrum is rugged and gives attachment to various muscles and ligaments covering it. It has a median crest representing the fused upper 4 spinous processes; the 5th spinous process is usually missing where there is an opening called the sacral hiatus. There is a second longitudinal elevation lateral to the median crest, called the intermediate crest, which is formed by the fusion of the articular processes of the sacral vertebrae. A third longitudinal elevation on the posterior surface of the sacrum, called the lateral longitudinal crest, is formed by the fusion of the transverse processes of the sacral vertebrae. Between the intermediate and lateral crests there are 4 openings, called the posterior sacral foramina, which are traversed by the posterior primary rami of the sacral nerves and blood vessels. As previously mentioned, an appreciable portion of the local anesthetic injected caudally escapes through the anterior and posterior sacral foramina.

The Sacral Hiatus

The laminae of the 5th sacral vertebra fail to grow and fuse in the midline, thus creating a gap called the sacral hiatus. The

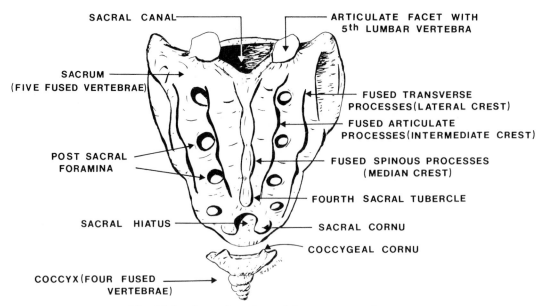

SACRAL CANAL

ARTICULATE FACET WITH
5th LUMBAR VERTEBRA

SACRUM
(FIVE FUSED VERTEBRAE)

FUSED TRANSVERSE
PROCESSES (LATERAL CREST)

FUSED ARTICULATE
PROCESSES (INTERMEDIATE CREST)

POST SACRAL
FORAMINA

FUSED SPINOUS PROCESSES
(MEDIAN CREST)

FOURTH SACRAL TUBERCLE

SACRAL HIATUS

SACRAL CORNU

COCCYGEAL CORNU

COCCYX (FOUR FUSED
VERTEBRAE)

Fig. 13-2.   Posterior view of the sacrum and coccyx.

sacral hiatus looks like an inverted "v" or an inverted "u." Its length is 2 cm. and its widest part is 1.5 cm. (Fig. 13-3). The articular processes of the 5th sacral vertebra forming the caudad end of the intermediate longitudinal crest are prominent and prolonged in the form of two rounded processes on each side of the sacral hiatus, called the sacral cornua. However in 10 per cent of the population there are variations from this classic picture,[91] and in 5 per cent the hiatus is less than 2 mm. in diameter, making caudal analgesia extremely difficult or even impossible.[33]

The Sacral Canal

The portion of the vertebral canal that lies inside the sacrum is called the sacral canal (see Figs. 13-2 and 13-4A). Cephalad, it is continuous with the lumbar portion of the vertebral canal. Caudad, it is closed by the posterior sacrococcygeal ligament, which is 1 to 3 mm. thick. This ligament attaches the 5th sacral vertebra to the first coccygeal segment and covers the sacral hiatus. The posterior sacrococcygeal ligament is covered by skin and subcutaneous tissue containing variable amounts of fat. Usually it lies 1 to 2 cm. from the skin surface. In some toxemic parturients the subcutaneous tissue may be edematous. The thickness of fat and/or edema makes identification of the sacral hiatus difficult. The sacral canal is about 10 cm. long, triangular in shape in its upper part, and oval in its lower part. It is narrower caudad where its anteroposterior diameter is only 2 to 3 mm., while it is 2 to 3 cm. in the cephalad portion. Its anterior surface is formed by the fused sacral vertebral bodies which are covered by the posterior longitudinal ligament. The fusion of the bodies may form slight transverse ridges which can be felt during the advancement of the caudal catheter through the canal. The posterior surface of the canal is formed by the fused laminae of the sacral vertebra. The canal has a smooth inner surface compared with the rough posterior surface of the sacral bone. Such a difference helps in confirming the position of the caudal catheter or needle. The anterior and posterior sacral foramina, traversed mainly by the sacral nerves and vessels, are found on the lateral wall of the sacral canal.

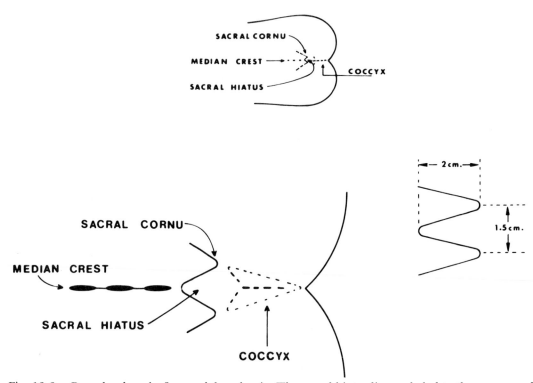

Fig. 13-3. Bony landmarks for caudal analgesia. The sacral hiatus lies cephalad to the coccyx and at the caudal end of the median crest. The sacral cornua lie at its lateral borders. It is only 2 cm. long and 1.5 cm. wide.

Contents of the Sacral Canal

The sacral canal contains the following structures:

1. *The sacral and coccygeal nerves* that extend from the end of the spinal cord at the second lumbar vertebra to their corresponding exit at the sacral foramina.

2. *The dura and arachnoid maters* that extend down to the second sacral vertebra where they terminate forming a cul-de-sac (Fig. 13-4A). The average distance between the posterior sacrococcygeal ligament and the termination of the subarachnoid space is 43 mm., with extremes of 19 and 75 mm.[33] If a needle is advanced too far into the caudal canal, especially when the dura extends more than usual, the dura may be punctured inadvertently, with the potential danger of extensive subarachnoid block and the possibility of post-lumbar-puncture cephalgia.

3. *The filum terminale* that extends from the end of the spinal cord through the dural cul-de-sac, sacral canal, and posterior sacrococcygeal ligament to be attached to the posterior surface of the first coccygeal segment (Fig. 13-4A)

4. *The blood vessels of the sacral canal,* mainly veins, which are part of the internal vertebral venous plexus. Owing to the compression of the inferior vena cava by the gravid uterus, these thin-walled veins are distended. Consequently, the possibility of traumatizing one or more of these veins by the caudal needle, or even a catheter, is higher than in the nonpregnant state.

5. *Lymphatic vessels and a variable quantity of fatty areolar tissue* that fill the remaining part of the sacral canal. The lymphatic vessels leave the sacral canal with the blood vessels and nerves through the sacral for-

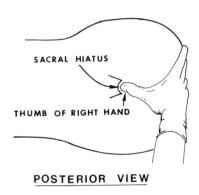

POSTERIOR VIEW

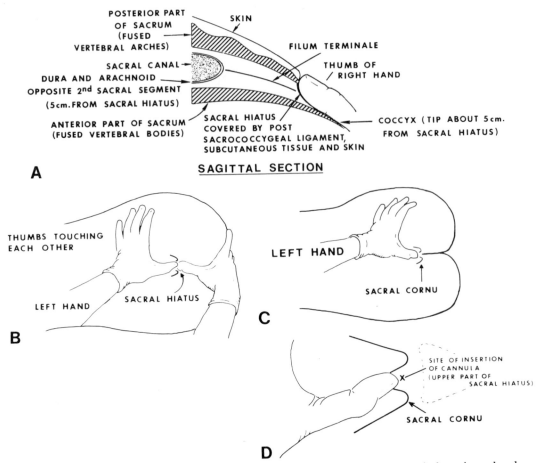

SAGITTAL SECTION

A

B

C

D

Fig. 13-4. Feeling the landmarks at the sacrococcygeal region. In the saggital section, the dura ends opposite the second sacral bony segment, about 5 cm. from the sacral hiatus. The filum terminale extends through the dural cul-de-sac and the posterior sacrococcygeal ligament to be attached to the posterior surface of the coccyx. *A.* The thumb of the right hand fits snuggly into the gap formed at the sacral hiatus, in line with the patient's back, and in contact with the skin covering the posterior sacrococcygeal ligament and the coccyx. *B.* The tips of the two thumbs touch each other at the sacral hiatus. *C.* The right hand is removed leaving the left thumb in touch with the sacral hiatus. *D.* Local infiltration at the upper part of the sacral hiatus.

amina. The fatty areolar tissue forms a depot for the fat-soluble local anesthetics.

LANDMARKS RELEVANT TO CAUDAL ANALGESIA

In order to perform caudal analgesia successfully and atraumatically, visualization of the anatomy of the sacrum, coccyx, sacral canal, and hiatus is a prerequisite. One should also be familiar with the landmarks, which should be identified before inserting any needle in the caudal area. Otherwise, the patient will suffer from the operator's repeated attempts, and the operator will be frustrated by failure to achieve a task. Also, the complication rate will be high (e.g., injury to the maternal rectum and/or fetal head).

The sacral hiatus lies at the cephalad end of the anal cleft. If the patient is on her side, the hiatus may be felt a few millimeters from the midline toward the upper hip, *but never toward the lower one.* This is due to gravity causing sagging of the anal cleft. The lumbosacral fascia covers the sacrospinal muscle and gives origin to the gluteus maximus muscle. The fasciae of both sides join in the midline at the sacral hiatus. Therefore, if the patient is muscular and/or slim, the junction of the two lumbosacral fasciae helps to localize the sacral hiatus (Fig. 13-5). The distance from the tip of the coccyx is quite variable. The attempt to locate the sacral hiatus by measuring 5 cm. from the tip of the coccyx is thus unreliable and may cause contamination of the field. If the thumb of the right hand is passed caudad on the middle line of the sacrum of a patient lying on her left side, the median crest suddenly stops at the sacral hiatus and branches into the two sacral cornua. There is usually a change of direction from the sacrum to the coccyx, and the absence of the 5th sacral spine allows the thumb to fit snuggly into the gap thus created (Fig. 13-4A).

In thin individuals the groove between the median and intermediate crests is sometimes mistaken for the sacral hiatus, each crest being

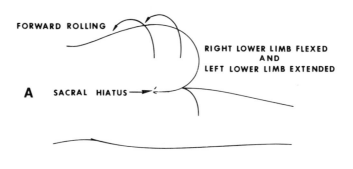

Fig. 13-5. Positions for caudal analgesia. The sacral hiatus lies at the cephalad end of the anal cleft, a few mms. from the mid-line toward the upper hip, and at the junction of lumbosacral fasciae. *A.* Sim's position. *B.* the semiprone flexed position.

misinterpreted as a sacral cornu. The absence of the cephalad junction of the two crests should help to preclude such a mistake.

The landmarks of the area can be simulated by extending the interphalangeal joints of the left hand and semiflexing the metacarpophalangeal joints (Fig. 13-6). If the thumb of the right hand is inserted in the gap between the knuckles of the left index and middle fingers, the gap feels like the sacral hiatus and the knuckles like the sacral cornua. The change of direction from the metacarpal to phalangeal bones simulates the change from the sacrum to the coccyx.

DRUGS USED FOR CAUDAL ANALGESIA

In our institute, many drugs have been used for caudal analgesia (e.g., lidocaine, mepivacaine, bupivacaine, chloroprocaine). Recently only two drugs, namely chloroprocaine and bupivacaine, are used exclusively.

Chloroprocaine

Chloroprocaine (Nesacaine), 2 per cent, is used when delivery is expected within 30 minutes because of its fast onset of action and its duration of about one hour.[70] The short duration of action of chloroprocaine

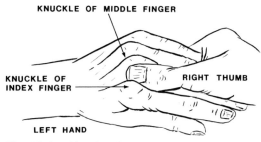

Fig. 13-6. Simulated sacral hiatus and cornua. The knuckles of index and middle fingers simulate the sacral cornua, and the gap between them the sacral hiatus. The change of direction from metacarpals to phalanges simulates the change from sacrum to coccyx.

is important because, for safety reasons, our patients are not allowed to leave the recovery room as long as they have a residual effect of epidural or caudal block. With 8,000 deliveries per year, the recovery room can be jammed if the local anesthetic used at the time of delivery has too long a duration of action. Moreover, the use of bupivacaine for the delivery prolongs the insensitivity of the urinary bladder, thus requiring catheterization and increasing the risk of infection. Because of chloroprocaine hydrolysis by the maternal plasma and placental cholinesterase, a minimum amount of drug is expected to be transmitted to the fetus.[54] For this reason it is recommended to use chloroprocaine throughout labor and delivery.[60] But since our policy is that an anesthesiologist or a physician should perform every "refill" and stay with the patient until adequate analgesia has been established without complications, the use of chloroprocaine from the first stage of labor would require too much manpower and becomes too expensive. Therefore, for the first stage of labor we prefer to use a longer-acting drug.

Bupivacaine

Bupivacaine (Marcaine) is our drug of choice for the first stage of labor or cesarean section because:

1. It has excellent analgesic properties. It is superior to etidocaine, which has short, poor analgesic properties with marked, prolonged motor paralysis causing the patient an unpleasant feeling, similar to poliomyelitis.[66]

2. It has as fast an onset of action as lidocaine or mepivacane, but a 2 to 3 times longer duration of action.

3. Its motor effects can be easily regulated by changing its concentration, e.g., if no motor weakness is required 0.25 per cent is used, whereas 0.75 per cent will produce profound muscular relaxation required for cesarean section.[65]

4. It has no depressant effect on the

cardiovascular system even in doses that produce seizures.[68]

5. Its maternal blood level and duration of effect are not significantly changed by the addition of epinephrine.[78] Thus, the use of another drug which has its own inherent problems is excluded.

6. It is minimally transferred to the fetus compared to lidocaine or mepivacaine, mainly due to its higher binding capacity to the maternal plasma proteins.[79] Thus, with bupivacaine the neurobehavioral responses of the neonates are comparable to those of neonates delivered under "natural childbirth."[82]

7. It is clinically safer for both the mother and the fetus than lidocaine or mepivacaine. Although both the toxicity and potency of bupivacaine are 4 times those of the other two drugs, *the rates of metabolism and excretion of the three drugs are equal.*[61] Since bupivacaine has a longer duration of action and will be injected less frequently, the probability of a rise of its blood level with repeated administration is much less than with either of the other two drugs.

Both 0.25 per cent and 0.5 per cent bupivacaine are used for vaginal delivery. The higher concentration has a superior analgesic property, a faster onset of action, and less association with tachyphylaxis. However, the 0.25 per cent concentration is preferred in the following situations:

1. When the mother's ability to push is the important factor for delivery and any degree of motor paralysis is inadvisable (e.g., with breech delivery, borderline disproportion, multiple gestations).

2. When preservation of the muscle tone of the pelvic floor plays a major role for fetal head rotation (e.g., with occipitoposterior position of the fetus).

3. When labor is too early, the cervix is dilated 2 or 3 cm., and dysrhythmic uterine contractions with much pain and little progress are present. A dilute concentration of bupivacaine, caudally or epidurally administered, together with in-

travenous infusion of oxytocin will improve the situation.

4. When caudal analgesia has to be repeated following failure to inject the drug into the sacral canal. The 0.25 per cent concentration should be used, otherwise toxic drug levels could be reached.

Crawford[30] recommends the use of 0.375 per cent bupivacaine, with which the advantages of both the 0.25 per cent and 0.5 per cent concentrations are obtained without their disadvantages. Cunningham and Kaplan[32] and Villa and Marx[98] recommended the use of a combination of chloroprocaine and bupivacaine for surgery and obstetrics respectively. They state that the onset of action with the combination is faster than with chloroprocaine alone; moreover, since chloroprocaine is metabolized by cholinesterase, and bupivacaine by the hepatic microsomal enzymes, these different metabolic patterns increase the safety of the block.

TECHNIQUES

The technique of caudal analgesia is modified according to whether it is used for vaginal delivery or cesarean section. One rule applies in all cases: *do not use force.*

CAUDAL ANALGESIA FOR VAGINAL DELIVERY

Caudal analgesia for vaginal delivery can be performed by either injecting the local anesthetic once called *single-dose (one shot) caudal analgesia,* or continuously, called *continuous caudal analgesia.*

Single-Dose Caudal Analgesia

Single-dose caudal analgesia is usually performed when delivery is expected within 30 minutes. The technique and the expected changes in the patient's sensations following the block are explained to the patient. An intravenous cannula is inserted in her hand or forearm, an infusion is started, and the pulse and blood pressure are measured. Then the patient is positioned. The main purposes of the assumed position are: (1) the relaxation of the patient's gluteal muscles, since their contraction makes it difficult to identify the landmarks; (2) the accessibility of the sacral hiatus and the convenient direction of the caudal canal to the movement of the performer's hand; e.g., if he is right-handed the patient lies on her left side (left lateral position) and vice versa; and (3) the placement of the patient in a decent and comfortable position. The semiprone position with the patient extending her dependent lower limb and flexing the other is commonly used. It is called a modified Sim's position (Fig. 13-5A). The main disadvantage of this position is that the gluteal muscles of the extended limb can contract, making it difficult to feel and identify the landmarks and to visualize the plane of the sacral canal. Therefore, as an alternative, the author uses the semiprone flexed position (Fig. 13-5B). This position is achieved by flexing both lower limbs, with the dependent thigh slightly less flexed to allow forward rolling of the patient. By bringing the patient's hips to the edge of the bed, the usual sagging of the central part of the mattress helps to achieve this position as the patient rolls forward. The landmarks are felt to make sure of the feasibility of performing atraumatic caudal block before proceeding further.

The caudal tray is opened. This author prefers to use a hospital-prepared tray in all blocks because it is less expensive, easier to dispose of, and made to the satisfaction of the hospital staff. However, ready-made disposable trays purchased from a manufacturer can be used if the number of blocks performed is small and the hospital lacks experienced personnel to prepare the trays. Wearing a face mask and a cap, the anesthesiologist opens the tray which contains one 20-ml. glass syringe, one 5-ml. glass syringe, two 3.8-cm. 19-gauge hypodermic needles and one 1.9-cm. 24-gauge hypodermic needle, a metal cup, 4 × 4 sponges, a sponge holder, and 4 towels, all placed on a metal tray and presterilized by autoclaving (Fig. 13-7). Then the gloves are put on. Since delivery is usually expected within a short time, the drug of choice is 2 per cent chloroprocaine. This drug deteriorates if autoclaved, and therefore, an assistant should hold the unsterilized vial while the performer aspirates its contents into the 20-ml. syringe. The drug is then transferred into the metal cup. If the patient is a primi-gravida and a longer-acting drug is preferred, 0.5 per cent bupivacaine is the drug of choice. Bupivacaine will not deteriorate by autoclaving and the presterilized 50-ml. vial can be added to the tray. The 20-ml. syringe is lubricated and filled with part or all of the estimated therapeutic dose. The dose is 20 ml. for a patient who is 150 cm. (5 feet) tall; for each 2.5 cm. (inch) above or below this height the dose is increased or decreased by 1 ml., e.g., 26 ml. for a patient who is 165 cm. (5'6") tall. The assistant is then asked to put a 4 × 4 sponge between the patient's buttocks to protect the sensitive mucous membrane of the rectum and the vagina from any possible irritant action of the antiseptic solution. A wide area of the patient's back is sterilized twice using Betadine or Prepodyne solution, the excess of solution is removed from the expected site of puncture, and drapes are applied to isolate the sacral area from the rest of the body.

The area at the cephalad end of the anal cleft and the junction of the lumbosacral fasciae is palpated with the right hand if the performer is right-handed. The right thumb, with its tip directed cephalad, is placed in the area between the two sacral cornua (Fig. 13-4A). The left thumb is placed on the patient's back, in the opposite direction, cephalad to the right thumb with the tips touching each other (Fig. 13-4B). The right thumb is then removed. The left thumb is kept in place (Fig. 13-4C) until the caudal canal is entered by needle

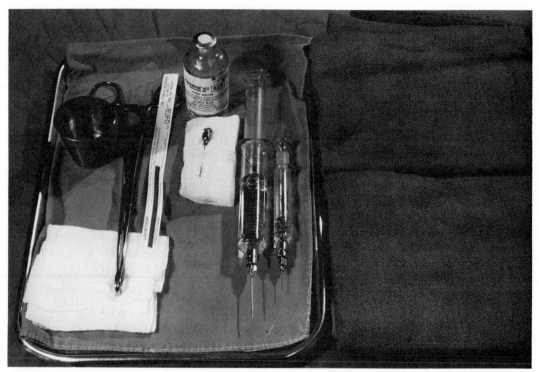

Fig. 13-7. Single-dose caudal analgesia tray showing sterilization indicator strip, metal cup, local anesthetic vial bupivacaine (Marcaine), 0.5%, 5-ml. syringe for local infiltration and exploration, 20-ml. syringe containing local anesthetic for therapeutic dose, and 4 towels.

or cannula. The area of skin opposite the upper part of the sacral hiatus just distal to the middle of the left thumb is infiltrated with the local anesthestic using the 24-gauge hypodermic needle (Fig. 13-4D). The needle is advanced to infiltrate the posterior sacrococcygeal ligament. It is not unusual to feel the fine 1.9-cm. needle piercing the ligament and reaching the caudal canal. In fact, this is usually sought. A 19-gauge needle is inserted into the infiltrated area with an angle of 45 degrees to the patient's back (Fig. 13-8A). It is gently advanced until the sudden loss of resistance is felt as it pierces the posterior sacrococcygeal ligament. The hub of the needle is then anteriorly pushed so that it forms an angle of 30 degrees with the patient's back and the needle is advanced forward for 1 to 2 cm. more (Fig. 13-8B). If the sacral canal is shallow the anterior

smooth surface of the canal may be touched by the needle following the "give" of the posterior sacrococcygeal ligament. In such a case the needle is withdrawn just enough to disengage its tip from the periosteum. The angle the needle forms with the patient's back is changed as mentioned above and the needle is advanced for only 1 to 2 cm. more.

The operator should watch for any blood or cerebrospinal fluid that might appear at the hub of the needle. In the absence of blood or fluid, the well-lubricated 5-ml. syringe is attached and 3 ml. of air is injected through the needle while placing the flat of the left hand on the patient's back over the expected tip of the needle (Fig. 13-9). The needle is considered to be in the proper position if no resistance or crepitus is felt and the plunger of the syringe does not bounce

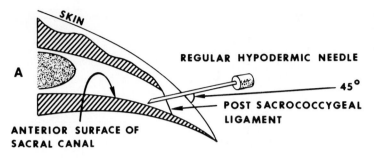

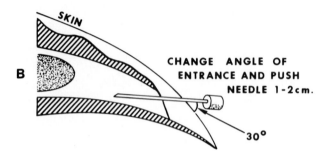

Fig. 13-8.   Insertion of the needle in single-dose caudal analgesia. *A*. The needle pierces the posterior sacrococcygeal ligament and enters the caudal canal at a 45° angle with the patient's back. *B*. The angle of entry is changed to 30° and the needle is advanced in the canal for 1 to 2 cm.

back following injection. No more than 3 ml. of air is injected at one time; otherwise it will escape through the posterior sacral foramina and a crepitus will be felt causing a false position sign. This is especially liable to occur in thin individuals.

After verifying the proper location of the needle the 5-ml. syringe loaded with the test dose (4 ml.) is attached to the hub of the needle. Aspiration is done. The absence of aspirate, whether cerebrospinal fluid or blood, is essential before injecting

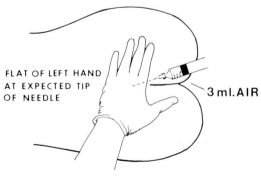

Fig. 13-9.   Feeling for air crepitus or fluid tumefaction.

any local anesthetic. The test dose is slowly injected. No tumefaction should be felt during injection of the local anesthetic. Immediately following injection reaspiration is performed and no blood or cerebrospinal fluid should be obtained. Verbal contact with the patient is maintained and she is asked if she has any abnormal sensation to exclude intravascular or intrathecal injection.

If the abdominal pain persists and no change in the patient's sensorium occurs, the 20-ml. syringe is attached and the therapeutic dose is slowly injected at the rate of 1 ml. per second. Rapid injection can cause the patient to feel cramps in both legs, and although this confirms the position of the needle, it may cause temporary discomfort. Aspiration is repeatedly performed during and at the end of injection to exclude intravascular injection. The absence of resistance during injection also confirms the proper position of the needle. During injection the hand holding the hub of the needle is kept steady against the patient's back and the verbal contact with the patient is continued to determine any change in her sensorium and to reassure her.

After completing injection of the therapeutic dose, the needle is removed, the patient is turned on her back, and the uterus is pushed to the left, e.g., by placing a folded sheet or pillow under the right hip. In cases of hydramnios or twin pregnancy, the patient is kept on her left side for 5 to 10 minutes, then turned to the right.

Manifestations of caudal analgesia are looked for as they develop, the first of which is loss of the urge to bear down if the patient had this feeling before injection of the local anesthetic. Thereafter, the following signs and symptoms usually occur in this order: loss of anal reflex (in about 5 minutes); hypalgesia of the perineum, numbness and tingling of the toes, vasodilatation of the lower limbs, and dryness and warmth of the feet (in 5 to 15 minutes); gradual diminution of uterine pain, and analgesia to pinprick extending from the perinuem to the lower limbs and lower abdomen (in about 10 to 20 minutes). If 2 per cent chloroprocaine, 1.5 per cent lidocaine, 1.5 per cent mepivacaine, or 0.5 per cent bupivacaine is used, the tone of the anal sphincter is lost and the lower limbs become weak as evidenced by the difficulty of flexing the hip with the knee extended (in about 10 to 20 minutes). If lower concentrations of local anesthetics are used (e.g., 0.25% bupivacaine), the motor power will remain intact. Owing to the effect of gravity, all these manifestations will start first on the side on which the patient was lying at the time of injection. Fifteen minutes following injection of the therapeutic dose, if the patient still has the urge to push and/or the anal reflex is still intact, a fault in the technique has occurred and other methods of analgesia should be considered depending on the circumstances at the time. Injection of a local anesthetic to produce caudal analgesia once more after such a short interval is not advisable, lest the highest permissible dose be exceeded and a toxic reaction occur. Subarachnoid block is preferable if the patient is ready for delivery.

Management of Complications That Might Occur During the Procedure. If after inserting the needle in the caudal canal *blood appears at the hub,* the needle should be removed. The procedure is repeated using a regular intravascular cannula No. 18, as described in the continuous technique. The cannula is gently advanced as far as possible so that its tip is further away from the injured blood vessel. Aspiration is performed before, during, and after injection; then the solution is slowly injected.

If cerebrospinal fluid appears at the hub of the needle, the management depends on the stage of labor. If the patient is about to deliver, the technique can be converted into a subarachnoid block by injecting hyperbaric lidocaine or tetracaine (see Chap. 15, Subarachnoid Block). The patient is turned on her back and her hips are kept flexed for a few minutes to obliterate the lumbar lordosis, thus allowing adequate cephalad flow of the local anesthetic. If the patient is still in the first stage of labor, the needle is removed and continuous lumbar epidural technique can be substituted through a cephalad-directed catheter. Owing to the developed communication between the epidural and subarachnoid spaces; the local anesthetic should be injected in small increments until the required level of anesthesia is achieved.

Continuous Caudal Analgesia

Since October 1973, the Teflon intravascular cannula technique described by Owens and coworkers[73] has been used at Magee-Womens Hospital with satisfactory results. It is mainly utilized for continuous caudal analgesia, but sometimes for one-dose caudal block. It gives the operator better tactile sensation with less chance of puncturing the dura or a blood vessel than the conventional caudal needle technique.

Following will be a description of continuous caudal analgesia using the Teflon intravascular cannula technique as used in this institute. However, if such a cannula is not available, a thin-walled No. 18 caudal needle can be substituted.

The procedure and the expected changes in sensations are explained to the patient who is then placed in the proper position. The caudal tray is opened. A standard intravascular No. 16-gauge 6.2 cm. Teflon cannula with needle stylet (Abbocath), a continuous No. 20-gauge 91.5-cm. (36 inches) epidural caudal catheter,* Neosporin ointment and the local anesthetic (e.g., 0.5% bupivacaine) are added to the tray (Fig. 13-10).

The operator proceeds as described in the single-dose caudal analgesia technique

*The catheter used in our institute is the Desert Radiopaque Teflon Epidural Catheter, manufactured by Desert Pharmaceutical Co., Sandy, Utah, 84070.

until the skin and posterior sacrococcygeal ligament are infiltrated with the local anesthetic using the 24-gauge needle. The No. 16-gauge intravascular cannula is inserted into the patient's back in the sagittal plane, with a 45-degree angle to the skin, until the sudden loss of resistance occurs as the posterior sacrococcygeal ligament is pierced (Fig. 13-11A). If the patient feels pain and resistance is encountered before the sudden "give" is felt, the cannula is outside the sacral canal and touching the sensitive periosteum. In such a case the needle is withdrawn, the landmarks are felt again, and the site and/or the angle of insertion are changed. Once the "snap" of the posterior sacrococcygeal ligament is felt, the needle and cannula are pushed further for 1 cm. to ensure their intrasacral position. *At this step the proper position of both the cannula and the needle is suggested by:*

1. The sudden loss of resistance follow-

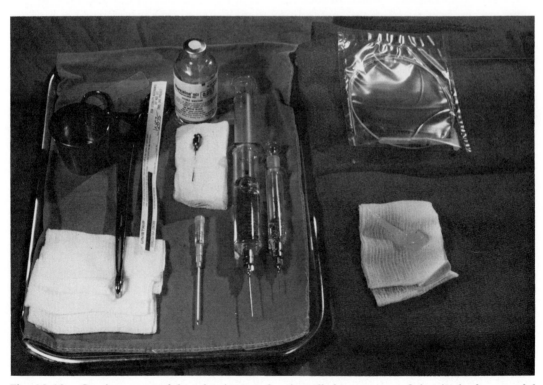

Fig. 13-10.   Continuous caudal analgesia tray showing all the contents of the single-dose caudal analgesia tray plus 16-gauge Teflon cannula (Abbocath), 20-gauge epidural catheter with adapter in the plastic bag, and antibiotic ointment.

ing the piercing of the posterior sacro-coccygeal ligament.

2. The cephalad direction of the cannula and the needle being maintained in the sagittal plane. If they skid the sacral hiatus, the median sacral crest deviates them to one side or the other.

3. The maintenance of the 45-degree angle with the patient's back while entering the sacral canal. If the cannula and the needle fail to enter the canal they become superficial to the sacral bone and rather parallel to the patient's back.

4. The feeling of the smooth anterior surface of the sacral canal. This is different from that of the rugged posterior surface of the sacrum, which is covered by muscles and ligaments.

After the operator is confident that the intravascular cannula is in the sacral canal, the stylet needle is withdrawn about 0.5 cm., the cannula is pushed cephalad for about 2 cm., and then the stylet needle is removed, leaving the cannula *in situ* (Fig.13-11B).

At this step the proper site of insertion is confirmed by:

1. The absence of resistance to the advancement of the cannula

2. The absence of crepitus when 3 ml. of air is injected

3. The absence of resistance during air injection

4. The absence of reflux of air into the syringe following injection

If no blood or cerebrospinal fluid is seen at the hub of the cannula or in the syringe following aspiration, the 20-gauge caudal catheter is threaded through the 16-gauge cannula (Fig. 13-11C). If there is a wire stylet inside the catheter, it should be removed before insertion of the catheter into the caudal canal to minimize the chances of injury to blood vessels, nerves, or dura. *Confirmation of the proper position of the caudal catheter at this step is determined by:*

1. The absence of resistance to the advancement of the caudal catheter

2. The patient's feeling of an "electric

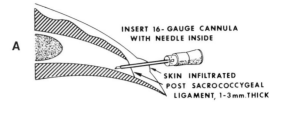

A   INSERT 16-GAUGE CANNULA WITH NEEDLE INSIDE

SKIN INFILTRATED

POST SACROCOCCYGEAL LIGAMENT, 1-3mm.THICK

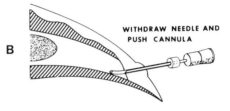

B   WITHDRAW NEEDLE AND PUSH CANNULA

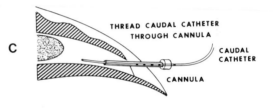

C   THREAD CAUDAL CATHETER THROUGH CANNULA

CAUDAL CATHETER

CANNULA

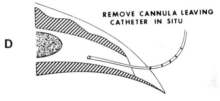

D   REMOVE CANNULA LEAVING CATHETER IN SITU

Fig. 13-11. Insertion of the cannula and threading of the catheter through it in continuous caudal technique.

twitch" in one of the hips due to the catheter touching one of the sacral nerve roots. The patient should be warned against the possibility of such a sensation beforehand, and reassured if it occurs.

3. The operator's experience of a special tactile sensation as the catheter advances along the smooth surface of the sacral canal

4. The operator's feeling of the catheter as it crosses the transverse ridges that sometimes occur at the unions of the sacral vertebrae, similar to driving on the high-

way and feeling the bumps between sections of concrete.

After advancing the caudal catheter to a reasonable length, the cannula is withdrawn over it. The markings on the catheter help to estimate the length of the portion left in the caudal canal (Fig. 13-11D). The catheter, if necessary, is pulled out to the required length. If caudal analgesia is intended to be part of the double-catheter technique, the distance from the catheter tip to the skin level is about 8 cm. Thus, the catheter tip lies among the sacral nerves. If continuous caudal technique is the only method used, then this distance should be about 14 cm. Thus, the catheter tip lies in the vicinity of the lumbosacral joint, thereby reducing the total dose of the local anesthetic injected and ensuring adequate cephalad spread of the solution.

The adapter is attached to the free end of the catheter. Aspiration is gently done to exclude intrathecal or intravascular position of the catheter. A test dose of 4 ml. of the local anesthetic is injected, and aspiration is performed immediately following. There should be no resistance to injection, and no blood or cerebrospinal fluid upon aspiration. Neosporin ointment is applied at the entrance of the catheter into the skin which is covered with sterile gauze. The catheter is brought to the side of the lower abdomen and fixed to the skin using 3-inch adhesive tape. With a ballpoint pen the word "caudal" is written on the tape covering the distal part of the catheter close to the adapter. The patient is turned on her back and the uterus is allowed to fall to the left by bringing the patient to the right edge of the bed and/or placing a folded towel under the right hip. After 5 minutes has lapsed from injection of the test dose, and in the absence of spinal block or intravascular injection of the local anesthetic, the therapeutic dose is injected. If the catheter is used as a part of the double-catheter technique, 6 to 8 ml. is injected. If continuous caudal is the only method to be used for analgesia and a large segment of catheter is left in the epidural space, the volume recommended for single-dose caudal is reduced by 5 ml., i.e., 15 ml. for a patient 150 cm. (5 feet) tall and 21 ml. for a patient 165 cm. (5'6") tall. Injection should always be performed slowly, with the patient in the horizontal position if possible. Aspiration should be performed before, during, and after injection, and verbal contact with the patient should be maintained.

The follow-up of patients after the initial and repeated injection is more or less similar to that of epidural analgesia. The difference is that with caudal block, perineal analgesia is the first to occur and the last to disappear. In 1943, when continuous caudal analgesia was still in its infancy, patients were kept on their sides.[48] Occasionally when analgesia rose to a higher level on the dependent side, the patient was turned to the opposite side. This lateral positioning was for a purpose other than avoiding inferior vena caval or aortic compression, namely to avoid dislodging or breaking of the caudal needle which was left *in situ*. However, it was a bonus and demonstrates the feasibility of its use. It cannot be overemphasized that all women, whether having regional analgesia or not, should labor on their sides; at least the right hip should be raised by bringing the patient to the right edge of the bed and/or by placing a folded bedsheet, a pillow, or a wedge underneath.

A few hours following the initial dose of local anesthetic the patient starts to feel uncomfortable again and a refill dose through the catheter is required. Aspiration is performed before and after injecting 4 ml. of the local anesthetic as a test dose. In the absence of intravascular or subarachnoid injection, the refill dose is given, guided by the level of analgesia obtained by the first dose, i.e., if too high a block was obtained with the first dose reduce the following dose and vice versa. In order to reach the same segmental block the refill dose should be the same or just a few milliliters less than the initial dose. Too much delay between refills is not advisable, not only because the patient should not be allowed to suffer unnecessarily, but also to avoid tachyphylaxis. On the other hand, the author does not recommend periodical administration of the anesthetic drug before the patient feels any discomfort because the duration of action of a drug differs in different patients.

CAUDAL ANALGESIA FOR CESAREAN SECTION

Caudal analgesia is not advisable for routine use in elective cesarean section. However, if continuous caudal technique has been used for trial labor that failed, and a large segment of the catheter has been left in the sacral canal, caudal analgesia can be utilized for cesarean section. Analgesia to the T5 level is then achieved by injecting a volume of local anesthetic equivalent to that producing analgesia to the T10 level plus 5 ml. The concentration is increased to 0.75 per cent bupivacaine in order to produce adequate abdominal relaxation and maximum analgesia. Such a high dose for cesarean section should not be injected before 2 hours from the last local anesthetic dose; otherwise a toxic reaction may occur. If cesarean section cannot be delayed for such a period, a lumbar epidural block is used to supplement the caudal analgesia in order to minimize the total dose of the local anesthetic drug. Analgesia to the T5 level can be achieved by injecting about 10 ml. of 0.75 per cent bupivacaine at the L2 to L3 interspace with the patient in the Trendelenburg position and the bevel of the Tuohy needle directed cephalad. It should be remembered that the maximum permissible dose of bupivacaine is 3 mg./kg. without epinephrine and 3.5 mg./kg. with epinephrine and that such a dose should not be repeated before 2 to 3 hours.

COMPLICATIONS ASSOCIATED WITH CAUDAL ANALGESIA

To avoid the complications associated with caudal analgesia a trainee performing a caudal block should always be supervised by an experienced physician until he is adequately trained. Thereafter, a supervisor should always be available for consultation. The complications of caudal analgesia can be divided into two groups, maternal and fetal.

MATERNAL COMPLICATIONS

Infection

Infection is a serious complication. It is stated that infection is more liable to occur with caudal than with epidural analgesia, because of the proximity of the caudal site to the rectum and perineum. In 1943, Hingson reported 1 case out of 10,000 cases of caudal analgesia that died from infection.[48] He also reported 6 cases that had infections at or around the sacral and gluteal area, which cleared under sulfonamide therapy. In 1959, Bush reported 1 case of septic meningitis out of 1,813 cases of caudal analgesia.[21] However, this case was preceded by respiratory infection in a patient who had myasthenia gravis. It was not associated with epidural abscess and the dura was intact. To avoid possible infection the attachment of a bacterial filter to the terminal end of the caudal catheter is recommended.[27] However peridural abscesses can occur spontaneously.[9,29] Moreover a bacterial filter attached to the extradural catheter did not prevent the development of an epidural abscess following systemic infection.[30] Sepsis secondary to caudal or epidural block should be of historic interest. The only way to prevent infection is to consider these techniques as major surgical procedures requiring the necessary sterility precautions. They should not be used in a patient with generalized systemic infection. The author recommends the use of a bacterial filter only if the dura was inadvertently punctured, the patient is diabetic or debilitated, and/or the catheter has to be used for several days, e.g., for the treatment of chronic pain.

Toxic Reaction

In the literature, the incidence of toxic reaction following caudal analgesia varies; e.g., it has been reported as 1:1200,[6] 2:1000,[33] and 3:600.[66] In Magee-Womens Hospital 2 cases of convulsions followed caudal analgesia in 1,342 patients, one after single-dose caudal and the other after continuous caudal technique (Table 13-1). In both cases the use of a test dose was omitted. To avoid this complication certain precautions should be followed:

1. The label on the vial or ampule should be read to make sure of the name and concentration of the drug.

2. It should be remembered that the doses of local anesthetic drugs used for caudal analgesia are close to the maximum permissible dose. Therefore, repetition of the dose within a short time should be avoided even if failure to produce adequate analgesia has occurred.

3. The local anesthetic should be injected slowly to avoid a sudden rise of the blood level of the drug.

4. The test dose (4 ml.) should precede the therapeutic dose. Verbal contact with the patient should continue, asking her to report any abnormal sensation and watching for her reaction. If the patient complains of a metallic taste, ringing in her ears, or blurred vision, even though no blood is obtained on aspiration, the needle or catheter is removed, the situation is reevaluated, and the site of injection or the technique is changed. There is a tendency to rush things in the delivery room and the anesthesiologist tends to omit the test dose. It should be remembered that "safety first" is the rule under all circumstances. Aspiration should be done before, during, and after each injection.

5. A catheter can be in a blood vessel and yet no blood is aspirated, because the catheter tip can be against the vessel wall (Fig. 13-12A). In such a case, aspiration following injection of 2 ml. of solution is more liable to obtain a sanguineous aspirate than prior to injection, because the injectate distends the vein and separates the catheter tip from the vessel wall (Fig. 13-

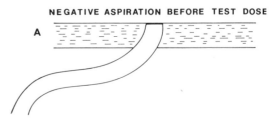

Table 13-1. The Incidence of Major Complications Associated With Caudal Analgesia in 1,342 Cases

Complication	Incidence with Single-Dose Technique No. Out of 611 Cases	%	Incidence with Continuous Technique No. Out of 731 Cases	%
Toxic reaction	1	0.16	1	0.13
Dural puncture	0	0	1	0.13
Residual effect (48 hours)	0	0	1	0.13
Infection	0	0	0	0
Hypertension	0	0	0	0
Hypotension (More than 20%)	22	3.6	21	2.8

Fig. 13-12. Intravascular position of the epidural or caudal catheter. *A.* Before injecting the test dose, the tip of the catheter is against the vessel wall preventing aspiratin of blood. *B.* After injecting the test dose, distention of the vein and separation of the catheter from the vessel wall allow aspiration of blood.

12B). However, as mentioned before, aspiration can be negative even if the catheter tip lies in a blood vessel. Therefore, aspiration is only important when positive, and the only reliable sign that the catheter is inside a blood vessel is the reaction of the patient to the test dose.

6. All drugs and equipment necessary for resuscitation should be available before injecting local anesthetics for any procedure. Diazepam, mephentermine, thiopental and succinylcholine should be available close to the patient, as well as facilities for intubation and artificial ventilation with oxygen.

7. A refill dose should be administered only by a person who can deal with convulsions, total respiratory paralysis, severe hypotension, and cardiac arrest.

8. In addition to the anesthesiologist, the presence of a second person (physician or nurse) is mandatory to assist promptly if toxic reaction occurs.

Dural Puncture

The possibility of puncturing the dura following caudal analgesia is less than following epidural analgesia. This is because the distance between the dural sac and the posterior wall of the epidural space is about 10 times greater in the caudal area than in the lumbar region. The dura can be punctured by a needle, catheter, or both. In 13,639 cases of caudal analgesia the dura was punctured 171 times (1.2%).[33] Unrecognized dural puncture leading to an accidental spinal occurred 9 times in 6,334 cases (0.1%). The use of the Teflon cannula instead of the caudal needle tends to minimize the chances of dural puncture. In 1,342 cases of caudal analgesia performed at Magee-Womens Hospital, the dura was accidentally punctured in one case, not by the needle or cannula but by the 20-gauge Teflon caudal catheter without the stylet. A catheter may perforate the dura after being in the epidural space for several hours. This can be both misleading and serious. Previous injections through the catheter causing a segmental block may give a false sense of security and the second or third injection may be followed by total subarachnoid block.[12,64] The incidence of such a complication is about 1:4000. The perforation could be due to the pistonlike movement of the catheter against the end of the dural sac during the patient's movement in bed. Subsequently the dura is eroded and the catheter gains access to the subarachnoid space.

Total subarachnoid block may follow the test dose and can occur in less than 1 minute.[51] This is because local anesthetics used for epidural or caudal blocks are usually hypobaric compared to the cerebrospinal fluid. Therefore, the patient should not be in a sitting position during the injection of the test dose.

There are cases of total spinal block occurring with the therapeutic dose of the local anesthetic, in spite of a negative test dose.[28,41,66] Thus, the test dose may give a false sense of security, especially if the dose is too small or the interval between it and the therapeutic dose is too short. To make the test dose through an epidural or caudal catheter more reliable, the amount of local anesthetic injected should be 4 ml. and the interval between the test dose and the definitive dose should be at least 5 minutes.[1] When drugs are injected through a needle, either for caudal or epidural analgesia, the most important precaution to avoid total spinal block is not the test dose, but rather to keep the hand holding the needle steady against the patient's back to prevent the tip of the needle from advancing and puncturing the dura. The duration of apnea following total spinal block varies with the drug used (with bupivacaine it is usually 3 hours). No harmful effect on the fetus will occur if the maternal respiration and circulation are maintained at normal values. The possibility of total subarachnoid block is another reason that refill doses with epidural and caudal blocks should be taken more seriously and be injected only by a person capable of dealing with total respiratory paralysis, severe hypotension, and even cardiac arrest. Moreover, if epidural and/or caudal are used in the labor suite, it cannot be overemphasized that facilities for adequate resuscitation should be available in the patient's room each time refill doses are administered.

Hypotension

In the literature, the incidence of hypotension following caudal analgesia for vaginal delivery is 2.2 per cent.[39] In our series the incidence of hypotension was 3.6 per cent with the single-dose caudal, and 2.8 per cent with the continuous caudal technique (Table 13-1). The difference between the incidence of hypotension in the literature and in our series is probably due to the definition of hypotension. The author considers hypotension to have occurred if the systolic blood pressure drops more than 20 per cent of the original level irrespective of the absolute value. Dehydration and/or narcotics potentiate the sympathetic blockade caused by caudal or epidural analgesia.[30] Therefore it is recommended that patients who had prolonged labor should be infused with 1 or 2 liters of fluid before initiating the block. The causes and management of hypotension with caudal analgesia are similar to those discussed with epidural analgesia (see also Chaps. 5, Effects of Vertebral Blocks on the Cardiovascular System and 14, Epidural Analgesia).

Hypertension

In the literature, the incidence of hypertension with caudal analgesia is 0.5 per cent.[21] In general to avoid hypertension the following precautions are advised:

1. The usage of epinephrine should be avoided because accidental intravenous injection can lead to hypertension.

2. The usage of ergot alkaloids should be avoided except as a life-saving measure

to control postpartum hemorrhage and then only by the intramuscular route.

3. The name and dose of the vasopressor should be checked before its injection.

4. It should be remembered that toxemic and/or hypertensive patients are particularly sensitive to vasopressors.

Nausea and Vomiting

The incidence of nausea and vomiting with caudal analgesia is 3.1 per cent.[21] The main cause of nausea and vomiting is hypotension, which must be excluded and corrected before taking any other measure or administering an antiemetic drug. Other possible causes of nausea and vomiting are opiates, anxiety and other psychologic problems, hypertension, hypoxia and/or hypercapnia, and blocking of the sympathetic fibers leading to predominantly vagal autonomic effects.

Shivering

The incidence of shivering with caudal analgesia for obstetrics is 8.4 per cent.[39] Shivering can be due to: (1) loss of heat following peripheral vasodilation in the lower part of the body, infusion of fluids at room temperature, and exposure of the patient; (2) nervousness, since some patients even under "natural childbirth" develop shivering; (3) access of minute amounts of amniotic fluid into the maternal circulation;[77] (4) reaction to the local anesthetics, especially if given in large doses; (5) reaction to epinephrine. If the patient develops shivering, overdosage of local anesthetics should be excluded and the patient should be reassured and watched closely. Before delivery 2.5 mg. of diazepam and after delivery 50 mg. of mepheridine may be helpful.

Backache

Backache following caudal analgesia occurred in 176 out of 2,310 patients (7.6%).[33] It is 4 times more common after caudal than after epidural. The laxity of ligaments caused by pregnancy and the supine position associated with relaxation of the lower back cause a strain on the joints of the lower back. This is one reason for keeping mothers on their side during labor (see also Chaps. 5, 14, and 15).

Coccygodynia

In 102 out of 1,828 patients,[21] pain at the site of injection following caudal analgesia was sufficiently severe to require analgesic drugs during the hospital stay. However, an important cause of coccygodynia is the delivery itself, because the coccyx has to give way for the oncoming fetal head.

Leg Pains

Leg pains, lasting from one to several days, occur in about 1 per cent of patients after caudal analgesia. The pains can be due to a residual effect of the caudal technique or from trauma to the nerves within the pelvis caused by the delivery or the forceps. They may also be due to pressure on the nerves during lithotomy position.

Residual Effect

In our series, one out of 1,342 cases had residual effect of caudal analgesia. This case was a 32-year-old patient who was gravida II, para 1. When the cervix was 7 cm. dilated, she had continuous caudal block for labor. She had paresthesia of the right hip when the catheter was inserted, and injections of 20 ml. of 0.5 per cent bupivacaine caused a block on the right side only. Two hours later the same dose was injected with the patient in the left lateral position. Thirty minutes later the analgesia remained localized to the right side, and the patient was ready for delivery. The caudal analgesia was supplemented with left pudendal nerve block. During the postpartum period the patient had paresis, numbness, and hypalgesia of the right lower limb, which lasted for 48 hours. She was reassured and complete recovery occurred 24 hours later.

Bladder Dysfunction

Overdistention of the bladder should not be allowed to occur during labor, not only because it interferes with the fetal head rotation but also because it predisposes to postpartum bladder atony. Obstetric trauma can itself cause bladder and urethral dysfunction. The patient is advised to empty her bladder before caudal block is initiated, and before each refill dose if required.

Problems Associated With Caudal Catheters

A caudal catheter can be sheared off by the sharp edge of the caudal needle, particularly if the catheter is pulled out while the needle is in place. This complication should not occur if the caudal catheter is inserted through the Teflon cannula as described. A caudal catheter can make a knot in the sacral canal which could tighten, and even the catheter may break if force is used in pulling it out at the termination of delivery.[24] It is the author's opinion that the caudal or epidural catheter should be removed by an anesthesiologist, preferably the one who inserted it, or an experienced nurse anesthetist. There should be no force exerted during its removal. The removed catheter should be examined carefully lest any of its parts are missing; the marks on the catheter tip help in ruling this out. If a part of the catheter is left inside the caudal canal the patient should be informed, and whether to remove it surgically or not depends on the individual case and any associated symptoms (see also Chap. 14, Epidural Analgesia, Problems With the Use of Catheters).

Breakage of Needles

This problem is reported to occur in 1.4 per cent of single-dose caudal blocks.[33] With increased experience and adhering to the previously mentioned rule, "do not use force," it should not occur. If a part of the needle is left inside the body, the patient should be informed and it should be removed surgically as soon as feasible.

FETAL COMPLICATIONS

Fetal bradycardia may occur secondary to caudal analgesia.[4] The possible mechanisms are:

1. *Maternal arterial hypotension produced by sympathetic blockade and accentuated by inferior vena caval compression* may cause a decreased uterine blood flow with subsequent fetal hypoxia, acidosis, and bradycardia.[56] Every precaution should be taken to avoid hypotension and to correct it immediately when the drop in blood pressure exceeds 20 per cent of the original level.

2. *Compression of the maternal abdominal aorta by the gravid uterus* may cause a decreased uterine blood flow without a reduction of arterial pressure as measured in the brachial artery.[35] This can be prevented by left uterine displacement (e.g., keeping the patient on her side).

3. *The local anesthetic drug injected accidentally into the fetal head* leads to fetal intoxication and bradycardia. Such an accident has been reported in 4 cases and caused severe neonatal bradycardia, apnea, and convulsions. Death occurred in two of the cases.[38,87] The other two babies survived, but required exchange transfusion. This mishap should be prevented by identifying the landmarks of the caudal hiatus before attempting caudal analgesia, if possible inserting the caudal catheter when the fetal head is high, not using force, and doing rectal examination in doubtful cases.[64]

4. *The local anesthetic drug injected directly into a maternal vein or near to a lacerated one* may lead to a dangerously high plasma concentration of the drug in the mother, a large blood-placental gradient, and fetal central nervous system depression and bradycardia. In such a case the mother will develop symptoms or signs of drug toxicity, caudal analgesia will not be accomplished, and the maternal plasma concentration of the local anesthetic at the time of fetal distress will be high.

5. *The local anesthetic inadvertently injected into the sacral bone*[34,58] may lead to a dangerously high maternal blood level of the drug with maternal and fetal toxic reaction. The sudden give of the periosteum covering the sacral bone can be mistaken for that of the posterior sacrococcygeal ligament. To avoid such a complication, no force should be used and gentle aspiration should always precede injection. The aspiration of thick blood which on microscopic examination shows bone marrow cells is diagnostic. If there is resistance to air or fluid injection, the needle should be removed.

6. *Accidental intrathecal injection* can lead to total spinal block with respiratory paralysis, severe hypotension, and subsequently, fetal hypoxia.

7. *Vasodilation of the lower limbs before paralysis of the sympathetic nerves supplying the uterine blood vessels may "steal" blood from the placenta.* Temporary loss of baseline variability of the fetal heart rate occurs in 53 per cent of cases 4 to 18 minutes following epidural analgesia.[11] Moreover there is a tendency for the slowing of the fetal heart rate between 10 and 40 minutes following epidural analgesia.[56] This may be the result of a decrease in uterine blood flow. Since the sympathetic outflow to the lower limb vasculature is from segments L1 and L2, and that to the uterus is from T10 to L2,[92] there may occur an initial period in which there is vasodilation in the lower limbs accompanied by uterine vasoconstriction. This can temporarily lead to decreased uterine blood flow with subsequent loss of baseline variability of fetal heart rate or fetal bradycardia. As the block extends to T10, the uterine blood vessels dilate and the problem is usually corrected.

8. *A coincidental factor* may cause fetal bradycardia, e.g., cord compression. Marked variable decelerations at the second stage of labor have been more noticeable since routine electronic monitoring has been instituted. In such cases, at the time of delivery a tight loop of umbilical cord is usually found around the fetal

neck. The Apgar scores of these infants are usually good and no significant fetal acidosis is present. The cause of the fetal bradycardia can be due to cord compression, and also increased intracranial pressure secondary to obstruction of venous return from the head as the umbilical cord tightens around the neck during uterine contractions and fetal descent. Favoring this theory is the fact that these decelerations become more pronounced when the mother bears down.

The increased uterine tone occurring either spontaneously or due to excessive oxytocin administration interferes with the uteroplacental circulation. This can lead to fetal hypoxia and bradycardia.

9. *Multiple factors* may cause fetal bradycardia, e.g., ascending sympathetic blockade, a systemic drug effect, increased uterine tone, and cord compression.[3] Each of these factors by itself may be insufficient to cause fetal bradycardia.

INDICATIONS FOR USE OF CAUDAL ANALGESIA

Caudal analgesia can be used if a patient has pain during parturition and no contraindication for its use is present. It is especially indicated in the following conditions:

Delivery of Preterm Infant

In cases of delivery of a preterm infant caudal analgesia has the following advantages:

1. With caudal analgesia *there is a minimal trauma to the fetal head* due to relaxation of the birth canal and perineum. The expulsive force associated with strong pushing and sudden release of pressure as the head passes through the introitus is replaced by voluntary controlled pushing and gentle delivery of the head by the obstetrician.

2. With caudal analgesia *there is no need for narcotics or tranquilizers* in the first stage of labor, *nor for general anesthesia* in the second stage. All these drugs cross the blood-placental barrier to the fetus, with possible resulting fetal and neonatal depression, a situation particularly undesirable in the premature infant since its brain is especially sensitive to central nervous system depressants[67] and its respiratory center is underdeveloped.

3. With caudal analgesia *there is decreased maternal stress* owing to loss of pain. Stressful conditions of the mother can lead to fetal hypoxia,[69] and excessive catecholamines decrease uterine blood flow.[80]

Maternal Cardiac Disease

For the following reasons caudal analgesia, preferably as a part of the double-catheter technique, is the ideal method of pain relief for labor and delivery of a cardiac patient:

1. Pain during labor increases the cardiac output and the pulse rate.[71] By relieving pain, caudal analgesia saves an already diseased heart from an added strain.[63]

2. Caudal analgesia causes sympathetic blockade. Thus the peripheral resistance and the cardiac work diminish.[13]

3. Bearing down during the second stage of labor decreases the venous return to the heart, and subsequently, the cardiac output falls. In patients with limited cardiac output, such as in mitral stenosis, this may be serious. Moreover, during bearing down, the patient holds her breath and can easily become hypoxic. Therefore, elimination of Valsalva maneuver is essential in the management of cardiac patients, and can best be accomplished by caudal analgesia.

4. Cardiac arrhythmias are initiated or worsened during labor and delivery in cardiac patients.[5] Pain relief as achieved by caudal analgesia is beneficial in these cases.

5. The most common time for onset of acute heart failure or pulmonary edema is during the fourth stage of labor.[94] After delivery the heart is suddenly faced with a decreased circulatory bed due to the uterine retraction and increased blood

volume due to the relief of inferior vena caval compression. Caudal and/or epidural methods of analgesia produce sympathetic blockade which results in vasodilation of the lower limbs. This vasodilation acts as a reservoir for the increased blood volume until the heart adjusts to the new hemodynamics and diuresis occurs. In the postpartum period, the caudal catheter can be left *in situ* for 24 to 36 hours to achieve this if required. The team work of the obstetrician, cardiologist, and anesthesiologist is essential in these cases.

6. Epidural and/or caudal methods of analgesia are also beneficial to the fetus which is usually compromised and delivered prematurely. With these techniques of analgesia there is minimal fetal depression and less acidosis during labor, and the pelvic relaxation prevents fetal trauma during delivery.

In cardiac patients hypotension should be avoided, especially in patients with a circulatory shunt, e.g., patent ductus, interatrial septal defect, interventricular septal defect, Fallot's tetralogy or Eisenmenger's complex.[7,31] If systemic blood pressure drops, a left-to-right shunt can be reversed or a right-to-left shunt can be accentuated, leading to hypoxia and acute heart failure. Therefore, when vertebral analgesia such as caudal block is used, the level of the block should be gradually titrated by using the continuous technique, and preferably combining epidural and caudal where catheters are inserted close to the target and minimal local anesthetic drugs are injected. No epinephrine should be used because it decreases the mean arterial blood pressure[50] and causes tachycardia.

The cardiac patient under caudal and/or epidural analgesia should labor on her side or at least have a pillow placed under her right hip, with elevation of the legs, and humidified oxygen should be administered through a transparent face mask. If hypotension occurs, it should be corrected immediately by using a vasopressor. The kind of vasopressor and the dose are selected and titrated by monitoring the blood pressure, pulse rate, and electrocardiogram. Hypotension should be corrected expeditiously with minimal change in pulse rate. For example, although phenylephrine (0.25 mg.) may decrease the uteroplacental blood flow, this is of secondary importance under these circumstances, and this drug is indicated to correct hypotension associated with maternal tachycardia. In cardiac patients who are under anticoagulant therapy, vertebral methods of analgesia, namely spinal, epidural, or caudal, are contraindicated.

Toxemias of Pregnancy

Caudal analgesia has the following beneficial effects in toxemic patients:

1. As mentioned previously, pain increases the cardiac output, and caudal analgesia, by eliminating pain, *prevents further rise of the blood pressure.* Moreover, the hypertension can be controlled by caudal analgesia alone or with minimal use of vasodilator drugs.[60]

2. Toxemia is associated with generalized vasoconstriction and a decreased blood volume. *Caudal and/or epidural blocks cause vasodilation,* and if the blood volume is corrected by fluid administration, the uterine blood flow will increase provided hypotension is avoided.[19b]

3. With caudal analgesia the placental and renal blood flow improve markedly,[49] the urine output increases, and the urine specific gravity decreases, due to the sympathetic blockade and the relief of the vasoconstriction.[93] If toxemia is associated with disseminated intravascular coagulopathy and the patient shows bleeding manifestations, all vertebral methods of pain relief are contraindicated because of fear of bleeding causing compression of the spinal cord and subsequently paraplegia.[10]

Induction of Labor

Induced labor with oxytocin can be quite painful. Since uterine contractions and fetal heart rate are monitored, the dangers of combining epidural and/or caudal analgesia with oxytocin are minimal because of their early detection. Provided hypotension due to caudal analgesia and hypertonus due to oxytocin are avoided, the combination of induced labor and caudal or epidural analgesia is a pleasant, fast, and convenient way of delivery for all concerned.[22]

Multiple Gestations

The anesthetic management of cases with multifetal gestation has a vital role in the outcome of the mother and fetuses. The infants are usually premature, small for gestational age,[57] and may be anemic.[77] Sometimes intrauterine manipulation or immediate interference may be required. Caudal block is safe for the babies and provides adequate analgesia for the mother without interfering with her consciousness or ability to push.[3]

History of Precipitous Labor

Caudal analgesia changes the bearing-down reflex from an involuntary to a voluntary act. Therefore in a patient who has had a history of precipitous labor, caudal analgesia is beneficial because it changes delivery into a more controllable process. Thus the mother and fetus are protected from the trauma associated with precipitous labor.

Breech Presentation

Caudal and epidural blocks have been successfully used for breech delivery.[15,16,42] They are accompanied by less mortality and morbidity than nonepidural techniques. In our institute caudal analgesia using 0.25 or 0.375 per cent bupivacaine, either alone or preferably as a part of the double-catheter technique, is the anesthetic method of choice for breech delivery. The adequate analgesia during both labor and delivery combined with the ability of the mother to bear down are the merits of caudal analgesia in such cases.

Moreover, the removal of reflex spasm of the pelvic floor helps the descent of the fetus.

Uterine Dyskinesia

When a patient with dyskinetic uterine contractions, prolonged labor, and ruptured membranes fails to respond to oxytocics, there is a potential danger of amnionitis. In these cases, if continuous epidural or caudal analgesia is instituted, uterine contractions become regular and strong, and vaginal delivery is usually accomplished within 2 to 6 hours.[6] Denervation of the sympathetic fibers to the uterus by caudal analgesia will stop the dysrhythmic contractions, and the uterus will subsequently respond in a bettter way to the oxytocic drug. The increase in placental circulation following caudal analgesia is also an important factor.[49]

Operative Vaginal Delivery Such as Forceps Rotation or Forceps Delivery

Epidural, caudal, or spinal block provides excellent conditions for operative vaginal deliveries without the risk of aspiration pneumonitis. The parents, moreover, enjoy watching the delivery, and this may have a significant impact on the psychologic relationship between the mother and her baby.[52]

Diabetes Mellitus

In nondiabetic patients there is less maternal and fetal acidosis with regional analgesia than without it.[74,75,89,90] This may also be the case in a diabetic patient. However, owing to the large size of the fetus and the associated hydramnios, the anesthesiologist should take all precautions to prevent supine hypotensive syndrome.

Intrauterine Growth Retardation

With intrauterine growth retardation there is chronic placental insufficiency and the intrauterine environment is inadequate. For these fetuses, the use of epidural and/or caudal analgesia is the best technique of pain relief because it does not interfere with the uterine blood flow provided hypotension is prevented, and does not depress the fetus as occurs with paracervical block. The small size of the uterus is an advantage since inferior vena caval compression is less than with normal gestation. The administration of oxygen to the mother can be advantageous to the fetus.

Rh-Sensitization

The Rh-sensitized fetus is usually premature and anemic. Therefore, the anesthetic technique should not cause any further depression of the fetus. There is an associated hydramnios and all precautions should be taken to avoid inferior vena caval compression.

Sickle Cell Disease

The pregnant patient with sickle cell disease is anemic and her cardiac output is increased; any further increase due to pain is not advisable. Factors leading to acidosis, hypoxia, hypothermia, and sludging should be avoided. Administration of oxygen to the mother is advisable.

Maternal Hypertension

Epidural analgesia is accompanied with the least cardiovascular changes compared to general anesthesia or subarachnoid block.[94a] The blood pressure with general anesthesia may show excessive rise whereas it may drop more precipitously with spinal analgesia. With caudal analgesia, the cardiovascular changes are expected to be comparable to epidural analgesia rather than to spinal or general anesthesia.

CONTRAINDICATIONS FOR THE USE OF CAUDAL ANALGESIA

The contraindications for use of caudal analgesia are shown in the list below and most of them are discussed with epidural analgesia. The following conditions require further clarification:

Pilonidal Sinus or Infected Cyst

A pilonidal sinus or infected cyst is an *absolute* contraindication for caudal analgesia because of the danger of introducing infection into the caudal canal. Previous pilonidal cystectomy is a *relative* contraindication to caudal block because the scarring of the area may render the technique relatively difficult.

Obscure Landmarks Due to Fat, or Edema Over the Sacrococcygeal Area

Unless landmarks are adequately identified, caudal analgesia should not be performed. Moreover, if after attempting

---

Contraindications to Caudal Analgesia

Absolute Contraindications	*Relative Contraindications*
1. Anticoagulant or bleeding diatheses	1. Cephalopelvic disproportion unless for trial labor or cesarean section
2. Acute hypovolemia	2. Previous cesarean section
3. Shock	3. Patient's choice
4. Increased intracranial pressure, e.g., space-occupying lesion	4. Inexperience of the team

5. Infection
  a. At the site
  b. Systemic
  c. Meningitis
	5. History of coccygodynia

6. Tumor at the site	6. Previous pilonidal cystectomy
7. Poor landmarks	7. Incomplete or faulty development of the sacral hiatus
	8. Active central nervous system disease, except epilepsy

caudal analgesia a hematoma is formed, obscuring the landmarks, no further trials are allowed. That is why the best chance to have a successful caudal puncture is the first attempt.

As a rule caudal analgesia should not be tried more than three times on the same patient. This is not only because of the physical and psychologic trauma to the patient, but also because it is an indication that the landmarks are difficult to identify and/or the operator has lost the anatomical orientation of the sacral hiatus and canal.

Previous Cesarean Section

Some feel that following cesarean section a patient can safely deliver vaginally under caudal or epidural analgesia if no disproportion exists.[62,30] Tactile palpation of the scar tissue during vaginal examination can give an early warning of dehiscence.[62] Yet most obstetricians, especially in the United States, find performing cesarean section is safer for both the mother and the baby because the incidence of ruptured uterus with vaginal delivery following a previous cesarean section is 2.1 per cent with classical and 0.5 per cent with lower segment incision.[36] However, if a patient who has had a previous cesarean section arrives at the hospital at the end of the first stage of labor with no disproportion and the obstetrician feels that she can be delivered vaginally, the author considers epidural and caudal methods of analgesia to be contraindicated, and other methods such as pudendal nerve block should be utilized. This decision is based on many facts including the difficulty to palpate the site of the uterine scar if the fetal head is down.[43] With ruptured uterus under epidural or caudal analgesia, the abdominal pain may be diffuse, poorly localized, and could be mistaken for failure of the block.[36] Pain may even be completely absent and the patient may have complete rupture of the uterus with extrusion of the fetus and placenta into the abdominal cavity before the condition is diagnosed.[43] *In conclusion, it is too risky to allow a mother who* *has had a previous cesarean section to labor, and the administration of epidural or caudal analgesia increases this risk.*

History of Coccygodynia Especially Following Caudal Analgesia

If a patient has a history of coccygodynia, other methods of pain relief should be considered (e.g., epidural or subarachnoid block).

Brain Tumor

Patients with brain tumors should not be allowed to bear down because of the associated rise of intracranial pressure. Epidural, caudal or paracervical plus pudendal nerve block can obtund the perineal reflex and provide adequate analgesia for forceps delivery, episiotomy, and repair. Crawford[27] considers caudal analgesia to be the method of choice in patients with brain tumors because the possibility of dural puncture is much less than with epidural analgesia.

Although the rise in cerebrospinal fluid pressure with caudal injections is minimal compared with that following lumbar epidural,[97] any further increase of intracranial pressure in patients with a brain tumor can be detrimental. In our department, in 2 patients with brain tumor, injection of 22 and 24 ml. of 1.5 per cent lidocaine resulted in apnea, total loss of consciousness, and severe bradycardia, lasting for 5 and 6 minutes. This episode was followed by adequate analgesia lasting for about 90 minutes, thus excluding intravascular injection of the local anesthetic. Therefore, caudal analgesia is also contraindicated in cases of increased intracranial pressure, and the method of choice is pudendal nerve block.

Cephalopelvic Disproportion

Caudal and/or epidural methods of analgesia should not be used to relieve pain of cephalopelvic disproportion unless the patient is watched carefully and cesarean section is considered if labor fails to progress.

Incomplete or Faulty Development of the Sacrum

Malformations of the sacrum cause abnormal landmarks and caudal analgesia becomes a difficult or even a risky procedure because of the possible injury to the mother's rectum or to the fetus.

ROLE OF CAUDAL ANALGESIA

ADVANTAGES OF CAUDAL ANALGESIA

Advantages Over Epidural Technique

1. *Perineal analgesia* is obtained in a few minutes with caudal analgesia, without resorting to any special position. On the other hand, with continuous epidural block, perineal analgesia may be incomplete either due to the large size of some of the sacral foramina and escape of the local anesthetic or obliteration of the epidural space near the lumbosacral joint. With epidural block, the time interval between injection of the refill dose and the development of adequate perineal analgesia may be too long. Moreover the sitting-up position for achieving perineal analgesia with epidural block is not greatly welcomed by some obstetricians, because the fetal head is crowning and pushed against the bed. They prefer either the horizontal position or a position with a slight head-up tilt.

2. *The analgesia is uniform and bilateral* with caudal analgesia. The problem of unilateral analgesia due to deviation of the catheter, such as encountered with lumbar epidural,[51,96] is rarely seen with caudal analgesia. With the epidural technique the catheter has to change its direction almost 90 degrees as it enters the epidural space. With caudal technique the catheter continues cephalad with a gentle curve and thus tends to remain in the median plane.

3. There is less danger of inadvertently puncturing the dura with caudal than with epidural technique, because the distance from the dura to the sacral hiatus is usually 10 times longer than from the dura to the ligamentum flavum.

4. *It is easier to maintain the patient in the proper position* while performing the technique with caudal than with epidural block, particularly if the patient is uncooperative and has severe pains with the uterine contractions.

Advantages Over Subarachnoid Block

1. *There is almost no chance of post-lumbar-puncture cephalgia with caudal block.* Following spinal analgesia the incidence of headache varies between 2 per cent[1] and 18 per cent.[34] Therefore, if analgesia is required during the late first stage or during the second stage of labor, it is worth examining the caudal area. If the landmarks are easily identified, the author believes that single-dose caudal analgesia is preferable to subarachnoid block.

2. *Caudal block provides analgesia during both labor and delivery,* whereas subarachnoid block is only utilized for the actual delivery. With a change from subarachnoid block to epidural and/or caudal, the labor suite has become quite a pleasant place at least for patients and their relatives.

3. *With caudal analgesia the mother can bear down easily when required.* This has made delivery a more controlled process. Thus, there is no need for rushing to the delivery room a patient who cannot stop the urge to push and trying to administer a spinal block to her under the most unfavorable circumstances.

Advantages Over Paracervical Block

1. *The incidence of neonatal depression* following paracervical block is high, and thus paracervical block is contraindicated in a compromised fetus. The use of paracervical block more than twice during labor is unadvisable because it is associated with higher perinatal mortality.[72,81]

2. *Paracervical block does not provide perineal analgesia.*

3. *Paracervical block cannot be used once the cervix is fully dilated and effaced.*

Advantages Over Pudendal Nerve Block

1. The caudal technique relieves *the uterine pain* during the first and second stages of labor, whereas pudendal nerve block causes only perineal analgesia.

2. *The success rate* is higher with caudal than with pudendal nerve block, because although the pudendal is the main nerve supplying the perineum, it is not the only one. Moreover, aberration of the inferior hemorrhoidal nerve occurs in 50 per cent of patients,[53] making its block unpredictable.

Advantages Over General Anesthesia for Vaginal Delivery

1. *Caudal analgesia can be used during the first as well as the second stage of labor,* whereas general anesthesia is utilized only for the delivery itself.

2. The danger of *aspiration* under general anesthesia is too high a risk to take for analgesia during childbirth.

3. Neonatal depression following general anesthesia is higher than with conduction anesthesia.

4. With general anesthesia the parents are deprived of *the joy of watching their baby delivered,* as well as hearing and seeing him in the delivery room. The touch and eye-to-eye contact between the mother and her baby at this stage is important for affectional bonding between them.[52]

5. *There is no excessive blood loss with caudal analgesia.* In 3,500 consecutive patients, the average blood loss with vaginal delivery was 225 ml.[39]

Advantages Over the General Analgesia Techniques

The analgesia produced by caudal block is superb, with minimal maternal, fetal, or neonatal depression. There is less maternal and fetal acidosis with regional analgesia than without it.[74,75,89,90]

DISADVANTAGES OF CAUDAL ANALGESIA

The alleged disadvantages of caudal analgesia are:

1. *Caudal block is technically difficult.* It is stated that caudal block is the most difficult technique of the regional and general anesthesia methods of pain relief in obstetrics. The incidence of anatomical variations in the sacral region is 10 per cent, and while the patient has only one caudal hiatus, yet 5 lumbar interspaces are available. The associated failure rates restrain many anesthesiologists from even thinking about caudal analgesia as a method of pain relief, or even attempting to feel the caudal area. The failure rate is between 1.5 per cent and 10 per cent.[12,21,33,39,48,62,66] The success rate varies from one center to another, and even among anesthesiologists at the same center. At Magee-Womens Hospital the failure rate is low (1.1%) because of (1) *the proper selection of patients,* i.e., if the landmarks are doubtful other techniques of analgesia are considered; (2) *the 24-hour coverage* by obstetric anesthesiologists; and (3) *the use of higher concentrations of drugs,* i.e., 0.25 per cent or 0.5 per cent bupivacaine rather than 0.125 per cent and 2 per cent chloroprocaine rather than 1 per cent. With increased experience caudal analgesia can sometimes be easier and less risky than epidural analgesia. The obstetric anesthesiologist should be capable of performing either or both techniques efficiently.

2. *A large dose of local anesthetic is required to produce caudal analgesia.* For first-stage analgesia the segments to be blocked are only T10 to L1. In order to reach a level of T10 by the caudal route, the dose of local anesthetic needed is 2 or 3 times the dose of anesthetic needed for epidural block. In order to minimize the dose of the local anesthetic and the chances of failure, the author recommends the double-catheter technique whenever feasible, where epidural is utilized to relieve the uterine pain and the caudal to deaden the perineal pain (see also Chap. 14, Epidural Analgesia).

3. *The area is close to the mother's rectum and the fetal head.* As stressed before, proper surgical sterile technique should be

adopted with caudal analgesia. No attempt at caudal analgesia should be made if landmarks are poor or no longer identifiable. If in doubt, the rectum is examined to ensure that the needle did not pierce it. However, the author is against the routine use of rectal examination because of the possibility of contamination of the field. It is stated that in order to avoid fetal trauma, caudal analgesia should be avoided when the fetal head is low.[64] This policy will unfortunately limit the use of caudal analgesia, particularly the single-dose technique. The best way to avoid fetal trauma is to know the anatomy, use caudal analgesia only when the landmarks are felt and supervise properly the trainee until adequate experience is gained.

4. *The course of labor is prolonged with the caudal technique.* This is still debatable, and there is evidence to the contrary. To reduce such a possibility: (1) caudal analgesia should only be used when labor is active; (2) 0.25 per cent bupivacaine rather than 0.5 per cent bupivacaine is used in early labor; (3) maternal hypotension should be avoided and immediately corrected; (4) preferably double-catheter technique is utilized when epidural is used for relief of the uterine pain. However, if for any reason labor is slow, oxytocin is administered by using the Harvard pump, and the uterine contractions and the fetal heart rate are electronically monitored. The obstetric team should accept the use of oxytocin when required and not contraindicated, rather than argue whether caudal or epidural analgesia has slowed down labor, which is difficult to prove or disprove.

5. *Caudal analgesia may cause a higher incidence of persistent occipitoposterior position of the fetal head.* An adequate tone of the perineal muscles is important to allow for rotation of the fetal head. If too high a concentration of the local anesthetic is used, relaxation of the perineal muscles may occur with resultant failure of the fetal head to rotate spontaneously. This problem can be prevented by using 0.25 per cent bupivacaine in the first stage of labor until the position of the fetal head is confirmed to be in the anterior position.

CONCLUSION

Caudal block, preferably as a part of a double-catheter technique, is a valuable method for obstetric analgesia which, when used intelligently and by experienced personnel, adds to the comfort and safety of the mother and fetus.

REFERENCES

1. Abouleish, E.: [Correspondence] The inadvertent continuous spinal continued. Br. J. Anaesth., *46*:628, 1974.
2. ——: Evaluation of a tapered spinal needle. Anesth. Analg., *53*:258, 1974.
3. ——: Caudal analgesia for quadruplet delivery. Anesth. Analg., *55*:61, 1976.
4. ——: Foetal bradycardia during caudal analgesia: a discussion of possible causative factors. Br. J. Anaesth., *48*:481, 1976.
5. Adams, J. Q.: Management of the pregnant cardiac patient. Clin. Obstet. Gynecol., *11*:910, 1968.
6. Arens, J. F.: Epidural and caudal anesthesia for complicated obstetrics. South. Med. J., *63*:44, 1970.
7. Asling, H., and Fung, D. L.: Epidural anesthesia in Eisenmenger's syndrome: a case report. Anesth. Analg., *53*:965, 1974.
8. Asling, H., et al.: Paracervical block anesthesia in obstetrics. II. Etiology of fetal bradycardia following paracervical block anesthesia. Am. J. Obstet. Gynecol., *107*:626, 1970.
9. Baker, A. S., et al.: Spinal epidural abscess. N. Engl. J. Med., *293*:463, 1975.
10. Beechman, J. B., Watson, W. J., and Clapp, J. F.: III Eclampsia preeclampsia and disseminated intravascular coagulation. Obstet. Gynecol., *43*:576, 1975.
11. Boehm, F. H., Woodruff, L. F., Jr., and Growdon, J. H., Jr.: The effect of epidural anesthesia on fetal heart rate baseline variability. Anesth. Analg., *54*:779, 1975.
12. Bonica, J. J.: Principles and Practice of Obstetric Analgesia and Anesthesia. Vol. 1, p. 579. Philadelphia, F. A. Davis, 1967.
13. ——: Anesthesia in the pregnant cardiac patient. Clin. Obstet. Gynecol., *11*:940, 1969.
14. Bowen-Simpkins, P., and Fergusson, I. L. C.: Lumbar epidural block and the breech presentation. Br. J. Anaesth., *46*:420, 1974.
15. Boyson, W. A., and Simpson, J. W.: Breech man-

agement with caudal anesthesia. Am. J. Obstet. Gynecol., *79*:1121, 1960.

16. Bromage, P. R.: Spinal Epidural Analgesia. Edinburgh, E. & S. Livingstone, 1954.

17. ———: Spread of analgesia solutions in the epidural space and their site of action: a statistical study. Br. J. Anaesth., *34*:161, 1962.

18. ———: Aging and epidural dose requirements: segmental spread and predictability of epidural analgesia in youth and extreme age. Br. J. Anaesth., *41*:1016, 1969.

19. ———: Lower limb reflexes changes in segmental epidural analgesia. Br. J. Anaesth., *46*:504, 1974.

19a. ———: Mechanism of action of extradural analgesia. Br. J. Anaesth., *47*:199, 1975.

19b. Brotanek, V., *et al.*: The influence of epidural anesthesia on uterine blood flow. Obstet. Gynecol., *42*:276, 1973.

20. Burn, J. M., Guyer, P. B., and Langdon, L.: The spread of solutions injected into the epidural space: a study of using epidurograms in patients with the lumbosciatic syndrome. Br. J. Anaesth., *45*:338, 1973.

21. Bush, R. C.: Cuadal analgesia for vaginal delivery. II. Analysis of complications. Anesthesiology, *20*:186, 1959.

22. Caseby, N. G.: Epidural analgesia for the surgical induction of labour. Br. J. Anaesth., *46*:747, 1974.

23. Cathelin, F.: A new route of spinal injection: a method for epidural injections by way of the sacral canal; application to man. C. R. Soc. Biol. (Paris), *53*:452, 1901.

24. Chun, L., and Karp, M.: Unusual complications from placement of catheters in caudal canal in obstetrical anesthesia. Case report. Anesthesiology, *27*:96, 1966.

25. Cohen, E. N.: Distribution of local anesthetic agents in the neuraxis of the dog. Anesthesiology, *29*:1002, 1968.

26. Corbin, K. B., and Gardner, E. D.: Decrease in number of myelinated fibers in human spinal roots with age. Anat. Rec., *68*:63, 1937.

27. Crawford, J.: Principles and Practice of Obstetric Anaesthesia. Ed. 3. Oxford, Blackwell Scientific Publications, 1972.

28. ———: The strange case of the (inadvertent) continuous spinal. [Letter] Br. J. Anaesth., *46*:82, 1974.

29. ———: Pathology in the extradural space. Br. J. Anaesth., *47*:412, 1975.

30. ———: Patient management during extradural anaesthesia for obstetrics. Br. J. Anaesth., *47*:273, 1975.

31. Crawford, J. A., Mills, W. G., and Pentecost, B. L.: A pregnant patient with Eisenmenger's syndrome. Case report. Br. J. Anaesth., *43*:1091, 1971.

32. Cunningham, N. L., and Kaplan, J. A.: A rapid onset, long-acting regional anesthetic technique. Anesthesiology, *41*:509, 1974.

33. Dawkins, C. J.: An analysis of the complications of extradural and caudal block. Anaesthesia, *24*:554, 1969.

34. DiGiovanni, A. J.: Inadvertent intraosseous injection—a hazard of caudal anesthesia. Anesthesiology, *34*:92, 1971.

35. Eckstein, K. L., and Marx, G. F.: Aortocaval compression and uterine displacement. Anesthesiology, *40*:92, 1974.

36. Eckstein, K. L., Oberlander, S. G., and Marx, G. F.: Uterine rupture during extradural blockade. Can. Anaesth. Soc. J. *20*:566, 1973.

37. Ellis, H., and McLarty, M.: Anatomy for Anaesthetists. P. 114. Philadelphia, F. A. Davis, 1963.

38. Finster, M., *et al.*: Accidental intoxication of the fetus with local anesthetic drug during caudal anesthesia. Am. J. Obstet. Gynecol., *92*:922, 1965.

39. Fox, L. P., Weller, W. J., and Wilder, H.: Obstetrical caudal anesthesia in a community hospital: a satisfactory plan. West. J. Med., *120*:189, 1974.

40. Galindo, A., *et al.*: Quality of spinal anaesthesia: the influence of spinal nerve root diameter. Br. J. Anaesth., *47*:41, 1975.

41. Gillies, I. D., and Morgan, M.: Accidental total spinal analgesia with bupivacaine. Anaesthesia, *28*:441, 1973.

42. Gunther, R. E., and Harer, W. B., Jr.: Single injection caudal anesthesia: report on 531 deliveries with 1.5 percent mepivacaine. Am. J. Obstet. Gynecol., *92*:305, 1965.

43. Hargrove, L.: Discussion. *In* Crawford, J. S.: Patient management during extradural anesthesia for obstetrics. Br. J. Anaesth., *47*:273, 1975.

44. Hehre, F. W., Yules, R. B., and Hipona, F. A.: Continuous lumbar peridural anesthesia in obstetrics. III: Attempts to produce spread of contrast media by acute vena cava obstruction in dogs. Anesth. Analg., *45*:551, 1966.

45. Hingson, R. A.: Anesthesia for obstetric delivery and for operations on and through the perineum. J. Int. Coll. Surg., *40*:37, 1963.

46. ———: Obstetrics and anesthesiology, Anesthesiology, *26*:378, 1965.

47. Hingson, R. A., and Edwards, W. B.: Continuous caudal anesthesia during labor and delivery. Anesth. Analg., *21*:301, 1942.

48. ———: Continuous caudal analgesia: an analysis of the first ten thousand confinements thus managed with the report of the author's first thousand cases. J.A.M.A., *123*:538, 1943.

49. Johnson, T., and Clayton, C. G.: Studies in placental action during prolonged and dysfunctional labours using radioactive sodium. J. Obstet. Gynecol. Br. Commonw., *62*:513, 1955.

50. Kennedy, W. F., *et al.*: Cardiorespiratory effects of epinephrine when used in regional anaesthesia. Acta Anaesthesiol. Scand. [Suppl.], *23*:320, 1966.

51. Kim, Y., Mazza, N. M., and Marx, G. F.: Massive spinal block with hemicranial palsy after a "test dose" for extradural analgesia. Anesthesiology, *43*:370, 1975.

52. Klaus, M. H., and Kennell, J. H.: Maternal-Infant Bonding. St. Louis, C. V. Mosby, 1976.

53. Klink, E. W.: Perineal nerve block. Anatomical and clinical study in the female. Obstet. Gynecol., *1*:137, 1953.

54. Lenson, G., and Shnider, S. M.: Placental trans-

fer of local anesthetics: clinical implications. *In* Marx, G.: Parturition and Perinatology. P. 177. Philadelphia, F. A. Davis, 1973.

55. Lund, P. C.: Peridural Analgesia and Anesthesia. Springfield, Ill., Charles C Thomas, 1966.

56. McDonald, J. S., Bjorkman, L. L., and Reed, E. C.: Epidural analgesia for obstetrics: a maternal, fetal and a neonatal study. Am. J. Obstet. Gynecol., *120*:1055, 1974.

57. McFee, J. G., *et al.*: Multiple gestations of high fetal number. Obstet. Gynecol., *44*:99, 1974.

58. McGown, R. G.: Accidental marrow sampling during caudal anaesthesia. Br. J. Anaesth., *44*:613, 1972.

59. Macintosh, R. R., and Mushin, W. W.: Observations on the epidural space. Anaesthesia, *2*:100, 1947.

60. Marx, G. L.: Personal communication.

61. Mather, L. E., Long, G. J., and Thomas, J.: The intravenous toxicity and clearance of bupivacaine in man. Clin. Pharmacol. Ther., *12*:935, 1971.

62. Meehan, F. P., Moolgaoker, A. S., and Stallworthy, J.: Vaginal delivery under caudal analgesia after caesarean section and other major uterine surgery. Br. Med. J., *2*:740, 1972.

63. Metcalfe, J.: Rheumatic heart disease in pregnancy. Clin. Obstet. Gynecol., *11*:1010, 1968.

64. Moore, D. C.: Caudal anesthesia in obstetrics. N. Engl. J. Med., *274*:749, 1966.

65. Moore, D. C.: *et al.*: Bupivacaine. A review of 2077 cases. J.A.M.A., *214*:713, 1970.

66. ———:Caudal and epidural blocks with bupivacaine for childbirth. Report of 657 parturients. Obstet. Gynecol., *37*:667, 1971.

67. Moya, F., and Thorndike, V.: The effects of drugs used in labor on the fetus and newborn. Clin. Pharmacol. Ther., *4*:628, 1963.

68. Munson, E. S., *et al.*: Etidocaine, bupivacaine and lidocaine seizure thresholds in monkeys. Anesthesiology, *42*:471, 1975.

69. Myers, R. E.: Maternal psychological stress and fetal asphyxia: a study in the monkey. Am. J. Obstet. Gynecol., *122*:47, 1975.

70. Nellermoe, C. W., *et al.*: A clinical appraisal of 2-chloroprocaine in continuous caudal obstetrical anesthesia. Anesthesiology, *21*:269, 1960.

71. Niswonger, J. W., and Langmade, C. F.: Cardiovascular changes in vaginal deliveries and cesarean sections. Am. J. Obstet. Gynecol., *107*:337, 1970.

72. Nyirjesy, I., *et al.*: Hazards of the use of paracervical block anesthesia in obstetrics. Am. J. Obstet. Gynecol., *87*:231, 1963.

73. Owens, W. D., *et al.*: A new technique of caudal anesthesia. Anesthesiology, *39*:451, 1973.

74. Pearson, J. F., and Davies, P.: The effect of continuous lumbar epidural analgesia on maternal acid-base balance and arterial lactate concentration during the second stage of labour. J. Obstet. Gynecol. Br. Commonw., *80*:225, 1973.

75. ———:The effect of continuous lumbar epidural analgesia on the acid-base status of maternal arterial blood during the first stage of labour. J. Obstet. Gynaecol. Br. Commonw., *80*:218, 1973.

76. Petrie, R. H., *et al.*: Placental transfer of lidocaine following paracervical block. Am. J. Obetet. Gynecol., *120*:791, 1974.

77. Rausen, A. R., Seki, M., and Strauss, L.: Twin transfusion syndrome. A review of 19 cases studied at one institution. J. Pediatr., *66*:613, 1965.

78. Reynolds, F.: The influence of adrenaline on maternal and neonatal blood levels of local analgesic drugs. Pp. 31–40. Proceedings of the Symposium on Epidural Analgesia in Obstetrics. Kingston Hospital, Kingston-upon-Thames, March 18, 1971.

79. Reynolds, F., and Taylor, G.: Maternal and neonatal concentrations of bupivacaine. A comparison with lignocacne during continuous extradural analgesia. Anaesthesia, *25*:14, 1970.

80. Rosefield, C. R., Barton, M. D., and Meochia, G.: Circulatory effects of epinephrine in the pregnant ewe. Am. J. Obstet. Gynecol., *124*:156, 1976.

81. Rosefsky, J. B., and Petersiel, M. E.: Perinatal deaths associated with mepivacaine paracervical block anesthesia in labor. N. Engl. J. Med., *278*:530, 1968.

82. Scanlon, J. W., Brown, W. N., and Ostheimer, G. W.: Neurobehavioral response of newborns after maternal epidural anesthesia with bupivacaine. Anesthesiology, *45*:400, 1976.

83. Shantha, T. R., and Evans, J. A.: The relationship of epidural anesthesia to neural membranes and arachnoid villi. Anesthesiology, *37*:543, 1972.

84. Shnider, S. M., *et al.*: Paracervical block anesthesia in obstetrics. 1. Fetal complication and neonatal morbidity. Am. J. Obstet. Gynecol., *107*:619, 1970.

85. Sicard, A.: Les injections medicamenteuses extratdurales par voie sacrococcygienne. C. R. Soc. Biol. (Paris), *53*:396, 1901.

86. Sicard, A., and Forestier, J.: Roentgenolig exploration of the central nervous system with iodized oil (Lipiodol). Arch. Neurol. Psychiat., *16*:420, 1926.

87. Sinclair, J. C., *et al.*:Intoxication of the fetus by a local anesthetic. An newly recognized complication of maternal caudal anesthesia. N. Engl. J. Med., *273*:1173, 1965.

88. Stoeckel, D.: Sakrale anasthesia. Zentralbl., Gynaekol., *33*:3, 1909.

89. Thalme, B., Raabe, N., and Belfrage, P.: Lumbar epidural analgesia in labour. II. Effects on glucose, lactate, sodium, chloride, total protein, haematocrit and haemoglobin in maternal, fetal and neonatal blood. Acta Obstet. Gynecol. Scand., *53*:113, 1974.

90. Thalme, B., Belfrage, P., and Raabe, N.: Lumbar epidural analgesia in labour. Acta Obstet. Gynecol. Scand., *53*:27, 1974.

91. Trotter, M., and Letterman, G. S.: Variations of the female sacrum; their significance in continuous caudal anesthesia. Surg. Gynecol. Obstet., *78*:419, 1944.

92. Truex, R. C., and Carpenter, M. B.: Human Neuroanatomy. Ed. 6, p. 221, Baltimore, Williams & Wilkins, 1969.

93. Turner, H. B., and Houck, C. R.: Renal hemodynamics in the toxemias of pregnancy. Alterations of kidney function by regional nerve block. Am. J. Obstet. Gynecol., *60*:126, 1950.

94. Ueland, K., and Hansen, J. M.: Maternal cardiovascular dynamics: III. Labor and delivery under local and caudal analgesia. Am. J. Obstet. Gynecol., *103*:8, 1969.

94a. Ueland, K., *et al.*: Maternal cardiovascular dynamics. VI. Cesarean section under epidural anesthesia without epinephrine. Am. J. Obstet. Gynecol., *114*:775, 1972.

95. Urban, B. J.: Clinical observations suggesting a changing site of action during induction and recession of spinal and epidural anesthesia. Anesthesiology, *39*:496, 1973.

96. Usubiaga, J. E., Reis, A., and Usubiaga, L. E.: Epidural misplacement of catheters and mechanisms of unilateral blockade. Anesthesiology, *32*:158, 1970.

97. Usubiaga, J. R., *et al.*: Effect of saline injections on epidural and subarachnoid space pressures and relation to postspinal anesthesia headache. Anesth. Analg., *46*:293, 1967.

98. Villa, E. A., and Marx, G. F.: Chloroprocaine-bupivacaine sequence for obstetric extradural analgesia. Can. Anaesth. Soc. J., *22*:76, 1975.

14

Epidural Analgesia

Ezzat Abouleish, M.D.

DEFINITION

Epidural analgesia is that form of vertebral block produced by injecting a local anesthetic drug into the lumbar epidural space. The terms lumbar epidural, peridural, extradural, and spinal epidural are all synonymous.

HISTORY

In 1885, Corning produced the first epidural block. In an attempt to anesthetize the spinal cord, he injected cocaine between the spinous processes of dogs which resulted in anesthesia of their hind legs. In 1921, an epidural block was used clinically for surgery by Pages. In 1931, a catheter placed through a needle into the epidural space was first used in obstetrics by Aburel. It is through the efforts of pioneers like Dogliotti, Hingson, Cleland, Bromage, Moore, Bonica, Lund, Crawford, and other anesthesiologists and obstetricians that the epidural technique has become an established, well-refined, and splendid method of pain relief in obstetrics.

ANATOMY AND PHYSIOLOGY RELATIVE TO EPIDURAL ANALGESIA

BORDERS OF THE EPIDURAL SPACE

At the base of the skull, the two layers of the cranial dura mater fuse with each other as well as with the outer periosteal layer of the skull. Then the inner layer of the cranial dura extends caudad as the spinal dura mater. The spinal epidural space extends from the foramen magnum down to the sacral hiatus where it ends at the posterior sacrococygeal ligament. Thus the cranial and vertebral subarachnoid spaces are continuous while the epidural spaces are separate. Therefore, if the cranial nerves are paralyzed following an attempted lumbar epidural block, the dura must have been inadvertently punctured and the drug must have been injected into the subarachnoid space. Anteriorly, the epidural space is limited by the posterior longitudinal ligament covering the bodies of the vertebrae and intervertebral disks (Figs. 14-1 and 14-2). Posteriorly, it is bordered by the ligamentum flavum and the vertebral laminae. The ligamentum flavum is a thick ligament which is rich in elastic fibers, hence its name the yellow ligament. It extends from the inner surface of the lamina above to the outer surface of the lamina below, and is thickest in the midline, about 5 mm., and thinnest laterally, about 2 mm. (Fig. 14-1). *The ligamentum flavum is the most important landmark for identifying the epidural space* because as the ligamentum flavum is pierced and the epidural space is entered a sudden loss of resistance, a "snap," is felt and air or fluid can be easily injected. Laterally, the epidural space is connected to the paravertebral spaces by the intervertebral foramina through which

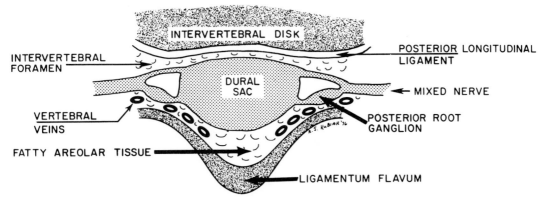

Fig. 14-1. Diagrammatic cross section of the vertebral canal showing the contents of the epidural space. **Note:** 1. The ligamentum flavum is thickest in the midline. 2. The epidural space is widest in the midline. 3. The nerves and blood vessels are in the anterolateral part of the epidural space.

segmental nerves and blood vessels traverse. The epidural space is widest posteriorly, being about 5 mm. in diameter, while it is shallow laterally. Therefore, if the epidural needle crosses the ligamentum flavum laterally, the epidural space is less easily identified owing to the thinness of the ligament in its lateral part. Then, if the needle is further advanced for a short distance, the dura is easily punctured owing to the shallowness of the epidural space in its peripheral portion.

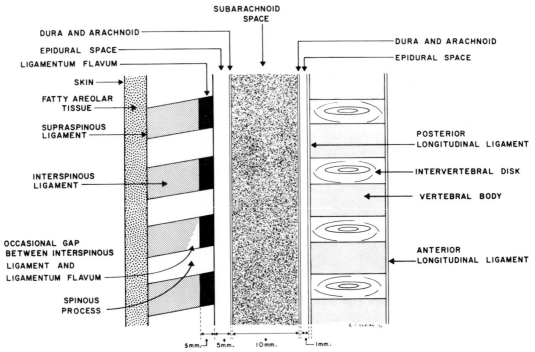

Fig. 14-2. Diagrammatic sagittal section of the back at the lumbar region. Notice, the structures that have to be traversed by the needle from skin to epidural space; the slightly caudad direction of the spinous processes; the thickness of the ligamentum flavum and the diameters of the epidural and subarachnoid spaces; and the occasional gap between the interspinous ligament and ligamentum flavum.

The median approach is the safest and the easiest way to identify the epidural space in the lumbar region.

CONTENTS OF THE EPIDURAL SPACE

The epidural space surrounds the dural sac and contains the following structures:

The Anterior and Posterior Nerve Roots With Their Covering Sheaths

The nerves unite together at the corresponding intervertebral foramina to form the segmental nerves which pass laterally outside the vertebral column. The union of the nerve roots in the epidural space makes them less movable and more liable to trauma by the needle or catheter than in the subarachnoid space. Therefore, if during continuous epidural the tip of the needle lies in the lateral part of the epidural space, the introduction of the catheter may be difficult or impossible because the catheter tip impinges on the nerve root, and the patient may feel paresthesia. This is one more reason why it is better to puncture the ligamentum flavum in the midline.

Blood Vessels

Arteries. The arterial blood supply of the spinal cord consists of:

The Radicular Arteries. These arteries arise from the aorta or its branches. On their way to the spinal cord they accompany the posterior and anterior nerve roots. They supply the lateral parts of the spinal cord.

The Anterior Spinal Artery. This artery arises from the two vertebral arteries at the foramen magnum and descends down the spinal cord in the midline. It supplies the anterior part of the spinal cord.

The Two Posterior Spinal Arteries. These arteries arise from the vertebral arteries at the side of the medulla oblongata and descend down the spinal cord at the junction of the posterior roots with the spinal cord. They supply the posterior column.[113]

The radicular arteries are the only arteries that cross the epidural space. However, a space-occupying lesion in the epidural space, such as a hematoma or abscess, can compress the spinal cord and cause enough ischemia to produce paralysis.

Veins. The vertebral veins drain the vertebral column and the nervous tissue, and form the vertebral venous plexus. They are present mainly in the anterolateral part of the epidural space. This venous plexus is a primitive valveless system, easily distensible and thin-walled. The vertebral veins communicate cephalad with the cranial veins, caudad with the pelvic veins, and laterally with the pelvic, abdominal, and thoracic veins. They form an anastomosis between the inferior and superior vena cavae. In the nonpregnant state, 10 per cent of the cardiac output passes through them.[21] During pregnancy, the gravid uterus compresses the inferior vena cava and obstructs the flow through it. Therefore, blood is shunted through the vertebral veins to the superior vena cava, leading to marked distention of these veins. The changes in this venous plexus during pregnancy have tremendous clinical effects which influence and modify vertebral blocks:

1. *The dose of the local anesthetic is reduced.* A large portion of the spinal canal becomes occupied by the distended vertebral veins, leading to shrinkage of the cerebrospinal fluid volume. Therefore, for a subarachnoid block, a patient at term requires one-third less of the anesthetic drug than in the nonpregnant state. During an epidural block, escape of the local anesthetic through the intervertebral foramina is reduced due to distention of these veins. Therefore, the solution spreads more longitudinally than laterally, leading to a more extensive block. Also, the distention of these veins limits the potential space available for the local anesthetic, thus causing more spread of the epidural block.

2. *The technique for epidural analgesia has*

to be modified. The negative epidural pressure in the lumbar region becomes positive owing to the distention of the vertebral veins.[48] Therefore, in obstetrics, signs depending on the negative pressure as a method of identifying the epidural space are unreliable (e.g., the hanging-drop technique).

3. A vertebral block becomes a more delicate procedure. The dilated thin veins can be easily traumatized by an epidural or a spinal needle, or even by a soft epidural catheter. Injury to these veins leads to a breach in the circulation, with a subsequent higher rate of access of the local anesthetic into the bloodstream, hence increasing toxicity and diminishing the duration of analgesia. Furthermore, an epidural catheter can easily enter one of these veins, causing subsequent convulsions in the patient if a large dose of the local anesthetic drug is injected. These are some of the reasons why the midline should be adhered to during insertion of the epidural needle, and the stylet should be removed from the catheter before its advancement into the epidural space.

Fatty Areolar Tissue

This tissue lies between the nervous and vascular structures in the form of loculi. Lipid-soluble local anesthetics are stored in the fatty tissue of the epidural space, forming a reservoir adjacent to the nerves and thus prolonging the duration of the block. If after penetrating the ligamentum flavum the tip of the needle is introduced into one of these loculi, injection of air leads to distention of this loculus, and thus the plunger of the syringe bounces when pressure on it is released. A novice in epidural technique may think that the tip of the needle is still in the ligaments, and may advance the needle further, with subsequent inadvertent dural puncture. This mistake can be avoided if the following are kept in mind: (1) the needle is kept in the midline where the ligamentum flavum is thickest and the sudden change of

pressure is quite evident; (2) the operator's feeling of injection of air into the loculus is different from that of injection into the ligaments of the back, the injection being met with minimal resistance in the former situation; (3) the bouncing of the plunger when the tip of the needle is in such a loculus is slow and gentle whereas it is fast and abrupt if air is injected into the ligaments; and (4) the injection of a few milliliters of fluid into the epidural space is met with almost no resistance, whereas if injected into the back ligaments, the pressure rapidly builds up and much resistance is encountered.

PRESSURE IN THE EPIDURAL SPACE

The epidural space pressure is usually subatmospheric, especially in the thoracic and cervical regions. The possible causes of this negative pressure are:

1. *Tenting of the Dura.* In 1926 Janzen was the first to observe that the epidural pressure is negative. He thought the pressure change was due to indentation of the dura by the advancing needle.

2. *Difference in Growth Between the Vertebral Column and the Spinal Cord.* In 1928 Heldt and Moloney thought the negative epidural pressure was created by the higher rate of growth of the vertebral column compared with that of the spinal cord.

3. *Flexion of the Back.* In 1936 Odom claimed that acute flexion of the back increases the capacity of the epidural canal, thus causing the negative pressure.

4. *Falling Forward of the Intestines.* As the intestines fall anteriorly, they pull on the mesentery, thus creating a negative pressure in the paravertebral space which is transmitted through the intervertebral foramina to the epidural space.[129]

5. *Transmission of the Negative Intrathoracic Pressure.* In 1947 Macintosh found that the negative epidural pressure is due to the transmission of the negative intrathoracic pressure through the inter-

vertebral foramina. The negative pressure is best recorded in the thoracic portion of the epidural space, and is maximal in the sitting position. This negative pressure is progressively less evident away from the thoracic region especially toward the caudal end of the epidural space.

In nonpregnant patients, the epidural pressure has been found to be negative in 90.2 per cent of cases.[115] At term and during parturition, it changes from negative to positive[48] while the cerebrospinal fluid pressure remains constant.[58,71,74] Displacement of the uterus off the inferior vena cava reduces the positive pressure encountered at term.[48]

Owing to the negative epidural pressure in the thoracic region, local anesthetics injected into the lumbar region spread more readily cephalad than caudad.[24]

Following injection of a fluid into the epidural space, the pressure rise extends to only a few segments and is more manifest in the sitting than in the lying position. The pressure created is directly proportionate to the rate of injection and the volume of the solution injected, and inversely proportionate to the capacity of the epidural space. Therefore, if there is much dripping of fluid from the hub of the needle following injection of a certain volume, this means that the capacity of the epidural space is limited and/or the escape of fluid through the intervertebral foramina is reduced, and subsequently the level of the block will be higher.[115]

THE STRUCTURES BETWEEN THE SKIN AND THE EPIDURAL SPACE (FIG. 14-2)

The structures which have to be transversed by the epidural needle are:

1. The skin
2. The subcutaneous tissue. This is of a variable thickness depending on the amount of fat.
3. The supraspinous ligament. This is a longitudinal ligament covering the spinous processes of the vertebrae.

4. The interspinous ligament. This is the ligament filling the gap between the spinous processes. It usually extends from the tips of the spinous process to the ligamentum flavum. However, the interspinous ligament occasionally stops short of the ligamentum flavum. In this case if the loss of resistance using air is applied to identify the epidural space, the gap between the two ligaments may be mistaken for the epidural space. This can be differentiated by the injection of fluid. Since this gap is localized to one space, resistance rapidly builds up after the injection of a few milliliters of fluid. If the tip of the needle is in the epidural space, the injection of this small volume will not be followed by increased resistance.

5. The ligamentum flavum. This is the last and most important structure the needle pierces before reaching the epidural space.

DETERMINING THE LEVEL OF EPIDURAL BLOCK

Dermatomal Distribution as a Method for Determining the Level of a Block

The part of the skin supplied by each spinal segment is called a dermatome. By identifying the surface area which is anesthetized, the sensory level of the block can be determined. Remember that autonomic blockade extends one to two segments above the sensory level whereas the motor paralysis extends four segments below the sensory level.

Certain points on the body are chosen to help determine the level of a block (Fig. 14-3):

1. *The cheek,* for testing cranial nerve V
2. *Supraclavicular fossa,* for testing C3 and C4. The supraclavicular nerves supply the skin of the shoulder and neck down to and including the first intercostal space.
3. *Lateral side of the upper arm,* for testing C5
4. *Lateral side of the forearm,* for testing C6

Fig. 14-3. Pinprick points for determining analgesia level. *A*. General view. *B*. Detailed view. **Note:** 1. The dermatomal distribution is as follows: face is supplied by trigeminal nerve; neck and upper part of chest to the second intercostal space by cervical nerves; upper limb by lower cervical and T-1; chest and abdomen by thoracic nerves; lower limbs by lumbar except outer part of the foot (S-1); and perineum by sacrals and coccygeal nerve. 2. Only one pinprick site per dermatome is selected to determine whether such a segment is blocked or not. 3. Testing the level of block on the abdomen should be close to the midline owing to the slanting distribution of each dermatome.

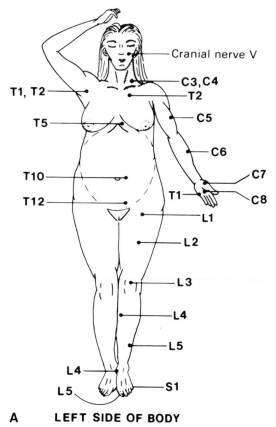

A   LEFT SIDE OF BODY

XIPHISTERNAL JUNCTION

T5
T6
T7
T8
T9
UMBILICUS — T10
T11
T12

LEFT SIDE OF ABDOMEN

B

S2
L1
S2,3,4
S4,5
CO

PERINEUM
(LEFT SIDE)

L5 — S1

SOLE OF LEFT FOOT

T1
C6 — C8
C7

PALM OF LEFT HAND

5. *Palm of the hand,* the lateral side for testing C7, the middle for testing C8, and the medial side for testing T1

6. *The axilla,* for testing T1 and T2

7. *The medial sides of the upper arm, forearm, and hand,* for testing T1

8. *Second intercostal space,* for testing T2

9. *Each subsequent intercostal space,* for testing the corresponding thoracic segment

10. *Xiphisternal junction,* for testing T5

11. *From xiphisternum to umbilicus,* for testing from T5 to T10 segments

12. *From umbilicus to symphysis pelvis,* for testing from T10 to T12 segments

13. *Upper third of the thigh,* for testing L1

14. *Middle third of the thigh,* for testing L2

15. *Patella,* for testing L3

16. *Medial side of the leg and medial malleolus,* for testing L4

17. *Lateral side of the leg and lateral malleolus,* for testing L5

18. *Lateral toes and lateral two-thirds of the sole,* for testing S1

19. *Popliteal fossa and middle of the back of the thigh,* for testing S2

20. *Around the vulva,* for testing S3 and S4

21. *Around the anus,* for testing S4 and S5

22. *Behind the anus,* for testing the coccygeal segment

Method of Choice for Determining the Level of a Block

There are many methods for determining the level of a block, e.g., pinprick, temperature, and others. The commonest and the most practical method is to compare the sensation to pinprick felt in the unblocked part of the body to that in the blocked. The proper way to utilize this method is to follow these rules: *first, determine the normal sensation to pinprick* by applying it to an area far away from the expected block, e.g., for vertebral analgesia in obstetrics, the sensation to pinprick at the tip of the shoulder or the neck is tested. *Second, proceed from the dermatomal level corresponding to the site of injection of the local anesthetic on the dependent side,* e.g., for lumbar epidural start at the middle of the thigh and proceed up, testing the level on the abdomen, then down the lower limb, and lastly the perineum. Ask the patient to report only when the sensation to pinprick is felt to be of the same intensity as that in the control area. *Third, apply pinprick only at certain chosen points.* Since there is some overlap of dermatomes there is no need to prick the patient along each millimeter of her body. Certain points (Fig. 14-3) can be chosen intelligently to provide adequate information about the extent of the block quickly, efficiently, and with minimal discomfort to the patient. *Fourth, follow the same steps on the other side of the body* to determine the extent of the block. *Fifth, record both the upper and lower levels of the block for each side.*

SITE OF ACTION OF LOCAL ANESTHETIC DRUGS FOLLOWING EPIDURAL ANALGESIA

See Chapter 13, Caudal Analgesia.

FACTORS CONTROLLING THE SPREAD OF LOCAL ANESTHETICS INJECTED INTO THE EPIDURAL SPACE

See Chapter 13, Caudal Analgesia.

EFFECT OF EPIDURAL ANALGESIA ON THE COURSE OF LABOR

Epidural analgesia may give the impression of prolonging the course of labor. The main reason for this wrong impression is that epidural analgesia is frequently administered to patients with difficult prolonged labor but not to those with easy labor.

On an individual basis, epidural analgesia may increase, decrease, or cause no change in the uterine activity.[68] On the whole, the first stage of labor is shortened with epidural analgesia, especially in nulliparae.[30,92] On the other hand, the second stage of labor is increased from 46 to 58 minutes in nulliparae, and from 19 to 38 minutes in multiparae.[30] The overall effect of properly administered epidural analgesia on the course of labor is insignificant.[20,23,30,63]

Any depressant effect of epidural analgesia on the course of labor can be due to:

1. *The interruption of the motor fibers supplying the uterus.* The motor fibers to the uterus are the sympathetic efferent fibers arising from T5 to T10 segments. Therefore, if the block extends much higher than the T10 level, interruption of these fibers early in labor can cause depression of uterine contractions. Later on as labor progresses, the intrinsic uterine activity plays a more important role than these nerve fibers, with the result that any depressant effect of epidural analgesia disappears. Accordingly, it has been shown that epidural analgesia may cause uterine depression for 20 to 30 minutes with the initial dose of drug administered. Subsequent injections are devoid of such an effect.[125,126]

2. *Hypotension.* If hypotension occurs with epidural analgesia, the uterine blood flow decreases, causing acute ischemia and subsequent decrease of uterine muscle activity. Correction of the hypotension brings the uterine contractions to the preepidural level.[23,118,119] In practice this is the most important factor; measures to prevent and correct hypotension are essential.

3. *The local anesthetic drug itself.* The amide-type drugs may cause more depression of uterine contractions than the ester-type because the latter are rapidly hydrolyzed.[27] Lidocaine has been found to cause temporary depression of the uterine contractions for 10 to 30 minutes, even after pudendal nerve block.[68,124] This action is only manifest with the first injection. Such a depressant effect may be specific to lidocaine, since another amide, prilocaine, shows much less effect on uterine activity.[68] Since at the present time bupivacaine is widely used for epidural analgesia, its ef-

fect on uterine contractions should be evaluated.

4. *The beta vasopressors.* These drugs are well-known inhibitors of spontaneous and induced uterine activity.[130] Lidocaine with 1:200,000 epinephrine causes significantly more depression of uterine contractions than plain lidocaine.[125] The decrease in the uterine activity is mainly due to depression of the intensity rather than the frequency of uterine contractions.[75] This is one of the reasons for avoiding the use of epinephrine in obstetrics.

5. *Interference with the rotation of the fetal head due to paralysis of the pelvic floor.* This occurs when large doses and high concentrations of the local anesthetic drugs are given in the first stage of labor.

6. *Inability of the mother to bear down during the second stage of labor.* If the perineal reflex is interrupted due to the involvement of the sacral nerves by the epidural block, the patient has no feeling of the perineal pressure associated with the uterine contractions. Therefore, the reflex bearing mechanism is lost. However, she can still push voluntarily if the abdominal muscles are not paralyzed. Therefore, if an experienced nurse is not beside the patient to tell her when a contraction occurs and to encourage her to push, or if the patient has received too much narcotics and/or sedatives rendering her uncooperative, the second stage of labor is prolonged.

In conclusion, although epidural analgesia has a potential depressant effect on the uterine contractions, if properly administered, the effect is insignificant. In cases of dysrhythmic contractions the course of labor may even be shortened (see below, Indications for the Use of Epidural Analgesia).

EFFECT OF EPIDURAL ANALGESIA ON THE UTERINE BLOOD FLOW

At term, the normal uterine blood flow is about 500 to 700 ml./min. (see Chap. 3, The Placenta and Placental Transfer of Drugs at Term).

The uterine blood flow is different from cerebral blood flow in that it is not sensitive to variations in maternal $PaCO_2$ level.[67] However, hypocapnia causes a shift in the maternal oxygen-hemoglobin dissociation curve to the left, umbilical vasoconstriction, and a possible increase in the intraplacental shunting, all leading to fetal hypoxia and acidosis.[67,80]

Increase in maternal PaO_2 does not affect the uterine blood flow. The uterine blood flow is very sensitive to vasoconstrictors and sympathetic stimulation. Normally there is uterine vasodilatation,[52] and vasodilators do not increase normal uterine blood flow. During preeclampsia, there is uterine vasoconstriction and the uterine blood flow is reduced.

The changes in uterine blood flow under epidural analgesia can be due to:

Effect of the block. On the whole, epidural analgesia in humans does not decrease the uterine blood flow.[23] If maternal hypotension occurs, there is a proportionate decrease in uterine blood flow which is corrected by treating the fall in maternal blood pressure. Sometimes, especially in toxemic patients, the uterine blood flow is increased following epidural analgesia.[23] Therefore, if the blood pressure is maintained during epidural analgesia, the uterine blood flow is not adversely affected and may even improve. The uterine blood vessels are very sensitive to catecholamines[97] and sympathetic stimuli.[67] Stressful conditions of the mother can lead to fetal hypoxia.[82] Therefore, by relieving pain, epidural analgesia can have a beneficial effect on the fetus by preventing the possible decrease in the uterine blood flow associated with the stress of labor and delivery.

Effect of epinephrine. Epinephrine used with the local anesthetic not only depresses the uterine contractions, but also reduces the uterine blood flow in the following manner:

1. The mean arterial blood pressure is lower when epinephrine is added to the local anesthetic owing to the decreased total peripheral resistance and lowered diastolic pressure.[13]

2. Even with no change in blood pressure there is redistribution of the cardiac output following administration of epinephrine, resulting in increased muscle blood flow and diminished uterine blood flow.[97]

3. The combination of 1:100,000 epinephrine with 1.5 per cent chloroprocaine for epidural analgesia causes a transient 14 per cent decrease in uterine blood flow as compared with chloroprocaine alone.[120]

Epinephrine does not significantly prolong the duration of action of bupivacaine[95] and has potential harmful effects, such as hypertension and arrhythmias, if inadvertently injected into the circulation. For all these reasons, the use of epinephrine in obstetrics is not recommended.

Effect of the vasopressors (discussed in detail in Chap. 5, Effects of Vertebral Blocks on the Cardiovascular System). In summary, the use of vasopressors to correct maternal hypotension should follow these rules:

1. Vasopressors should only be used if hypotension occurs despite left lateral displacement of the uterus and the rapid administration of 500 to 1,000 ml. of fluid.

2. There is no need for prophylactic administration of vasopressors because they may reduce the uterine blood flow;[93] moreover, they may not be required in the first place.

3. Vasopressors should be intravenously administered as soon as hypotension occurs. If injected intramuscularly, their effect may be too slow and may extend too much into the postpartum period, thus, when combined with ergot preparations, they may cause severe hypertension.[25]

4. Alpha stimulants, such as phenylephrine or metaraminol, cause significant uterine vasoconstriction to negate the effects of increased blood pressure; hence, the uterine blood flow is decreased and

fetal acidosis occurs.[59,107] Beta stimulants, such as ephedrine or mephentermine, raise the blood pressure mainly by increasing the cardiac output, thus improving the uterine blood flow. Therefore, alpha stimulants should not be used unless adequate doses of beta stimulants fail to raise the blood pressure and there is associated marked tachycardia. In such a situation, minute quantities of alpha stimulants lead to marked increase in the blood pressure. Therefore, following administration of a beta stimulant and intravenous fluids, alpha stimulants, if required, should be titrated to reach only the required blood pressure level. A safe method of administering an alpha stimulant under these circumstances is by diluting the drug and giving it in small increments while the blood pressure is almost continuously measured.

Effect of the local anesthetic drug used. Recently much interest in the vasoactivity of the local anesthetic drugs has been expressed. These drugs can directly produce either vasoconstriction or vasodilatation depending on their concentration and type (see Chap. 16, Paracervical Block, and Chap. 4, Local Anesthetic Drugs). Their action on the vasculature is particularly significant when injected into the vicinity of uterine vessels such as with paracervical block. With epidural analgesia the effect would probably be less significant. However, this aspect requires further investigation.

EFFECTS OF EPIDURAL ANALGESIA ON THE FETUS AND NEONATE

Administration of epidural analgesia results in lower lactate concentrations in the parturients and their babies compared with conventional obstetric analgesia.[110] The fetal acidosis seen in "nonepidural" cases may be secondary to the maternal lactacidemia due to hyperventilation and increased catecholamines.[110] The relief of pain by epidural analgesia is responsible for the lower lactate levels in both maternal

and fetal blood during labor and in the first 20 minutes of neonatal life.[110] In the "nonepidural" babies the postnatal lactate rise is higher and it takes about 1 hour for their lactate level to drop to that of the "epidural" babies. This beneficial effect of epidural analgesia on the metabolism of the mother and fetus has also been confirmed by other investigators.[125,126] There is more metabolic acidosis of the mother and fetus in the nonanesthetized group as well as in those having pudendal block than in the epidural group. Therefore, although the second stage of labor may be prolonged with epidural analgesia, the fetus is in a better metabolic condition than the one whose mother has not received epidural analgesia.

Following epidural analgesia the commonest abnormality is a temporary decrease in the fetal heart rate variability which occurs in 20 to 53 per cent of cases.[8,10,54] Its time of onset is early, usually about 10 minutes after administration of the drug, and it lasts for only 10 minutes.[92] There is no correlation of this decrease in fetal heart rate variability with fetal blood level of bupivacaine, fetal blood pH, or maternal blood pressure.[8] It may be due to the initial vasodilatation of the lower limbs following epidural block and corrected by the sympathetic blockade of the uterine blood vessels as the level extends more cephalad.[3]

With epidural analgesia, serious fetal deceleration can occur in about 14 per cent of cases,[125] a figure very similar to the nonanesthetized patients.[104] However, if maternal hypotension occurs, especially when associated with hypertonia due to oxytocin infusion, the incidence may be as high as 40 per cent[104,128] (see also Chap. 13, Caudal Analgesia).

In conclusion, provided no major complications occur, lumbar epidural analgesia is safe for the fetus. Fetal distress following epidural analgesia has almost always been associated with maternal hypotension, supine position, and/or uterine hypertonia. Attention to the prevention and early adequate treatment of these factors are the main safeguards against the fetal stressful effects of epidural analgesia.

Neurobehavior tests are recent complex tests that take into consideration many parameters, such as awake and alert status, response to pinprick, muscle tone, rooting, sucking, Moro's reflex, and responses to light and sound. These tests are more of a research value than the Apgar score. They may prove to be significant in terms of early neonatal adjustments. The development of maternal-infant relationships and the implication, if any, for future growth and development remain to be elucidated. The reader who wishes to know more details on the subject should refer to the articles by J. W. Scanlon *et al.*[101a,102]

The tests have shown that for 8 hours postpartum, babies delivered from mothers having epidural analgesia under lidocaine or mepivacaine are alert but their muscle tone is diminished compared to those delivered under nonepidural techniques. In both groups the Apgar scores are the same and both are discharged from the hospital in good condition.[101a] When bupivacaine instead of lidocaine or mepivacaine is used to produce the epidural analgesia, there is no difference between the babies from the epidural and nonepidural groups.[102] This has been attributed to the decreased fetal transmission of bupivacaine compared to mepivacaine or lidocaine.

EQUIPMENT AND DRUGS USED FOR EPIDURAL ANALGESIA

The main equipment for epidural analgesia is included on the epidural tray which is usually sterilized by autoclaving. Disposable trays may be used if the number of epidural blocks performed at the institution is small. Whether the tray is prepared and sterilized in the hospital or commercially, it should contain a sterilization indicator which should be checked before the technique is started. The tray (Fig. 14-4) contains: one Tuohy needle; two 5-ml. syringes, one 10-ml. syringe, and one 20-ml. syringe; two 24-gauge needles, two 19-gauge needles, and one 16-gauge needle; 2 metal cups, one for the local anesthetic and the other for the degerming solution; 4 × 4 swabs; a sponge forceps; and 4 towels; all placed on a metal tray.

A preautoclaved bupivacaine vial or ampule is added to the tray. In case chloroprocaine is to be used, the vial cannot be autoclaved; therefore, an assistant helps the operator to empty the contents of the vial into the metal cup without contamination. In case of continuous epidural block, a disposable Teflon, 20-gauge 91.5-cm. catheter is added to the tray (Fig. 14-4).

Bupivacaine, 0.5 per cent, is used during the first stage of labor because of its prolonged duration of action, superb analgesic property, and minimal effect on the fetus. For the second stage of labor, 2 per cent chloroprocaine is used because of its rapid onset and short duration, thus minimizing the mother's period of stay in the recovery room and reducing the need for urinary catheterization with subsequent danger of infection. For cesarean section, 0.75 per cent bupivacaine is our drug of choice because of its good analgesic property, adequate muscular relaxation, and prolonged action. (For more details see Chap. 4, Local Anesthetic Drugs, and Chap. 13, Caudal Analgesia.)

For skin preparation, it was found that Zephiran tincture (1:750 benzalkonium chloride in 50% alcohol) was inferior to Prepodyne; therefore, the use of Zephiran for skin preparation should be discontinued.[3] Thus, the patient's skin should be prepared using an organic iodine compound such as 1 per cent Prepodyne or Betadine solution. They are water-soluble

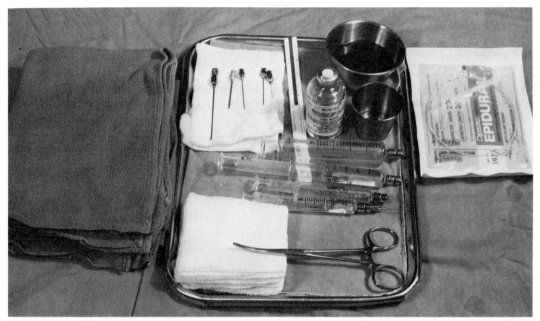

Fig. 14-4. Continuous epidural analgesia tray, showing sterilization indicator strip, a 5-ml. syringe containing local anesthetic for skin infiltration, a 5-ml. glass syringe for identifying the epidural space, 10-ml. and 20-ml. syringes for drug administration, a 17-gauge Tuohy needle, a 15-gauge needle for skin puncture, other needles for withdrawing the drug, the vial of local anesthetic, metal cup for local anesthetic, metal cup for degerming solution, sponge forceps, epidural catheter, sponges, and 4 towels.

and effective against gram-negative, gram-positive, aerobic and anaerobic organisms, fungi, yeast, and tubercle bacilli. Most of the organisms are killed within 30 seconds of contact with the solution.[116] There is no need to use the tincture, thus avoiding irritation of the vaginal or anal mucosa. The allergic and toxic reactions to the organic forms of iodine are much less in comparison to the inorganic iodine.[28]

Facilities for cardiovascular resuscitation should be available for immediate use. This includes oxygen, bag and mask, endotracheal tube, laryngoscope, suction machine and catheters, succinylcholine, diazepam, and vasopressors such as ephedrine, mephentermine, and epinephrine. All should be in good working condition. A cart having all these necessary drugs and equipment can be rolled into the patient's room before starting the block.

TECHNIQUES

Trainees in anesthesiology should be taught the epidural technique on suitable cases in the operating room; then when considered competent, they are allowed to perform epidurals in obstetrics under supervision. *Epidural analgesia is more difficult in a parturient* because of the uterine pains rendering the patient less cooperative, the inability to flex the back optimally owing to the gravid uterus, the softness of the ligaments, and the tendency for edema or fat in the lumbar region.

Epidural technique can be for either vaginal delivery or cesarean section, and in each situation it can be either single-dose or continuous. One rule applies to all: *do not use force,* whether inserting the epidural needle or the catheter. *To achieve a successful safe epidural block, meticulous attention to details is required.*

EPIDURAL ANALGESIA FOR VAGINAL DELIVERY

Single-Dose Epidural Block

There are many techniques for performing an epidural block. The technique to be described is not the only one, but reflects the author's preference and has proven to be simple and efficient.

Timing. Single-dose epidural is performed when delivery is expected within 30 minutes. It is usually performed in the delivery room. This is important because it is inadvisable to move the patient from the labor suite to the delivery room while the block is not yet fixed; otherwise, hypotension may occur unnoticed during transportation, with serious sequelae to the mother and/or fetus.

Explanation of the Technique to the Patient. The patient has usually been interviewed during the third trimester or when first admitted to the labor suite. Her height, weight, past medical history, and experiences with anesthesia or analgesia for previous deliveries or operations have been recorded. The purpose of the block, the steps of the procedure, the expected position of the patient, the importance of her cooperation, and the changes in her sensorium following the block are all explained to her. This step is important because it establishes good rapport between the anesthesiologist and the patient, a milestone in achieving cooperation and pain relief.

Intravenous Fluid Administration. An intravenous cannula is inserted into a vein in the upper limb and securely taped (Fig. 14-5). The fluid administered depends on the condition of the patient; usually 5 per cent dextrose in water, with or without salts solution e.g. lactated Ringer's solution, is satisfactory. Dehydration and metabolic acidosis can result from strenuous labor. *It is our advice that every patient admitted to the labor suite should have fluids through an intravenous cannula whether she is going to have anesthesia or not.* This is important not only to prevent dehydration and metabolic acidosis, but also to administer drugs if required, e.g., oxytocics, and to combat any sudden complication during the course of parturition, e.g., hemorrhage or amniotic fluid embolism.

Maternal and Fetal Monitoring. The patient's pulse and blood pressure are measured (Fig. 14-5).

Monitoring of the uterine contractions and fetal heart rate before and during epidural analgesia is an important advance in the technique because of the following:

1. Epidural analgesia usually gives the impression that it slows labor because the patient gradually feels less pain and ultimately she may become unaware of the contractions. If she is obese, it may be difficult or impossible to palpate these contractions. Identifying the beginning and end of each of the uterine contractions is important for the timing of the bearing down during the second stage. Moreover any diminution in the intensity and/or frequency of uterine contractions can be accurately detected and thus corrected by oxytocin.

2. The fetal heart rate pattern before epidural analgesia should be obtained. Any change in the form of fetal distress can be accurately identified and adequately corrected by the help of the continuous fetal monitor. Oxytocin to improve uterine contractions can be safely used and regulated; any deleterious effect on the fetus secondary to the drug can be diagnosed early and corrected.

Positioning the Patient. The patient is positioned either in the lateral or the sitting position. The author prefers the lateral position because it is more comfortable for the patient. However, in case of difficulty, *the sitting position* is better because in this position the median furrow of the back coincides with the vertebral spines, whereas in the lateral position the furrow sags due to gravity toward the dependent side. Moreover, in the sitting position there is better flexion of the back if the

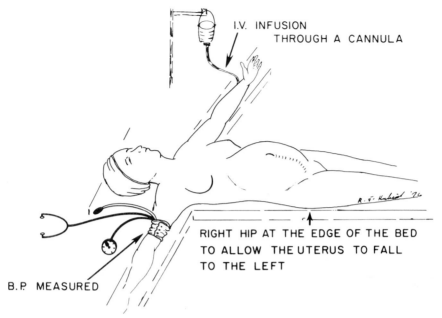

I.V. INFUSION
THROUGH A CANNULA

RIGHT HIP AT THE EDGE OF THE BED
TO ALLOW THE UTERUS TO FALL
TO THE LEFT

B.P. MEASURED

Fig. 14-5. Blood pressure measurement and intravenous fluid administration before performing the epidural technique.

shoulders are allowed to drop, the lower limbs are bent so that the knees are further apart while the feet just cross ("Indian position"), and the head is flexed. Both shoulders should be at the same level and the patient is asked to arch her back like "an angry cat" or "letter C." This widens the interlaminar space and makes the technique easier. An assistant holds the patient to prevent sudden movement. Better relaxation of the extensor muscles of the back, thus better flexion, is obtained if the patient voluntarily assumes and maintains the position. In *the lateral position* the patient lies in the left lateral position if the operator is right-handed. The patient's shoulders and pelvis are brought to the edge of the bed. Both the shoulders and the pelvis are parallel to each other and perpendicular to the bed. Especially if the bed is sagging, there is usually a tendency for the patient to fall forward, which can be prevented by placing a folded towel or a small pillow under the flexed knees. If the independent shoulder falls forward while the pelvis is perpendicular to the bed,

twisting of the back occurs at the lumbar region, thus tending to close the interlaminar space and rendering epidural puncture either difficult or impossible. A pillow under the head makes it easier to achieve the optimum position of the shoulders (Fig. 14-6A). The knees are voluntarily brought as far as possible toward the chin and the patient's back is arched. An assistant helps to maintain the patient in position throughout the procedure. Remember that without proper positioning, epidural analgesia can be difficult, even impossible, to perform.

Feeling the Landmarks. A line joining the highest levels of the iliac crests usually crosses the fourth lumbar vertebra (Fig. 14-6A). If the spinous processes are not felt, the technique is contraindicated.

Preparing the Epidural Tray. The operator, wearing a mask, opens the tray, then puts on sterile gloves and prepares the contents. The anesthetic solution is poured into the special cup and is used to thoroughly lubricate all the syringes. One 5-ml. syringe is filled with the local anes-

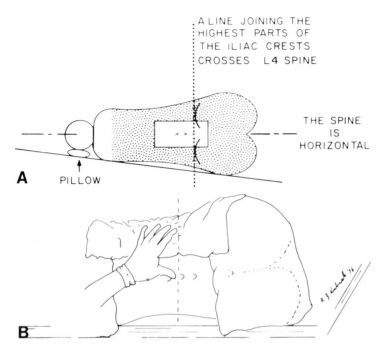

A LINE JOINING THE HIGHEST PARTS OF THE ILIAC CRESTS CROSSES L4 SPINE

THE SPINE IS HORIZONTAL

A   PILLOW

B

Fig. 14-6. *A.* Positioning of the patient and selecting the interspace for epidural puncture. **Note:** 1. A pillow is placed under the patient's head. 2. Although the head of the bed or table is slightly elevated, the vertebral column is horizontal because the female pelvis is wider than her shoulders. 3. The shoulders and pelvis are perpendicular to the edge of the bed or table. *B.* Choosing the L3 to L4 interspace. The index finger is positioned on the highest part of the iliac crest and the thumb is placed on the third lumbar spine.

thetic; the other one is filled with 3 ml. of air for identifying the epidural space (Fig. 14-4). The 10-ml. syringe is filled with the local anesthetic for the test and the therapeutic doses. The degerming solution (1% Prepodyne or Betadine) is poured into the other cup. One should make sure that the degerming solution is not spilled, contaminating the local anesthetic, needles, or syringes, since these antiseptic solutions are neurotoxic and can cause nerve damage if they reach the epidural space.

Preparing the Patient's Back. Using the degerming solution, the patient's back is widely prepared twice and the excess is removed, especially from the area of injection.

Draping. The area of the lumbar region is isolated from the rest of the body by using the sterile towels. The patient's shoulders are kept exposed to make sure that they remain parallel during the procedure (Fig. 14-6A).

Choosing the Interspace. The highest part of the iliac crest is felt with the fingers of the left hand while the thumb palpates

the fourth lumbar spine. To ensure adequate perineal analgesia at the expected time, the L3 to L4 interspace or preferably L4 to L5 interspace is chosen. The thumb of the left hand is placed in the interspace in contact with the limiting cephalad spine (Fig. 14-6B). The proposed needle entry is just distal to the middle of the thumb, exactly in the midline.

Infiltrating the Skin. At the selected point the 24-gauge needle is inserted almost parallel to the skin which is infiltrated. Then the needle is inserted a little further to infiltrate the subcutaneous tissue. There is no need to infiltrate the ligaments of the back because there is little discomfort unless the needle is pushed against the periosteum.

Puncturing the Skin. Using the sharp 15-gauge needle, the skin is punctured at the selected point (Fig. 14-7).

Inserting the Epidural Needle. The Tuohy needle is inserted into the back with its opening directed cranially. The needle is introduced exactly in the midline, just distal to the upper spinous process, and

Fig. 14-7. Local infiltration of the skin and subcutaneous tissue followed by skin puncture with the sharp 15-gauge needle.

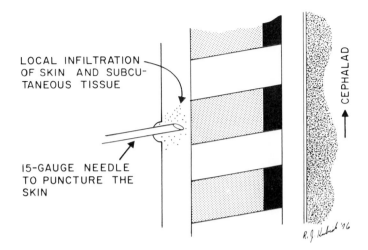

LOCAL INFILTRATION OF SKIN AND SUBCU-TANEOUS TISSUE

15-GAUGE NEEDLE TO PUNCTURE THE SKIN

CEPHALAD

advanced forward with a little cephalad inclination, to remain parallel to the spinous processes. When the operator feels that the needle is held in position by the interspinous ligament, the stylet is removed and the well-lubricated glass syringe containing 3 ml. of air is attached.

Identifying the Epidural Space. The back of the operator's left hand lies in contact with the patient's back while the needle hub is held by the fingers. The right hand holds the syringe near the plunger entrance (Fig. 14-8A). The position of the needle in the interspinous ligament is confirmed by gently "tapping" the plunger, with the rapid bouncing of the plunger verifying the position. The needle is gently advanced for a few millimeters, using both hands, while any sudden jerk is controlled by the left hand. The air test is performed and the process is repeated until the ligamentum flavum is reached when the resistance and the bouncing of the plunger become quite evident. The advancement of the needle in increments of a few millimeters is continued until the sudden "snap" of puncturing the ligamentum flavum and the sudden loss of resistance upon entering the epidural space are felt (Fig. 14-8B).

At this point there should be a pause of a few seconds in the technique. If the needle inadvertently pierces a blood vessel or the dura, blood or cerebrospinal fluid will quickly appear through the wide-bore 17-gauge needle. Aspirating in 4 directions and rotating the needle are not required and can only do harm by increasing the possibility of dural or venous puncture.

Injecting the Local Anesthetic. The dose of local anesthetic required for vaginal delivery primarily depends on the patient's height, position, the site of entry, and the rate of injection. To ensure adequate perineal spread, the head of the bed should be elevated if the patient is in the lateral position. The dose is usually 15 ml. if the patient's height is 150 cm. (5 feet), and 1 ml. is added or subtracted for each 2.5-cm. (1-inch) variation. At this stage, a large dose and a relatively high block will not affect the uterine contractions, but rather will only ensure the needed adequate analgesia, especially if episiotomy, repair, and forceps are required. The drug injected depends on the expected time of delivery. Since no catheter is inserted and unexpected delay may occur, the author prefers 0.5 per cent bupivacaine to 2 per cent chloroprocaine especially in a nullipara. The rate of injection is 1 ml./sec. Too rapid injection causes a transient rise of cerebrospinal fluid pressure leading to a short period of dis-

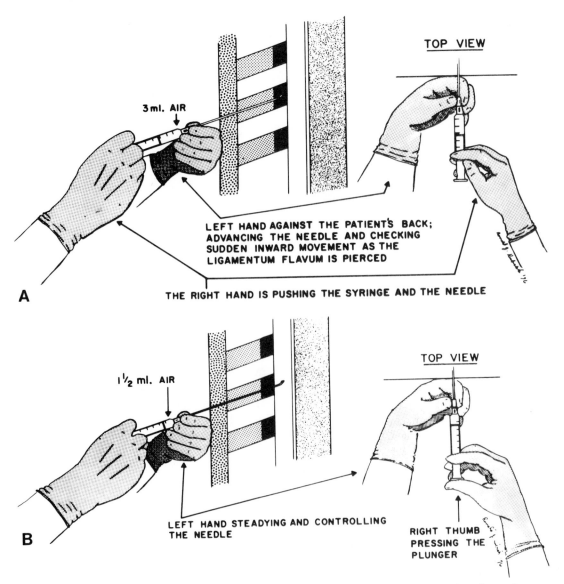

Fig. 14-8. The position of the hands. *A.* Advancing the epidural needle. *B.* Testing for resistance to air injection.

comfort and dizziness.[115] After administering the first 4 ml., the injection is temporarily halted and the patient is asked about any abnormal sensations. In the absence of evidence of intravascular administration, the injection is continued. Gentle aspiration every 4 to 5 ml. is important to detect inadvertent intravascular injection. *The main factors for avoiding subarachnoid injection are the steady hands of the operator and the constant contact of the operator's left hand with the patient's back, thus preventing the epidural needle fron advancing during the injection* (Fig. 14-7). Continuous verbal contact with the patient during and after the administration of the drug not only reassures the patient, but also helps detect early manifestations of toxic reactions.

Maintaining the Head-Up Position. Following injection, the patient is turned onto her back with the right hip on the edge of the bed. This causes left lateral displacement of the uterus owing to the elevation of the right hip due to the sagging of the middle part of the bed. If this tilt is inadequate a folded towel is placed under the right hip or even a lateral displacement device is used (Fig. 14-9). In case of multiple gestations, the patient is turned from one side to another until adequate equal spread occurs, at which point she remains in the left lateral position until time of delivery. The head of the bed is kept elevated to ensure adequate perineal analgesia. The pulse and blood pressure are measured and recorded every 1 minute for 20 minutes, then every 5 minutes. In case hypotension occurs and vasopressors are administered, the blood pressure should be followed more closely.

The fetal heart rate and uterine contractions are monitored and the cooperation of the obstetrician is essential. If fetal bradycardia occurs, the patient is tilted to the left, the blood pressure is measured, any maternal hypotension is corrected, and oxygen is administered. If uterine contractions decrease, oxytocin infusion using a Harvard pump is started.

Checking the Efficiency of the Block. If at the time of the drug injection the patient was in the lateral position, all the symptoms and signs of analgesia will start on the dependent side.

The symptoms of epidural block are usually in this order: first, in about 5 to 10 minutes the patient feels a tingling sensation in the lower limbs. Then the uterine contractions

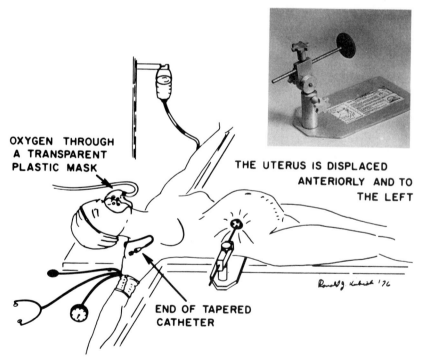

OXYGEN THROUGH
A TRANSPARENT
PLASTIC MASK

THE UTERUS IS DISPLACED
ANTERIORLY AND TO
THE LEFT

END OF TAPERED
CATHETER

Fig. 14-9.   Left uterine displacement device. The lateral displacement of the uterus by the device, the administration of oxygen, and bringing the epidural catheter tip to the patient's shoulder are routinely used with epidural analgesia for cesarean section.

become less painful; the pains are felt only at the peak of the contractions. Analgesia occurs in about 10 to 20 minutes following the injection of the drug. There is a variable degree of weakness of the lower limb and a sensation of warmth. If the patient has the urge to push, this is lost in about 15 to 20 minutes, and the perineal pain gradually becomes rather a feeling of pressure and is usually lost in 20 minutes.

The signs of epidural block are: first, dryness and warmth of the feet when the block extends to L1 segment and paralyzes the sympathetic fibers of the lower limbs (L1 and L2). Second, using pinprick, the limits of the block are determined once the patient feels comfortable or in 15 minutes following injection of the drug. *Premature testing of the block levels is useless and confusing;* moreover, it may erode the patient's confidence.

Once perineal analgesia is obtained, the obstetrician can apply forceps and do the episiotomy. Premature obstetrical procedures are unfair to the patient and the anesthesiologist. Therefore, timing of the initiation of block and the cooperation of the obstetrician are essential for the favorable outcome of epidural analgesia. The manifestations of adequate perineal analgesia are loss of the urge to push, loss of the anal reflex, obtundation of pinprick sensation, and rectal sphincter relaxation. *Perineal analgesia is the last step to occur with epidural analgesia for the following reasons:*

1. The negative intrathoracic pressure favors the cephalad spread of the local anesthetic.[24]

2. The trabeculae anchoring the dura to the lumbosacral joint may be thick enough to interfere with the caudal spread of the local anesthetic.

3. The S1 nerve root is much thicker than the other nerves and more difficult to block.[47]

Continuous Epidural Block

Timing. Presently the accepted time for injecting the local anesthetic drug is when the patient feels pain, irrespective of the stage of labor. It was commonly stated that the cervix should have reached a certain degree of dilation, e.g., 5 to 6 cm. in a primigravida and 4 to 5 cm. in a multipara, before injecting the drug. However, pain itself and dysrhythmic uterine contractions may be the cause of failure of labor to progress. Therefore, relief of pain is not only humane but also can improve the uterine contraction pattern (see Indications for the Use of Epidural Analgesia). Regarding the time for inserting the epidural catheter, there are two schools of practice. According to one school the time to insert the epidural catheter is when the patient is first admitted to the labor suite even before the onset of labor, but withholding the local anesthetic injection until labor has become established.[30] According to the other school the epidural is performed when the patient asks for pain relief. The author belongs to this second school because it is difficult to predict the need for analgesia or to decide beforehand the best method to be used at the time of need. Once the patient feels uncomfortable, the condition of the mother and the labor pattern and its progress, as well as the status of the fetus are evaluated. Then the type of analgesic technique is decided. For example, if a multipara starts to feel pain when the cervix is almost fully dilated, a subarachnoid block at the time of delivery or even local infiltration of the perineum may be a better choice of analgesic technique than inserting the epidural catheter early but not having enough time to achieve good perineal analgesia with the epidural technique. Inserting an epidural catheter before onset of pain or discomfort exposes the patient to the risk of the complications of the procedure without any sure beneficial effect. Also, when epidural block starts early in labor before any discomfort or pain, a nullipara does not usually appreciate the analgesic effect of the technique and complains of the numbness of her legs. On the other hand, waiting too long before administering epidural to a patient who has been in pain may mean that the block is performed in a restless patient, thus increasing the technical difficulty. Moreover, following epidural analgesia the patient may become stuporous owing to pain relief and the previous administration of large doses of narcotics and/or tranquilizers. Thus, she becomes unable to cooperate and bear down during the second stage of labor. Therefore, timing of the epidural is important and availability of the anesthesiologist is essential.

Procedure. The steps described in the single-dose technique are followed until the epidural space is identified. Then, a 20-gauge, 91.5-cm., epidural Teflon catheter without a stylet is introduced through the Tuohy needle (Fig. 14-10A). The patient may feel an "electric shock" in one of her legs as the catheter touches one of the sensory nerve roots in the epidural space. The patient must be warned against such a possibility and reassured that it only indicates the correct position of the catheter. After introducing the catheter the needle is then withdrawn, leaving about 3 cm. of the catheter in the epidural space (Fig. 14-10B). The marks on the catheter help to estimate the length of the segment in the epidural space. The catheter is then taped to the patient's back and brought to the patient's abdomen. If the double-catheter technique is used, in which both epidural and caudal blocks are utilized, the epidural catheter is taped above the caudal catheter and both are marked by a pen to avoid any confusion on subsequent injections. For vaginal delivery, the author prefers to

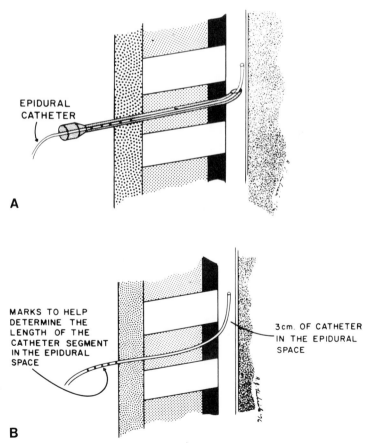

EPIDURAL CATHETER

A

MARKS TO HELP DETERMINE THE LENGTH OF THE CATHETER SEGMENT IN THE EPIDURAL SPACE

3cm. OF CATHETER IN THE EPIDURAL SPACE

Fig. 14-10. *A*. Insertion of the epidural catheter through the Tuohy needle. *B*. The epidural catheter *in situ*.   B

bring the epidural catheter to the abdomen rather than the shoulder to avoid the patient's discomfort as the tape is removed at the end of the procedure. Once the patient is in the supine position with the right hip on the edge of the bed, a test dose of local anesthetic is injected. To exclude the intravascular or subarachnoid position of the catheter, it is essential to aspirate, inject 4 ml. of 0.5 per cent bupivacaine, and aspirate again. The absence of both blood aspiration and abnormal sensations is suggestive of the extravascular position of the catheter. If the catheter has been in the subarachnoid space, the test dose should have caused analgesia within 5 minutes, loss of motor power in the lower limbs, and complete perineal analgesia. Injection of 4 ml. into the epidural space has a limited

spread and the action is manifest only after several minutes (Fig. 14-11). After excluding subarachnoid and intravascular position of the catheter, 6 to 10 ml. of 0.5 per cent bupivacaine is injected slowly (1 ml./ sec.), with aspiration before and after injection. Verbal contact with the patient, fetal and maternal monitoring, and post-injection evaluation of the block are all performed as in the single-dose technique.

The timing of the refill doses is important. They should not be administered on an hourly basis because the duration of action of a local anesthetic drug varies in different patients. On the other hand, to avoid tachyphylaxis the injection should be performed once the patient feels discomfort with the uterine contractions. The test dose is essential (4 ml.) before each refill

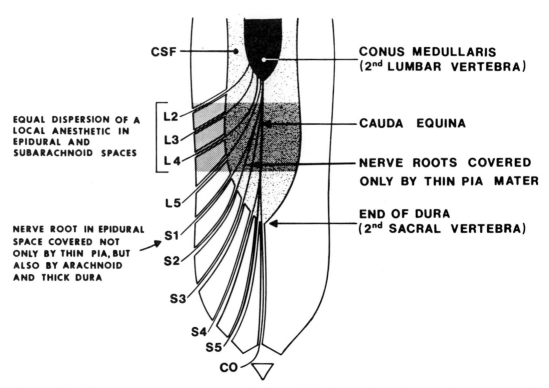

Fig. 14-11.   Diagrammatic explanation of the limited blocking effect of epidural compared with spinal analgesia. The nerves leave the subarachnoid space to the epidural space shortly before their exit through the corresponding intervertebral foramina. Therefore, an equal spread of a local anesthetic in the two spaces at the lumbar region causes an extensive block in the subarachnoid space (from L-2 through coccygeal nerve) and a limited block in the epidural space (L-2 to L-4).

dose. Aspiration before and after injection is important. After 5 minutes, the therapeutic dose is administered. The volume of the drug injected is determined by the extent of the block produced by the first injection.

Before injecting the final dose for delivery, the extent of the block should be determined. Often there is adequate analgesia, including the perineum, already present and a refill dose is not required. However, if the patient is uncomfortable or perineal analgesia is inadequate, a final dose is required. The volume of such a dose is determined by the extent of the block with each previous dose; usually 13 to 17 ml. are required and the drug of choice is 2 per cent chloroprocaine. The drug is injected slowly with the patient in the semisitting position, and that position should be maintained until perineal analgesia is obtained.

Problems With the Use of Catheters. The use of epidural catheters is associated with many problems and difficulties. However, proper visualization and understanding of the mechanisms of these problems are essential to minimize failures and frustrations. These problems are:

Problems Associated With Catheters

1. Difficulty in advancing the epidural catheter
2. Unilateral anesthesia
3. Kinking of the catheter
4. Leakage of the catheter
5. Extrusion of the catheter out of the epidural space
6. Compression of the catheter between vertebrae
7. Knotting of the catheter
8. Shearing of the catheter
9. Unpredictability of the direction of the catheter
10. Perforation of the dura mater by the catheter

---

1. *Difficulty in advancing the epidural catheter through the Tuohy needle.* This may occur at either the tip of the needle or after the catheter has passed the needle bevel. The markings on the catheter determine the site of obstruction, e.g., in the Deseret catheter when the first mark is at the nee-

dle hub, the tip of the catheter is at the needle bevel, while if one or more marks disappear, the tip of the catheter has passed the needle. If obstruction occurs at the tip of the needle, then most probably the needle opening is restricted because the ligamentum flavum is not completely penetrated. The remedy for this problem is to gently and cautiously advance the needle for a few millimeters. If the obstruction is beyond the tip of the needle, then the catheter may be against the dura, blood vessel, or a nerve root. The use of force or stylet is not advisable because it only leads to complications, i.e., penetration of the dura or a blood vessel, or trauma to a nerve. To avoid such a complication one should adhere to the midline during insertion of the Tuohy needle where the epidural space is widest and the blood vessels and nerve roots are further away. If such a problem is encountered, paresthesia can help in directing the needle bevel away from the affected side. If no paresthesia is felt, the needle is rotated 20 to 40° and the catheter is advanced. Counterclockwise rotation is safer than clockwise rotation, because in case of the latter the needle has a tendency to advance and nick the dura. If these maneuvers fail, the needle and catheter should be removed and the procedure should be repeated. The catheter should never be withdrawn while the needle is in place, otherwise it will be sheared.

2. *Unilateral anesthesia.* In obstetrics, the incidence of unilateral anesthesia with the continuous epidural technique has been reported to be as high as 30 per cent.[26,37] If a too long segment of the catheter is inserted into the epidural space, it tends to be deflected by blood vessels and nerve roots that lie in its path.[19,79] Even when only 5 to 10 cm. of the catheter is inserted, it curls or doubles on itself in almost 50 per cent of the cases.[81,100] A catheter may even leave the epidural space through an intervertebral foramen, leading to a spotty block.[111] If there is resistance to the

cephalad or caudal advancement, the catheter may deviate laterally to reach the anterolateral compartment of the epidural space (Fig. 14-12A). The spread of the injected local anesthetic to the other side is hampered posteriorly by the dilated vertebral veins and anteriorly by the anterior trabeculae connecting the dura to the posterior longitudinal ligament. Since fluid takes the route of the least resistance, it spreads longitudinally on the ipsilateral side and escapes through the corresponding intervertebral foramina, leading to unilateral analgesia.[65,114] Positioning the patient on the unanesthetized side and administering more drug fail to correct the problem, but rather only reinforce and extend the block on the anesthetized side. To avoid such a complication, only a short segment of the catheter (about 3 cm.) is introduced into the epidural space, the median plane is used, and the ligamentum

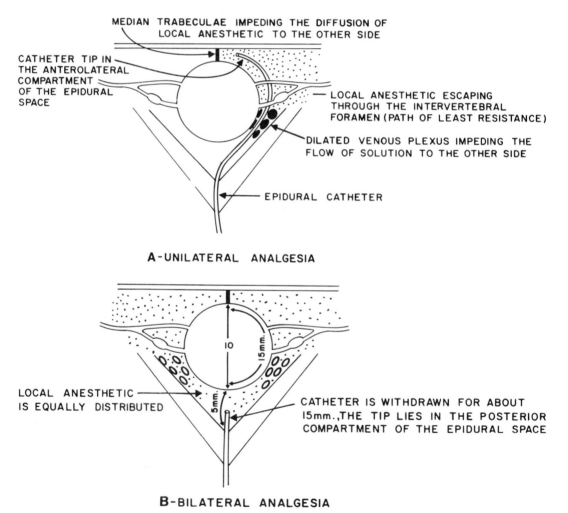

Fig. 14-12.   Mechanism and treatment of unilateral analgesia with continuous epidural technique. *A.* Unilateral analgesia is caused by the catheter tip being in the anterolateral compartment of the epidural space, with local anesthetic escaping through the intervertebral foramen. *B.* The catheter is withdrawn about 15 mm. so that the tip lies in the posterior compartment of the epidural space. Bilateral analgesia is accomplished because the therapeutic dose of the local anesthetic is equally distributed when the tip of the catheter is in the posterior compartment.

flavum is punctured in the midline. The diameter of the dural sac in the lumbar region is 10 to 15 mm., and thus its circumference is 30 to 45 mm. (Fig. 14-12). It takes only 1.5 to 2 cm. of the catheter to reach the anterior compartment of the epidural space. Therefore to treat unilateral analgesia, the patient lies on the unanesthetized side, the catheter is withdrawn for about 1.5 to 2 cm. in order to bring its tip to the posterior portion of the epidural space, and a full therapeutic dose (8 to 10 ml.) is administered (Fig. 14-12B). The patient is kept in this position until manifestations of adequate analgesia develop on the dependent side.

Very rarely adhesions limit the spread of the anesthetic[108] or a congenital median septum divides the epidural space into two separate compartments.[14]

Unilateral analgesia due to improper position of the catheter differs from the unequal spread of analgesia secondary to injection of a small volume (4 to 6 ml.) while keeping the patient on one side. In the latter situation there is restricted spread on both sides which is more limited on one. Such a problem can be prevented by injecting a relatively large volume of local anesthetic (8 to 10 ml.) while the patient is in the supine position. It can be corrected by positioning and administering a booster dose without need to pull out the catheter.

It is important to remember that the incidence of unilateral analgesia is far more frequent with continuous epidural than with subarachnoid or continuous caudal block. This is because the catheter has to change direction, almost 90°, as it leaves the Tuohy needle and advances into the epidural space. This sudden change in direction tends to deviate the catheter. On the other hand, with caudal analgesia, the catheter leaves the cannula and advances into the caudal canal almost in a straight line. Moreover, there is a median groove in the posterior wall of the sacral canal which makes a good bed for the catheter and

permits it to advance in the midline. In subarachnoid block, mixing of the local anesthetic with the cerebrospinal fluid allows for a uniform distribution of the drug if prolonged lateral position of the patient following injection is avoided.

3. *Kinking of the catheter.* Catheters used for epidural analgesia must be fine and soft, and this makes them liable to kinking and occlusion. Usually this occurs when the catheter is compressed between the bed and a bony portion, e.g., in cesarean section when the catheter is brought to the shoulder, it may be compressed by the scapula or the spine. To avoid this, the catheter is not allowed to cross to the other side but passes in the furrow between the scapula and the spinous processes and must be tested while the patient is on the operating table before the start of surgery. If difficulty in injection occurs during epidural analgesia for vaginal delivery, the patient is tilted to one side and injection is attempted again. This usually solves the problem. However, one may have to partially or completely remove the tape that holds the catheter and follow the catheter to discover and correct the kink which may occur at the entrance of the catheter through the skin. In such a case, the catheter is pulled out for a few millimeters and straightened by the operator, who is wearing sterile gloves, while the assistant is injecting the local anesthetic.

4. *Leakage of the catheter.* In case of prolonged recumbency, a Teflon catheter may partially break at the site of the kink at the skin level (Fig. 14-13).[2] This may cause leakage of the local anesthetic and failure of epidural analgesia. Therefore, if the catheter has been in place for many hours, e.g., when used the next day for postpartum tubal ligation, the catheter should be pulled out for a few millimeters while an assistant is injecting the drug to detect any leakage. If the catheter is leaking, the site of the hole is gently compressed between a sterile-gloved thumb and index finger while injection is resumed.

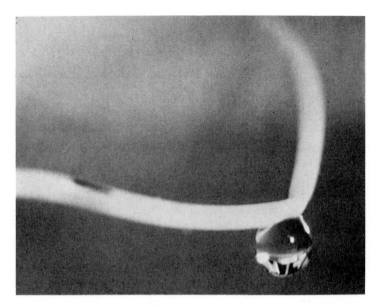

Fig. 14-13.   Partial breaking of the epidural catheter. (Abouleish, E.: Preventing and detecting leakage in epidural catheters. Anesth. Analg., *53*:474, 1974).

5. *Extrusion of the catheter out of the epidural space.* In prolonged recumbency, especially with much movement of the patient, the catheter may be pulled out of the epidural space, causing failure of subsequent doses of the local anesthetic to produce analgesia. The problem can be avoided by securely fixing the catheter with good-quality adhesive tape. The use of tincture of benzoin in patients with greasy skin or in case of expected prolonged insertion of the catheter helps to prevent such a problem. If inadequate analgesia occurs on subsequent injections, the problem should be suspected and the catheter should be exposed.

6. *Compression of the catheter between two vertebrae.* Especially if the patient has osteoarthritis, the catheter may be compressed between the spinous processes[64] or the laminae of two adjacent vertebrae. This makes injection of the local anesthetic or removal of the catheter difficult with the back extended, and this is only possible with flexion of the spine. In such a case, at the termination of anesthesia gentle removal of the catheter should be attempted with the back flexed; no force should be used, otherwise the catheter is severed.

7. *Knotting of the catheter.* If a long segment of the catheter is introduced and then pulled out, a knot may form[55] making its removal impossible. This is a rare condition and can be avoided by introducing a short segment. Again, no force should be used in pulling out the catheter.

8. *Shearing of the catheter.* Pulling out the catheter after advancing it through the Tuohy needle can lead to cutting of the catheter by the bevel of the needle. Also, at the termination of epidural analgesia, using force in removal of the catheter can lead to its breaking. To avoid such a complication, first, once the catheter tip passes the bevel of the needle, the catheter alone should not be pulled out. Second, no force should be used. Third, the catheter should be removed only by an experienced person and examined to exclude any missing part. If such an accident occurs, the obstetrician as well as the patient should be notified. The use of radiopaque catheters makes their identification in the epidural space easy. The catheter usually causes no reaction even after many years[11,38] and no treatment except reassurance of the patient is required. However, if neurologic manifestations such as bladder dysfunc-

tion, paresthesia, and loss of motor power in the lower limbs occur, surgical removal is required.

9. *Difficulty in predicting the direction of the catheter.* In only 23 per cent of cases the catheter goes up or down the extradural space according to the intention of the anesthesiologist.[17,100] In 6 per cent it emerges through an intervertebral foramen. Most of these problems occur if a too long segment of catheter is introduced into the epidural space.

10. *Perforation of the dura mater.* The dura was perforated by the catheter in 18 out of 3,132 cases.[38]

DOUBLE-CATHETER TECHNIQUE

Whenever feasible, a combination of epidural and caudal analgesia (double-catheter technique) is utilized; the epidural block is used for the uterine pain, and the caudal block for the perineal pain. The *advantages of the double-catheter technique over either epidural or caudal alone are:*

1. *The total dosage of the injected local anesthetic is reduced* because the tips of the catheters in double-catheter technique are close to the nerves to be blocked. If caudal alone is used from the first stage of labor, the sacral and lower lumbar nerve roots have to be unnecessarily blocked to reach segments T10 to L1 in order to produce adequate analgesia. If epidural alone is used, the lumbar segments have to be blocked to reach the sacral nerves and provide analgesia for the second stage of labor.

2. *Analgesia is faster* because the catheters are at the strategic points. With epidural alone, sometimes there is not sufficient time to sit the patient up and wait for 20 minutes to obtain perineal analgesia.

3. *Analgesia is more adequate* because the nerves to be blocked are surrounded with sufficient quantities of the local anesthetic. With epidural alone, the spread of the drug to the sacral roots may be inadequate due to the impedance caused by the trabeculae at the lumbosacral region. Also, the S1, being thickest and further from the site of injection, may be insufficiently anesthetized, leading to inadequate analgesia. It sometimes happens that by increasing the dose of the drug injected through the epidural catheter and sitting the patient up, the level of analgesia spreads even to the T4 or T5 level while perineal analgesia is still inadequate. Also, with caudal analgesia, due to the difficulty of spread at the lumbosacral region there may be inadequate cephalad spread as most of the solution escapes through the wide sacral foramina.

4. *Incidence of hypotension is less* with double-catheter technique than with either epidural or caudal. The reason is the predictability of the level of the block with the double-catheter technique compared to either single technique alone.

5. *The problems such as unilateral analgesia or intravascular position of the catheter can be easily handled.* Sometimes no time is available to repeat the technique if blood is aspirated from the epidural catheter or one is faced with persistent unilateral analgesia. In such a case the catheter in the caudal canal is used to produce the required analgesia.

However, the ideal anatomical conditions for the utilization of the double-catheter technique are not always present. Therefore, a choice between epidural and caudal techniques is made depending on the prominence of the landmarks, the stage of labor, and the cooperation of the patient. As a rule, the lumbar epidural is used unless: (1) delivery is expected within one hour; (2) the landmarks in the sacral region are better felt than in the lumbar region, which is a rare situation; (3) the patient is quite restless and will not flex her back; and/or (4) in multiple gestations where there is marked lordosis making epidural difficult. In these cases caudal alone is used.

EPIDURAL ANALGESIA FOR CESAREAN SECTION

Cesarean section can be either elective or emergency.

Epidural Analgesia for Elective Cesarean Section

In the preoperative visit the epidural technique is explained to the patient and a hypnotic is administered to ensure adequate night sleep before surgery. Sixty minutes before surgery, 75 mg. of hydroxyzine hydrochloride (Vistaril) is injected intramuscularly. Thirty minutes before surgery the patient is transferred to the delivery room suite while lying on her left side. It is advisable to have a special room for induction of anesthesia. It is preferable to have all the cesarean sections performed in the delivery room suite which is equipped to handle all cases of cesarean section, whether elective or emergency. A delivery room next to the cesarean section room is utilized for induction of epidural analgesia. It is important to administer anesthesia early enough to ensure adequate spread and maximum action of the drug. The drug is injected about 20 minutes before the scheduled time of surgery.

Preloading with intravenous fluids is essential to prevent hypotension. Before the block is started, 500 to 1,000 ml. of fluid is rapidly administered intravenously through a 16-gauge cannula. The fluid is usually 5 per cent dextrose combined with lactated Ringer's solution. Dextrose is important to prevent metabolic acidosis because all patients due for elective cesarean section have been fasting since midnight. Prevention of this acidosis has a beneficial effect on the fetus.[110] If the patient is diabetic, glucose administration is postponed until the baby is delivered. Since glucose is transmitted through the placenta, it stimulates pancreatic secretion in the fetus with subsequent hypoglycemia in the neonatal period. One of the problems of the neonates of diabetic mothers is hypoglycemia,

and this reaction to the glucose administration makes it worse. On the other hand, the removal of the placenta with its anti-insulin effect causes postpartum maternal hypoglycemia. Therefore, the mother should not receive insulin on the day of surgery and requires dextrose administration once the baby is delivered. Both the maternal and neonatal blood sugar should be followed closely in the postpartum period. If the patient is preeclamptic, 500 ml. of 5 per cent albumin plus 500 ml. of 5 per cent dextrose in water are required before surgery in order to expand the constricted blood volume associated with toxemia.[106]

The technique of epidural analgesia for cesarean section is similar to what has been described before for vaginal delivery with a few exceptions that will be discussed in detail. The blood pressure is measured, the patient is positioned, and the tray is prepared as previously described. The interspace is then selected. The author prefers interspace L3 to L4 because it allows a better spread, both caudad and cephalad, than L4 to L5 or L2 to L3. The epidural space is identified and the drug is injected. The aim is to give a large enough dose to ensure adequate analgesia for the abdominal procedure by reaching the T5 level, and to obtain adequate muscle relaxation. The drug of choice is 0.75 per cent bupivacaine without epinephrine. The omission of epinephrine makes the cardiovascular system more stable.[112] The volume of the local anesthetic is calculated according to the patient's height, 15 ml. for a patient who is 150 cm. (5 feet) high, adding or subtracting 1 ml. of fluid for each 2.5-cm. (1-inch) variation. The drug is usually injected while the patient is in the left lateral position with the head of the bed elevated. After injection of the local anesthetic through the needle, an epidural catheter is threaded cephalad to be used in case there is unforeseen delay or too much prolongation of the operation. It may also be used for postpartum analgesia. After injection, the patient assumes the supine position with the right hip at the edge of the bed and the semisitting position is maintained. In 20 minutes the block is usually fixed. The upper and lower levels on both sides are determined. The blood pressure should be closely watched, and if hypotension occurs it should be immediately corrected. Hypotension is defined arbitrarily as a fall in the systolic blood pressure more than 20 per cent of the original level. Since the patient is already preloaded with fluid and the uterus is displaced, the only remaining method of remedy is administering a vasopressor. This should be administered intravenously as soon as hypotension occurs. Alpha stimulants such as methoxamine are contraindicated since they reduce the uterine blood flow.[59] The drug should be a beta stimulant, e.g., 25 mg. of ephedrine or 15 mg. of mephentermine. The blood pressure should be measured very closely and there should be no hesitation to repeat the dose if the blood pressure falls again. If no response to the first dose occurs, half this dose is readministered. The usual cause of resistant hypotension is delay in the treatment. After the level is fixed and the blood pressure is stable, the patient is transferred to the cesarean section room. She should be gently moved from the bed to the operating table, otherwise severe hypotension occurs. Once on the operating table, the uterus is displaced to the left either by tilting the table, using a wedge under the right hip,[44] or using the left uterine displacement device (Fig. 14-9); the latter technique (the device) has been found to be superior to the others.[12] It should be used to *lift the uterus up and to the left* and not merely to push the uterus to the side. The mother is given oxygen by a transparent plastic face mask since it has been found that having the mother breathe oxygen during cesarean section is better for the neonate than having her breathe only air.[46] Throughout the procedure, the vital signs are closely followed and verbal contact with the patient is maintained. *The conversation with the patient is the substitute for strong premedication.* After the baby is born, tranquilizers and/or narcotics can be administered if required.

With epidural analgesia for cesarean section, 17.5 per cent of the patients may experience pain during the pelvic manipulations.[47,112] This is probably due to the inadequate blockade of the sacral nerves, especially S1. That is why the author prefers to inject the dose through the needle rather than the catheter which can be one or more spaces higher, use the L3 to L4 interspace rather than the L2 to L3 interspace, keep the head of the bed elevated during and after injection, and allow perineal analgesia to develop (usually 20 minutes) before moving the patient to the cesarean section room.

Epidural Analgesia for Emergency Cesarean Section

If there is time for epidural analgesia to develop and continuous epidural has been utilized during labor, a refill dose through the catheter can be administered. The drug of choice is 0.75 per cent bupivacaine. The volume is determined by the degree of the spread of the previous doses; then 1 ml. is added for each additional segment to be blocked. Remember, for cesarean section blockage of 19 segments is required (T5 through coccygeal nerve). If no epidural catheter has been inserted before, then the technique for elective cesarean section is followed.

CONTINUOUS EPIDURAL INFUSION

Continuous infusion into the epidural space has been used either by a gravity drip of the local anesthetic[51] or by a Harvard constant infusion pump.[57,103] However, the author finds it safer and more efficient to use the intermittent injection technique rather than the continuous infusion. A catheter may insidiously pass into the subarachnoid space or into a blood vessel; the continuous administration of the local anesthetic under these circumstances can be hazardous. Moreover, the analgesia in many cases has been inadequate in spite of giving supplementary "top-up" doses.[122] With the continuous infusion technique the total dosage of the local anesthetic is higher than with the intermittent injections.[57,126] The patient during parturition is frequently connected to infusion lines, oxytocin pump, uterine catheters, and so on. The addition of another infusion line for the continuous epidural administration further complicates the picture, limits the patient's movement, and makes the possibility of error in connecting pumps or setting their rates quite dangerous without a significant proven advantage. The answer to the need for continuous smooth analgesia is to use a long-acting local anesthetic drug which should be injected as soon as the analgesia starts to fade, rather than the use of a continuous infusion.

COMPLICATIONS ASSOCIATED WITH EPIDURAL ANALGESIA
MATERNAL COMPLICATIONS

The use of epidural analgesia may be followed by complications in the mother and/or the fetus. Some of these complications following epidural analgesia have already been discussed in Chapter 13, Caudal Analgesia, and Chapter 4, Local Anesthetic Drugs. To avoid repetition, the complications as a whole will be mentioned here and the reader is referred to the corresponding chapter.

Hypotension

Hypotension is the commonest complication of epidural analgesia.

Incidence. The incidence of hypotension may be as low as 1.4 per cent and as high as 13 per cent.[6,26,91]

Mechanism. Hypotension is due to combined inferior vena caval compression and sympathetic blockade.[105] Dehydration and/or narcotics potentiate the hypoten-

---

Maternal Complications of Epidural Analgesia

1. Hypotension
2. Respiratory insufficiency
3. Toxic reaction to the local anesthetic drug
4. Dural puncture
5. Nausea and vomiting
6. Shivering
7. Hypertension
8. Prolonged labor
9. Need for operative delivery
10. Prolonged effect
11. Neurologic complications
12. Bladder dysfunction
13. Backache
14. Catheter problems
15. Infection
16. Introduction of a foreign body into the epidural space
17. Headache
18. Implantation dermoid
19. Horner's syndrome

---

sive effect of epidural analgesia.[34] However, the fall in blood pressure may represent a return to a normotensive level in an acutely anxious patient.[29,30]

Hypotension is more common in cesarean section than in vaginal delivery. Moreover, it is of higher incidence and severer degree in elective cesarean section than emergency cases who have been in labor (e.g., emergency cesarean section for disproportion).

The reasons for the low incidence of hypotension in vaginal delivery are:

1. Less compression of the inferior vena cava. This is due to rupture of the membranes, loss of the bulk of amniotic fluid, decreased size of the uterus, and descent of the fetus deep into the pelvis.

2. Increased venous return to the heart and diminished vascular bed with each uterine contraction. When the uterus contracts, it changes in configuration and lifts itself off the inferior vena cava, allowing more blood to return to the heart. Also, venous blood is squeezed out of the uterus. The uterine arterial blood supply is temporarily stopped; instead, 500 to 700 ml./min. is diverted into the systemic circulation.

3. Elevated cardiac output during labor.

Therefore the starting point from which the cardiovascular system changes following the block is already high.

4. The limited sympathetic blockade required for vaginal delivery compared to that for cesarean section. Therefore the compensatory vasoconstriction above the level of the block is better retained with vaginal delivery.

5. The elevation of the legs during vaginal delivery compared to cesarean section. Therefore venous return to the heart is better since there is less pooling of blood in the lower limbs with vaginal delivery.

For emergency cesarean section, the limited fall in blood pressure compared to elective cases can be explained by the diminished vena caval compression and the effects of labor, as in vaginal delivery.

The decrease in the maternal blood pressure is accompanied by a proportionate decrease in the uterine blood flow.[59] Therefore, if hypotension occurs it should be corrected promptly and efficiently.

Prophylaxis. The patient should stay on her side or at least the right hip should be elevated. She should be well hydrated, and fluid should be administered by rapid infusion before the block.

Treatment. The lower limbs are elevated if possible, intravenous fluids are continued at a fast rate, and a beta stimulant is administered.

Respiratory Insufficiency

Respiratory insufficiency is usually due to inadvertent dural puncture and massive subarachnoid block, ischemia of the respiratory center, or toxic reaction to the drug. This complication is explained in Chapter 6, Effects of Vertebral Blocks on the Respiratory System.

Toxic Reaction to the Local Anesthetic Drug

A toxic reaction can be due to intravascular injection, excessive dose, or decreased metabolism (see Chap. 4, Local Anesthetic Drugs). The commonest cause is inadvertent intravascular injection, especially through the catheter (see Chap. 13, Caudal Analgesia). Recognized vascular puncture during epidural attempt occurs in 2.8 per cent of cases.[38] To avoid the possibility of a toxic reaction, another interspace is used and the drug is injected slowly. A negative aspiration does not exclude the intravascular position of the catheter. A test dose is a must (4 ml.). Provided ventilation is adequately maintained, there should be no maternal or fetal mortality. Fortunately the local anesthetic drugs used today have no depressant effect on the cardiovascular system at or below doses that produce convulsions.[81a] Therefore, cardiovascular depression is mainly secondary to hypoxia and/or barbiturates when injected as an antidote to the local anesthetic (see Chap. 4, Local Anesthetic Drugs).

Dural Puncture

One of the major complications of epidural analgesia is dural puncture. The following factors predispose to such an accident:

1. Inexperience of the anesthesiologist. Dural puncture diminishes with increased skill of the operator. It usually occurs when a trainee performing the epidural has some confidence in himself, yet lacks the adequate experience. At an acceptable level of experience, dural puncture occurs only in one out of 200 cases of epidurals performed, or less.[22]

2. Piercing the lateral part of the ligamentum flavum

3. New sharp epidural needles. The chances of puncturing the ligamentum flavum without noticing the loss of resistance is higher with sharp needles.

4. Rotating the needle in the epidural space

5. The operator pushing the needle forward during injection of the therapeutic dose

6. Restless or uncooperative patient

7. Using a stiff epidural catheter or stiffening it with a stylet. This is especially important when force is used to overcome resistance to the catheter advancement.

Dural puncture occurs more frequently with the epidural needle than with the catheter, the ratio being 7 to 1.[30] The incidence of dural puncture varies from one center to another, usually between 0.5 per cent and 3 per cent.

The management of inadvertent dural puncture depends on whether it is recognized or not at the time of its occurrence.

Recognized Dural Puncture. In the management of such a situation, the following options are available:

1. *To use the technique as a spinal block* by injecting the local anesthetic through the needle. This is usually resorted to if the surgical procedure or the delivery can soon be started, e.g., for cesarean section when the surgeon and the operating room are ready.

2. To administer *general anesthesia* for the operation if there is no contraindication and much delay is expected.

3. *To try epidural puncture at a different space,* because if the same interspace is used the incidence of a spinal block is high (2:11) despite the negative aspiration of cerebrospinal fluid.[62] The bevel of the needle is directed away from the site of dural puncture, and then the catheter is introduced, hoping that its tip will be far from the site of the dural puncture. This option is usually followed if the indication for continuous epidural analgesia still exists and cannot be substituted by spinal or general anesthesia, e.g., pain in the first stage of labor.

By using the epidural technique in such a case, it must be kept in mind that certain changes have occurred: there is a communication between the epidural and subarachnoid spaces; as a result of leakage of cerebrospinal fluid into the epidural space, the volume and pressure of cerebrospinal fluid in the subarachnoid space are reduced; the local anesthetic drug injected into the epidural space is diluted and its volume is increased by the cerebrospinal fluid that has leaked. *These factors will lead to:*

1. A need for decreasing the dosage and volume of the local anesthetic injected into the epidural space

2. A possible combination of epidural and subarachnoid blocks, i.e., greater degree of motor paralysis and more common perineal analgesia than with epidural alone. Therefore, in the management of such a case a test dose is mandatory and adequate time should be allowed to observe the result of the test dose. Then, increments of 2 to 5 ml. of the local anesthetic are injected through the catheter and the extent of the block is evaluated. Usually the total dose is reduced by about 30 per cent. The local anesthetic drugs should be injected slowly to avoid excessive rise of epidural pressure with the possibility of shunting fluid into the subarachnoid space. Following delivery and complete recovery from the epidural block, 60 ml. of saline is injected through the catheter which is then removed. The patient is followed daily for the possibility of post-lumbar-puncture cephalgia which is treated according to its severity.

Unrecognized Dural Puncture. The dose to produce an epidural block is usually 10 times that needed for a subarachnoid block. Therefore, if the anesthesiologist is unaware of the dural puncture and the local anesthetic drug is injected in the dose commonly used for epidural analgesia, total spinal block occurs. To avoid this, a test dose is injected which should be sufficient (4 ml. rather than 2 ml.) to warn the anesthesiologist of the subarachnoid position of the catheter before injecting the therapeutic dose. However, test doses have been misleading in many circumstances because the dose was too small and/or the interval between the injection and the testing for subarachnoid block was too short.[105a,105b] That is why on several occasions total spinal block has occurred despite the test dose.[49]

The dura can be punctured without notice during single-dose or continuous epidural. *During single-dose epidural,* it is hard to conceive that dural puncture by a large bore needle such as the Tuohy's passes unnoticed. Most probably the dura is punctured during the injection of the therapeutic dose through the needle which is advanced during the injection.

Following continuous epidural, the mechanism of dural puncture is different. The needle could nick the dura unnoticeably during a difficult epidural attempt by an inexperienced person. Therefore, it may occur at a different space than the one through which the catheter is ultimately inserted. Thus, a 2-ml. test dose through the catheter may not show any indication of communication between the subarachnoid and epidural spaces. However, a full dose will result in an extensive anesthesia which is a mixture of epidural and subarachnoid block.[32] Very rarely the epidural catheter, after staying a long time against the dura, ultimately perforates it, as explained with caudal analgesia (Chap. 13). This leads to total spinal block following a refill dose, despite an epidural block through the catheter on previous doses. Therefore, with continuous epidural analgesia, a test dose (4 ml.) should always be administered before each refill dose and adequate time should elapse (at least 5 minutes) before the full dose is injected.[5] *The local anesthetic drugs used for epidural analgesia have low specific gravities at body temperature* and are potentially hypobaric compared to cerebrospinal fluid[73] (Table 4-1). Moreover, the specific gravity of cerebrospinal fluid is elevated by increased glucose content. Induced hyperglycemia increases the cerebrospinal fluid glucose level within 15 minutes, with a peak effect at 30 and 45 minutes.[66] Therefore, a test dose through the catheter should be administered with the patient in the horizontal position; otherwise, too much cephalad spread occurs leading to an extensive spinal block if the catheter tip has been in the subarachnoid space.[66]

The treatment of total spinal block is to maintain respiration and circulation. The former is best maintained by endotracheal intubation to ensure an adequate airway and prevent aspiration. One hundred per cent oxygen is administered. Too much positive-pressure ventilation is to be avoided because it decreases the cardiac output. Under general anesthesia, positive-pressure ventilation reduces the uterine blood flow because it increases the intrathoracic pressure and decreases the venous return to the heart; subsequently, the sympathetic tone is increased and uterine vasoconstriction occurs.[67] However, under total spinal block there is total sympathectomy and the reduction in uterine blood flow will only follow the degree of hypotension. Therefore, by maintaining the cardiovascular status as near normal as possible, there should be a minimal effect on the fetus. Monitoring of the fetus, the uterine contractions, and the maternal vital signs is essential.

Injection of local anesthetics should only be performed by persons capable of dealing with cardiorespiratory failure, and facilities for resuscitation should be readily available.

Table 14-1. Specific Gravity of Commonly Used Local Anesthetics for Epidural Analgesia

Drug Concentration	*Specific Gravity at 37°C.**
Bupivacaine	
0.25%	1.0058
0.5 %	1.0059
0.75%	1.0063
Chloroprocaine	
2%	1.0044

Mean cerebrospinal fluid specific gravity = 1.007.†

*Kim, Y. I., Mazza, N. M., and Marx, G. F.: Massive spinal block with hemicranial palsy after a "test dose" for extradural analgesia. Anesthesiology, *43*:370, 1975.

†Wolman, J. J., Evans, B., and Lasker, S.: The specific gravity of cerebrospinal fluid. Am. J. Clin. Pathol., *16*:33, 1946.

Nausea and Vomiting

Nausea and vomiting occur in about 12 per cent of patients under epidural analgesia. For the mechanism and treatment, see Chapter 13, Caudal Analgesia, and Chapter 15, Subarachnoid Block.

Shivering

Shivering occurs after both spinal and epidural analgesia.[86] The incidence with or without anesthesia is high (4 to 25%). The mechanism and treatment are discussed in Chapter 13, Caudal Analgesia.

Hypertension

Hypertension with epidural analgesia occurs in one out of 1000 cases.[30] It can be due to the inadvertent intravenous injection of the local anesthetic mixture containing epinephrine, injection of ergot alkaloids, and/or administration of vasopressor either in excessive dosage or injecting the wrong drug. For methods to avoid such a complication, see Chapter 13, Caudal Analgesia.

Prolonged Labor

That labor is prolonged by epidural analgesia is a misconception rather than a complication. A properly administered epidural block does not prolong labor and may even shorten it (see Effect of Epidural Analgesia on the Course of Labor, above).

Need for Operative Delivery

The introduction of a large-scale service has certainly not resulted in a marked increase in the demand for operative delivery.[29] On the contrary, epidural analgesia has led to a reduction in the requirement to intervene surgically during the first stage of labor, i.e., by reducing emergency cesarean section and vacuum extraction (ventouse delivery).[30]

Prolonged Effect

With bupivacaine, a prolonged action of the drug up to 60 hours may very rarely occur.[87] No treatment is required and the patient should be reassured that ultimately normal function will be restored.

Neurologic Complications

Neurologic complications are mainly post-lumbar-puncture cephalgia in case the dura has been punctured, and radicular nerve dysfunction. Post-lumbar-puncture cephalgia has been described in detail in Chapter 7, Effects of Vertebral Blocks on the Nervous System.

Radicular effect may occur in the form of pain, paresthesia, or anesthesia. It may last for 6 weeks and is usually followed by spontaneous recovery without any residual effect. The commonest form is an area of numbness on the outer aspect of the thigh,[30] occurring in one out of 1000 epidurals.[31] The cause of this radicular dysfunction is difficult to explain.[9] It may be due to trauma by the catheter, pressure on the nerve by the fetal head, posture during labor or delivery, and/or the obstetric manipulation. Paresthesia occurs in 13 per cent of cases of lumbar puncture[42] and in only 0.07 per cent of cases of epidural block.[113] The reason for the much higher incidence with spinal than with epidural is that the chances of encountering nerve roots are greater with lumbar puncture when the nerves hang from the cauda equina, while in the epidural space the nerves are localized laterally and correspond only to the individual segment (Fig. 14-11). Therefore, to avoid paresthesia during epidural block, the needle should be introduced in the median plane; with spinal, the dura should be punctured in the midline and the needle introduced into the subarachnoid space for only 2 to 3 mm. *If the patient feels paresthesia, the local anesthetic should not be injected before changing the position of the needle.* In the epidural space, if the drug is injected into the substance of the nerve, temporary or permanent damage may occur due to its compression and ischemia.[113] There is also the danger of centripetal spread causing damage to the spinal cord. The drugs usually injected for spinal block are markedly hypertonic due to the addition of dextrose. Thus, they carry an added danger if injected intramurally.

Serious neurologic complications are the result of gross negligence. If the contraindications are respected, the proper drugs injected, aseptic techniques followed, no force applied, and the physiology and the pharmacology understood, no case of paraplegia, cauda equina lesion, or brain damage should occur.

Bladder Dysfunction

Bladder dysfunction occurs in about 15 per cent of cases in the immediate postpartum period. It is mainly caused by the delivery and is unrelated to the regional block.[30,53,77] As expected, it is of higher incidence following forceps delivery than following spontaneous delivery, irrespective of the anesthetic technique.[53]

Following epidural analgesia with bupivacaine, the need for catheterization was significantly higher than following spinal block with lidocaine.[86] Bladder dysfunction can be due to overdistention of the bladder leading to its atony, or to inhibition of micturition caused by the abdominal incision in cesarean section or the perineal pain in vaginal delivery. *To avoid the need for catheterization and the possible introduction of infection, the following points are advised:*

1. The patient is encouraged to void before the start of the epidural block and before each refill dose, if possible.

2. A short-acting local anesthetic drug, such as chloroprocaine, is recommended for the delivery.

3. Analgesic drugs are administered once the patient complains of pain following recovery from the epidural analgesia.

Backache

During the hospital stay, backache is a common complaint among obstetric patients (about 32%).[30,53] In a study by Moir,[77] backache was recorded in 22 per cent of patients who had delivered under epidural block, and in 32 per cent of those who had received pudendal nerve block. Thus there is no substantiation of the belief that epidural puncture causes backache, even when performed with a 16-gauge needle. The incidence of backache is the same after general or conduction anesthesia, and the postpartum backache is usually caused by a faulty lithotomy position and the lordosis of pregnancy.[11] In a review of the complications of epidural analgesia, Dawkins[38] found the incidence to be 2 per cent in 9,107 cases. His figures probably indicate a long-term follow-up. The corresponding figure with caudal anesthesia was 7.6 per cent. When a very blunt needle (Cheng needle) was used for the epidural block, the incidence of backache was 30 per cent (see also Chap. 7).

To avoid backache, exercises during pregnancy help to build up the girdle muscles. Avoiding touching the periosteum, reaching the epidural space with a minimal number of attempts, and not using force are important points to minimize trauma to the back and subsequent backache. Also, during positioning of the patient from supine to lithotomy position and vice versa, both legs should be lowered simultaneously. Otherwise, twisting of the back combined with decreased muscle tone due to general or vertebral anesthesia puts a strain on the ligaments and predisposes to backache. The use of an abdominal binder to support the back in the postpartum period decreases the chances of developing backache (see also Chaps. 5 and 15).

Catheter Problems

Catheter problems have been discussed in detail with the technique.

Infection

Infection can lead to cellulitis, epidural abscess, arachnoiditis, myelitis, or a combination of two or more.[113] Because of the fear of infection a bacterial filter has been recommended in every case of continuous epidural analgesia for obstetrics.[36,40,60] However, such a recommendation has not been substantiated by a controlled study. Moreover, epidural abscesses have occurred despite the utilization of bacterial filters.[35,99] It is of interest to know that two of the most commonly used local anesthetic drugs in obstetrics, namely bupivacaine and chloroprocaine, have antibacterial actions.[45,60]

Adhering strictly to surgical aseptic techniques, utilizing a disposable adapter at the end of the epidural catheter, and using a disposable syringe for each injection[60] are important factors in lowering the incidence of contamination. The use of a filter is not a substitute for these rules. Moreover, in a controlled study using bacterial cultures from different segments of the epidural system (Fig. 14-14) it was found that the use of bacterial filters did not significantly lower the incidence of bacterial growth or the number of colonies.[3] Therefore, bacterial filters are not required for normal obstetric patients. In cases of prolonged use, e.g., for pain

therapy, especially in a diabetic or a debilitated patient, or when the dura has been inadvertently punctured, the use of bacterial filters may be of theoretical value and has to be evaluated. The above-mentioned bacteriological study has been substantiated with vast clinical experience since no infection has occurred in thousands of epidural blocks performed every year. In a close follow-up of 95 patients there was no clinical evidence of an epidural abscess or mass in the form of severe back pain and tenderness, inability to move the lower limbs, sensory disturbances, incontinence, rigor, and/or associated high fever.[3] In conclusion, although bacterial infection is a potential hazard, it takes gross breach in antiseptic techniques or a blood-borne infection to cause an epidural abscess. *In case such a complication arises,* surgical intervention is expeditiously required to relieve the pressure on the cord and stop the thrombophlebitis from interfering with its blood supply. Broad-spectrum antibiotics are administered until the cultures of the blood and/or the pus from the epidural

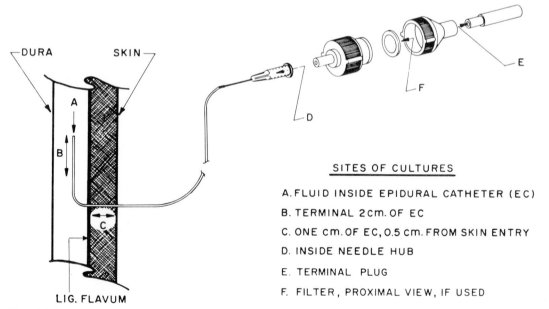

SITES OF CULTURES

A. FLUID INSIDE EPIDURAL CATHETER (EC)

B. TERMINAL 2 cm. OF EC

C. ONE cm. OF EC, 0.5 cm. FROM SKIN ENTRY

D. INSIDE NEEDLE HUB

E. TERMINAL PLUG

F. FILTER, PROXIMAL VIEW, IF USED

Fig. 14-14. Sites of cultures taken from the different segments of the epidural system. (Abouleish, E., et al.: Are bacterial filters needed in continuous epidural analgesia for obstetrics? Anesthesiology, *46*:351, 1977)

space determine the offending organism and the antibiotic sensitivity.

Introduction of a Foreign Body Into the Epidural Space

A foreign body in the epidural space may create a body reaction with the formation of a mass in the epidural space.[36] However, the use of a bacterial filter is not a guarantee against the access of foreign materials which can be introduced into the epidural space prior to the insertion of the filter,[36] e.g., a friable or shreddable material can be caught within the epidural needle and projected into the epidural space as the catheter is inserted. Moreover, the threads of the bacterial filter itself can be dislodged into the epidural space and become a nucleus for the formation of a space-occupying lesion. The only method of prevention of such a complication is vigilance and not bacterial filters.

Headache

In the absence of dural puncture, headache following epidural analgesia was not shown to be significantly different from that following pudendal nerve block.[77] In other comparative studies, the incidence of headache after general anesthesia was also the same as after pudendal nerve block.[121,123] On the whole, headache occurs in about 10 to 20 per cent of these procedures and is rarely severe. It is almost of the same incidence whether the patient delivers spontaneously or with forceps.[53] It differs from that following lumbar puncture by the fact that it is not worsened by the erect posture. Severe post-lumbar-puncture cephalgia following epidural analgesia, requiring epidural blood patch, occurs in about 1 per cent of cases[5] (see also Chap. 7).

Implantation Dermoid

The introduction of epidermal cells into the subarachnoid or epidural space can lead to the formation of a cyst causing pressure symptoms.[16] This is a very rare

complication and it takes several years for such a tumor to reach a size of clinical significance. To avoid such a problem, the use of an introducer with subarachnoid block is advisable. For epidural block, the use of a large sharp needle to cut the skin before inserting the Tuohy needle is recommended.

Horner's Syndrome

Extradural analgesia produces a high incidence of temporary myosis, ptosis, and enophthalmos.[76] The sympathetic outflow to the pupil leaves the spinal cord in the upper four thoracic nerves.[94] If these fibers are blocked, Horner's syndrome is produced and lasts for the duration of the block. It can occur on one side or bilaterally, and has no serious sequelae.

FETAL COMPLICATIONS

See Anatomy and Physiology Relative to Epidural Analgesia, above, Chapter 13, Caudal Analgesia, and Chapter 4, Local Anesthetic Drugs.

Mechanisms of Fetal Bradycardia Under Epidural Analgesia

1. Maternal hypotension
2. Compression of maternal abdominal aorta
3. Local anesthetic drug toxicity
   a. Local anesthetic inadvertently injected intravenously into the mother
   b. Fetal acidosis and "trapping" of the local anesthetic in the fetus
4. Accidental intrathecal injection in the mother: maternal hypoxia and hypotension
5. Sympathetic blockade of lower limbs vasculature before the uterines → "stealing" of blood from the placenta

---

INDICATIONS FOR THE USE OF EPIDURAL ANALGESIA

For vaginal delivery, epidural analgesia is indicated when the mother has pain and no contraindication is present.

In high-risk pregnancy epidural and/or caudal are especially indicated. These high-risk problems have been discussed in Chapter 13, Caudal Analgesia, and are listed as follows:

1. Delivery of a preterm infant
2. Maternal cardiac disease
3. Toxemias of pregnancy[60a,78,83]
4. Induction of labor
5. Multiple gestations[34,60b]
6. History of precipitous labor
7. Breech presentation[15,33]
8. Uterine dyskinesia
9. Operative vaginal delivery such as forceps rotation or forceps delivery
10. Diabetes mellitus[34]
11. Intrauterine growth retardation[29,30]
12. Rh-negative sensitization
13. Sickle cell disease[29,30]
14. Maternal hypertension

CONTRAINDICATIONS FOR THE USE OF EPIDURAL ANALGESIA

The anesthesiologist should be aware of the contraindications for the use of epidural analgesia, which are either absolute or relative.

Contraindications for the Use of Epidural Analgesia

Absolute Contraindications	Relative Contraindications
1. Anticoagulant therapy or bleeding diathesis	1. Cephalopelvic disproportion unless for trial labor or cesarean section
2. Hemorrhage	2. Previous cesarean section
3. Shock	3. Patient's choice
4. Infection	4. Inexperience of the team
5. Tumor at site of injection	5. Active central nervous system disease except epilepsy
6. Increased intracranial pressure	6. Backache
	7. Previous laminectomy
	8. Technical difficulties

ABSOLUTE CONTRAINDICATIONS

Anticoagulant Therapy or Bleeding Diathesis

If any vertebral block is attempted while the patient is under anticoagulant therapy or has a bleeding diathesis, a blood vessel may be injured, a hematoma is formed, the cord is compressed, and paraplegia occurs.[18,39,109,117] No anticoagulant therapy should be instituted while a catheter is in the epidural space. Movement of the catheter as the patient changes position in bed can injure a blood vessel and cause bleeding. Moreover, no patient should have anticoagulant therapy during the 24 hours following a vertebral block. There are cases of reported hematoma formation and paraplegia when such a therapy was instituted immediately following surgery under epidural analgesia.[113]

Hemorrhage

Cases of antepartum, intrapartum, or postpartum hemorrhage are contraindications to vertebral blocks, even if the blood pressure is normal. In such cases, the compensatory mechanisms of acute hypovolemia are increased sympathetic tone and vasoconstriction. Paralysis of the sympathetic fibers following a vertebral block can lead to severe hypotension which can endanger the mother's and/or the baby's lives.

Shock

Whatever the cause, shock is a contraindication to vertebral blocks because it can lead to cardiac arrest.

Infection

Infection can be:

1. *At the site of injection,* e.g., a boil or an abscess, or even active acne. There is the danger of introducing infection into the vertebral canal as the needle passes through the infected area, leading to an epidural abscess, osteomyelitis, or meningitis.

2. *Systemic infection such as septicemia.* If a blood vessel is injured in the vertebral canal, blood containing pathologic organisms is extravasated, forming ideal conditions for bacterial growth and abscess formation.

3. *Active meningitis.* The dura may be in-

jured, spreading the infection into the epidural space.

Tumor at the Site of Injection

In case of a tumor at the site of injection, there is the danger of introducing tumor cells into the epidural or subarachnoid spaces with the advancing needle.

Increased Intracranial Pressure

Epidural analgesia is contraindicated in cases of increased intracranial pressure because of the fear of further increase in the intracranial pressure or injury to the dura with sudden fall in pressure and cerebellar herniation (see also Chap. 13, Caudal Analgesia).

RELATIVE CONTRAINDICATIONS

Cephalopelvic Disproportion Unless for Trial Labor or Cesarean Section

See Chapter 13, Caudal Analgesia.

Previous Cesarean Section

See Chapter 13, Caudal Analgesia.

Patient's Choice

If the patient refuses a certain technique and efforts to change her mind fail, such a technique should not be forced upon her.

Inexperience of the Team

If the *anesthesiologist* is not familiar with a technique, he should not utilize it in an emergency situation. For example, if he is not used to the epidural technique and the management following it, not only is the failure rate high, but also the technique is difficult and hazardous. Such a situation can occur when an anesthesiologist with limited experience in obstetric anesthesia is asked to administer epidural to a highly recommended patient because the obstetrician has read that epidural analgesia is unequivocal. The prudent approach is that the anesthesiologist, under such a stressful situation, should use the method and drugs to which he is accustomed. However,

there should be a place for learning and practicing new techniques under adequate guidance and supervision.

If the *obstetrician* is not willing to cooperate, or if he lacks the experience to adequately monitor the fetus and the course of labor, to deal with such problems such as augmentation by oxytocin, or to use operative procedures such as forceps when required, then epidural technique should not be applied. If the *nursing staff* lacks interest and there is inadequate coverage to monitor the mother and coach her during the second stage of labor, epidural analgesia should not be used.

Active Central Nervous System Disease Except Epilepsy

For example, multiple sclerosis has spontaneous remissions and exacerbations, and if a patient with multiple sclerosis is administered an epidural block any flareup of the disease is bound to be attributed to the epidural block. However, in several such cases severe pain occurred during the first stage of labor requiring epidural analgesia. The technique was explained to the patients who accepted it, and thus the epidural block was administered with much gratitude by the patients and their relatives. Therefore, if the course of a disease is not expected to worsen because of the vertebral block, it should not be denied to the patient on just a medicolegal basis.

Backache

Backache is such a common condition that epidural or spinal should not be considered as contraindications because of its presence.[69] Also, the history of a prolapsed disk is not a contraindication to vertebral blocks which have been used by reputable anesthesiologists as the anesthetic techniques of choice.[69] Moreover, intrathecal, caudal, or epidural instillations of corticosteroids are used in the treatment of many syndromes in which sciatica and backache are common symptoms.

Previous Laminectomy

Following laminectomy, the landmarks may be difficult to feel and there may be adhesions between the dura and ligamentum flavum leading to increased chance of dural puncture and to inadequate spread of the local anesthetic. If the laminectomy is extensive in the lumbar region, a caudal or spinal block is preferable to epidural. If it is localized, an experienced anesthesiologist may attempt an epidural block at an intact interspace.

Technical Difficulties

Marked scoliosis, lordosis, and/or obesity constitute relative contraindications to vertebral blocks. However, with increased experience, these become lesser obstacles.

ROLE OF EPIDURAL ANALGESIA
ADVANTAGES OF EPIDURAL ANALGESIA

Skillfully administered epidural analgesia has many advantages both to the mother and fetus.

Advantage Over "Natural Childbirth"

1. There is less fetal and neonatal acidosis with epidural than with non-epidural cases.[88,89,110,125]

2. Based on the obstetric and anesthetic practice in Ontario, Canada, the neonatal mortality rate varied whether or not anesthesia was used.[98] For patients delivered without anesthesia, a neonatal mortality of 31.9 per thousand was recorded; with general anesthesia the neonatal mortality was 11.5 per thousand; and with epidural analgesia it was 8.2 per thousand live births.

3. There is decreased maternal oxygen consumption and lactic acidosis with epidural analgesia.[101]

Advantages Over General Analgesia

1. The use of narcotics supplemented by inhalation analgesia is the basis of pain relief in many countries today. Such a regimen even when administered conscientiously with close supervision by experienced medical staff can at the most provide satisfactory analgesia in less than 60 per cent of the parturients.[7] With epidural, the analgesia is superb, and in good hands the failure rate is negligible.

2. With epidural analgesia, the relaxed state of the pelvic floor makes maneuvers such as forceps rotation easier and much less traumatic for mother and fetus.

3. With epidural analgesia the incidence of nausea and vomiting is 12 per cent while with meperidine it is 23 per cent.

Advantages Over General Anesthesia

1. With epidural analgesia there is a lesser degree of fetal acidosis and better oxygenation than with general anesthesia.[46]

2. There is also less stress with epidural analgesia as evidenced by lower levels of plasma corticosteroid concentration than with general anesthesia.[50]

3. The danger of aspiration pneumonitis is markedly reduced by the use of epidural analgesia.

4. Epidural can be administered for both labor and delivery while general anesthesia is used only for the second stage.

5. With epidural, the mother is conscious and both parents can share and enjoy the moment of childbirth. This probably increases the attachment between parents and baby.

Advantages Over Subarachnoid Block

1. With epidural analgesia, the incidence and severity of hypotension is less than with subarachnoid block.[50a] This may be due to the fact that the sympathetic blockade with epidural is less than with subarachnoid block and the onset of hypotension is more gradual with epidural, thus giving the body systems and the anesthesiologist time to react.

2. The respiratory insufficiency with epidural is less than with spinal analgesia

because the degree and extent of muscular paralysis is less.

3. By varying the concentration of the local anesthetic, analgesia without muscular paralysis can be obtained more readily with epidural analgesia. Therefore, in cases such as breech presentation or multiple gestations this is advantageous since the mother can readily bear down.

4. The incidence of nausea and vomiting is less with epidural than with spinal analgesia, probably because of the decreased incidence and severity of hypotension with the former technique.

5. Epidural can be used for both labor and delivery while subarachnoid block is usually utilized for delivery only.

6. In the absence of dural puncture, epidural is not accompanied by post-lumbar-puncture cephalgia.

Advantages Over Paracervical Block

1. It is safer for the fetus and newborn to use epidural rather than paracervical block.

2. Paracervical block is limited to the first stage while epidural can be used throughout parturition.

3. Paracervical block does not relieve perineal pain.

Advantages Over Pudendal Nerve Block

1. Epidural analgesia can relieve both the uterine and perineal pain while pudendal nerve block only deals with the perineal nerves. Therefore, while epidural can be used for both the first and second stages of labor, pudendal nerve block is only used for delivery.

2. Epidural can be used for operative obstetric procedures such as forceps rotation; pudendal nerve block without supplementation is insufficient for such procedures.

3. The success rate with epidural analgesia is much higher than with pudendal nerve block.

4. The degree of fetal acidosis with epidural is less than with pudendal nerve block.[124]

DISADVANTAGES OF EPIDURAL ANALGESIA

Failure Rate

Failure to successfully complete an extradural block varies inversely with the skill of the anesthesiologist. In general, inability to achieve any kind of epidural analgesia is about 2 per cent.[38] If epidural has to be supplemented for delivery or cesarean section, this is considered unsatisfactory analgesia. With continuous epidural analgesia for vaginal delivery, sometimes additional treatment is required because the delivery is imminent or forceps extraction is necessary before the occurrence of adequate analgesia. For cesarean section, the inadequate analgesia usually is due to failure of blocking the sacral nerves. If surgery is started as soon as analgesia to pinprick on the abdomen develops, the analgesia may not always be adequate.

Increased Forceps Rate

Many obstetricians prefer the use of low-outlet forceps and episiotomy. They consider the episiotomy less traumatic to the mother than the stretching of the pelvic floor and the possibility of uncontrolled tears. It is also considered less traumatic to the fetus to be gently delivered by the outlet forceps rather than to allow the sudden release of the pressure on the fetal head as it comes out spontaneously through the unrelaxed perineum. In centers where spontaneous delivery is encouraged and the use of forceps is considered an obstetric interference, Doughty[41] found that in a 12-year period, although the number of deliveries under epidural had increased, the rate of forceps deliveries had decreased. Controlled studies have shown that even in nulliparae the rate of forceps deliveries is not higher with epidural than with nonepidural deliveries.[84,91] During the second stage of labor, although the patient does not push involuntarily, the expulsion effort can be sustained by the use of the auxiliary muscles. Blocking the sacral nerves inactivates the Ferguson reflex which normally guides the patient in her pushing. Nonetheless, the intelligent patient who is relieved of pain and properly coached is often better able to cooperate and push effectively during the expulsive phase.[90]

Unblocked Segment

Unblocked segment is defined as an area in which analgesia is absent while present above and below.[43] Pain in one groin is due to pulling on the round ligament and incomplete block of its nerve supply (T10 segment).[96] Therefore, although there is hypalgesia to pinprick, the pain relief is incomplete and this inadequacy becomes more evident as uterine contractions become stronger. Such a problem is less frequent with increasing experience of the anesthesiologist. It is due to insufficient dose of the local anesthetic or inadequate spread of the drug because of the effect of gravity or anterolateral position of the tip of the catheter. The problem can be avoided by administering adequate volume and concentration of bupivacaine, and limiting the length of the segment of the catheter in the epidural space. It can be corrected by treating the cause.

Problems Associated With the Catheter

Although the use of an epidural catheter is advantageous, catheters have their own problems, which have been discussed earlier. Therefore, if possible, reliance on the first dose injected through the needle is advisable, e.g., for cesarean section or if the patient is expected to deliver in about 1 hour. Then the catheter is inserted to be used for extending the duration of the block if required.

A Difficult Technique

The epidural block requires more skill and finesse than other techniques (e.g., subarachnoid block or general anesthesia). However, if the basic sciences are well un-

derstood, and proper training and supervision are provided, it is a safe, relatively easy, and reliable technique.

CONCLUSION

Epidural analgesia is not, and should not be, considered as the panacea for all patients in labor.[29,30] However, its judicious use during vaginal delivery can add to the parents' joy and the safety of mother and fetus. Should a cesarean section be required, analgesia can be undertaken by administering a refill dose through the catheter, thereby avoiding the risks of vomiting and aspiration associated with general anesthesia. The golden rule in obstetric anesthesia is that *if the patient has no pain, no analgesia is needed.*

A good medical center should be able to provide and use intelligently different methods of pain relief. In other words, anesthesia should be tailored to the patient rather than the other way around. Epidural and/or caudal blocks are up in the list of the requirements of any good obstetric hospital because of the superb relief of pain they provide during labor. At the present, with decrease in the use of paracervical block, there is much demand for epidural and/or caudal analgesia. The resentment against the use of these vertebral techniques stemming from assumptions and clinical impressions from limited clinical experience is harmful for the profession and the patient as well.

REFERENCES

1. Abouleish, E.: The inadvertent continuous spinal continued. Br. J. Anaesth. *46*:628, 1974.
2. ———: Preventing and detecting leakage in epidural catheters. Anesth. Analg. *53*:474, 1974.
3. Abouleish, E., Amortegui, T., and Taylor, F.: Are bacterial filters needed in continuous epidural analgesia for obstetrics? Anesthesiology, *46*:351, 1977.
4. Abouleish, E., Yamaoka, H., and Hingson, R. A.: Evaluation of a tapered spinal needle. Anesth. Analg. *53*:258, 1974.

5. Abouleish, E., *et al.*: Long-term follow-up of epidural blood patch. Anesth. Analg., *54*:459, 1975.
6. Aronski, A., *et al.*: Remarks on continuous epidural analgesia as a method of controlling pains during labour. Anaesth. Resusc. Intensive Ther., *1*:349, 1973.
7. Beagley, J. M., *et al.*: Relief of pain in labour. Lancet, *1*:1033, 1967.
8. Belfrage, P., *et al.*: Lumbar epidural analgesia with bupivacaine in labor. Am. J. Obstet. Gynecol., *121*:360, 1975.
9. Birkhan, P., and Heifetz, M.: Correspondence. The second thousand epidural blocks in an obstetric hospital. Br. J. Anaesth., *45*:334, 1973.
10. Boehm, F. H., Woodruff, L. F., Jr., and Growdon, J. H., Jr.: The effect of epidural anesthesia on fetal heart rate baseline variability. Anesth. Analg., *54*:779, 1975.
11. Bonica, J. J.: Principles and practice of Obstetric Anesthesia and Analgesia. P. 608. Philadelphia, F. A. Davis, 1967.
12. ———: Basic principles in obstetric anesthesia. *In* Shnider, S. M., and Moya, F. (eds.): The Anesthesiologist, Mother and Newborn. Pp. 3-19. Baltimore, Williams & Wilkins, 1974.
13. Bonica, J. J., *et al.*: Circulatory effects of peridural block. II. Effects of epinephrine. Anesthesiology, *34*:514, 1971.
14. Bose, N.: Unusual behavior of extradural analgesia. Br. J. Anaesth., *47*:806, 1975.
15. Bowen-Simpkins, P., and Fergusson, L. C.: Lumbar epidural block and the breech presentation. Br. J. Anaesth. *46*:420, 1974.
16. Brandus, V.: The spinal needle as a carrier of foreign material. Can. Anaesth. Soc. J., *5*:197, 1968.
17. Bridenbaugh, L. D., *et al.*: The position of plastic tubing in continuous block techniques: an x-ray study of 552 patients. Anesthesiology, *29*:1047, 1968.
18. Bridenbaugh, P. O.: Is administration of spinal anesthetic contraindicated in a patient with a normal coagulation profile, who will be systemically heparinized during the operative procedure? Anesth. Analg., *54*:507, 1975.
19. Bromage, P. R.: Spinal Epidural Analgesia. P. 92. Edinburgh and London, E. & S. Livingstone, 1954.
20. ———: Continuous lumbar epidural analgesia for obstetrics. Can. Med. Assoc. J., *85*:1136, 1961.
21. ———: Physiology and pharmacology of epidural analgesia. Anesthesiology, *28*:593, 1967.
22. ———: The incidence of dural puncture. Lancet, *1*:200, 1976.
23. Brotanek, V., *et al.*: The influence of epidural anesthesia on uterine blood flow. Obstet. Gynecol., *42*:276, 1973.
24. Burn, J. M., Guyer, P. B., and Langdon, L.: The spread of solutions injected into the epidural space: a study using epidurograms in patients with lumbosciatic syndrome. Br. J. Anaesth., *45*:338, 1973.
25. Casady, G. M., Moore, D. C., and Bridenbaugh, D. L.: Postpartum hypertension after use of vasoconstrictor and oxytocic drugs. J.A.M.A., *172*:101, 1960.
26. Caseby, N. G.: Epidural analgesia for the surgical induction of labour. Br. J. Anaesth., *46*:747, 1974.
27. Cibils, L. A., and Spackman, T. J.: Caudal analgesia in the first stage of labor: effect on uterine activity and the cardiovascular system. Am. J. Obstet. Gynecol., *84*:1042, 1962.
28. Close, A. S., *et al.*: Preoperative skin preparation with povidone-iodine. Am. J. Surg., *108*:398, 1964.
29. Crawford, J. S.: Lumbar epidural block in labour: a clinical analysis. Br. J. Anaesth., *44*:66, 1972.
30. ———: The second thousand epidural blocks in an obstetric hospital practice. Br. J. Anaesth., *44*:1277, 1972.
31. ———: Correspondence. Br. J. Anaesth., *45*:334, 1973.
32. ———: The strange case of the (inadvertent) continuous spinal. [Correspondence] Br. J. Anaesth., *46*:82, 1974.
33. ———: Lumbar epidural analgesia for the Singleton breech presentation. Anaesthesia, *40*:119, 1975.
34. ———: Patient management during extradural anaesthesia for obstetrics. Br. J. Anaesth., *47*:273, 1975.
35. ———: Pathology in the extradural space. Br. J. Anaesth., *47*:412, 1975.
36. Crawford, J. S., Williams, M. E., and Veales, S.: Particulate matter in extradural space. [Correspondence] Br. J. Anaesth., *47*:807, 1975.
37. Dauchot, P. J.: Unilateral analgesia after continuous epidural anesthesia in the obstetrical patient. Annual Meeting of the American Society of Anesthesiologists. Pp. 9–10. Washington, D.C., October 12–16. Abstracts of Scientific Papers, 1974.
38. Dawkins, M.: An analysis of the complications of epidural and caudal block. Anaesthesia, *24*:554, 1969.
39. DeAngelis, J.: Hazards of subdural and epidural anesthesia during anticoagulant therapy: a case report and review. Anesth. Analg., *51*:676, 1972.
40. Desmond, J.: The use of micropore filters in continuous epidural anaesthesia. Can. Anaesth. Soc. J., *19*:97, 1972.
41. Doughty, A.: Selective epidural analgesia and the forceps rate. Br. J. Anaesth., *41*:1058, 1969.
42. Dripps, R. V., and Vandam, L. D.: Long-term follow-up of patients who received 10,098 spinal anesthetics: failure to discover major neurological sequelae. J.A.M.A., *156*:1486, 1954.
43. Ducrow, M.: The occurrence of unblocked segments during continuous lumbar epidural analgesia for pain relief in labour. Br. J. Anaesth., *43*:1172, 1971.
44. Eckstein, K. L., and Marx, G. F.: Aortocaval compression and uterine displacement. Anesthesiology, *40*:92, 1974.

45. Foldes, F. F., and McNall, P. G.: 2-Chloroprocaine: new local anesthetic agent. Anesthesiology, *13*:287, 1952.

46. Fox, G. S., and Houle, G. L.: Acid-base studies in elective caesarean sections during epidural and general anaesthesia. Can. Anaesth. Soc. J., *18*:60, 1971.

47. Galindo, A., *et al.*: Quality of spinal extradural anaesthesia: the influence of spinal nerve root diameter. Br. J. Anaesth., *47*:41, 1975.

48. Gilbert, M. W., and Marx, G. F.: Extradural pressures in the parturient patient. Anesthesiology, *40*:499, 1974.

49. Gillies, I. D. S., and Morgan, M.: Accidental total spinal analgesia with bupivacaine. Anaesthesia, *28*:441, 1973.

50. Gordon, N. H., Scott, D. B., and Percy Robb, I. W.: Modification of plasma corticosteroid concentrations during and after surgery by epidural blockade. Br. Med. J., *1*:581, 1973.

50a. Gottschalk, W.: Regional anesthesia: I-Spinal, lumbar epidural, and caudal anesthesia. Obstet. Gynecol., Ann., *3*:377, 1974.

51. Green, R., and Massey, D.: Postoperative analgesia, the use of continuous drip epidural block. Anaesthesia, *21*:372, 1966.

52. Greiss, F. C.: A clinical concept of uterine blood flow during pregnancy. Obstet. Gynecol., *30*:595, 1967.

53. Grove, L. H.: Backache, headache, and bladder dysfunction after delivery. Br. J. Anaesth., *45*:1147, 1973.

54. Hehre, F. W., Hook, R., and Hon, E. H.: Continuous lumbar peridural anesthesia in obstetrics. VI. The fetal effects of transplacental passage of local anesthetic agents. Anesth. Analg., *48*:909, 1969.

55. Hehre, F. W., and Muechler, H. C.: Case history. Anesth. Analg., *44*:245, 1965.

56. Heldt, H. J., and Moloney, J. C.: Negative pressure in the epidural space. Am. J. Med. Sci., *175*:371, 1928.

57. Holmadahl, M. H., *et al.*: Clinical aspects of continuous epidural blockade for postoperative pain relief. Ups. J. Med. Sci., *77*:47, 1972.

58. Hopkins, E. L., Hendricks, C. H., and Cibils, L. A.: Cerebrospinal fluid pressure in labor. Am. J. Obstet. Gynecol., *93*:907, 1965.

59. James, F. M., Greiss, F. C., and Kemp, R. A.: An evaluation of vasopressor therapy for maternal hypotension during spinal anesthesia. Anesthesiology, *33*:25, 1970.

60. James, F. M., *et al.*: Bacteriologic aspects of epidural analgesia. Anesth. Analg., *55*:187, 1976.

60a. James, F. M., and Davies, P.: Maternal and fetal effects of lumbar epidural analgesia for labor and delivery in patients with gestational hypertension. Am. J. Obstet. Gynecol., *126*:195, 1976.

60b. James, F. M., *et al.*: Lumbar epidural analgesia for labor and delivery of twins. Am. J. Obstet. Gynecol., *127*:176, 1977.

61. Janzen, E.: Der negative Vorschlag bei Lumbalpunktion. Dtsch. Z. Nervenheilkd., *94*:280, 1926.

62. Kalas, D. B., and Hehre, F. W.: Continuous lumbar peridural anesthesia in obstetrics. VIII: Further observations on inadvertent lumbar puncture. Anesth. Analg., *51*:192, 1972.

63. Kandel, P. F., Spoerel, W. E., and Kinch, R. A. H.: Continuous epidural anaesthesia for labour and delivery: review of 1,000 cases. Can. Med. Asso. J., *95*:947, 1966.

64. Kaufman, R. D., and Reynolds, B. C.: Occlusion of an epidural catheter secondary to osteoarthritis. Anesthesiology, *44*:253, 1976.

65. Kim, J. M., and Robinson, J.: Uneven epidural analgesia—early diagnosis and correction: case reports. Anesth. Analg., *54*:593, 1975.

66. Kim, Y. I., Mazza, N. M., and Marx, G. F.: Massive spinal block with hemicranial palsy after a "test dose" for extradural analgesia. Anesthesiology, *43*:370, 1975.

67. Levinson, G., *et al.*: Effects of maternal hyperventilation on uterine blood flow and fetal oxygenation and acid-base status. Anesthesiology, *40*:340, 1974.

68. Lowensohn, R. I., *et al.*: Intrapartum epidural anesthesia. An evaluation of effects on uterine activity. Obstet. Gynecol., *44*:388, 1974.

69. Lund, P. C.: Is the presence of backache and sciatica a contraindication to spinal anesthesia. Anesth. Analg., *54*:505, 1975.

70. Lund, P. C., Cwik, J. C,, and Gannon, R. T.: Extradural anaesthesia: choice of local anaesthetic agents. Br. J. Anaesth., *47*:313, 1975.

71. McCaustand, A. M., and Holmes, F.: Spinal fluid pressure during labor. West. J. Surg., *65*:220, 1957.

72. Macintosh, R. R., and Mushin, W. W.: Observations on the epidural space. Anaesthesia, *2*:100, 1947.

73. Marx, G. F., and Orkin, L. R.: Cerebrospinal fluid proteins and spinal anesthesia in obstetrics. Anesthesiology, *26*:340, 1965.

74. Marx, G. F., Zemaitis, M. T., and Orkin, L. R.: Cerebrospinal fluid pressures during labor and obstetrical anesthesia. Anesthesiology, *22*:348, 1961.

75. Matadial, L., and Cibils, L. A.: The effect of epidural anesthesia on uterine activity and blood pressure. Am. J. Obstet. Gynecol., *125*:846, 1976.

76. Mohan, J., Lloyd, J. W., and Potter, J. M.: Pupillary constriction following extradural analgesia. Injury, *5*:151, 1973.

77. Moir, D. D., and Davidson, S.: Postpartum complications of forceps delivery performed under epidural and pudendal nerve block. Br. J. Anaesth., *44*:1197, 1972.

78. Moir, D. D., Victor-Rodrigues, L., and Willocks, J.: Epidural analgesia during labour in patients with pre-eclampsia. J. Obstet. Gynaecol. Br. Commonw., *79*:465, 1972.

79. Moore, D. C.: Regional Block. Ed. 4, p. 436. Springfield, Ill., Charles C Thomas, 1965.

80. Motoyama, E. K., *et al.*: Adverse effect of maternal hyperventilation of the foetus. Lancet, *1*:286, 1966.

81. Muneyuki, M., Shirai, K., and Inamoto, I.: Roentgenographic analysis of the positions of catheters in the epidural space. Anesthesiology, *33*:19, 1970.

81a. Munson, E. S., *et al.*: Etidocaine, bupivacaine and lidocaine seizure thresholds in monkeys. Anesthesiology, *42*:471, 1975.

82. Myers, R. E.: Maternal psychological stress and fetal asphyxia: a study in the monkey. Am. J. Obstet. Gynecol., *122*:47, 1975.

83. Mylks, G. W., Jones, K., and Douglas-Murray, G. M.: Acute fulminating eclampsia—management with prolonged epidural sympathetic block. Can. Med. Assoc. J., *82*:422, 1960.

84. Nash, T. G.: Epidural analgesia by the obstetrician: a personal series. Guys Hosp. Rep., *122*:313, 1973.

85. Odom, C. B.: Epidural anesthesia. Am. J. Surg., *34*:547, 1936.

86. Ostheimer, G. W.: Recovery room complications of epidural anaesthesia in the obstetric patient. Anaesthesia, *30*:120, 1975.

87. Pathy, G. V., and Rosen, M.: Prolonged block with recovery after extradural analgesia for labour. Br. J. Anaesth., *47*:520, 1975.

88. Pearson, J. F., and Davies, P.: The effect of continuous lumbar epidural analgesia on the acid-base status of maternal arterial blood during the first stage of labour. J. Obstet. Gynaecol. Br. Commonw., *80*:218, 1973.

89. ———: The effect of continuous lumbar epidural analgesia on maternal acid-base balance and arterial lactate concentrations during the second stage of labour. J. Obstet. Gynaecol. Br. Commonw., *80*:225, 1973.

90. Popper, P. J.: Evaluation of local anaesthetic agents for regional anaesthesia in obstetrics. Br. J. Anaesth., *47*:322, 1975.

91. Potter, N., and Macdonald, R. D.: Obstetrical consequences of epidural analgesia in nulliparous patients. Lancet, *1*:1031, 1971,

92. Printz, J. L., and McMaster, R. H.: Continuous monitoring of fetal heart rate and uterine contractions in patients under epidural anesthesia. Anesth. Analg., *51*:876, 1972.

93. Ralston, D. H., Shnider, S. M., and de Lorimer, A. A.: Effects of equipotent ephedrine, metaraminol, mephetermine, and methoxamine on uterine blood flow in the pregnant ewe. Anesthesiology, *40*:354, 1974.

94. Ray, B. S., Hinsey, J. C., and Geohegan, W. A.: Observations on the distribution of sympathetic nerves to pupil and upper extremity as determined by stimulation of anterior roots in man. Ann. Surg., *118*:647, 1943.

95. Reynolds, F.: The influence of adrenaline on maternal and neonatal blood levels of local analgesia drugs. *In* Symposium on Epidural Analgesia in Obstetrics. Pp. 31–40. London, H. K. Lewis, 1972.

96. Roberts, R. B.: The occurrence of unblocked segments during continuous lumbar epidural analgesia for pain relief in labour. Br. J. Anaesth., *44*:628, 1972.

97. Rosenfeld, C. R., Barton, M. D., and Meschia, G.: Circulatory effects of epinephrine in the pregnant ewe. Am. J. Obstet. Gynecol., *124*:156, 1976.

98. Russell, E. S.: Neonatal depression and mortality: influence of anaesthesia, sedation, and method of delivery. *In* Proceedings of the Fourth World Congress of Anesthesiologists. P. 35. International Congress Series, No. 168. Amsterdam, Excerpta Medica, 1968.

99. Saady, A.: Epidural abscess complicating thoracic epidural analgesia. Anesthesiology, *44*:244, 1976.

100. Sanchez, R., Acuna, L., and Rocha, F.: An analysis of the radiological visualization of the catheters placed in the epidural space. Br. J. Anaesth., *49*:485, 1967.

101. Sangoul, F., Fox, G. S., and Houle, G. L.: Effect of regional analgesia on maternal oxygen consumption during the first stage of labor. Am. J. Obstet. Gynecol., *121*:1080, 1975.

101a. Scanlon, J. W., *et al.*: Neurobehavioral responses of newborn infants after maternal epidural anesthesia. Anesthesiology, *40*:121, 1974.

102. Scanlon, J. W., *et al.*: Neurobehavioral responses and drug concentrations in newborns after maternal epidural anesthesia with bupivacaine. Anesthesiology, *45*:400, 1976.

103. Scarborough, C. D.: Continuous lumbar epidural anesthesia in obstetrical patient: administration by the mechanical constant infusion pump. South. Med. J., *65*:1134, 1972.

104. Schifrin, B. S.: Fetal heart rate patterns following epidural anaesthesia and oxytocin infusion during labour. J. Obstet. Gynaecol. Br. Commonw., *79*:332, 1972.

105. Scott, D. B.: Inferior vena cava occlusion during epidural block. *In* Proceedings of the Symposium on Epidural Analgesia in Obstetrics. Kingston Hospital, March 18, 1971.

105a. Scott, D. B.: Analgesia in labour. Brit. J. Anaesth., *49*:11, 1977.

105b. Scott, D. B.: Analgesia in labour. [Correspondence]. Brit. J. Anaesth., *49*:841, 1977.

106. Shnider, S. M.: Personal communication, 1976.

107. Shnider, S. M., de Lorimier, A. A., and Steffenson, J. L.: Vasopressors in obstetrics. III. Fetal effects of metaraminol infusion during obstetric spinal hypotension. Am. J. Obstet. Gynecol., *108*:1017, 1970.

108. Singh, A.: Unilateral epidural analgesia. Anaesthesia, *22*:147, 1967.

109. Sreerama, V., *et al.*: Neurosurgical complications of anticoagulant therapy. Can. Med. Assoc. J., *108*:305, 1973.

110. Thalme, B., Raabe, N., and Belfrage, P.: Lumbar epidural analgesia in labour. II. Effects on glucose, lactate, sodium, chloride, total protein, haematocrit and haemoglobin in maternal, fetal and neonatal blood. Acta Obstet. Gynecol. Scand., *53*:113, 1974.

111. Thornton, H. L., and Knight, P. F.: Emergency Anaesthesia. P. 153. London, Arnold, 1965.

112. Ueland, K., *et al.*: Maternal cardiovascular dynamics. VI. Cesarean section under epidural

anesthesia without epinephrine. Am. J. Obstet. Gynecol., *114*:775, 1972.

113. Usubiaga, J.: Neurological complications following epidural anesthesia. Int. Anesthesiol. Clin., *13*:3, 1975.

114. Usubiaga, J. E., Dos Reis, A., Jr., and Usubiaga, L. E.: Epidural misplacement of catheters and mechanisms of unilateral blockade. Anesthesiology, *32*:158, 1970.

115. Usubiaga, J. E., *et al.*: Effect of saline injections on epidural and subarachnoid space pressures and relation to postspinal anesthesia headache. Anesth. Analg., *46*:293, 1967.

116. Vander Wyk, R. W.: Killing efficiency of an iodophor: laboratory study of the microbicidal activity of povidone-iodine. Anesthesiology, *34*:371, 1967.

117. Varkey, G. P., and Brindle, G. F.: Peridural anaesthesia and anti-coagulant therapy. Can. Anaesth. Soc. J., *21*:106, 1974.

118. Vasicka, A., and Kretchmer, H.: Uterine dynamics. Clin. Obstet. Gynecol., *4*:17, 1961.

119. Vasicka, A., *et al.*: Spinal and epidural anesthesia: fetal and uterine response to acute hypo- and hypertension. Am. J. Obstet. Gynecol., *90*:800, 1964.

120. Wallis, K. L., *et al.*: Epidural anesthesia in the normotensive pregnant ewe: effects on uterine blood flow and fetal acid-base status. Anesthesiology, *44*:481, 1976.

121. White, C. W., *et al.*: Anesthesia and postpartum headache. Obstet. Gynecol., *20*:734, 1962.

122. Wilson, J.: Discussion. *In* Crawford, J. S.: Patient management during extradural anaes-

thesia for obstetrics. Br. J. Anaesth., *47*:273, 1975.

123. Winkler, W. P., Sherk, W. M., and Hale, R.: Postpartum spinal headache. Am. J. Obstet. Gynecol., *85*:500, 1963.

123a. Wolman, I. J., Evans, B., and Lasker, S.: The specific gravity of cerebrospinal fluid. Am. J. Clin. Pathol., *16*:33, 1946.

124. Zador, G., Lindmark, G., and Nilsson, B. A.: Pudendal block in normal vaginal delivery. Acta Obstet. Gynecol. Scand. [Suppl.], *34*:51, 1974.

125. Zador, G., and Nilsson, B. A.: Low dose intermittent epidural anaesthesia in labour. II. Influence on labour and foetal acid-base status. Acta Obstet. Gynecol. Scand. [Suppl.], *34*:17, 1974.

126. ———: Continuous drip epidural anaesthesia in labour. II. Influence on labour and foetal acid-base status. Acta Obstet. Gynecol. [Suppl.], *34*:41, 1974.

127. Zador, G., Willdeck-Lund, G., and Nilsson, B. A.: Continuous drip lumbar epidural anaesthesia with lignocaine for vaginal delivery. Acta Obstet. Gynecol. Scand. [Suppl.], *34*:31, 1974.

128. Zilanti, S. M.: Fetal heart rate and pH of fetal capillary blood during epidural analgesia in labor. Obstet. Gynecol., *36*:881, 1970.

129. Zorraquin, G.: Anesthesie metamerique peridurale. Pregr. Med., *44*(1):783, 1936.

130. Zuspan, F. P., Cibils, L. A., and Pose, S. V.: Myometrical and cardiovascular responses to alterations in plasma epinephrine and norepinephrine. Am. J. Obstet. Gynecol., *84*:841, 1962.

15

Subarachnoid Block

Ezzat Abouleish, M.D.

DEFINITION

Subarachnoid block is the reversible nerve block produced by injection of local anesthetic into the subarachnoid space. Subarachnoid block, spinal block, spinal analgesia, spinal anesthesia, and lumbar anesthesia are all synonyms.

HISTORY

In 1885, while J. Leonard Corning of the United States was experimenting with cocaine in dogs, he accidentally injected the drug into the subarachnoid space, thus producing the first spinal block in history. Later in the same year, he used subarachnoid block in man for the treatment of ailments such as premature ejaculation.

In 1899, Bier of Germany was the first to use subarachnoid block for anesthesia in surgery. In 1900, Kreis of Germany was the first to use subarachnoid block for pain relief in obstetrics.

Following the discovery of the analgesic value of subarachnoid block, the use of spinal anesthesia flourished and the technique was refined. However, since 1942 the use of muscle relaxants has tended to overshadow subarachnoid block.[73] The former drugs allowed better and safer control of general anesthesia by providing easy intubation and adequate muscle relaxation in association with light planes of anesthesia.

Recently, subarachnoid block has become a much safer technique than three decades ago because of the better understanding of its physiology, the introduction of reliable, safe, and potent local anesthetic drugs, the use of proper methods of sterilization of instruments, and the production of better equipment, especially fine spinal needles. The awareness of the danger of aspiration pneumonitis in association with general anesthesia, the better condition of the neonates with subarachnoid block, and the interest of parents to watch and enjoy the delivery process stabilized the use of subarachnoid block in obstetrics as an important and useful anesthetic armamentarium. In fact, subarachnoid block in the United States is mostly utilized in obstetrics rather than in surgery.

ANATOMY AND PHYSIOLOGY RELATIVE TO SUBARACHNOID BLOCK

ANATOMICAL CONSIDERATIONS

At birth, the spinal cord extends from the foramen magnum to the third lumbar vertebra (L3) while in adults it usually ends at the upper part of the L2 vertebra. With flexion of the back, the spinal cord terminates at the lower part of the L1 vertebra. The subarachnoid space extends caudad to the second sacral vertebra (S2). Therefore,

305

by introducing the spinal needle below the L2 vertebra, lumbar puncture or subarachnoid block can be safely performed without trauma to the spinal cord.

The spinal cord is surrounded by the meninges, which are the spinal dura, the arachnoid mater, and the pia mater. The spinal dura is a continuation of the inner layer of the cranial dura and forms the outer layer of the sac containing the cerebrospinal fluid. Internally the dura is lined by the smooth endothelial layer called arachnoid mater, which is very thin and closely attached to the dura; therefore, once the dura is punctured, the arachnoid is usually punctured as well. The third investing layer is the pia mater, which closely surrounds the brain and the spinal cord and is separated from the arachnoid mater by cerebrospinal fluid (see Fig. 7-1).

As the nerves extend from the spinal cord to the periphery, they are covered by these three investing layers. During their passage through the subarachnoid space the nerves are covered only by the thin pia mater; thus they are easily and rapidly blocked by the local anesthetic drugs. In the epidural space, the nerves have arachnoidal and dural sleeves as well; therefore, the local anesthetics have difficulty in reaching them. The meningeal sleeves usually end and fuse with epineurium at the intervertebral foramina where the anterior and posterior nerve roots unite. However, they may rarely extend outside the vertebral column. Thus, during a paravertebral block the needle may enter one of these pockets and the injected drug may thus gain access to the subarachnoid space causing a subarachnoid block.

In addition to nerves, the subarachnoid space is traversed by arteries and veins on their way to and from the spinal cord. These blood vessels are surrounded by microscopic spaces called the perivascular spaces which are extensions of the subarachnoid space and advance into the substance of the spinal cord. Local anesthetics administered into the subarachnoid space can diffuse along these spaces to reach the spinal cord, thus causing blockade of the structures in the neuraxis.[87] Therefore, a spinal or an epidural block can start by a radicular blockade, causing a slanting segmental distribution on the body surface. With time, this distribution of the blockade changes to one that is almost transverse, denoting intraspinal action of the drug. Because of the difference in rates of anesthetic uptake and elimination, the cord blockade becomes clinically apparent as the block of the nerve roots wears off, i.e., it is detected during recession of the subarachnoid or epidural blockade.

The line joining the highest parts of the iliac crests usually, but not always, crosses the fourth lumbar spinous process (see Fig. 14-6A). The lumbar spinous processes are broad, extending posteriorly from the bodies of the vertebrae almost at a right angle with slight caudad direction. Thus the tip of each spinous process, as felt by palpation through the skin of the back, corresponds with the lower part of its vertebral body (see Fig. 14-2).

If the vertebral column of a supine or standing person is laterally viewed, a series of alternating curvatures is observed, i.e. cervical lordosis, thoracic kyphosis, lumbar lordosis, then sacral kyphosis (Fig. 15-1). In the supine position, the highest point of the vertebral canal is at the fourth lumbar vertebra and the lowest point is at the fifth thoracic vertebra. If a local anesthetic with a specific gravity higher than that of the cerebrospinal fluid (hyperbaric solution) is injected into the subarachnoid space caudad to L4 (i.e., between L4 and L5 or L5 and S1), it becomes very hard for it to spread cephalad. This is one reason for failure to reach an adequate level of block following subarachnoid block for cesarean section. On the other hand, having all other factors constant, injection of the local anesthetic at L2 to L3 can cause a marked cephalad spread, not only because L2 to L3

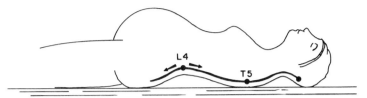

Fig. 15-1. The spinal curvatures. Notice the alternating curvatures of the spine. The highest part of the curvatures is L4 and the lowest part is T5. Injection of a hyperbaric solution caudad to L4 tends to spread caudad rather than cephalad, and vice versa.

is closer to the thoracic segments than L3 to L4, but also because it is on the cephalad slope of the lumbar curve.

The lumbar lordosis varies with different individuals and in different races, being more exaggerated in Negroes than in Caucasians. In order to balance for the protruding abdomen, lumbar lordosis is also increased by obesity and by full term pregnancy, particularly with twins or hydramnios. Exaggerated lumbar lordosis makes lumbar puncture more difficult.

Theoretically, a hyperbaric solution cannot spread beyond the fifth thoracic vertebra because this is the most dependent part of the spinal canal when the patient is in the supine position. Practically this is not the case with the hyperbaric solution injected into the lumbar region. As it spreads further from the site of injection a hyperbaric solution becomes diluted and

more or less isobaric, thus easily reaching beyond T5.

The subarachnoid space can be reached by inserting the needle between the spinous processes and then through the interlaminar space. Flexion of the back widens not only the interspinous gap but also the interlaminar space (Fig. 15-2). Although the lordosis of pregnancy and the enlarged uterus do not allow for optimum flexion of the back and widening of the interlaminar space, in a cooperative patient this is usually sufficient to allow for the median approach to the subarachnoid space. In cases of abnormal lordosis or calcification of ligaments of the back, the paramedian approach is preferred. The needle is inserted just lateral to the spinous process and directed medially, anteriorly, and cephalad (Fig. 15-3), thus avoiding the obstacle caused by the spinous processes and their

Fig. 15-2. The importance of back flexion during epidural or subarachnoid block. Back flexion widens, not only the interspinous space but also the interlaminar space.

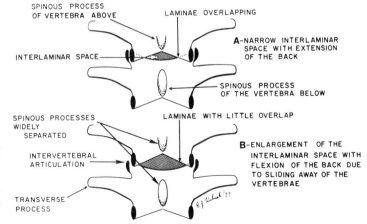

SPINOUS PROCESS OF VERTEBRA ABOVE
LAMINAE OVERLAPPING
INTERLAMINAR SPACE
A-NARROW INTERLAMINAR SPACE WITH EXTENSION OF THE BACK
SPINOUS PROCESS OF THE VERTEBRA BELOW

SPINOUS PROCESSES WIDELY SEPARATED
LAMINAE WITH LITTLE OVERLAP
INTERVERTEBRAL ARTICULATION
B-ENLARGEMENT OF THE INTERLAMINAR SPACE WITH FLEXION OF THE BACK DUE TO SLIDING AWAY OF THE VERTEBRAE
TRANSVERSE PROCESS

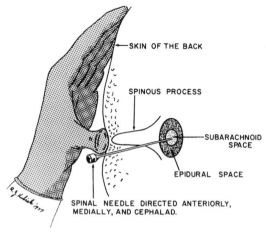

SKIN OF THE BACK

SPINOUS PROCESS

SUBARACHNOID SPACE

EPIDURAL SPACE

SPINAL NEEDLE DIRECTED ANTERIORLY, MEDIALLY, AND CEPHALAD.

Fig. 15-3. The paramedian approach to the subarachnoid space. Although the needle punctures the skin to one side of the midline, the dura is penetrated at the midline. By using the paramedian approach, the spinous process and the ligaments attached to it are avoided.

ligaments. Flexion of the back should be performed as much as possible whether the median or paramedian approach is followed in order to widen the interlaminar space.

In the *median approach*, the tissues that a spinal needle has to pass through before reaching the subarachnoid space are: the skin, subcutaneous tissue, supraspinous ligament, interspinous ligament, ligamentum flavum, epidural space, dura and arachnoid (see Fig. 14-2). Using the *paramedian approach*, the tissues to be traversed are: the skin, subcutaneous tissue, lumbar aponeurosis, ligamentum flavum, epidural space, dura and arachnoid (Fig. 15-3).

The nerve supply of the abdominal contents is shown in Figure 15-4 and explained in the accompanying legend. Pulling on the peritoneum and exploring the abdomen require the blocking of all the splanchnic nerves. Therefore, for any intra-abdominal surgery, including cesarean section, the level of the block should reach T5 to ensure adequate analgesia. However, traction on the omentum or viscera may cause distressing unpleasant sensation due to stimulation of the intact vagus nerve. The surgeon and his assistants should realize this fact and be as gentle as possible.

FACTORS CONTROLLING THE SPREAD OF THE LOCAL ANESTHETIC DRUG IN THE SUBARACHNOID SPACE

Dosage

The larger the dose of the drug injected, the more extensive the block becomes. The volume of the injection plays a minor role compared to the total dose.

Specific Gravity of the Injected Local Anesthetic

The specific gravity of cerebrospinal fluid varies between 1.003 and 1.009, with an average of 1.007 at 37° C. compared to water at the same temperature. A local anesthetic is considered hyperbaric if its specific gravity is higher than 1.011 and hypobaric if it is less than 1.003.[38] The further the specific gravity of the injectate is from that of the cerebrospinal fluid, the more controllable the direction of flow and the more predictable the level of the block. That is one of the reasons the author prefers 5 per cent lidocaine in 7.5 per cent dextrose (specific gravity, 1.032) to 0.5 per cent tetracaine in 5 per cent dextrose (specific gravity, 1.018).

Position of the Patient, Especially During Injection

If a hyperbaric solution is injected while the patient is sitting and the patient is kept in this position for 3 minutes following injection, the solution gravitates caudad and tends to be limited to the lower lumbar and sacral regions, leading mainly to perineal analgesia, the so-called saddle block. When the patient is in the lateral position, the direction of the vertebral column is not necessarily parallel to the direction of the table. In females in whom shoulders are narrower than the pelvis, the spine is more

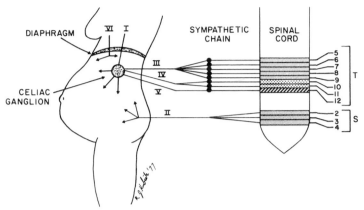

Fig. 15-4. Nerve supply of the abdominal contents.
Parasympathetic System:
  I. Vagus nerve. Relays in celiac ganglion. It supplies abdominal viscera to and including the transverse colon and omentum.
  II. Pelvic parasympathetic (S2–S4). Supplies splenic flexure of the colon, descending colon, and pelvic organs.
Sympathetic System:
  III. Greater splanchnic nerve (T5–T9)
  IV. Lesser splanchnic nerve (T10–T11)
  V. Least splanchnic nerve (T12)
All sympathetic fibers relay in the celiac ganglion before distribution to abdominal and pelvic contents.
  VI. Phrenic nerve (C3, C4, C5); motor and sensory (e.g., abdominal surface of diaphragm usually not blocked by spinal)

in a Trendelenburg position if the table is horizontal. Therefore, hyperbaric solutions tend to spread more cephalad in this position. During the induction of subarachnoid block, attention should be paid to the direction of the patient's vertebral column rather than to the position of the table (See Fig. 14-6A). Following injection there is a certain period during which changing the patient's position affects the level of the block. This period is usually 5 minutes and can extend up to 10. The later the change of posture, the less the effect on the block level, because more and more of the local anesthetic has become fixed by the neural tissues and absorbed through circulation. In fact, after about 5 minutes, putting the patient in the Trendelenburg position to correct inadequate levels of analgesia with cesarean section does not significantly increase the level of analgesia.

It only causes more cephalad spread of a dilute anesthetic solution which is sufficient to block only the sympathetic fibers, thus causing hypotension.

When a hyperbaric solution is injected while the patient is in the lateral position, the anesthesia starts in the dependent side, and then ultimately both sides will be equally anesthetized. Therefore, to test for the level of analgesia in the first few minutes following injection, it is logical to do so in the dependent side because analgesia may be quite limited or may even not have started on the other side.

Volume of Cerebrospinal Fluid

Owing to the increased blood volume in the spinal canal due to dilatation of the vertebral veins, the volume of cerebrospinal fluid is reduced in late pregnancy. Therefore to obtain the same level of block, the ratio of the dose for a parturient compared to that for a nonpregnant female is 2 to 3. This is the main reason some anesthesiologists who are acquainted only with subarachnoid block for cesarean section achieve inadequate block if they use the same dose for abdominal hysterectomy in a nonpregnant patient.

The volume of cerebrospinal fluid is also affected by the degree of hydration, being reduced if the patient is dehydrated.

Height of the Patient

The dose of a local anesthetic used for subarachnoid block is determined by the patient's height rather than her weight. For example, the doses used for cesarean section are shown in Table 15-1, and are determined by the patient's height.

Site of Injection

As explained earlier, owing to the curvature of the spine the site of injection plays a major role in determining the level of the subarachnoid block. As the solution spreads away from the site of injection, two things happen: the solution is taken up by the nerves en route, and the solution becomes more dilute. This has the following results: first, close to the site of injection the block starts earlier, is most solid, and lasts longer than at the periphery; second, since the autonomic fibers are the smallest in diameter and have the largest relative surface area, they are the most widely affected fibers, followed by the sensory, and then the motor fibers.

Rate and Force of Injection

Rapid and forceful injection of the local anesthetic tends to spread it widely by causing turbulent currents. Although by using a fine spinal needle, 25- or 26-gauge, the speed of injection is limited, yet it still can affect the level of the block. The usual rate of injection is 5 to 10 seconds for vaginal delivery and 10 to 15 seconds for cesarean section.

Barbotage

During the administration of the local anesthetic, the process of the repeated alternating aspiration and injection of cerebrospinal fluid is called barbotage. It creates eddies which carry the local anesthetic far away from the site of injection. The level of the block thus reached is unpredictable and can be dangerously high. Therefore, the use of barbotage to spread the local anesthetic block is not advisable. The aspiration of a small volume of cerebrospinal fluid (0.1 ml.) just before injection and immediately after termination to verify the correct position of the needle is not harmful and not considered barbotage.

Increased Intra-abdominal Pressure

Coughing, pushing, and vomiting increase the intrathoracic and intra-abdominal pressures and further distend the vertebral veins. Therefore they tend to squeeze the cerebrospinal fluid and the local anesthetic and widely extend the block. The local anesthetic injection is pre-

Table 15-1.   Doses of Local Anesthetic Drugs for Cesarean Section Under Subarachnoid Block

Drug	Dose According to Patient's Height			
	150 cm. *(5 ft.)*	*157.5 cm.* *(5 ft. 3 in.)*	*165 cm.* *(5 ft. 6 in.)*	*172.5 cm.* *(5 ft. 9 in.)*
Tetracaine	6 mg.	7 mg.	8 mg.	9 mg.
Lidocaine*	50 mg.	60mg.	70 mg.	80 mg.

*Epinephrine, 0.2 mg., is added to lidocaine routinely. The addition of epinephrine to tetracaine is only required if surgery is expected to last more than 2 hours.

ferably done between contractions when the patient is not bearing down. If delivery is imminent, the drug is injected even while the patient is pushing, but other factors should be used to compensate for the expected increased spread of the block, e.g., by modifying the table position. In obese patients or in case of a large fetus, hydramnios, or multiple gestations, the intra-abdominal pressure is higher than usual; thus, the dose should be reduced.

Direction of the Needle Bevel

With regular spinal needles the direction of the bevel does not influence the extent of the block. It is only with the Whitacre needle that the direction of the opening affects the spread of the anesthetic;[50] the Whitacre needle is a special needle which has a closed tapering pencil-like tip with an opening to one side 2 mm. from the tip.

PHYSIOLOGICAL CHANGES IN THE MOTHER AND/OR BABY PRODUCED BY SUBARACHNOID BLOCK

MATERNAL EFFECTS OF SUBARACHNOID BLOCK

Cardiovascular Effects

The main danger as well as the major maternal effect of subarachnoid block is maternal hypotension. This complication can seriously affect the mother and/or baby. Therefore, it should be avoided if possible and properly treated if it occurs (see Chap. 5, Effects of Vertebral Blocks on the Cardiovascular System).

With subarachnoid block especially for cesarean section, the following measures are recommended: proper fluid administration, e.g., 500 to 1,000 ml. within 10 minutes of the block, left uterine displacement, and the immediate use of a beta-stimulant vasopressor in adequate dosage as soon as the systolic blood pressure falls below 80 per cent of the original level. Either ephedrine or mephentermine can be used since they are capable of restoring both the maternal blood pressure and the uterine blood flow.[31,77] The use of alpha stimulants such as methoxamine or phenylephrine is not advised because, although these drugs can correct the maternal hypotension, they fail to improve the uterine blood flow, leading to fetal hypoxia and acidosis. They also increase the uterine tone, thus reducing the perfusion of the intervillous space. However, if the administration of an adequate dosage of a beta stimulant, e.g., two 15-mg. doses of mephentermine, fails to restore the maternal blood pressure and is accompanied by maternal tachycardia, then there is a need for an alpha-stimulant drug. The latter is administered intravenously in dilute amounts and in small increments while the blood pressure is carefully recorded until the blood pressure is restored. Under these circumstances of having a fluid load of at least one liter and a relatively large dose of a beta-stimulant drug, the patient is very sensitive to the administration of alpha stimulants and care should be taken to avoid excessive elevation of the blood pressure.

To prevent hypotension, the prophylactic intramuscular administration of vasopressors is not advisable. Following delivery, there is an increase of 80 to 100 per cent in the cardiac output which is compensated for by decreased peripheral resistance, thus keeping the blood pressure more or less normal.[7] If an alpha stimulant has been given intramuscularly, the peak of action occurs at that time, offsetting the compensatory peripheral vasodilatation and leading to severe hypertension. If a beta stimulant has been injected intramuscularly, it may not be needed since the fall in blood pressure is not always predictable, and in the pregnant woman there is no correlation between the level of anesthesia and the degree of hypotension[85]; moreover, its peak of action may occur when it is undesirable, i.e., after delivery. Therefore, the best policy is to monitor the blood pressure very closely, especially with elective cesarean section, and to correct it as soon as it falls below 80 per cent of the original level with intravenous drugs in adequate dosage.

Respiratory Effects

Details of respiratory effects have been explained in Chapter 6, Effects of Vertebral Blocks on the Respiratory System. It is sufficient to mention here that the main cause of respiratory arrest is ischemia of the respiratory center due to hypotension. The thickly myelinated phrenic nerves are resistant to the block by the local anesthetic which is much diluted as it reaches the cervical region.[27] By maintaining the blood pressure, inadequacy of ventilation is usually of short duration and the respiration improves as soon as the fetus is delivered. *No subarachnoid block is to be performed unless the operator is familiar with cardiopulmonary resuscitation and the required equipment and drugs are readily available. The patient should be closely monitored following the induction of the block.*

Nervous Effects

Nervous effects have been explained in detail in Chapter 7, Effects of Vertebral Blocks on the Nervous System. If the blood pressure is kept within normal limits, usually no dangerous effect occurs on the central nervous system. The essential points contributing to the safety of subarachnoid block include: (1) proper sterilization of equipment, with the avoidance of detergent solutions; (2) strict aseptic techniques; (3) respect of contraindications; (4) the choice of the lumbar puncture site; (5) the use of fine needles; (6) stopping of the injection of any drug into the subarachnoid space and checking the label on the used ampule if the patient is complaining of pain during the injection; and (7) the dexterity of the operator in performing lumbar puncture.

As stated in Chapter 7, drowsiness is common with epidural analgesia due to the central nervous system depressant action of the local anesthetic drug absorbed into the circulation. With high spinal analgesia, drowsiness is mainly due to reducing the afferent impulses to the central nervous system from a large part of the body. If the block is extensive, the local anesthetic reaching the brain stem can paralyze the reticular activating system. Even dilute concentrations of the local anesthetic, insufficient to cause respiratory or vasomotor center paralysis, can affect the reticular activating system. Being polysynaptic and rich in nerve cells, the latter is very susceptible to the action of local anesthetics. Another contributing factor to central nervous system depression with high spinal block is hypotension.[42] These factors can also contribute to the central nervous system depression associated with epidural analgesia.

In cesarean section when large doses of local anesthetics have been administered, it has been the author's experience to observe drowsiness with epidural analgesia. However, with subarachnoid block patients are usually alert and their reactions almost as good as before the block. The only exception with spinal analgesia occurs when the patient has had a long, hard labor and/or large doses of narcotics have been administered; the relief of pain by the subarachnoid block sometimes puts the patient to sleep.

Gastrointestinal Effects

Nausea and vomiting under spinal anesthesia are usually symptoms of hypotension.[12,67] Correction of the hypotension relieves the symptoms and the administration of oxygen decreases their incidence.[72] Other factors causing nausea and vomiting include psychological problems, hyperacidity, narcotics, intra-abdominal manipulations such as pulling on the omentum, and autonomic imbalance due to paralysis of the sympathetic fibers while the parasympathetic remain intact. The incidence of nausea and vomiting is higher with subarachnoid block than with epidural analgesia, and more with cesarean section than with vaginal delivery. To prevent this complication, the blood pressure should be closely monitored and hypotension should be immediately corrected. Routine oxygen administration is advised with cesarean section where the incidence of hypotension and the possibility of respiratory insufficiency are high.

If nausea and vomiting persist despite the adequacy of the blood pressure, 1.25 mg. (0.5 ml.) of droperidol, which can be repeated once, is usually beneficial. It must be remembered that although this drug's antiemetic property is 800 times that of chlorpromazine,[76] it is also an alpha blocker; therefore, the blood pressure should be maintained before its administration and closely checked thereafter.

Under subarachnoid block the intestines are usually well contracted due to the produced autonomic imbalance. This has been a long-noticed advantage of spinal anesthesia for abdominal surgery and was used to treat paralytic ileus.

Hepatic Effects

If the blood pressure is maintained near its original level, subarachnoid block has no harmful effect on the liver.[27,81]

Renal Effects

As applies to all parenchymatous organs, if the blood pressure is well maintained, subarachnoid block has no deleterious effects on the kidneys.

Metabolic Effects

In the absence of hypoxia and/or marked hypotension, subarachnoid block has minimal effects on metabolism. Thus, it is indicated in diabetic patients.

Effects on Uterine Contractility

During Pregnancy. In regard to the developing fetus, because of the negligible amount of drug administered subarachnoid block is one of the safest techniques of anesthesia for surgery during gestation. If subarachnoid block has any effect at this stage on uterine contractility, it causes a decrease in the intensity, duration, and tonus of the uterine contractions. Therefore, subarachnoid block does not have an abortive effect.[51]

During the First and Second Stages of Labor. There was much controversy in regard to the effect of subarachnoid block on uterine activity. Some considered it to increase uterine muscle tone, and thus it was contraindicated in cesarean section, especially in case of a compromised fetus or obstructed labor. Others considered it to stop labor and arrest delivery. These unjustified conclusions were based on clinical impressions and were not substantiated with any accurate measurements of uterine activity.

In 1930, for the first time Mohan used external hysterography for evaluating the effects of subarachnoid block on uterine contractions. However, the utilization of external monitors for such a measurement[69] does not provide accurate information because the external monitors are influenced by the tone and contraction of the abdominal muscles which can be paralyzed by the subarachnoid block.

Neme[52] studied the effects of continuous subarachnoid block during the various stages of labor in the same patient, at various levels of blocks and during their regression. He directly and simultaneously measured the intra-amniotic pressure and the intramyometrial pressures in the upper, mid, and lower uterine segments (Fig. 15-5). His results have shown that subarachnoid block does not cause any remarkable alterations in the uterine activity irrespective of the stage of labor or the level of the block up to the T2 segment. If any change does occur after subarachnoid block, it is a tendency of a slight increase in intensity and duration of contraction with a decrease in frequency. Therefore, there

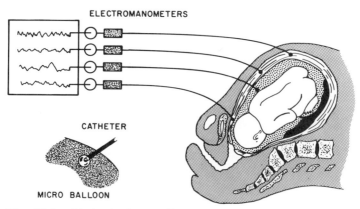

Fig. 15-5. Method of recording the amniotic pressure and simultaneously the intramyometrial pressure in the fundus, median, and lower parts of the uterus. (Neme, B.: Effects of spinal anesthesia on pregnant human uterine contractility. Matern. Infanc., *30*:189, 1971)

is no danger to the fetus from sustained uterine contractions. The difficulty encountered during a cesarean section is attributed to attempts to deliver the baby during a uterine contraction rather than to a tetanic contracture of the uterus. On the other hand, spinal anesthesia is not the method of choice if relaxation of the uterus is required for intrauterine manipulation, e.g., internal podalic version. Although subarachnoid block has no direct effect on uterine contractions, it can indirectly influence uterine activity by changing the blood pressure. Vasicka and Kretchner[90] have shown that subarachnoid block, even up to the T1 level, does not change the uterine contractions except if hypotension occurs, in which case significant reduction in uterine activity results. On the other hand, hypertension associated with subarachnoid block is followed by increased uterine contractions. In this study, however, the hypertension was iatrogenically produced by the administration of alpha-adrenergic stimulants, which are known to have a direct oxytocic effect. Therefore, the increase in uterine contractions is not necessarily due to the hypertension.

The paralysis of the pelvic floor due to subarachnoid block can interfere with the spontaneous rotation of the fetal head. However, the perineal relaxation and the adequate analgesia allow manual rotation to be easily performed. Owing to the loss of the perineal reflex, the mother does not have the usual urge to push. Therefore, unless she is cooperative and well coached, the second stage of labor is prolonged. However, a low forceps delivery can be easily accomplished if required.

During the Third Stage of Labor and the Immediate Postpartum Period (Fourth Stage). By using intrauterine and intramyometrial pressure recordings, Neme[53] found that despite a block up to the T8 level, spinal analgesia does not significantly change the uterine contractibility during the third stage of labor or in the first 24 hours postpartum.

FETAL AND NEONATAL EFFECTS OF
SUBARACHNOID BLOCK

Subarachnoid block offers the best anesthetic technique in regard to the direct effects of drugs on the fetus. With other regional techniques, including pudendal nerve block, local anesthetics are transmitted to the fetus, with potential fetal depression depending on the total dose, the type of drug, and the fetal condition before the block. Also, general anesthesia causes fetal and neonatal depression proportionate to the duration and depth of anesthesia. With subarachnoid block the dose of the local anesthetic is so small that the maternal and subsequently the fetal blood levels of the drug are negligible. This advantage has been proven by the good condition of the neonates following subarachnoid block in everyday practice as well as in controlled studies by Apgar,[5] Moya,[49] Phillips,[59] and many others. However, subarachnoid block may cause a major problem, maternal hypotension, which if uncorrected can lead to perinatal hypoxia.[65,82] Prolonged moderate hypotension, e.g., a fall of systolic blood pressure from 120 to 90, is more serious than severe hypotension which is properly and immediately corrected.[49] Persistent maternal hypotension causes delayed decelerations of the fetal heart rate.[26,30] Therefore, every effort should be made to prevent hypotension following subarachnoid block, especially in cesarean section where the incidence and severity of hypotension are much higher than in vaginal delivery, and to treat it quickly and efficiently if it occurs.

DRUGS USED FOR SUBARACHNOID BLOCK

Many drugs have been used for subarachnoid block. Some of the commonly used drugs are described below.

Local Anesthetic Drugs

In comparison to the specific gravity of the cerebrospinal fluid, local anesthetic drugs can be either hypo-, iso-, or hyperbaric.

Isobaric Solutions. An example of isobaric solutions is 1:200 cinchocaine (Nupercaine). Since the specific gravity of cerebrospinal fluid is variable, the effect of this solution is unpredictable and its use is not recommended.

Hypobaric Solutions. An example of hypobaric solutions is when 2 ml. of 1 per

cent tetracaine solution is added to 18 ml. of distilled water.[38] The resulting solution contains 1 mg. of tetracaine per milliliter and has a specific gravity of 1.003. Some authorities believe that the cephalad spread is not due to the hypobaric character of the solution, having a specific gravity very close to that of cerebrospinal fluid, but rather to the volumetric displacement of cerebrospinal fluid.[42]

As mentioned in Chapter 14, Epidural Analgesia, local anesthetics used for such a block are hypobaric at body temperature. Therefore in injecting the test dose the patient should not be in the reverse Trendelenburg position; otherwise, extensive cephalad spread can occur if the dura has been inadvertently punctured.[34]

Hyperbaric Solutions. The commonly used drugs for subarachnoid block are lidocaine and tetracaine.

Five Per Cent Lidocaine in 7.5 Per Cent Dextrose. This solution is available in sterile 2-ml. ampules. The specific gravity is 1.032. It can be autoclaved with the rest of the spinal tray without loss of potency. Lidocaine is the drug of choice for vaginal delivery because of its rapid onset of action and short duration. For low spinal (saddle block) a dose of 30 mg. is used; for mid spinal the dose is 40 to 50 mg.; and for cesarean section the doses are shown in Table 15-1. The block usually lasts for 1 hour.

Half Per Cent Tetracaine in 5 Per Cent Dextrose. Tetracaine hydrochloride ampules may be sterilized once by autoclaving. The ampules of tetracaine should be examined closely before use; cloudy or discolored solutions or solutions containing crystals must not be used. Tetracaine solutions have the disadvantages of undergoing slow hydrolysis, resulting in precipitation of butylaminobenzoic acid crystals. Ampules of tetracaine hydrochloride should be protected from light and should be stored at 2 to 8° C. Ampules that have passed their expiration date should be discarded. Just before injection, equal volumes of 1 per cent tetracaine and 10 per cent dextrose from separate ampules are mixed together to form the hyperbaric solution. The specific gravity of the solution is 1.018. For low subarachnoid block the dose is 3 to 4 mg. of tetracaine; for mid subarachnoid block the dose is usually 5 mg.; and for cesarean section the doses are shown in Table 15-1.

Although lidocaine is the drug of choice for vaginal delivery, opinions vary in regard to the drug to be used for cesarean section. Some prefer tetracaine to lidocaine because of its longer duration of action. However, with the addition of 0.2 mg. of epinephrine to lidocaine, the duration of analgesia extends to 90 minutes which is sufficient for cesarean section. If cesarean section hysterectomy is to be performed, tetracaine plus epinephrine is preferable since analgesia lasts for 135 minutes instead of 90 minutes. Lidocaine has the advantages over tetracaine of being more stable and having no expiration date, as well as being a superb analgesic.

One Per Cent Bupivacaine in 5 Per Cent Dextrose. Although bupivacaine has been extensively used for epidural analgesia, its use for subarachnoid block has been limited.[58,63,66,83] In a recent comparison between tetracaine and bupivacaine, the two drugs in the same dosage were shown to have essentially the same clinical effects, including the same onset and duration of action. The only exception is that there is more motor paralysis associated with tetracaine.[58]

Vasopressor Drugs

In subarachnoid block, the addition of 0.2 mg. of epinephrine or 2 mg. of phenylephrine to the local anesthetic drug improves the quality of the block and prolongs its duration by 50 to 70 per cent respectively, without delaying the onset of action.[56] Increasing the dose of epinephrine to 0.5 mg. does not increase the benefit and is not recommended. There is no danger of ischemia of the blood supply of the cord by the addition of these vaso-pressors.[2,11,44] The main danger to the cord is prolonged hypotension and/or surgical interference with its blood supply.

The mechanism of action of vasopressors in prolonging the duration of subarachnoid block is not yet clear. The possible mechanisms are:

1. Allowing more uptake of the local anesthetic agent by the nervous tissue due to vasoconstriction.

2. Having a local anesthetic action.

3. Interfering with the clearance of the local anesthetic from the nervous tissue.

These vasoconstrictor drugs have little or no systemic effect because of the very slow absorption rate from the subarachnoid space.[38] If a systemic reaction to the local anesthetic in the form of tachycardia and hypertension is accompanied by little or no anesthesia, then the drug was injected elsewhere than into the subarachnoid space, probably intravascularly.

EQUIPMENT USED FOR SUBARACHNOID BLOCK

The equipment required for performing a subarachnoid block is simple. The following items are required:

1. *Spinal Needles.* Many kinds of spinal needles have been used, e.g., regular, Whitacre, tapered, Greene, or Quincke-Babcock needle. The *Whitacre needle* has been previously described (p. 311).

The *tapered needle* (Fig. 15-6) has a 20-gauge shaft; its terminal part near the bevel tapers to 25-gauge. The tapered needle is claimed to have a greater maneuverability owing to the thick proximal part of the shaft while its tapering end ensures a small hole in the dura. By comparing cases in which the tapered needle was used with cases in which a regular needle which is uniform throughout was used, the former needle was found to be associated with a higher incidence and greater severity of headache than the latter.[1] Owing to the nonuniform thickness of the tapered

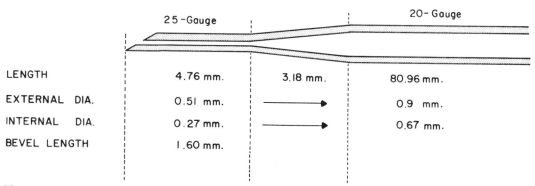

	25-Gauge		20-Gauge
LENGTH	4.76 mm.	3.18 mm.	80.96 mm.
EXTERNAL DIA.	0.51 mm.	$\longrightarrow$	0.9 mm.
INTERNAL DIA.	0.27 mm.	$\longrightarrow$	0.67 mm.
BEVEL LENGTH	1.60 mm.		

Fig. 15-6.   The tapered spinal needle. (Abouleish, E., Yamaoka, H., and Hingson, R. A.: Evaluation of a tapered spinal needle. Anesth. Analg., *53*:258, 1974)

needle, the tactile perception of the three important structures, the ligamentum flavum, the dura, and the subarachnoid space, is poor. Thus, there is a tendency to advance the needle too far and puncture the dura with the thick part of the shaft, causing a larger hole and subsequently more headache (see Fig. 7-3).

The *Greene needle* has a special point with a rounded noncutting bevel which is designed to produce a small dural hole because it tends to separate rather than cut the dural fibers.

The commonly used needle is a regular needle with a short bevel and either a Greene tip or a *Quincke-Babcock* tip which has a sharp cutting bevel. The author prefers a *26-gauge disposable regular needle with a short (1 mm.) bevel* (Fig. 15-7). The non-disposable needles are difficult to clean, especially number 26-gauge because of its

fine lumen, and the tip may become serrated or blunt with repeated use. The use of a fine needle is important because the smaller the size of the needle, the lower the incidence of post-lumbar-puncture cephalgia.

2. *Introducers.*   The spinal needle can be introduced either directly or through a large-bore needle inserted into the interspinous ligament. Using the introducer has the following advantages: (1) the spinal needle does not touch the skin, and thus there is less likelihood of contamination. (2) The introducer supports the fine 26-gauge spinal needle by acting as a scaffold. (3) Because the introducer is short and strong, the angle of the insertion can be easily changed while the introducer is still in the ligaments. If an attempt is made to change the direction of the fine spinal needle used without an introducer while it

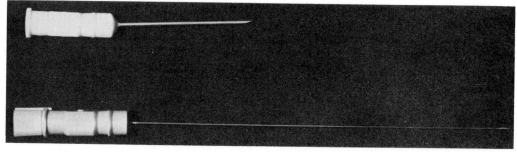

Fig. 15-7.   Disposable 20-gauge introducer and a 26-gauge spinal needle.

is in the back ligaments, the needle will bend without changing the position of the terminal part. If a spinal needle is used without an introducer, it should be pulled out to the subcutaneous tissue before attempting to change its direction. (4) If blood appears in the spinal needle or if it is desired to change to another size needle, the original needle is removed and the other needle is inserted through the introducer without causing another skin puncture. (5) If a 26-gauge spinal needle is used without the introducer, in order to be able to introduce it through the skin it is usually first held by the shaft. By using the introducer, the needle is held by the hub and can be easily inserted without touching the shaft, thus decreasing the possibility of contamination.

The distance to which the introducer is advanced varies, of course, with the size of the patient. The intention is to introduce it into the interspinous ligament and not into the epidural space. Attempts to introduce it that far have resulted in inadvertent dural puncture and severe headache because of the large bore of the introducer.[24] The author prefers the 20-gauge introducer shown in Figure 15-7 because it is disposable, short (3.2 cm.), and it is easy to insert the needle through it since the interior of its hub is conical.

3. *Syringes.* Two 3-ml. syringes are required, one for the local infiltration of the skin and the other for the spinal block. At least one of them should be made of glass so that aspiration of cerebrospinal fluid can be easily seen.

The Spinal Tray

The spinal tray can be either disposable or reusable. Disposable trays are more expensive and of inferior quality, but they are recommended if the number of subarachnoid blocks performed at the institution is limited and/or the institution lacks experienced personnel to prepare the trays. If one decides to prepare his own spinal trays, precautions should be taken not to contaminate them with bacteria or chemical substances. The syringes should be cleaned with water, then ether, and finally rinsed with distilled water; the use of detergents is prohibited because they can produce neurologic damage. Each tray should contain a sterilization indicator which should be checked before administering the block (Fig. 15-8). The trays can be either gas-sterilized or autoclaved for 30 minutes at a pressure of 20 pounds per square inch. The author prefers autoclaving the trays because autoclaving allows for immediate use without the need for a period of aeration. The spinal tray contains a sterile towel, 4 × 4 gauze sponges, a sponge forceps, two 3-ml. glass syringes, 1 ampule containing 2 ml. of 5 per cent lidocaine in 7.5 per cent dextrose, a 24-gauge hypodermic needle for local infiltration of the skin, and a 19-gauge needle for aspiration of lidocaine, all placed on a stainless steel tray (Fig. 15-8). After opening the tray, the presterilized disposable introducer and spinal needle are added without contamination. Autoclaving these with the tray is not necessary, adds more work, and may cause damage to the cement attaching the metallic shafts to the plastic hubs.

TECHNIQUE

Types of Subarachnoid Block

In obstetrics, there are three levels of subarachnoid block and each fulfills a certain requirement.

1. *Low Spinal Block, "Saddle Block."* Low spinal block provides perineal analgesia only, without relief of abdominal or back pains. It is indicated if there is imminent danger of hypotension, the anesthesiologist does not have much experience with subarachnoid block and/or no operative delivery is anticipated.

2. *Mid Spinal Block.* In mid spinal block, the analgesia level extends to and includes the T10 segment. It provides complete relief of pain during vaginal delivery, explo-

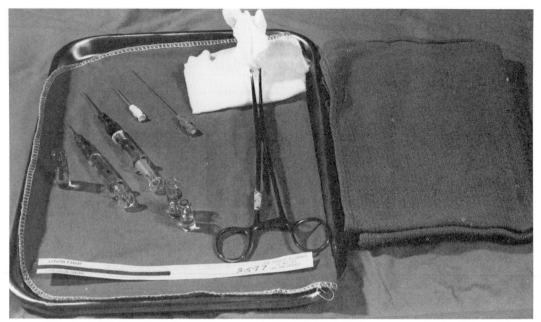

Fig. 15-8.   Spinal tray showing sterilization indicator strip, sponge forceps, 26-gauge disposable spinal needle, disposal introducer, a 3-ml. glass syringe containing lidocaine (Xylocaine) with epinephrine for subarachnoid injection, and another syringe containing 1 per cent procaine (Novocain) for skin infiltration.

ration of the uterus, or manual removal of the placenta. It is ideal for forceps delivery or vacuum extraction. However, it does not cause relaxation of the uterus to permit version extraction. It is the commonly used spinal block for vaginal delivery because it offers more analgesia than a true saddle block. The danger of hypotension with this technique has been unjustifiably exaggerated.

3. *High Spinal Block.* The block in such a case extends to T_5 segment to provide adequate analgesia for cesarean section.

Mid Spinal Block

The technique for mid spinal block will be explained in detail, and then the required modifications to produce a low or a high spinal block will be described.

Explanation of the Technique to the Patient. If possible, the technique is described to the patient as well as what is expected of her and what she will feel following the block. The time for such an expla-

nation is preferably during a prenatal office visit or when the patient is in early labor. This not only establishes good rapport with the patient, but also helps ensure her cooperation during the procedure, thus making the block atraumatic, easy, and fast.

Preliminary Steps on Arrival of the Patient at the Delivery Room. The patient's chart is reviewed, an intravenous infusion using a plastic cannula is started, and the blood pressure is measured. An assistant is of great help in a busy obstetric service, because he or she can start the intravenous infusion, hold the patient during the block, and monitor her vital signs following induction.

The Position of the Patient. Proper positioning is essential for performing subarachnoid or epidural block. Subarachnoid block can be induced while the patient is in the lateral or sitting-up position. The lateral position is preferred for the following reasons:

1. It is more comfortable for the patient.

2. It is more rapidly accomplished without disturbing the intravenous tubing and the connections to the monitors.

3. There is less possibility of postural hypotension that might occur with the sitting position, especially when narcotics and/or tranquilizers have been administered.

4. There is no resistance to the progress of the fetal head by the delivery table, and therefore less possible trauma than with the sitting position.

5. There is more predictability of the analgesic level, especially with cesarean section, due to the minimal change in the horizontal axis as the patient is turned to the supine position.

In obese patients, however, the median furrow of the back does not correspond to the spinous processes. This plus the difficulty in feeling the landmarks predispose to errors in performing the lumbar puncture in the lateral position. The sitting position is preferred in case of anticipated or encountered difficulties. For proper positioning either in the lateral or the sitting position, see Chapter 14, Epidural Analgesia, and Figure 14-6A. The patient's back should be well flexed to open the interlaminar space, i.e., to increase the size of the target through which the spinal needle will penetrate to reach the subarachnoid space. The shoulders and pelvis should be parallel to each other and perpendicular to the table. Twisting of the back takes place in the lumbar region and tends to close the interlaminar space; this is why the shoulders and pelvis should be parallel and drooping of one shoulder or the other is not allowed.

The assistant keeps the patient in position, prevents sudden movement of the patient, and constantly reassures her.

The Position of the Table. During and following induction, the position of the table depends on the type of block required. In case of mid spinal block for vaginal delivery with the patient in the left lateral position, the table is put in the reverse Trendelenburg position. The angle is about 15 to 20 degrees to ensure limited cephalad spread of the hyperbaric solution, and to allow for a more rapid flow of the cerebrospinal fluid through the narrow needle.

Preparing the Spinal Tray. The tray is opened; the disposable spinal needle and introducer are added. The operator, who is masked and capped, puts on sterile gloves before touching the contents of the tray. Strict attention should be paid to what is called the "no-touch" technique; i.e., the shafts of the introducer and the spinal needle, the plungers, and the inner sides of syringes should not be touched to avoid any possibility of introducing infection especially into the subarachnoid space. Local anesthetic solutions or vasopressors showing change of color or precipitation of crystals should not be used. Fifty mg. (1 ml.) of hyperbaric lidocaine is aspirated in the glass syringe for the subarachnoid block. Using the hyperbaric lidocaine for skin infiltration is not advisable because sloughing of the skin can occur due to the cell damage produced by the hypertonic solution. About 0.5 ml. of 1 per cent procaine is aspirated into the other syringe for local infiltration of the skin and subcutaneous tissue (Fig. 15-8). The local infiltration of the skin at the site of puncture may be omitted in vaginal delivery because of the distraction of the patient's mind by the uterine pains. This is why procaine ampules are not always included in the tray and can be added in the form of presterilized ampules stored in autoclaved test tubes.

The Position of the Operator. The operator should be comfortably seated on a stool, the level of which can be modified so that the operator's line of vision is as close as possible to the horizontal plane at the site of puncture. Being comfortable, the operator is more relaxed and in a better condition for concentration. If the

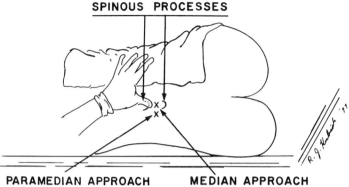

SPINOUS PROCESSES

PARAMEDIAN APPROACH   MEDIAN APPROACH

Fig. 15-9. The landmarks and points of entry for paramedian and median approaches of subarachnoid block. Notice that the thumb is touching the spinous process limiting the cephalad end of the interspace. The site of entry for the median approach is just distal to the thumb at the midline. The site of entry for the paramedian approach is just distal to the lateral border of the thumb.

operator's line of vision is close to the horizontal plane at the site of puncture, sideways deviation of the needle, which is a common mistake, is less likely to occur.

Preparing the Patient's Skin. The patient's back is prepared using an iodophor compound such as 1 per cent Betadine or Prepodyne solution and the excess of fluid is removed from the area of injection.

Draping of the Patient. A sterile towel is placed on the patient's side to cover the iliac crest (see Fig. 14-6B). The patient's shoulders should remain exposed to ensure their being parallel to the pelvis during the procedure.

Choosing the Interspace. The highest part of the iliac crest is palpated by the operator's fingers while the thumb feels the spinous processes in the lumbar region (See Fig. 14-6B). The spine opposite the highest part of the iliac crest is the fourth spine and the space chosen for mid and high spinal block is L3 to L4. The thumb is placed on the interspace in contact with the limiting cephalad spine.

Local Infiltration of the Skin and Subcutaneous Tissue. Local infiltration for the median approach to the subarachnoid space is performed in the midline between the two spinous processes just distal to the middle of the thumb (Fig. 15-9).

Inserting the Introducer. Proper insertion of the introducer is essential because the spinal needle will just follow its direction. The introducer is inserted exactly in the midline of the interspace and directed anteriorly with slight cephalad inclination. The aim is to pass it parallel to and between the lumbar spinous processes (Fig. 15-10A); the caudad angle it forms with the skin of the back is about 80 degrees. If it is 90 degrees, the spinal needle as it passes through will encounter the lamina of the vertebra below; if it is 70 or 60 degrees, it will encounter the lamina of the vertebra above. If the introducer deviates to one side, the needle will meet bony resistance caused by the laminae on that side. It should never be inserted with a caudad direction because the subarachnoid space cannot be reached in this direction. The introducer is inserted only to a certain depth which varies from one patient to another. The purpose, as mentioned before, is to insert it into the interspinous ligament; the end point is when the operator feels that the introducer "catches" and its movement becomes restricted.

Inserting the Spinal Needle. At the same time the left hand holds the introducer, the right hand holds the spinal needle at its hub like a dart and passes it through the introducer. Its bevel should be directed laterally in order to separate rather than cut the longitudinal fibers of the dura. During the steady advancement of the needle, the operator should pay attention to three things: (1) the sudden loss of resistance as the needle passes through the ligamentum flavum; (2) the sudden loss of resistance as the dura and arachnoid are punctured; and (3) the smooth feeling of the needle moving in fluid as it advances in the subarachnoid space. (Fig. 15-10B) The distinct feeling of these three elements is present in most cases, and their separate identification increases with experience. By advancing the needle for 2 to 3 mm. in the subarachnoid space, one ensures that the bevel is totally in the subarachnoid space. This is the end point at which the stylet is removed and cerebrospinal fluid is watched for. Since the needle used is a very fine one, the cerebrospinal fluid will appear only after a few seconds inside the hub as a shining drop of dew. The reverse Trendelenburg position of the table tends to accelerate the process.

Each time the anesthesiologist performs a subarachnoid block he is also performing an epidural puncture since the needle has to traverse the latter space first. If attention is paid to the feeling of tissues during a lumbar puncture, the anesthesiologist develops his tactile sensations, which are required not only for subarachnoid block but also for epidural and caudal blocks.

Injecting the Local Anesthetic. The

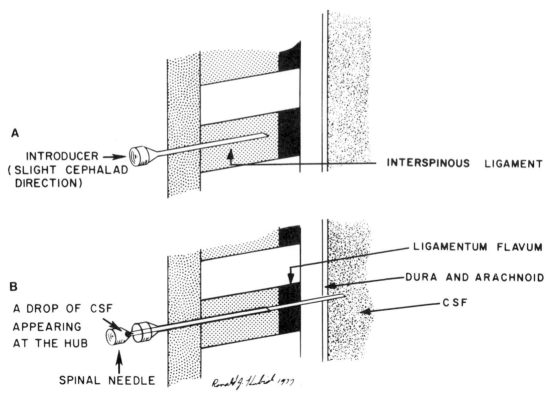

Fig. 15-10. Introducer and spinal needle *in situ* (sagittal section of the back at the lumbar region). *A.* The introducer is inserted into the interspinous ligament parallel to the spinous processes. *B.* The operator should pay attention to the sensations of penetrating ligamentum flavum, the dura and the arachnoid, and the smooth feeling of the needle moving in fluid (cerebrospinal fluid).

glass syringe containing lidocaine is attached to the needle. Caution should be taken not to change the position of the needle while the syringe is attached; otherwise, its tip can leave the subarachnoid space. Gentle aspiration is performed and cerebrospinal fluid will enter the syringe as a fine streak. The solution is injected in 5 to 10 seconds. At the end of injection, 0.1 ml. of cerebrospinal fluid is aspirated and reinjected to verify the proper position of the needle. The introducer, needle, and syringe are all simultaneously removed and the patient is gently turned on her back.

Positioning the Patient Following Injection of Local Anesthetic. The patient's legs are elevated and supported in stirrups. This ensures a better venous return to the heart and safeguards against hypotension. Immediately following injection, the position of the table is modified to limit the extent of the block to the T10 level. If the patient is 165 cm. (5′ 6″) tall, the table is placed horizontally; if the patient is 150 cm. (5′) tall, the 20-degree head-up tilt of the table is maintained; if the patient's height is in between the above heights, the level of the table is adjusted accordingly.

Determining the Level of Analgesia. The level of the block is checked on the dependent side close to the midline. The relief of abdominal and/or back pain is a reassurance that the block has at least reached the T10 level.

Monitoring the Patient. The patient's pulse and blood pressure are measured. The blood pressure is recorded every 1 minute for 10 minutes, then every 5 minutes. Verbal contact with the patient is maintained to reassure her and to detect any difficulty in breathing, discomfort, or nausea.

Monitoring the Fetus. Before and after the block, the fetal heart rate is determined either by auscultation or by using an ultrasonic device. This is also of medicolegal importance. If the fetal heart sounds could not be detected before the subarachnoid block, fetal demise cannot be blamed on the block.

Difficulties That May Be Encountered During Spinal Block

Encountering Bone. This can be due to:

1. *Inadequate flexion of the back.* With inadequate flexion, the laminae are close together and the interlaminar space is very narrow. This can be corrected by properly flexing the back.

2. *Improper angle of the introducer with the sagittal plane.* This can be corrected by withdrawing the spinal needle into the lumen of the introducer, changing the angle by moving the introducer, and then readvancing the needle.

3. *Lateral insertion of the introducer.* If the introducer is not inserted in the midline of the interlaminar space, the needle advancing directly anteriorly will encounter one of the two laminae on that side. To correct this, the introducer is redirected so that the tip of the needle is advanced more medially, or both are removed, the landmarks are rechecked, and then the introducer is reinserted exactly in the midline. This problem is usually due to removing the thumb from the interspace while doing local infiltration of the skin. To avoid this, once the thumb is in the correct place it should be kept there until the introducer is inserted in the right direction.

4. *Lateral deviation of the introducer.* The point of entry of the introducer is in the midline of the interlaminar space, but, while advancing, it deviates laterally. This problem usually arises when the operator's vision is far from the horizontal plane, e.g., performing lumbar puncture with the patient in the lateral position and the operator standing up. To correct this, the needle and introducer are partially withdrawn, the introducer is redirected toward the midline, and then the needle is advanced.

5. *Too far insertion of the needle.* The re-

sistance encountered in such a case is the posterior surface of the body of the vertebra or the intervertebral disk, covered by the posterior longitudinal ligament. This is liable to occur in a thin individual where the subarachnoid space is superficial. The operator, not paying attention to the sensations as the needle punctures the ligamentum flavum, the dura, and the subarachnoid space, or inserting the introducer too far into the epidural space, pushes the needle all the way across the subarachnoid space and the anterior epidural space. To correct this, the needle is withdrawn for 3 to 4 mm. to bring its tip back into the subarachnoid space.

Paresthesia. When the needle touches a sensory nerve root, the patient feels paresthesia, usually in one thigh. It is very difficult for the needle to touch one of the nerve roots in the subarachnoid space because the nerves are mobile. Paresthesia is usually due to touching the posterior nerve root in the lateral epidural space where it is anchored by its union with the anterior nerve root. If paresthesia occurs, the patient is asked whether it is left or right and the needle is partially withdrawn and then redirected away from that side to puncture the dura in the midline. The site of paresthesia should be recorded on the patient's chart because sometimes during the postpartum period the patient may complain of paresthesia and/or weakness due to nerve injury by other factors such as forceps application, pressure by the stirrup, or pressure by the fetal head. The patient's subsequent complaint may prove to be in a different limb or in a different part other than where paresthesia initially occurred. Subarachnoid block has been unjustifiably blamed for all the neurologic complications that follow its use.

"Bloody Tap." This is usually due to lateral deviation of the spinal needle. The lateral epidural space is rich with dilated veins which can be easily traumatized. To avoid such a problem, the needle is inserted exactly in the midline of the inter-laminar space and, once the dura is punctured, it is advanced for only 2 to 3 mm. If a "bloody tap" occurs, the needle is partially withdrawn, the introducer is redirected toward the midline, and the needle is gently reinserted. If blood appears again another interspace is chosen, preferably one that is more cephalad than caudad because blood gravitates more caudally. Once the operator feels the needle is in the subarachnoid space, the first part of the cerebrospinal fluid may be mixed with blood. Aspiration into a dry syringe is performed until the cerebrospinal fluid becomes almost clear before injecting the local anesthetic. If the cerebrospinal fluid contains much blood, part of the local anesthetic combines with the plasma proteins, thus decreasing the dose left for nerve blockade.

Failure of Cerebrospinal Fluid Aspiration. Sometimes cerebrospinal fluid appears at the needle hub but cannot be aspirated probably due to a nerve root or an arachnoid trabecula occluding the bevel of the needle. To correct this, the needle is rotated 90 degrees and reaspiration is done. If no cerebrospinal fluid appears, the stylet is added, the needle is advanced or withdrawn for 1 mm., the stylet is removed, and aspiration is repeated. If still no cerebrospinal fluid can be aspirated, it is better to try lumbar puncture at another interspace.

Failure of Cerebrospinal Fluid to Appear Despite Adequate Feeling of Puncturing the Ligamentum Flavum and the Dura, and Being in the Subarachnoid Space. The needle tip can be occluded by a nerve root or an arachnoid trabecula. The management is the same as above. Very rarely the operator feels the "give" due to puncture of the ligamentum flavum and the dura but not the smooth feeling of the cerebrospinal fluid. This is due to the needle being directed laterally and passing tangentially through the dura. Partially withdrawing the needle and redirecting it toward the midline corrects this problem.

Paramedian Approach of Lumbar Puncture

This technique is resorted to mainly when there is calcification of the supraspinous and interspinous ligaments. The introducer is inserted just lateral to the thumb (as shown in Fig. 15-9) near the dependent side and directed medially, anteriorly, and slightly cephalad. The needle is inserted through the introducer. The first ligamentous resistance met by the needle is the ligamentum flavum which is pierced and the needle is advanced, as in the median approach, to reach the subarachnoid space (see Fig. 15-3).

To learn lumbar puncture, the median approach is much simpler because there are fewer axes to handle than with the paramedian approach.

Low Spinal Block, "Saddle Block"

The term "saddle block" was introduced in 1946 by Adriani to describe this block in which the analgesia produced is limited to the inner thighs and perineum. To obtain such a block the dose of the local anesthetic is reduced to 30 mg. of hyperbaric lidocaine. The needle is inserted at the L4 to L5 interspace, while the patient is in the sitting or the lateral position with the head of the table elevated. In the sitting position, the patient is kept seated for 3 minutes. In the lateral position, she is turned on her back and the legs are elevated in stirrups while retaining the head-up position.

High Spinal Block

This block is used for cesarean section. The following modifications in mid spinal technique are required for high spinal block:

1. The intravenous fluid is administered through a wide-bore cannula.

2. Five hundred to 1,000 ml. of fluid is infused within 10 minutes from the induction.

3. The table is adjusted so that the vertebral column is horizontal.

4. Local infiltration of the skin and subcutaneous tissue is done in elective cases.

5. The L3 to L4 interspace is chosen. If difficulty is encountered, the L2 to L3 interspace is used provided the operator is aware that too high a level of block may occur; thus he must adjust the position of the table and/or the rate of injection.

6. The doses are higher than with mid spinal block (see Table 15-1). Epinephrine (0.2 mg.) or phenylephrine (2 mg.) is added as a routine to hyperbaric lidocaine and in special cases to hyperbaric tetracaine.

7. The rate of injection is about 10 to 15 seconds.

8. Oxygen by a clear plastic mask is administered to the parturient as soon as the drug is injected and she is turned to the supine position. This improves the oxygenation of the fetus, reduces nausea, and ensures good oxygen supply to the patient's vital organs and centers.

9. The uterus should be displaced to the left (see Fig. 14-9).

10. Hypotension should be anticipated and if it occurs should be corrected immediately and adequately.

11. The patient needs more reassurance, e.g., the marked extent of the block can lead to dyspnea in spite of adequate ventilation (for details see Chap. 6, Effects of Vertebral Blocks on the Respiratory System).

12. After the delivery of the fetus, a narcotic and/or tranquilizer can be administered if required.

13. Following delivery, the patient may feel shoulder pains that cause much discomfort. This is due to irritation of the undersurface of the diaphragm by blood and amniotic fluid. Suction of the peritoneal cavity usually cures the condition. If the blood pressure is adequate, tilting the table to the head-up position facilitates the suction.

Use of Hypobaric Tetracaine for Cesarean Section

Most authorities[10,17,43,48,61] prefer to use hyperbaric drugs in methods more or less as described above. However, one other technique deserves description, the technique using hypobaric tetracaine.[38] This technique has the advantage of having the patient in the Trendelenburg position during and after injection, thus ensuring better venous return to the heart and better control of blood pressure than when the table is in the horizontal or slight head-up tilt position.

The preparation of the solution has been described earlier. The lumbar puncture is performed in the usual manner at L3 to L4 interspace with the patient in the lateral position and the table in a slight Trendelenburg position. According to the patient's height, 9 to 11 ml. of the 0.1 per cent tetracaine solution is injected at a rate of 0.5 ml./sec. The patient is turned on her back and the table is maintained in position. The onset of anesthesia is rapid, within a few minutes, and lasts for 1.5 to 2 hours.

Continuous Subarachnoid Block

Continuous subarachnoid block was introduced primarily for surgery in 1940 by Lemmon. A malleable silver needle was placed into the subarachnoid space in the lumbar region, then bent and affixed to the skin with tape over an opening in a special mattress. Repeated injections can thus be performed while surgery is in progress. In 1947, Saklad and coworkers reported segmental spinal anesthesia by applying a urethral catheter through a Tuohy needle. In 1951, Carpenter and coworkers reported a continuous subarachnoid drip of procaine for labor and delivery. In 1964, Bizzarri and coworkers used a special No. 21-gauge spinal needle with a curved tip to direct the fine soft vinyl catheter inserted through it. The needle was removed, leaving the catheter for continuous administration of local anesthetics. In 1970, Elam used intermittent injection of hyperbaric lidocaine through a subarachnoid catheter to achieve segmental block during labor and delivery in 14 patients. In 1972, Giuffrida, Bizzarri, and their associates used the same technique introduced in 1964 for cesarean section in 75 patients.

Advantages. The above authors report that continuous subarachnoid block has the following advantages:

1. Being a continuous technique, it can be used during both labor and delivery.

2. Differential block can be easily obtained depending on the concentration of the drug injected. Sensory blockade can be achieved during labor; then both sensory and motor blockade can be obtained during delivery if required.

3. There is no fetal depression due to drug administration since the doses are very small.

4. For cesarean section, increments of the drug are injected to achieve the required level. Therefore, the level of the block can be accurately reached with minimal chance of hypotension.

Disadvantages. Continuous subarachnoid block has the following disadvantages:

1. There is a possibility of spinal cord or nerve injury by the catheter, even if made of Teflon, because the spinal cord and nerves are only covered by thin pia mater. In contrast, with continuous epidural analgesia, the nerve roots are covered by the pia, arachnoid, and the thick dura; the cord is separated from the epidural catheter by these layers as well as by the cerebrospinal fluid.

2. There is a possibility of infection because the catheter creates a fistula between the subarachnoid space and the outside.

3. There is a high incidence of headache following continuous subarachnoid block owing to the large dural rent.

Role. Continuous subarachnoid block can be an alternative to continuous epidural block for elderly poor-risk surgical patients in whom the incidence of headache is small and the risks of the technique may be less than the alternatives. In the obstetric patient, continuous subarachnoid block in its present form is unacceptable. If in the future a very fine catheter outside the lumbar puncture needle can be introduced into the subarachnoid space, continuous subarachnoid block may be useful.

When to Administer the Subarachnoid Block

For cesarean section the answer is simple: subarachnoid block is administered just before surgery. For vaginal delivery, there are two schools of thought. One school advises the use of subarachnoid block when the cervix is dilated 5 to 6 cm. in a multipara or 8 to 9 cm. in a nullipara.[10,38,43] The other school, to which the author belongs, recommends the administration of the subarachnoid block only when the patient is ready for delivery, e.g., when the fetal head is "crowning" in a nullipara; in a multipara, depending on the course of labor, subarachnoid block is required when the cervix is fully dilated or when the fetal head has descended to the perineum without perineal bulge.[60] The advantage of the first policy is that the patient gets pain relief for some time before delivery. The disadvantages are that the analgesia may wear off before parturition is completed, thus requiring a second block. This predisposes the patient to a higher incidence of headache. Moreover, the early administration of subarachnoid block may lead to inability of the patient to push due to paralysis of the abdominal muscles, or to her disinterest to bear down resulting from the obtundation of the perineal reflex and the relief of pain. Therefore, unless a "true saddle block" is administered, ensuring full motor power of the abdomen and feeling of the uterine contractions, the second stage of labor may be prolonged.

The advantage of the second policy is

that there is no prolongation of labor, and analgesia is optimum when most needed for the delivery, episiotomy, and repair. The disadvantages are: (1) it does not provide pain relief except for a short time during the course of labor; and (2) the presence of the anesthesiologist in the delivery room suite is essential for the timing and execution of the block without panic.

Success Rate of Spinal Analgesia

Spinal analgesia carries the highest success rate of any regional block technique in obstetrics. With an operator with average experience the success rate can be as high as 97 per cent.

Causes of Failure of Spinal Analgesia

Injection of the Local Anesthetic Drug Outside the Subarachnoid Space. This is by far the main cause of failure of subarachnoid block and its incidence decreases with increased experience of the operator. To avoid this complication the following steps should be taken:

1. Pay attention to the tactile feelings during advancement of the needle, the end point being the sensation of the gentle movement of the needle in a fluid medium.

2. Aspirate before and after injection of the local anesthetic.

3. Attach the loaded syringe to the needle without changing the position of the latter.

4. Keep the left hand against the patient's back to prevent the needle from moving during injection (see Fig. 14-8B).

With modern spinal needles, the bevel of the needle is made short to avoid the simultaneous position of the needle opening in both the epidural and subarachnoid spaces. With a long needle bevel, aspiration may cause the appearance of cerebrospinal fluid while injection allows the anesthetic solution to be deposited into both spaces, leading to inadequate analgesia.

Injection of the local anesthetic into the

subdural space is another cause of failure of subarachnoid block. The subdural space is only a capillary space filled with serous fluid and present between the dura and arachnoid. It is anatomically distinct from the subarachnoid space [74]. Rarely, there is cerebrospinal fluid in the subdural space owing to developmental defects in the arachnoid membrane or following traumatic perforation of the arachnoid by the needle during a difficult lumbar puncture.[18] However, with the spinal needle in the subdural space, the flow of cerebrospinal fluid is not free. Advancing the needle for 2 to 3 mm. after dural puncture ensures the penetration of the arachnoid as well; the free flow of cerebrospinal fluid following aspiration indicates the presence of the needle in the subarachnoid space.

During the connecting of the syringe to the spinal needle or while injecting the local anesthetic, the needle may move to penetrate a blood vessel or reach the epidural space. The injection of all or part of the dose causes inadequate analgesia.

The Administration of Impotent Drug. If tetracaine or any other local anesthetic is injected after its expiration date, analgesia may not develop.

Inadequate Spread of the Local Anesthetic That Has Been Injected Into the Subarachnoid Space. The analgesia does not reach the expected level if the dose was miscalculated in relation to the patient's height or position of the table, the injection site was too low, the drug was injected too slowly into the subarachnoid space, or part of the solution was lost during injection due to a leakage at the junction of the needle with the syringe.

If no signs of block occur in 10 minutes and if time allows, lumbar puncture should be repeated, preferably in another interspace, an amide drug should be used because of its stability, and free flow of cerebrospinal fluid should be obtained.

Too Alkaline Cerebrospinal Fluid. Normally the pH of cerebrospinal fluid is 7.3 to 7.4.[64] In case the pH is much higher, the local anesthetic drug may be precipitated before acting on the nerves, thus becoming inactive.[19] This is a very rare situation.

Unexplained Failure. It has been reported that despite the proper placement of a catheter in the subarachnoid space for continuous spinal analgesia, on two occasions the injection of tetracaine was unsuccessful. The cerebrospinal fluid pH was within normal range, and no explanation for such failures could be given.[92] Such a condition is extremely rare.

One should not quote these cases to explain failures due to faulty techniques.

COMPLICATIONS ASSOCIATED WITH SUBARACHNOID BLOCK

The complications of subarachnoid block are listed in the outline below. Most of these complications will be briefly discussed since they have been described in details in other parts of the book (e.g., Chap. 5, Effects of Vertebral Blocks on the Cardiovascular System; Chap. 6, Effects of Vertebral Blocks on the Respiratory System; Chap. 7, Effects of Vertebral Blocks on the Nervous System; Chap. 13, Caudal Analgesia; and Chap. 14, Epidural Analgesia). Some of the complications have also been mentioned in the sections dealing with the maternal, fetal, and neonatal effects of subarachnoid block, page 311. On the whole, the complications of subarachnoid block can be divided into two groups: maternal and fetal.

MATERNAL COMPLICATIONS

These can occur early, i.e., while the block is effective, or late, i.e., after recovery from the block.

EARLY COMPLICATIONS

Cardiovascular Complications

Cardiovascular complications are discussed in more detail in Chapter 5, Effects

Complications of Subarachnoid Block

I. *Maternal Complications*
  A. Early complications
    1. Cardiovascular
       a. Hypotension
       b. Bradycardia
       c. Hypertension
    2. Respiratory insufficiency
       a. Ischemia of the respiratory centers
       b. Paralysis of phrenic nerves
    3. Death or permanent neurologic damage due to uncorrected severe hypotension and/or respiratory insufficiency
    4. Gastrointestinal: nausea and vomiting
    5. Hiccups
    6. Broken needle
    7. Course of labor
       a. Prolonged second stage
       b. Need for forceps delivery
  B. Late complications
    1. Neurologic complications
       a. Variable degrees of brain damage due to early hypoxia and/or hypotension
       b. Paraplegia
       c. Post-lumbar-puncture cephalgia
       d. Cranial nerve palsy
       e. Radicular pain, atrophy and/or paresthesia
       f. Subarachnoid or epidural dermoid cyst
    2. Urinary retention
    3. Backache
II. *Fetal Complications*
  Potential fetal hypoxia and acidosis secondary to maternal hypotension and/or respiratory insufficiency

of Vertebral Blocks on the Cardiovascular System.

Hypotension. This is mainly due to compression of the inferior vena cava plus the sympathetic blockade produced by the subarachnoid block. Sympathetic blockade leads to decrease of the peripheral resistance and pooling of blood in the dilated veins, especially those of the lower limbs. If the block extends above T4, the sympathetic supply to the heart (T1 through T4) is interrupted and the autonomic imbalance thus produced augments the hypotension.

Bradycardia. This is due to:

1. Paralysis of the cardiac sympathetic fibers which occurs if the block level extends above T4.

2. Reflex bradycardia which can occur whether the block level extends above or below T4. It is secondary to hypotension and decreased venous return to the heart. The hypotension initiates a reflex, called Marey's reflex, which tends to produce tachycardia. The baroreceptors in the aortic arch and carotid sinus send impulses mainly by way of the glossopharyngeal nerve to the cardiac centers in the medulla. The efferent impulses are carried to the heart by way of the vagus and the sympathetic accelerator nerves, diminishing and increasing their tone respectively and leading to tachycardia. Meanwhile, the decreased venous return to the heart initiates another reflex, called Bainbridge reflex, which regulates the heart rate according to the pressure in the right atrium and the large thoracic veins. If the venous return is excessive, the heart rate is increased to cope with the extra load, and vice versa. With subarachnoid block, as a result of the decreased venous return to the heart, this reflex is initiated. The impulses are carried to the medullary centers by way of the vagus nerve and down to the heart through the vagus and sympathetic nerves, increasing and decreasing their tones respectively, thus causing bradycardia.[28] The balance between Marey's and Bainbridge's reflexes determines the heart rate.

3. In contrast to subarachnoid block, hemorrhage leads to hypotension associated with tachycardia despite the decreased venous return to the heart. With hemorrhage, the sympathetic system is intact leading to increased catecholamine release with subsequent tachycardia. On the contrary, with spinal anesthesia extending above T-10 level, the sympathetic nerve fibers including those to the adrenal medulla (T-10 to T-12) are blocked.

Bradycardia is commonly associated with nausea and hypotension. The treatment of the three conditions is by administration of a beta stimulant, e.g., ephedrine or mephentermine. Atropine usually corrects only the bradycardia and causes maternal discomfort due to dryness of the mouth. Therefore, in the author's opinion, the drug of choice for the treatment of bradycardia associated with subarachnoid block is a beta stimulant, e.g. 15 mg. mephentermine intravenously injected.

Hypertension. This complication is not due to the subarachnoid block, but to the improper management or fault in the technique. Examples are:

1. The use of a large dose of epinephrine or phenylephrine with the local anesthetic when injected intravenously instead of into the subarachnoid space

2. The use of an intramuscular prophylactic vasopressor together with a failed or limited block

3. The use of ergot preparations

4. The combination of more than one of the above factors.

To avoid such a complication, one should use only 0.2 mg. of epinephrine or 2 mg. of phenylephrine; prophylactic administration of a vasopressor should be avoided but rather hypotension should be treated when it occurs; and no ergot preparation should be used unless as a lifesaving measure to control postpartum hemorrhage, and then administered by the intramuscular route.

The treatment of hypertension depends on the severity, the cause, and any underlying cardiovascular disease. For the first example cited above, no treatment is usually required except careful monitoring and reassurance of the patient. For the second example, the hypertension usually does not endanger the patient's life if a beta stimulant has been used. For the third example, slow intravenous injection of up to 15 mg. of chlorpromazine is recommended. Hydralazine infusion has also been effective because it causes generalized vasodilatation, particularly of the renal vessels.[14]

Respiratory Insufficiency

Respiratory insufficiency is mainly due to maternal hypotension. Also, the phrenic nerves, although resistant to paralysis, can be partially or completely paralyzed. For details see Chapter 6, Effects of Vertebral Blocks on the Respiratory System, and Maternal Effects of Subarachnoid Block, page 311.

Death or Permanent Neurologic Damage

Recent studies[9,22,40,62,70] have exonerated subarachnoid block from being a direct cause of death or serious neurologic complications such as higher cortical damage, hemiplegia, or paraplegia. However, if monitoring of the patient and early adequate correction of hypotension and/or respiratory insufficiency are not performed, fatalities and serious central nervous system damage will continue to occur. *The fault is not in the technique itself, it is in the operator.* Since the technique of subarachnoid block is so simple that anyone who can do a lumbar puncture can administer a spinal block, it is tempting to use it, especially when there is a shortage of personnel. *It is again stressed that subarachnoid block should not be applied without proper understanding of the physiologic changes it can produce and without the adequate capabilities to prevent and correct these changes.* Cardiac arrest under subarachnoid block is due to negligence until proven otherwise. Usually the reasons are either the anesthesiologist did not respect the contraindications, injected too much of the drug relative to the patient's need, administered the wrong drug, did not monitor his patient adequately, or did not correct the complications properly and in time. If an obstetrician is willing to administer the subarachnoid block himself, he should not start scrubbing for the delivery until 10 minutes from the administration of the block. During that 10-minute period he should be checking the vital signs and the level of the block, and correcting hypotension if it occurs. After 10 minutes, an assistant capable of accurately monitoring the blood pressure and detecting and correcting changes in the vital signs should be in charge. A nurse anesthetist or an intensive care nurse is of great help in this respect.

Gastrointestinal Complications

The main and the most frequent gastrointestinal complication associated with subarachnoid block is nausea and vomiting. This has been previously discussed.

Hiccups

Hiccups are usually encountered in upper abdominal surgery but very rarely in vaginal delivery or cesarean section. Local infiltration around the terminal part of the esophagus to block the vagi is helpful. Sometimes hiccups are very resistant to treatment even when the patient is under general anesthesia and completely curarized. Various lines of treatment from instillation of ether into the nasal cavity to the use of ketamine have been tried.[75] Until the etiology and the mechanism are properly understood, hiccups cannot be effectively relieved and the treatment cannot be standardized.

Broken Needle

This should not occur if a good-quality product is used and no force is applied in doing lumbar puncture. If the needle is broken, it should be immediately removed.

Course of Labor

The second stage of labor can be prolonged following subarachnoid block. This may necessitate the use of forceps in delivery.[32]

LATE COMPLICATIONS

Neurologic Complications

Neurologic complications vary in severity according to the initial insult produced to the nervous system and the subsequent management. Dramatic reports of their occurrence have influenced the use of subarachnoid block in many countries, especially the United Kingdom and the Commonwealth.[73,93] The complications are listed above and all except the last one have been discussed in Chapter 7, Effects of Vertebral Blocks on the Nervous System.

Introduction of a Skin Core Into the Subarachnoid or Epidural Space. A hollow needle, especially if blunt or with a nonfitting stylet, can produce coring of the skin. If this needle is then introduced into the epidural or subarachnoid space and flushed by injecting fluid through it, the skin core can be dislodged into the space, leading to infection or epidermoid cyst.[21,46,89] To prevent such a complication, the use of an introducer is advised and the manufacture of good-quality spinal needles with well-fitting stylets, especially at the bevel, is recommended.

Urinary Retention

Urinary retention is mainly due to the surgical procedure.[72] In obstetrics, the pain associated with the episiotomy or the abdominal incision rather than the block itself can be responsible for urinary retention. Overdistension of the bladder or trauma to the bladder and urethra by the delivery process or the obstetric manipulation can be contributing factors. During prolonged labor, the bladder can be distended and reach the suprapubic region even without any block. This occurs especially when the fetal head is compressing the urethra, excessive intravenous fluid is being administered, and uterine pains are overshadowing any desire to micturate.

Evacuation of the bladder before the block, the use of a short-acting local anesthetic drug such as lidocaine, and good nursing care such as encouraging the patient to empty the bladder before its overdistension are important.

Backache

The incidence of backache following subarachnoid block varies between 0.7 per cent[88] and 2.7 per cent.[62] Under subarachnoid block the many causes responsible for backache include:

1. Relaxation of the back muscles. This may explain the higher incidence of backache with caudal than with either epidural or subarachnoid block (see Chap.

7, Effects of Vertebral Blocks on the Nervous System). A study to evaluate the influence of weakness of the muscles on the incidence of backache by comparing cesarean section using general anesthesia with muscle relaxants to subarachnoid block is needed.

2. Trauma to the nerve roots. This can be due to pressure by the fetal head or the obstetric manipulation.

3. Trauma by the needle. However, it has not been proven that the incidence of backache is higher with multiple attempts at lumbar puncture than with a single puncture or with epidural than with subarachnoid block.

4. The changes in the spinal curvature with pregnancy and delivery. These changes are important factors in explaining the higher incidence of backache in obstetrics.

5. Softening of ligaments and weakness of muscles due to pregnancy and lack of exercise. They can contribute to backache due to the strain on the ligaments.

Measures to Avoid Backache. To avoid backache under subarachnoid or other vertebral blocks, the following points should be considered:

Antepartum. Proper antenatal care to improve postural defects and muscle tone is advised.

Intrapartum.

1. The anesthesiologist should be gentle and should avoid too many repeated attempts to perform a subarachnoid block.

2. Attention should be paid to posture during the block to prevent twisting of the back and inducing a strain on the ligaments. This includes posturing in bed, turning the patient from one side to the other during transportation to and from the delivery table, and putting the legs in or out of the stirrups. For example, the two legs should be simultaneously elevated or lowered to prevent twisting of the back. This rule should be followed whether the patient is under general or vertebral anesthesia.

Postpartum. The use of an abdominal binder and the performance of exercises are advised.

In conclusion, subarachnoid block, without proof, has been unjustifiably accused of increasing backache. Backache is such a common condition that patients should not be denied spinal or epidural anesthesia because of its presence. Spinal and epidural blocks are commonly used as anesthetic techniques for the surgical removal of prolapsed intervertebral lumbar disks.[39] Moreover, subarachnoid, caudal, or epidural instillations of methylprednisolone are used in the treatment of postlaminectomy syndrome, radiculitis, and radiculopathies associated with sciatica. Therefore, it should be explained to the patient that subarachnoid block will not worsen the situation, and may even improve it by interrupting the vicious circle of pain.

FETAL COMPLICATIONS

Mismanaged subarachnoid block can produce fetal hypoxia, acidosis, or even death, if persistent maternal hypotension and/or respiratory insufficiency are produced.

INDICATIONS FOR THE USE OF SUBARACHNOID BLOCK

In obstetrics, subarachnoid block is indicated when the patient is ready for delivery by vaginal or abdominal route and there is no contraindication.

CONTRAINDICATIONS FOR THE USE OF SUBARACHNOID BLOCK

Most of the contraindications for the use of spinal analgesia are similar to those for epidural and caudal blocks. For detailed descriptions the reader is referred to Chapters 13 and 14. The contraindications for subarachnoid block are listed below.

Contraindications for the Use of Subarachnoid Block

I. Maternal contraindications	*II. Fetal contraindications*

A. Absolute contraindications
 1. Anticoagulant therapy
 2. Hemorrhage
 3. Shock
 4. Infection
   a. At the site
   b. Systemic
   c. Meningitis
 5. Tumor at the site of lumbar puncture
 6. Increased intracranial pressure
 7. Severe headache following previous lumbar puncture
 8. Absence of facilities for resuscitation or adequate monitoring
	A. Absolute contraindications
	        Cesarean section for acute fetal distress

B. Relative contraindications 1. Patient's choice 2. Inexperience of the team 3. Active central nervous system disease 4. Technical difficulties including previous laminectomy 5. "Rough" surgeon 6. Cardiac disease, especially limited cardiac output or congenital heart disease (cesarean section) 7. Toxemias of pregnancy (cesarean section)	B. Relative contraindication Compromised fetus (cesarean section)

Only those which have not been discussed before or need special consideration in relation to subarachnoid block are described.

Hemorrhage

Significant blood loss is a contraindication for subarachnoid block. However, if placenta previa is diagnosed by sonography prior to bleeding, spinal or epidural can be administered. The well-contracted uterus after delivery is an asset in these techniques. With abruptio placentae, the intrauterine bleeding and retroplacental hematoma are difficult to estimate and hypotension may jeopardize the compromised fetus. Therefore, general anesthesia is the method of choice.

Blood Coagulation Diathesis or Anticoagulant Therapy

As explained with epidural and caudal analgesia, subarachnoid block is contraindicated if the patient has a blood coagulation diathesis or is on anticoagulant therapy because of fear of hematoma formation. However, if general anesthesia is contraindicated and heparinization of the patient can be postponed for at least 30 minutes following lumbar puncture, subarachnoid block can be administered.[13] In such a case, experience is very important to achieve lumbar puncture with one trial using a 25- or 26-gauge needle and staying at the midline to avoid injury of the vertebral vessels.

Post-Lumbar-Puncture Cephalgia

If the patient has a history of severe headache following lumbar puncture for any cause, subarachnoid block should be avoided and other techniques, such as epidural or caudal, should be used.

Central Nervous System Diseases

Apart from increased intracranial pressure or active meningitis, central nervous system diseases are not a contraindication for subarachnoid block. The harm produced by a well-conducted subarachnoid block is no more than that produced by a lumbar puncture which is a procedure commonly used to investigate and follow up many of these diseases.

Cardiac Diseases, Especially Congenital Heart Disease

The occurrence of hypotension in congenital heart disease can be hazardous because it may initiate or increase the right to left shunt. In case of restricted cardiac output, such as with mitral stenosis, the decreased venous return to the heart following subarachnoid block can dangerously reduce the cardiac output. Therefore, general anesthesia is better than vertebral blocks, including subarachnoid block, for cesarean section. However, if the patient is ready for vaginal delivery, a carefully administered subarachnoid block is better than general anesthesia. It allows midforceps delivery, thus avoiding the Valsalva maneuver. A limited block for vaginal delivery plus the elevation of the legs and the descent of the fetus into the pelvis resulting in reduction of the uterine size, make the possibility of hypotension rare and, if it does occur, easily correctable. The vasopressor to correct hypotension, as explained in Chapter 13, depends on the pulse rate. If the patient is tachycardic, an alpha stimulant is used; if the patient is bradycardic, a beta stimulant is injected.

Toxemias of Pregnancy

With respect to maternal and fetal welfare, subarachnoid block is an excellent technique *for vaginal delivery* in the toxemic patient.[79,80]

For cesarean section many authors prefer epidural or general anesthesia.[86] The main reason why many physicians decide to avoid subarachnoid block in such cases with low plasma volume and generalized vasoconstriction is the danger of sympathetic blockade causing hypotension and endangering the fetus. However, the administration of 5 per cent albumin before the block tends to correct the discrepancy between the plasma volume and the vascular bed produced by the subarachnoid block. Moreover, it has been found that after an extensive spinal block, up to the T1 level, the blood pressure is well maintained in the toxemic patient, even better than in the normal gravida (Fig. 15-11).[6] This has been attributed to the possibility of a circulating humoral factor in the toxemic patient causing vasoconstriction[78,94] and compensating for the sympathetic blockade.[6] Also, continuous subarachnoid block was used for the treatment of toxemic patients without harmful effects on the fetus.[15,33,37,41] When muscle relaxants, especially the nondepolarizing group, are used in the presence of magnesium sulfate, their dose should be reduced because of their potentiation by the magnesium ion.[24a] By utilizing subarachnoid block instead of general anesthesia, the use of muscle relaxants and their inherent problems, especially in the presence of magnesium sulfate, are avoided. If the patient has eclampsia, general anesthesia is the method of choice for cesarean section; for vaginal delivery the method of anesthesia depends on the situation. If toxemia is associated with fetal distress as evidenced by delayed decelerations of the fetal heart rate, or with fetal compromise as shown by positive stress test, subarachnoid block for cesarean section is contraindicated because of the dangerous effects of possible hypotension.

"Rough" Surgeons

For cesarean section, if the surgeon or his assistant is known to be "rough," the patient will have a lot of discomfort because not all the nerves supplying the abdomen are blocked by spinal anesthesia. In such a situation, if there is no contraindication to general anesthesia, the latter technique is a better choice than subarachnoid or epidural block.

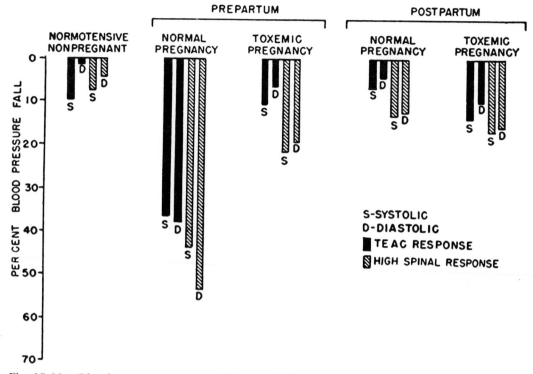

Fig. 15-11.   Blood pressure response with tetraethylammonium chloride and high spinal block in nonpregnant, pregnant, toxemic and postpartum patients. (Assali, N. S., and Prystowsky, H.: Studies on autonomic blockade; comparison between effects of tetraethylammonium chloride (TEAC) and high selective spinal anesthesia on blood pressure of normal and toxemic pregnancy. J. Clin. Invest., *29*:1354, 1950)

Technical Difficulties, Including Laminectomy

Technical difficulties, such as obesity, scoliosis, kyphosis, and others, are relative contraindications which diminish with increased experience of the operator. Laminectomy is more a contraindication to epidural block than to subarachnoid block. With epidural block there may be adhesions between the ligamentum flavum and the dura, thus increasing the possibility of inadvertent dural puncture and limiting the spread of the anesthetic. With subarachnoid block these are not handicaps since the adhesions are outside the subarachnoid space and the intention is to perform dural puncture. In fact, many patients who have had a laminectomy have

been successfully delivered under subarachnoid block. To perform the lumbar puncture one usually chooses a space higher or lower than the site of laminectomy because of the relatively undisturbed landmarks.

ROLE OF SUBARACHNOID BLOCK

The recognition of aortocaval compression and the proper prophylactic and curative correction of hypotension have made subarachnoid block a safe and valuable technique of analgesia for the parturient.

There are 4 million deliveries in the United States each year. Since at present most women deliver in hospitals, about 90 per cent of them receive some kind of anesthesia or analgesia. Anesthesiologists cover only about 14 per cent of vaginal deliveries[20] but the majority of obstetric anesthesia has been performed by nurse anesthetists.[29] Aspiration pneumonitis is a major cause of maternal death and it is the leading anesthetic factor in maternal deaths during general anesthesia. Therefore, to reduce this complication there should be more use of regional blocks than at present. This can be accomplished by either increasing the interest of anesthesiologists in obstetrics or properly training nurse anesthetists to perform these blocks. Since spinal block is the easiest and the least complicated procedure of the vertebral blocks, the author recommends that the nurse anesthetists perform subarachnoid block provided they have proper education and supervision by a qualified anesthesiologist at least until they master the technique. In some states nurse anesthetists are allowed to use paralyzing doses of muscle relaxants, give drugs that can cause cardiac arrest, and deliberately lower the blood pressure if desired, but they are not allowed to perform a spinal block. This restriction is cynical and not the best policy for utilizing manpower. Under certain circumstances, such as in obstetrics, if subarachnoid block is safer than general anesthesia, and the nurse anesthetist is trained and competent, she or he should not be prevented from performing the safer technique.

ADVANTAGES OF SUBARACHNOID BLOCK

The main advantages of subarachnoid block over other techniques for analgesia in obstetrics are:

Simplicity

Subarachnoid block is much simpler than epidural, caudal, or general anesthesia. The end point, i.e., the appearance of cerebrospinal fluid, is a clear-cut identifying mark compared to epidural or caudal analgesia, which makes the success rate with subarachnoid block higher than is the case with either of two techniques.

Rapidity of Onset

The onset of action with subarachnoid block is almost immediate. The waiting time of about 20 minutes which is required with epidural or caudal analgesia is not needed.

Absence of Toxic Drug Reaction

With subarachnoid block the amount of local anesthetic drug injected is so small that if it is inadvertently injected intravascularly, no untoward reaction occurs in the mother or fetus.

Superiority of Analgesia

The analgesia produced by subarachnoid block is excellent and uniform without patchy distribution or unilateral block.[45,73]

Adequacy of Duration of Analgesia

On the whole, subarachnoid block for cesarean section or vaginal delivery adequately covers the obstetric procedure.

Muscular Relaxation

Muscular relaxation is not a major advantage in obstetrics and may be a disadvantage under certain circumstances for vaginal delivery. However, the excellent abdominal relaxation produced by subarachnoid block associated with spontaneous adequate ventilation is an asset for lower abdominal surgery,[68] including cesarean section.

Minimal Bleeding

The well-contracted uterus and the spontaneous breathing with the maintenance of the negative intrathoracic pressure during subarachnoid block result in less blood loss than under general anesthesia.

Preservation of Patient's Consciousness

The patient remaining conscious has two advantages:

1. Subarachnoid block is much safer than general anesthesia because the airway reflexes are intact; thus, aspiration pneumonitis is very rare. However, under a high subarachnoid block, if there is lack of adequate observation of the patient who cannot cough, and if the patient has had a great amount of central nervous system depressants that obtund the laryngeal reflexes, this catastrophe can occur.

2. Both parents may share the joy of their baby's delivery. During vaginal delivery, both the father and the pain-free mother greatly appreciate being able to watch the delivery through a mirror. During cesarean section and before the surgery is over, the sight and the touch of the neonate as well as hearing the neonate's cries are a great relief to the mother, especially when there were doubts about the fetal condition. The value of the presence of the husband in the delivery room during cesarean section is under investigation.

Minimal Interference With Metabolism

Minimal interference with metabolism is particularly important in toxemic or diabetic patients. If hypotension and respiratory insufficiency are prevented or corrected, subarachnoid block does not cause derangement of the maternal physiology or a potential strain on the liver or the kidneys. There is no doubt that for vaginal delivery, especially when forceps or vacuum extraction is required, subarachnoid block is the best method of analgesia.

Allowance of Oxygen Administration

This is beneficial to the mother by decreasing the incidence of nausea and vomiting and may compensate for respiratory embarrassment. It has also been demonstrated both in animals and in humans that a rise of the maternal Po_2 is accompanied by a rise of the fetal Po_2.[4,35,47,54,57,84] For vaginal delivery, oxygen by a transparent mask is used only if there is maternal and/or fetal distress, while it is routinely administered in all cesarean sections, at least until the baby is delivered.

Minimal Fetal Drug Depression

A negligible amount of drug is transmitted to the fetus following subarachnoid block compared to general anesthesia, epidural, caudal, paracervical, or pudendal nerve block.

Minimal Cost

Subarachnoid block is the least expensive method of anesthesia. This may not be an important factor in rich countries, but in underprivileged parts of the world it is a major factor in deciding the choice of anesthesia.

Rapid Return to Oral Feeding

Unlike general anesthesia, subarachnoid block allows rapid return to oral feeding. The patient in the recovery room feels well and is free of nausea and vomiting.

DISADVANTAGES OF SUBARACHNOID BLOCK

Limited Duration of Action

Because of its limited duration of action, subarachnoid block is mainly used for delivery. Some authorities state that continuous subarachnoid block can be used for both labor and delivery, but as explained before, the actual and potential complications are so high that the technique is not commonly used. Others state that subarachnoid block can be repeatedly administered during the course of labor, using tetracaine and epinephrine to produce the longest possible duration of block. This technique, however, has the disadvantage of producing multiple dural punctures with the possibility of a higher incidence of post-lumbar-puncture cephalgia.

Muscular Paralysis

Following the usual techniques of subarachnoid block, there is complete muscular paralysis. This interferes with the ability of the mother to bear down, especially if the block extends above the T10 level. However, there have been attempts to inject low concentrations of local anesthetics (1.5% lidocaine instead of 5% lidocaine) into the subarachnoid space to produce sensory without motor paralysis. The value of such a technique in obstetrics has to be further investigated.

Neurologic Sequelae

As explained in Chapter 7, Effects of Vertebral Blocks on the Nervous System, the neurologic complications of spinal anesthesia have been excessively exaggerated. In a recent review of 78,746 cases of spinal anesthesia, no permanent neurologic sequelae were found.[55] The only practical drawback of subarachnoid block is post-lumbar-puncture cephalgia. With the use of fine spinal needles (25- or 26-gauge) and proper techniques, the severity and incidence of post-lumbar-puncture cephalgia are very low.

Hypotension

Hypotension is the major disadvantage of subarachnoid block and the main cause of serious complications. Compared with epidural, subarachnoid block causes more hypotension. In unpremedicated human volunteers the cardiovascular effects of T5 epidural block using lidocaine with or without epinephrine were compared with the cardiovascular effects of subarachnoid block. Using each subject as his own control, Ward[91] found that the degree of hypotension, the decrease in cardiac output, the decrease in total peripheral resistance, and the increase in heart rate were highest with epidural with epinephrine, lowest with epidural without epinephrine, and intermediate with subarachnoid block. The degree of experience of the anesthesiologist plays a major role in preventing and treating hypotension efficiently, thus deciding the safety of subarachnoid block.

It is important to know that the autonomic fibers are the first to be blocked and to recover following epidural or subarachnoid block.[33a,69a]

Respiratory Insufficiency

As explained in Chapter 6, Effects of Vertebral Blocks on the Respiratory System, in cesarean section the respiratory insufficiency associated with spinal is higher than with epidural analgesia.

REFERENCES

1. Abouleish, E., Yamaoka, H., and Hingson, R. A.: Evaluation of a taper spinal needle. Anesth. Analg., 53:258, 1974.
2. Adriani, J.: Intrathecal vasoconstrictors. Int. Anesthesiol. Clin., 1:789, 1963.
3. Adriani, J., and Roman-Vega, D.: Saddle block anesthesia. Am. J. Surg., 71:12, 1946.
4. Althabe, O., Jr., et al.: Effects on fetal heart rate and fetal Po₂ of oxygen administration to the mother. Am. J. Obstet. Gynecol., 98:858, 1967.
5. Apgar, V., et al.: Comparison of regional and general anesthesia in obstetrics: with special reference to transmission of cyclopropane across the placenta. J.A.M.A., 165:2155, 1957.
6. Assali, N. S., and Prystowsky, H.: Studies on autonomic blockade; comparison between effects of tetraethylammonium chloride (TEAC) and high selective spinal anesthesia on blood pressure of normal and toxemic pregnancy. J. Clin. Invest., 29:1354, 1950.
7. Berges, P. U.: Regional anesthesia for obstetrics. In Bonica, J. J. (ed.): Regional Anesthesia. Pp. 14-166. Philadelphia, F. A. Davis, 1971.
8. Bizzarri, D., et al.: Continuous spinal anesthesia using a special needle and catheter. Anesth. Analg., 43:393, 1964.
9. Bonica, J. J.: Management of Pain. Philadelphia, Lea & Febiger, 1953.
10. ———: Principles and Practice of Obstetric Analgesia and Anesthesia. Philadelphia, F. A. Davis, 1967.
11. Bonica, J. J., Backup, P. H., and Pratt, W. H.: The use of vasoconstrictors to prolong spinal anesthesia. Anesthesiology, 12:431, 1951.
12. Borison, H. L., and Wang, S. C.: Physiology and pharmacology of vomiting. Pharmacol. Rev., 5:193, 1953.
13. Bridenbaugh, P. O.: Is administration of spinal anesthetic contraindicated in a patient with a normal coagulation profile who will be systemically heparinized during the operative procedure. Anesth. Analg., 54:506, 1975.

14. Browning, D. J.: Serious side effects of ergometrine and its use in routine obstetric practice. Med. J. Aust., *1*:957, 1974.

15. Bryce-Smith, R., and Williams, E. O.: Treatment of eclampsia (imminent or actual) by continuous conduction analgesia. Lancet, *1*:1241, 1955.

16. Carpenter, S. L., Ceravolo, A. J., and Foldes, F. F.: Continuous-drop subarachnoidal block with dilute procaine solution for labor and delivery. Am. J. Obstet. Gynecol., *61*:1277, 1951.

17. Clark, R. B., Thompson, D. S., and Thompson, C. H.: Prevention of spinal hypotension associated with cesarean section. Anesthesiology, *45*:670, 1976.

18. Cohen, C. A., and Kallos, T.: Failure of spinal anesthesia due to subdural catheter placement. Anesthesiology, *37*:352, 1972.

19. Cohen, E. N., and Knight, R. T.: Hydrogen ion concentration of spinal fluid and its relation to spinal anesthetic failures. Anesthesiology, *8*:594, 1947.

20. Committee on Maternal Health: National Study of Maternity Care. Survey of Obstetric Practice and Associated Services in the Hospitals in the United States. A Report of the Committee, American College of Obstetricians and Gynecologists, Chicago, 1970.

21. DiGiovanni, A. J.: A critical evaluation of disposable spinal anesthesia needles. Anesthesiology, *34*:88, 1971.

22. Dripps, R. D., and Vandam, L. D.: Long-term follow-up of patients who received 10,098 spinal anesthetics; failure to discover major neurological sequelae. J.A.M.A., *156*:1486, 1954.

23. Elam, J. O.: Catheter subarachnoid block for labor and delivery: a differential segmental technic employing hyperbaric lidocaine. Anesth. Analg., *49*:1007, 1970.

24. Frumin, M. J.: Fine lumbar puncture needle (modification of technique). Anesthesiology, *17*:504, 1956.

24a.Ghoneim, M. M., and Long, J. P.: The interaction between magnesium and other neuromuscular blocking agents. *32*:23, 1970.

25. Giuffrida, J. G., *et al.*: Continuous procaine spinal anesthesia for cesarean section. Anesth. Analg., *51*:117, 1972.

26. Gomez-Rogers, G., Faundes-Latham, A., and Garrido, J.: Influence of spinal and caudal anesthesia on the FHR of human fetus. *In* Caldeyro Barciak, R. (ed.): Effects of Labor on the Fetus and Newborn. New York, Pergamon Press, 1967.

27. Greene, N. M.: Physiology of Spinal Anesthesia. Baltimore, Williams & Wilkins, 1967.

28. Guyton, A. C.: Textbook of Medical Physiology. Ed. 5, p. 272. Philadelphia, W. B. Saunders, 1976.

29. Hehre, F.: Observations, philosophic and opinionated, on obstetric anesthesia coverage. *In* Safar, P. (ed.): Public Health Aspects of Critical Care Medicine and Anesthesiology. Pp. 323-333. Philadelphia, F. A. Davis, 1974.

30. Hon, E. H., Reid, B. L., and Hehre, F. W.: The electronic evaluation of fetal heart rate: II. Changes with maternal hypotension. Am. J. Obstet. Gynecol., *79*:209, 1960.

31. James, F. M., III, Greiss, F. C., Jr., and Kemp, R. A.: An evaluation of vasopressor therapy for maternal hypotension during spinal anesthesia. Anesthesiology, *33*:25, 1970.

32. Johnson, W. L., *et al.*: Effect of pudendal, spinal, and peridural block anesthesia on the second stage of labor. Am. J. Obstet. Gynecol., *113*:166, 1972.

33. Jones, G. R., *et al.*: Continuous spinal anesthesia in the treatment of severe preeclampsia and eclampsia. South. Med. J., *45*:34, 1952.

33a.Kim, J. M., LaSalle, A. D., and Parmley, R. T.: Sympathetic recovery following lumbar epidural and spinal analgesia. Anesth. Analg., *56*:352, 1977.

34. Kim, Y. I., Mazza, N. M., and Marx, G. F.: Massive spinal block with hemicranial palsy after a "test dose" for extradural analgesia. Anesthesiology, *43*:370, 1975.

35. Kirschbaum, T. H., *et al.*: The dynamics of placenal oxygen transfer. I. Effects of maternal hyperoxia in pregnant ewes and fetal lambs. Am. J. Obstet. Gynecol., *98*:429, 1967.

36. Lemmon, W. T.: A method for continuous spinal anesthesia; a preliminary report. Ann. Surg., *111*:141, 1940.

37. Lund, P. C.: The role of conduction anesthesia in the management of eclampsia. Anesthesiology, *12*:693, 1951.

38. ———: Principles and Practice of Spinal Anesthesia. Springfield, Ill., Charles C Thomas, 1971.

39. ———: Is the presence of backache and sciatica a contraindication to spinal anesthesia? Anesth. Analg., *54*:505, 1975.

40. Lund, P. C., and Cwik, J. C.: Modern trends in spinal anaesthesia. Can. Anaesth. Soc. J., *15*:118, 1968.

41. McElrath, P. J., *et al.*: Continuous spinal anesthesia in the treatment of severe pre-eclampsia and eclampsia. Am. J. Obstet. Gynecol., *58*:1084, 1949.

42. Macintosh, R., and Lee, J. A.: Lumbar Puncture and Spinal Anesthesia. Ed. 3. Edinburgh, Churchill Livingstone, 1973.

43. Moore, D. C.: Anesthetic Techniques for Obstetric Anesthesia and Analgesia. Springfield, Ill., Charles C Thomas, 1964.

44. Moore, D. C., *et al.*: Prolongation of spinal blocks with vasoconstrictor drugs. Surg. Gynecol. Obstet., *23*:983, 1966.

45. ———: Present status of spinal (subarachnoid) and epidural (peridural) block: a comparison of the two techniques. Anesth. Analg., *47*:40, 1968.

46. Morely, T. S.: The spinal-needle director. [Correspondence] Anesthesiology, *34*:580, 1971.

47. Motoyama, E. K., *et al.*: The effect of changes in maternal pH and pCO$_2$ of fetal lambs. Anesthesiology, *28*:891, 1967.

48. Moya, F., and Smith, B.: Spinal anesthesia for cesarean section: clinical and biochemical studies of effects on maternal physiology. J.A.M.A., *179*:609, 1962.

49. ———: Maternal hypotension and the newborn.

Proceedings of the Third World Congress of Anesthesiology, 2:38, 1964.

50. Neigh, J. L., Kane, P. B., and Smith, T. C.: Effects of speed and direction of injection on the level and duration of spinal anesthesia. Anesth. Analg., 49:912, 1970.

51. Neme, B.: Effects of spinal anesthesia on pregnant human uterine contractility. I. Effects during pregnancy. Matern. Infanc., 30:189, 1971.

52. ———: Effects of spinal anesthesia on pregnant human uterine contracility. II. Effects during labor (first and second stages). Matern. Infanc., 30:189, 1971.

53. ———: Effects of spinal anesthesia on pregnant human uterine contractility. III. Effects during labor (third stage) and immediate postpartum (fourth stage). Matern. Infanc., 30:203, 1971.

54. Newman, W., et al.: Oxygen transfer from mother to fetus during labor. Am. J. Obstet. Gynecol., 99:61, 1967.

55. Noble, A. B., and Murray, J. G.: A review of the complications of spinal anesthesia with experience in Canadian teaching hospitals from 1959 to 1969. Can. Anaesth. Soc. J., 18:5, 1971.

56. Park, W. Y., Balingit, P. E., and MacNamara, T. E.: Effects of patient age pH of cerebrospinal fluid, and vasopressors on onset and duration of spinal anesthesia. Anesth. Analg., 54:455, 1975.

57. Parker, H. R., and Purves, M. J.: Some effects of maternal hyperoxia and hypoxia on the blood gas tensions and vascular pressures in the foetal sheep. Q. J. Exp. Physiol., 52:205, 1967.

58. Pflug, E. A., Aasheim, G. M., and Beck, H. A.: Spinal anesthesia: bupivacaine versus tetracaine. Anesth. Analg., 55:489, 1976.

59. Phillips, K. G.: The relative effects of obstetrical anesthesia and analgesia upon the promptness of neonatal respiration. Am. J. Obstet. Gynecol., 77:113, 1959.

60. Phillips, O. C.: Personal communication.

61. Phillips, O. C., Goddard, J. E., and Millstein, J.: Obstetric Analgesia and Anesthesia, Surgical Specialties. Philadelphia, F. A. Davis, 1967.

62. Phillips, O. C., et al.: Neurologic complications following spinal anesthesia with lidocaine: a prospective review of 10,440 cases. Anesthesiology, 30:284, 1969.

63. Pietrobono, P., and Maggi, U.: Spinal anesthesia with hyperbaric bupivacaine: an old technique for a modern anaesthesia (observation on 300 cases). Acta Anaesthesiol. Scand., 22:461, 1971.

64. Plum, F., and Siesjo, B. K.: Recent advances in CSF physiology. Anesthesiology, 42:708, 1975.

65. Prystowsky, H.: Fetal blood studies. VII: The oxygen pressure gradient between maternal and fetal bloods of humans in normal and abnormal pregnancy. Bull. Johns Hopkins Hosp., 101:48, 1957.

66. Ramaioli, F., and Pagani, I.: Experience with hyperbaric 1% bupivacaine in 321 cases of spinal anesthesia for orthopedic and traumatological surgery. Minerva Anestesiol., 38:1, 1972.

67. Ratra, C. K., Badola, R. P., and Bhargaya, K. P.: A study of factors concerned in emesis during spinal anaesthesia. Br. J. Anaesth., 44:1208, 1972.

68. Ravin, M. B.: Comparison of spinal and general anesthesia for lower abdominal surgery in patients with chronic obstructive pulmonary disease. Anesthesiology, 35:319, 1971.

69. Reynolds, S. R., Harris, J. S., and Kaiser, I. H.: Clinical Measurement of Uterine Forces in Pregnancy and Labor. Springfield, Ill., Charles C Thomas, 1954.

69a. Roe, C. F. and Cohn, F. L.: Sympathetic blockade during spinal anesthesia. Surg. Gynecol. Obstet., 136:265, 1973.

70. Sadove, M. S., Lavin, M. J., and Rant-Sejdinaj, I.: Neurological complications of spinal anaesthesia. Can. Anaesth. Soc. J., 8:405, 1961.

71. Saklad, M., et al: Intraspinal segmental anesthesia: a preliminary report. Anesthesiology, 8:270, 1947.

72. Scarborough, R. A.: Spinal anesthesia from the surgeon's stand point. J.A.M.A., 168:1324, 1958.

73. Scott, D. B., and Thorburn, J. T.: Editorial: spinal anaesthesia. Br. J. Anaesth., 47:421, 1975.

74. Sechzer, P. H.: Subdural space in spinal anesthesia. Anesthesiology, 24:869, 1963.

75. Shantha, T. R.: Ketamine for the treatment of hiccups during and following anesthesia. A preliminary report. Anesth. Analg., 52:822, 1973.

76. Shephard, N. W.: The chemistry and pharmacology of dioperidol, phenoperidine and fentanyl. In Shephard, N. W. (ed.): The Application of Neuroleptanalgesia in Anesthetic and Other Practice. New York, Pergamon Press, 1965.

77. Shnider, S. M., et al.: Vasopressors in obstetrics. I. Correction of fetal acidosis with ephedrine during spinal hypotension. Am. J. Obstet. Gynecol., 102:911, 1968.

78. Simon, N. M., and Krumlovsky, F. A.: The pathophysiology of hypertension in pregnancy. J. Reprod. Med., 8:102, 1972.

79. Smith, B. E.: Guest discussion. In Lerner, S., et al.: Considerations for complicated obstetrics: II. Preeclampsia and hypertensive vascular disease. Anesth. Analg., 48:776, 1969.

80. Smith, B., Cavanaugh, D., and Moya, F.: Anesthesia for vaginal delivery of the patient with toxemia of pregnancy. Anesth. Analg., 45:853, 1966.

81. Smith, B. E., Moya, F., and Shnider, S.: The effects of anesthesia on liver function during labor. Anesth. Analg., 41:24, 1962.

82. Stenger, V., et al.: Spinal anesthesia for cesarean section: physiological and biochemical observations. Am. J. Obstet. Gynecol., 90:51, 1964.

83. Szappanyos, G. G.: The utilization of Marcaine (LAC-43) in spinal and epidural anesthesia. Anaesthetist, 18:330, 1969.

84. Tervila, L., et al.: The effect of oxygen ventilation and a vasodilator on uterine perfusion, foetal oxygen and acid-base balance. I. A study in health gravidae. Acta Obstet. Gynecol. Scand., 52:177, 1973.

85. Ueland, K., Gills, R. E., and Hensen, J. M.: Maternal cardiovascular dynamics. I. Cesarean section under subarachnoid block anesthesia. Am. J. Obstet. Gynecol., *100*:42, 1968.

86. Ueland, K., *et al.*: Maternal cardiovascular dynamics. VI. Cesarean section under epidural anesthesia without epinephrine. Am. J. Obstet. Gynecol., *114*:775, 1972.

87. Urban, B. J.: Clinical observations suggesting a changing site of action during induction and recession of spinal and epidural anesthesia. Anesthesiology, *39*:496, 1973.

88. Vandam, L. D., and Dripps, R. D.: Long-term follow-up of patients who received 10,098 spinal anesthetics: syndrome of decreased intracranial pressure (headache and ocular and auditory difficulties). J.A.M.A., *161*:586, 1956.

89. Van Gilder, J. C., and Schwartz, H. G.: Growth of dermoids from skin implants to the nervous system and surrounding spaces of the newborn rat. J. Neurosurg., *26*:14, 1967.

90. Vasicka, A., and Kretchmer, H.: Effect of conduction and inhalation anesthesia on uterine contractions. Am. J. Obstet. Gynecol., *82*:600, 1961.

91. Ward, R. J., *et al.*: Epidural and subarachnoid anesthesia: cardiovascular and respiratory effects. J.A.M.A., *191*:275, 1965.

92. Weiskopf, R. B.: Unexplained failure of a continuous spinal anesthetic. Anesthesiology, *33*:114, 1970.

93. Williams, B.: The present place of spinal subarachnoid analgesia in obstetrics. Br. J. Anaesth., *41*:628, 1969.

94. Zuspan, F.: Adrenal gland and sympathetic nervous system response in eclampsia. Am. J. Obstet. Gynecol., *114*:304, 1972.

16

Paracervical Block

Ezzat Abouleish, M.D.

DEFINITION

Paracervical block is a form of nerve block in which the local anesthetic is injected into the vicinity of the cervix to block nerve impulses from the uterine body and cervix.

HISTORY

The first report of a paracervical block was published in Germany by Gellert in 1926.[18] The first American publication concerning paracervical block was by Rosenfeld in 1945.[47] This method of pain relief in obstetrics did not become popular until ten years later.

TECHNIQUE
RECENT MODIFICATIONS IN THE TECHNIQUE

Following the recent discoveries of the fetal complications of paracervical block, certain modifications are recommended to make paracervical block a safer technique.

Drug Dosage

In the past the usual dose of local anesthetic drug for paracervical block has been 100 mg. of bupivacaine (20 ml. of the 0.5 concentration) or 200 mg. of mepivacaine, lidocaine, or prilocaine (20 ml. of the 1% concentration). Recently it has been stressed that the dose should be reduced to the minimal effective level. A dose of 25 mg. of bupivacaine (10 ml. of the 0.25% concentration) or 100 mg. of the other amides (10 ml. of the 1% concentration) was found to be adequate.[28]

The use of 1 per cent chloroprocaine instead of the amide drugs offers at least a theoretical advantage, that is, of being better handled by the fetus.[13]

Depth of Injection

Proper understanding of the maternal anatomy is important for the safety of paracervical block. The paracervical plexus lies in the areolar tissue between the folds of the uterosacral ligament in close proximity to the uterine artery, uterine venous plexus, and ureter. During pregnancy the uterine artery and the venous plexus are drawn cephalad to a higher level than the nervous plexus. The aim of injecting the local anesthetic for paracervical block is to deposit the drug as close to the nervous plexus as possible, and as far away from the uterine vasculature as possible. Therefore, to determine the best depth and site of the injection, a study was recently performed by Jagerhorn.[28] In 20 women who were admitted for abortion between 17 and 19 weeks of pregnancy, a mixture of contrast medium and local anesthetic was injected at various sites and depths paracervically in order to study the spread and absorption from this area during pregnancy. The study showed clearly that the injection depth is of the greatest importance in determining the spread of the injected solution. At a depth of 4 mm. or more, intravascular spread is rapid as shown by parametriographic follow-up. At a depth of 2 mm., which corresponds to the thickness of the vaginal mucosa, the anesthetic gradually diffuses laterally and cephalad with minimal intravascular spread, thus becoming more or less localized to the area of the paracervical plexus.

The work by Jagerhorn confirmed an earlier report by Bloom and coworkers[8] in 1972 which stressed the importance of injecting the local anesthetic superficially into the submucous layer rather than deeply into the parametrium. In the latter study, 51 patients were given 87 paracervical blocks using 16 ml. of 1 per cent prilocaine injected at 4 sites around the cervix, at 3, 4, 8, and 9 o'clock. The needle tip was inserted into the mucosa to a depth sufficient to get the needle bevel through the mucosa. The bolus was injected so superficially as to raise a palpable wheal. Using this technique the success rate was 92 per cent. Both reports found no maternal or fetal toxicity related to the paracervical block itself.

Sites of Injection

The local anesthetic is preferably injected at four sites rather than at two in order to avoid the risk of too large a single dose being accidentally injected into a blood vessel, the lower uterine segment, or the fetus. The sites used by Jagerhorn were 4, 5, 7, and 8 o'clock. The total volume was 10 ml. of 0.25 per cent bupivacaine injected in the ratio of 3:2:2:3 respectively.

Avoidance of Excessive Pressure at the Fornices Vaginae

No undue pressure should be applied at the fornices vaginae by the fingers or the needle guide; otherwise, the site of injection would be brought close to the paracervical blood vessels or the pelvic wall. (Fig. 16-1).

Separating the Fetal Head from the Site of Injection

If the right hand is introduced to feel the patient's right vaginal fornix, the back of the fingers will be toward the cervix and the fetal head, separating them from the needle guide and the needle (Fig. 16-1). In the same manner the left hand is introduced to feel the patient's left vaginal fornix.

Tangential Direction of the Needle to the Fetal Head

The site of injection should be kept as far as possible from the presenting part of the fetus and the lower uterine segment. Therefore the needle is introduced tangentially to the presenting fetal part.

ONE-DOSE TECHNIQUE

1. The obstetrical history of the patient and the progress of labor are evaluated.

2. Vaginal examination is performed to determine the degree of cervical dilatation and the position of the presenting part of the fetus. Paracervical block is best performed during the acceleration phase when cervical dilatation is 4 to 5 cm. in a multipara and 5 to 6 cm. in a nullipara.

3. The fetal heart rate tracing is recorded, preferably by an internal monitor. The rupture of membranes before paracervical block also helps to exclude meconium staining of the amniotic fluid. The maternal pulse and blood pressure are measured.

4. The paracervical block tray is opened. The tray has usually been prepacked and presterilized by autoclaving. There are disposable trays which are gas-sterilized and can be used as an alternative.

5. The operator puts on sterile gloves and unpacks the tray, which contains a

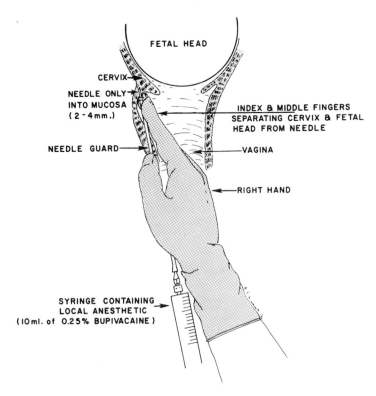

FETAL HEAD

CERVIX

NEEDLE ONLY
INTO MUCOSA
(2 - 4 mm.)

INDEX & MIDDLE FINGERS
SEPARATING CERVIX & FETAL
HEAD FROM NEEDLE

NEEDLE GUARD

VAGINA

RIGHT HAND

SYRINGE CONTAINING
LOCAL ANESTHETIC
(10 ml. of 0.25% BUPIVACAINE)

Fig. 16-1. Technique of paracervical block. Notice the position of the hand and fingers in relation to the cervix and fetal head; that no undue pressure is applied at the vaginal fornix by the fingers or the needle guide; and the shallow depth of the needle insertion.

10-ml. syringe., a 12-cm. 22-gauge needle, a needle guide (Iowa trumpet or Kobak needle), and a regular no. 19-gauge hypodermic needle (Fig. 16-2).

6. A presterilized local anesthetic vial is added to the tray except if chloroprocaine is to be used because the drug deteriorates when heat-sterilized.

7. The patient is placed in the lithotomy position. The perineum is carefully prepared. No special preparation is required for the vagina. The patient is draped as for vaginal examination.

8. The operator then introduces his index and middle fingers into the vagina, examines the cervix and the presenting part of the fetus, and places the two fingers in the fornix at the proposed site of injection.

9. The operator introduces the needle guide, along the interval between the two fingers, to the fornix.

10. The 12-cm. needle connected to the syringe containing the local anesthetic so-

lution is passed along the needle guide until its tip catches into the mucous membrane of the vagina. Then the needle is advanced for only 2 mm.

11. Aspiration is gently performed and, in the absence of blood, the dose of local anesthetic for this site is injected.

12. The same procedure is repeated at the other sites of injection.

13. The patient is turned onto her side and the vital signs are measured.

14. Fetal heart rate monitoring continues for at least 30 minutes.

Analgesia usually starts in a few minutes and lasts for about 1 to 2 hours depending on the drug used. Analgesia usually wears off rather abruptly.

CONTINUOUS PARACERVICAL BLOCK

Continuous paracervical block has been attempted[56] but the technique is rather complicated. The catheter used for the

Fig. 16-2. Paracervical tray showing the paracervical needle, the needle guard, and the local anesthetic.

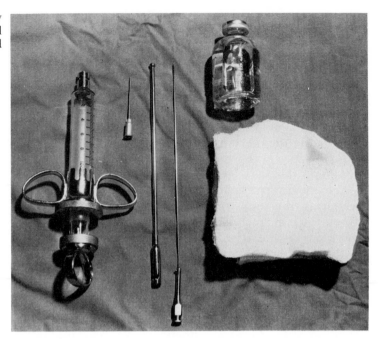

block tends to become dislodged, and the technique is rarely used.

USE OF THE SYRIJET ANESTHETIC GUN

Injection of local anesthetics by using high velocity to penetrate tissues instead of a needle point was performed successfully for paracervical and uterosacral blocks in gynecologic operations.[16,34] However, radiologic studies following paracervical injection of radiopaque material, even if the material was injected by needle, demonstrated immediate spread of the agent several centimeters in all directions, including toward the uterine fundus.[29,65] Therefore, the safety of these high-velocity jets to perform paracervical block in a pregnancy at term is questionable until it is proven that no direct spread of the local anesthetic to the fetus or placenta occurs.

COMPLICATIONS OF PARACERVICAL BLOCK

Paracervical block can lead to maternal and/or fetal complications.

MATERNAL COMPLICATIONS

Inadvertent Intravascular Injection of the Local Anesthetic

Inadvertent intravascular injection of the local anesthetic can lead to either mild or severe reactions. The mild reactions include dizziness, ringing in the ears, and/or strange aura which occur in about one out of 600 cases.[49] Severe toxic reactions causing convulsions can follow paracervical block for the termination of early pregnancy by dilatation and curettage at a rate of about one out of 3000 cases.[6] A similar incidence of seizures has been reported secondary to local or pudendal nerve block for delivery.[53] It has been demonstrated that during paracervical block the local anesthetic can gain direct vascular entry despite the failure to obtain blood upon aspiration prior to injection.[9] Perhaps this resulted from advancement of the needle tip into a blood vessel during injection. Convulsion following paracervical block can lead to maternal mortality.[6,20] To avoid such a complication, no undue pressure should be applied at the vaginal fornix;

otherwise, tenting would occur and the tip of the needle may approach and possibly enter the dilated thin-walled paracervical venous plexus. The needle should be inserted the shortest possible distance. Injection of the local anesthetic just beneath the mucosa by advancing the needle for only 2 mm. reduces the likelihood of inadvertent injection into the uterine vasculature.[8,28]

The author, as stated repeatedly throughout the text, shares with eminent anesthesiologists the belief that before administering the local anesthetic for any purpose including paracervical block, all equipment and drugs for resuscitation should be readily available and the operator should have experience in dealing with convulsions and cardiopulmonary collapse.[2a]

Extension of the Local Anesthetic to the Sacral Nerves Leading to Anesthesia of the Leg

If undue pressure is applied at the vaginal fornix, the distance between the vaginal wall and the pelvic wall becomes reduced to a few millimeters, and/or, if the needle is advanced too far, the local anesthetic can be injected into the vicinity of the sacral nerves. To prevent such a complication, no undue pressure should be used and the needle should be advanced for only 2 to 3 mm.

Sacral Neuritis

Several cases of sacral neuritis have been reported following the injection of neurolytic agents.[52]

Superficial Laceration of the Vagina by the Tip of the Needle

The incidence of this complication is 1:845.[51] With the proper use of a protective needle guide, it should rarely happen.

Bleeding from the Fornix

The incidence of bleeding from the fornix following paracervical block is 1:95.[5]

Maternal Hypotension

Maternal hypotension occurs in about one out of 600 cases and is due to compression of the inferior vena cava.[51] It is corrected by turning the patient onto her left side.

FETAL AND NEONATAL COMPLICATIONS

Fetal and neonatal complications of paracervical block are fetal bradycardia, fetal acidosis, neonatal depression, neonatal convulsions, and perinatal death.

FETAL BRADYCARDIA

Definition

Post-paracervical block fetal bradycardia is defined as a decrease in fetal heart rate to or below 120 beats/min. for more than 1 minute following the administration of paracervical block to the mother.

Incidence

The incidence of fetal bradycardia following paracervical block varies between 2 per cent and 70 per cent;[5] the average is 24 per cent.[40,51] This marked variation is due to the differences in the definition of bradycardia, the method used for its determination, the drug injected, the dose utilized, the technique applied, the cases selected, and the experience of the operator performing the paracervical block. For example, with continuous electronic recording of the fetal heart rate, fetal bradycardia is detected more frequently than with intermittent auscultation.[17]

Time of Onset

Fetal bradycardia usually starts within 1 to 12 minutes following paracervical block, the average time being 6 minutes.[15]

Duration

Fetal bradycardia usually lasts for between 2 and 32 minutes, the average duration being 8 minutes.[15]

Mechanisms

Fetal bradycardia can occur as a result of a direct effect of the local anesthetic drug, decreased placental blood flow, or reflex stimulation (Fig. 16-3).

Direct Effect of the Local Anesthetic on the Fetus. This is most probably the main cause of fetal bradycardia. It can be due to too much of the local anesthetic drug reaching the fetus, and/or increased fetal susceptibility.[61,62]

Too Much Local Anesthetic Reaching the Fetus. There is a correlation between the dose of the local anesthetic injected and fetal bradycardia. The incidence of fetal bradycardia is 20 per cent in patients receiving 200 mg. of mepivacaine, compared with an incidence of 70 per cent in those receiving 400 mg.[60]

There is a correlation between fetal bradycardia and the level of local anesthetic drug in the fetus.[19] With fetal blood levels of mepivacaine below 3 μg./ml., fetal bradycardia is rarely seen.[4] Ninety per cent of those fetuses developing bradycardia have a mepivacaine level of 3 μg./ml. or greater; in most of these cases, the mepivacaine level is higher in the fetus than in the mother. The fetal to maternal mepivacaine blood ratio in those who do not develop fetal bradycardia is 0.9 or less, while in those who do is above 2.[4]

With paracervical block, the dose may be proper, yet a large amount of the local anesthetic may reach the fetus due to any of the following:

1. *Direct injection into the fetus* causes an almost immediate fetal bradycardia which may lead to intrauterine or neonatal death.[10] The close proximity of the fetus to the site of paracervical injection makes such a complication quite possible.

2. *Injection into a low-lying placenta* causes almost immediate transfer of the local anesthetic to the fetus.

3. *Injection into the lower uterine segment* causes rapid access of the local anesthetic to the fetal circulation.

4. *Injection into the uterine artery* is espe-cially liable to occur if the drug is injected deeply into the paracervical tissue, no aspiration is done before administering the drug, and the hand is not kept steady during the injection.

5. *Injection into a uterine vein* causes a high maternal level of the local anesthetic. It is argued that this is probably not followed by fetal bradycardia, because the injection of a local anesthetic drug into the maternal antecubital vein was rarely followed by fetal bradycardia.[62] However, injection into a uterine vein is different because retrograde flow to the intervillous space may occur, especially if the injection is fast.

6. *Diffusion into a uterine artery* causes a high fetal blood level of the drug.[4] When paracervical block is followed by fetal bradycardia, the local anesthetic level in the fetus usually exceeds that in the mother.[4] Since there is no active transport of local anesthetic drugs across the placenta, it is unlikely in these cases that the fetus has received all of its local anesthetic drug through the maternal circulation. Therefore, the local anesthetic drug has to reach the fetus by a method bypassing the maternal circulation, which can be achieved by the drug diffusing through the wall of the uterine artery and directly to the intervillous space and the fetal circulation.[4] This theory is confirmed by the finding that mepivacaine readily diffuses across the femoral artery when injected around it.[54]

7. *Individual differences* affect the rate of absorption of the drug from the paracervical area. Maternal hemodynamics influencing the drug supply to the fetus include the time relationship between injection and uterine contractions; the arterial blood pressure; the venous return from the paracervical space and from the placenta as retarded by inferior vena caval compression; and differences in maternal body weight and placental function.

Increased Fetal Susceptibility. The toxic effects of local anesthetics can be more pronounced in the following fetal conditions:

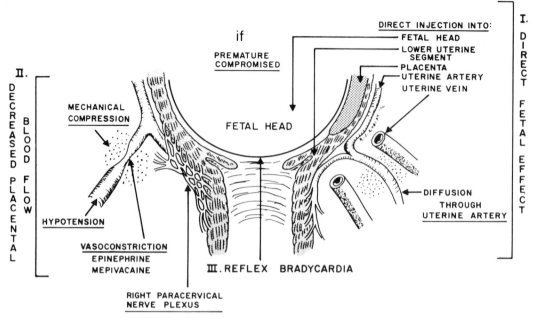

Fig. 16-3.   Mechanisms of post-paracervical block fetal bradycardia.

1. *Somatic Prematurity.* As a rule, the mother tolerates much higher levels of local anesthetics than does the fetus. This special sensitivity of the fetus is probably related to a lower level of somatic maturity. As a matter of fact, post-paracervical block fetal bradycardia is more common in premature fetuses.[49]

2. *Compromised Fetus.* For example, if the fetal scalp blood pH is 7.25 or less, the incidence and severity of fetal bradycardia is higher than if it is 7.30 or more.[22]

Decreased Placental Blood Flow. There are many possible causes for this:

Maternal Aortocaval Compression. Because of the lithotomy position of the mother during paracervical block, the uterus may cause aortocaval compression with subsequent decrease in the placental blood flow which leads to fetal hypoxia and bradycardia. This fetal bradycardia can easily be corrected by simply tilting the patient to one side (usually the left side).[28] However, post-paracervical block fetal bradycardia has been observed despite the lateral position of the parturient and the normal range of blood pressure.[58]

Mechanical Compression of the Uterine Blood Vessels. Decrease in uterine blood flow may be due to the volume of drug injected compressing the uterine blood vessels.[42] However, injection of the same volume of normal saline instead of mepivacaine does not cause significant changes in heart rate or blood pH of the fetus.[24]

Constriction of the Uterine Blood Vessels. This may be due to:

1. *Epinephrine.*[29] However, fetal bradycardia occurs both with and without epinephrine. Epinephrine is not recommended in obstetrics because it reduces the uterine blood flow, even in minute doses, which has no significant effect on the maternal arterial blood pressure.[46,49] This reduction in uterine blood flow following epinephrine can be due to redistribution of the cardiac output leading to the increased blood flow to other tissues such as the skeletal muscles.

2. *The Local Anesthetic Itself.* Mepivacaine,

is known to have a direct vasoconstrictor effect.[1,7] Recently both in vitro and in vivo studies, other drugs such as lidocaine, bupivacaine, and chloroprocaine are found to have a direct vasoconstrictive effect.[18a, 19a, 28a] The vasoconstrictive effect is most marked with lidocaine, slight with bupivacaine, and least with chloroprocaine. Moreover, in vitro, chloroprocaine produces an increasing vasodilator response with increasing gestational age.[28a]

Hypertonicity of the Uterus. Decrease of the uterine blood flow can be secondary to increased tonicity of the uterus and hyperactivity of the uterine muscle following paracervical block.[15,33] However, postparacervical block fetal bradycardia may be associated with decreased uterine activity.[40] Uterine contractions are usually not affected by paracervical block;[31] if they do change, they usually decrease.[13,42,64,66]

Reflex Bradycardia. Increased pressure on the fetal head during the vaginal manipulation increases vagal tone and fetal bradycardia. This fetal bradycardia should disappear once the manipulation has stopped.

FETAL ACIDOSIS

Fetal acidosis usually occurs if fetal bradycardia lasts more than 10 minutes.[15] The degree of fetal acidosis is proportionate to the severity and duration of fetal bradycardia. There is also a correlation between fetal acidosis and the fetal blood level of the drug.[4] This biochemical derangement is usually transient, and normal acid-base status is reached following restoration of normal fetal heart rate.

NEONATAL DEPRESSION

As evidenced by the Apgar scores and the time to sustained respiration, neonatal depression is significantly higher in those babies who showed fetal bradycardia compared to those who did not or those whose mothers had not received paracervical block.[51] In a series of 2,958 deliveries, fetal bradycardia following paracervical block occurred in 86 cases; low 1-minute Apgar scores (below 6) occurred in 16 cases; and low 5-minute Apgar scores occured in 5 neonates.[40] The neonatal depression is particularly evident when the delivery is accomplished within 30 minutes following paracervical block, and before restoration of the normal fetal heart rate.[15] There is a correlation between the neonatal blood levels of the local anesthetic and neonatal depression.[4]

NEONATAL CONVULSIONS

Neonatal convulsions following paracervical block are liable to occur if the drug is injected directly into the fetus, placenta, or lower uterine segment.[10,21,45] The immaturity of the fetal central nervous system renders it more vulnerable to the toxic injury by the local anesthetic than the adult's central nervous system.[21] These neonatal convulsions following paracervical block have a grave prognosis because they are associated with a high neonatal death rate.[10,45] A 5-year-old child who survived such an episode as a neonate still has residual effects of ataxia and dysarthria with poor motor skill and very limited verbal communication.[21]

PERINATAL DEATH

Direct injection of the local anesthetic into the fetus, placenta, or lower uterine segment can be followed by intrauterine fetal death.[38,45] As early as 1963 this hazard with the use of lidocaine has been pointed out by Nyirgesy. In one case in which the mother had severe preeclampsia, the fetal heart stopped 3 minutes after paracervical block and the infant was stillborn. Fetal and neonatal deaths also followed paracervical block using mepivacaine[45] and bupivacaine.[37,48]

PHARMACOLOGIC EFFECTS OF LOCAL ANESTHETICS ON THE FETUS

CARDIAC EFFECTS

Electrophysiologic Effects

Recently the electrocardiographic changes in the fetus during bradycardia have been studied.[15] Fetal bradycardia is usually associated with shortening of the PR interval and the development of nodal rhythm. Similar electrocardiographic changes have been found in adults under controlled hypotension using ganglion blockers. Secondary to hypotension, the pacemaker of the heart gradually descends from the head to the tail of the SA node, leading to shortening of the PR interval.[2] If hypotension progresses, the SA node is completely depressed, the AV node becomes the pacemaker, and nodal rhythm occurs. With fetal bradycardia following paracervical block as well as in adults under controlled hypotension, there are no significant changes in the width of the QRS complex; the ST segment and T waves do not show any consistent pattern. Therefore, these changes in the fetal electrocardiogram, which are similar to those in adult patients, may be secondary to the hypotension.

If the dose of the local anesthetic is excessive, e.g., when injected directly into the fetus, there is a direct cardiac depression, manifested by widening of the QRS complex and prolongation of the PR interval, which may be followed by complete cessation of all electrical activity of the heart.[15]

With continuous recording of the fetal heart rate, post-paracervical block fetal bradycardia usually follows a certain pattern. Initially, it is fixed, has no relation to the uterine contractions, and lasts for several minutes. This is followed by a period of late decelerations, and finally a phase of tachycardia.[59] The initial bradycardiac phase is due to the effect of the drug on the fetus. The late deceleration phase is the result of the supervening hypoxia which becomes exaggerated by the uterine contractions on a partially recovered fetus. The recovery of the fetus from the acute asphyxia is demonstrated by the tachycardiac phase. Of course, if fetal bradycardia continues, hypoxia and acidosis develop. This leads to more hypotension and myocardial depression, creating a vicious circle which may end in fetal death.[19,45,60]

Myocardial Effect

Studies have shown that local anesthetic drugs have a depressant effect on the fetal myocardium which is dose-dependent.[62] In the isolated human heart mepivacaine perfusion produces myocardial depression proportionate to the dose of the drug and the degree of acidosis.

CENTRAL NERVOUS SYSTEM EFFECTS

Local anesthetics depress the central nervous system at various levels and in various degrees:

1. Depression of the vasomotor center leads to hypotension.

2. Depression of the cardiac accelerator center leads to bradycardia.

3. Depression of the inhibitory higher center leads to neonatal convulsions.

4. Depression of the respiratory center leads to neonatal respiratory failure.

These results can lead to hypoxia, acidosis, and death. Therefore with excessive doses, central nervous system effects, myocardial depression, or both can cause death of the fetus or the neonate.

FETAL COMPLICATIONS AND SPECIFIC DRUGS USED FOR PARACERVICAL BLOCK

Both local anesthetic drugs and vasoconstrictors used for paracervical block are considered responsible for fetal bradycardia.

Local Anesthetic Drugs

Both amide- and ester-type local anesthetics are used for paracervical block. These drugs as well as their metabolites have potential effects on the fetus and neonate.

Amide-Type Anesthetics

Mepivacaine. This is the most studied drug in paracervical block in regard to its maternal-fetal ratio and its effect on the fetus and neonate.[4,10,15,19,21,40,49,50,60] The wide range of drug levels reported in babies, with or without symptoms, who survived or died is not surprising. The techniques and timing of blood samples were different and the methods of determination of the drug levels were variable, as was the acid-base status of mothers and babies. A fetal blood threshold of mepivacaine for bradycardia of 3 μg./ml. is suggested.[4] However, fetal blood levels of mepivacaine as high as 7.3 μg/ml. may not be associated with fetal bradycardia or neonatal symptoms or signs.[19] There are cases that develop fetal bradycardia following the first paracervical block but not after subsequent blocks.[15] This cannot be explained by the development of "tolerance" of the fetus to mepivacaine, but rather by a "fault" in the technique with the first block.

Prilocaine. Shnider[49] has compared prilocaine with lidocaine and mepivacaine, using the same dosage of 200 mg. and concentration of 1 per cent for all three drugs. The incidence of fetal bradycardia following paracervical block is 11 per cent with prilocaine and 22 per cent with either lidocaine or mepivacaine. This difference could be due to the inherently lower cardiac and central nervous system toxicity of prilocaine compared to the other two drugs,[11] or to the more rapid uptake and distribution of prilocaine.[49] However, the major disadvantage of prilocaine is the development of methemoglobinemia in the mother and the neonate.[3,23,43]

Lidocaine. Recently, serial fetal and maternal blood levels of lidocaine following paracervical block have been determined in 10 cases.[41] Following the injection of 200 mg. of lidocaine, the drug is detected in maternal blood in 1 minute and reaches its peak in 10 minutes. This rate of absorption of lidocaine following paracervical block is faster than following epidural block and is due to the high vascularity of the paracervical area. The drug is detected in fetal blood at the first sample, 3 minutes following paracervical block; the peak is reached in 9 minutes. Its fetal blood level usually reaches about 50 per cent that of the mother. *The mean uptake half-life* following paracervical block, which is the time required to reach half the maximum blood concentration of the drug, is 3 minutes for the mother and 5 minutes for the fetus. *The mean elimination half time* of the drug, which is the time required to reduce its blood concentration by one half, is 82 minutes for the mother and 95 minutes for the fetus. This confirms the slower elimination processes of the drug in the baby even *in utero*.

Bupivacaine. Using 50 to 100 mg. of bupivacaine for paracervical block, fetal bradycardia occurs with or without 1:200,000 epinephrine.[5,58,59] Using 25 mg. of bupivacaine (10 ml. of 0.25% solution) with 1:400,000 epinephrine and the technique that has been described (i.e., one-dose technique), there are no significant fetal effects attributed to the paracervical block.[28]

Ester-Type Local Anesthetics

Although the fetus cannot readily metabolize the amide-type local anesthetics because of its liver immaturity,[12] it has sufficient plasma cholinesterase to hydrolyze esters, such as local anesthetics.[22] This might explain the reason why no fetal or neonatal deaths have been associated with the use of procaine, chloroprocaine, or tetracaine.[13] In a study using 12 ml. of 1 per cent chloroprocaine with 1:200,000 epinephrine for paracervical block in 261 blocks, the results were better than many of those reported using amide-type local anesthetics.[13] Fetal bradycardia occurs in 5.8 per cent of cases and lasts less than 15 minutes (average, 7.6 minutes). Neonatal depression occurs in 5.2 per cent of cases. The success rate is 83 per cent, and analgesia lasts for 75 minutes.

The Metabolites of Local Anesthetics

The metabolites of local anesthetic drugs, whether amides or esters, may play an important role in fetal and neonatal complications.[32,41] For example, after paracervical block, monoethylglycin-exylidide (MEGX), a lidocaine metabolite, is found in equal amounts in the fetus and the mother while the fetal lidocaine level is about 50 per cent of the maternal level.[41] Para-aminobenzoic acid, a metabolite of procaine, is detected in the fetus in larger quantity than procaine itself.[63]

EPINEPHRINE

The use of epinephrine with the local anesthetic used for paracervical block is still controversial. Those who favor its use state that epinephrine prolongs the effect of the local anesthetic and adds to the safety of the fetus by reducing the absorption of the local anesthetic drug from the site of injection.[13,25,28] Those who oppose its use state that with epinephrine (1:200,000) there is a steady fall in fetal base excess[26] and increased incidence of fetal bradycardia,[29] probably due to a disturbing effect on the uteroplacental circulation.

PROPHYLAXIS OF FETAL AND NEONATAL COMPLICATIONS WITH PARACERVICAL BLOCK

It is essential to avoid the occurrence of fetal bradycardia following paracervical block because once it occurs there is little that can be done to correct it.

To avoid fetal bradycardia:
1. The fetal condition should be prop-
erly assessed before performing the paracervical block.

2. The fetal heart rate should be monitored for at least 10 minutes before the block.

3. The contraindications to paracervical block should be respected.

4. The number of paracervical blocks in a single patient should not exceed two.

5. The technical details, especially the recent modifications, should be followed.

TREATMENT OF FETAL AND NEONATAL COMPLICATIONS OF PARACERVICAL BLOCK

If in spite of the above precautions fetal bradycardia occurs:

1. The patient should be turned onto her left side to correct maternal aortocaval compression.

2. Oxygen by face mask should be administered and hypotension should be corrected if present.

Usually the bradycardia is transient and disappears within 20 minutes. If the fetal bradycardia lasts more than 20 minutes, the decision to interfere surgically depends on the severity and duration of the bradycardia and on any associated fetal acidosis and its degree. On the whole, there is a tendency for conservative treatment because if the neonate is born with a large bolus of the local anesthetic, it will not be able to efficiently metabolize it. The fetus *in utero* is better able to handle the circulating local anesthetic than the neonate[36] because the former transfers the drug to the mother to be metabolized and excreted. Once delivered, the neonate loses this placental clearance and must rely on its own liver to detoxify the local anesthetic; this is an inefficient process because of the well-known deficiency of the microsomal drug-metabolizing enzymes in the neonatal liver cells. The difficulty of metabolizing the local anesthetic drug by the neonate is even more pronounced in the premature fetus.[5] Similarly, if the uteroplacental or umbilical circulation is impaired, the rate of transfer from the fetus to the mother will be reduced and a high toxic level will be maintained in the fetus. If fetal acidosis supervenes, the local anesthetic that reaches the fetus becomes more ionized and thus not amenable for exchange with the maternal circulation. In a sense it becomes "trapped," not only in the fetal circulation, but more important in the fetal cells where it exerts its toxic effects.

If the baby is born depressed, support of respiration and circulation should continue until the state of depression is overcome. The duration and degree of resuscitation will depend on the severity of the condition. If convulsions occur, exchange transfusion will reduce the drug level in the neonate and may be lifesaving.[10] However, for exchange transfusion to be effective, it should be instituted early before a significant portion of the drug has been "trapped" in the central nervous system and heart.

INDICATIONS FOR THE USE OF PARACERVICAL BLOCK

In Obstetrics

Paracervical block is used for relieving pain during the first stage of labor. It is also effective in relieving uterine pain during the second stage provided the local anesthetic has been injected before the cervix, which is the main landmark, is fully dilated.

In Gynecology

Paracervical block is an effective method of analgesia for dilatation and curettage, especially for outpatient procedures.

CONTRAINDICATIONS FOR THE USE OF PARACERVICAL BLOCK

Paracervical block is contraindicated in the following conditions:

Fetal Prematurity

The incidence of fetal bradycardia with fetal prematurity is high. Moreover, if early delivery occurs, it will be difficult to detoxify the drug in the premature neonate.

Fetal Compromise

A compromised fetus, such as one associated with toxemia, diabetes, twins, essential or renal hypertension, or small for gestational age, is a contraindication for the use of paracervical block. The incidence and severity of fetal bradycardia and acidosis under such circumstances are high.[51]

Fetal Acidosis

Fetal acidosis is a contraindication for the use of paracervical block.[49]

Fetal Distress

Fetal distress as evidenced by abnormal fetal heart rate pattern or meconium staining of the amniotic fluid, even without acidosis, is a contraindication for the use of paracervical block.

Expected Delivery in Less Than One Hour

If the delivery is expected in less than 1 hour, a method of analgesia other than paracervical block should be chosen.

Inexperience of the Operator

Inexperience of the operator to perform the technique or to treat its maternal and/or fetal complications is a contraindication. As with any medical technique, to avoid complications proper teaching and adequate supervision of trainees are mandatory.

ROLE OF PARACERVICAL BLOCK
ADVANTAGES OF PARACERVICAL BLOCK

From the maternal point of view, paracervical block is safer than epidural block because of the possibility of hypotension and inadvertent dural puncture with the latter technique. It is also simpler and the landmarks are easily identified. There is minimal equipment required, and an anesthesiologist is not needed to perform the block. Also, the mother is in full control of her muscles to bear down.

DISADVANTAGES OF PARACERVICAL BLOCK

From the maternal point of view, paracervical block does not relieve the perineal pain and may not last to cover the uterine pain of the second stage of labor.

In regard to the fetus, there is always the risk of fetal bradycardia, fetal acidosis, neonatal depression, and even death.

CONCLUSION

The safety of paracervical block and its success rate depend mainly on the skill and experience of the operator performing the block. The recent modifications mentioned above help to reduce the mortality and morbidity from paracervical block. However, the effectiveness of these recommendations in the hands of the average obstetrician has to await the results of a large series of studies from different centers of the world. Therefore, at least for the time being, paracervical block should only be used when facilities preclude the use of epidural and/or caudal blocks.

REFERENCES

1. Aberg, G.: Studies in mepivacaine and its optically active isomers with special reference to its vasoactive properties. Thesis from the Department of Pharmacology, School of Medicine. Lindhoping, Sweden, 1972.
2. Abouleish, E.: Hypotensive anesthesia. Thesis in part fulfillment for the degree of M.D. *In* Anesthesia. Ain-Shams University, Cairo, Egypt, 1960.
2a. Alper, M. H.: Toxicity of local anesthetics. N. Engl. J. Med., *294*:1432, 1976.
3. Arens, J. F., and Carrera, A. E.: Methemoglobin levels following peridural anesthesia with prilocaine for vaginal deliveries. Anesth. Analg., *49*:219, 1970.
4. Asling, J. H., *et al.*: Paracervical block anesthesia in obstetrics. II. Etiology of fetal bradycardia following paracervical block anesthesia. Am. J. Obstet. Gynecol., *107*:626, 1970.
5. Baskett, T. F., and Carson, R. M.: Paracervical block with bupivacaine. Can. Med. Assoc. J., *110*:1363, 1974.
6. Berger, G. S., Tyler, C. W., and Harrod, E. K.: Maternal deaths associated with paracervical block anesthe ia. Am. J. Obstet. Gynecol., *118*:1142, 1974.
7. Blair, M. R.: Cardiovascular pharmacology of local anaesthetics. Br. J. Anaesth., *47*:247, 1975.
8. Bloom, S. L., Horswill, C. W., and Curet, L. B.: Effects of paracervical blocks on the fetus during labor: a prospective study with the use of direct fetal monitoring. Am. J. Obstet. Gynecol., *114*:218, 1972.
9. Chastain, G. M.: Acute blood levels of lidocaine following paracervical block. J. Med. Assoc. Ga., *58*:426, 1969.
10. Dodson, W. E., Hillman, R. E., and Hillman, L. S.: Brain tissue levels in a fatal case of neonatal mepivacaine (Carbocaine) poisoning. Pediatrics, *86*:624, 1975.
11. Englesson, S., and Matousek, M.: Central nervous system effects of local anaesthetic agents. Br. J. Anaesth., *47*:241, 1975.
12. Fouts, J. R.: Metabolism of drugs by livers from fetal and newborn animals. *In* Perinatal Pharmacology, Report of the 41st Ross Conference on Pediatric Research. P. 54. Columbus, Ohio, Ross Laboratories, 1961.
13. Freeman, D. W., and Arnold, N. I.: Paracervical block with low doses of chloroprocaine—fetal and maternal effects. J.A.M.A., *231*:56, 1975.
14. Freeman, D. W., Bellville, T. P., and Barno, A.: Paracervical block anesthesia in labor. Obstet. Gynecol., *8*:270, 1956.
15. Freeman, R. K., *et al.*: Fetal cardiac response to paracervical block anesthesia. Part I. Am. J. Obstet. Gynecol., *113*:583, 1972.
16. Frymire, L. J., and French, T. A.: The Syrijet anesthetic gun for paracervical and uterosacral block. Obstet. Gynecol., *44*:443, 1974.
17. Gabert, H. A., and Stenchever, M. A.: Continuous electronic monitoring of fetal heart rate during labor. Am. J. Obstet. Gynecol., *115*:919, 1973.
18. Gellert, P.: Aufhebung der Wehenschmerzen und Wehenüberdruck. Monatsschr. Geburtsh. Gynaek., *73*:143, 1926.
18a. Gibbs, C. P., and Noel, S. C.: Human uterine response to lidocaine. Abstracts of Scientific Papers. P. 537, American Soc. of Anesthesiologists, 1976.
19. Gordon, H. R.: Fetal bradycardia after paracervical block. N. Engl. J. Med., *279*:910, 1968.
19a. Greiss, F. C., Jr, Still, J. G., and Anderson, S. G.: Effects of local anesthetic agent on the uterine vasculatures and myometrium. Am. J. Obstet. Gynecol., *124*:889, 1976
20. Grimes, D. A., and Cates, W., Jr.: Deaths from

paracervical anesthesia used for first-trimester abortion. N. Engl. J. Med., *295*:1397, 1976.

21. Guillozet, N.: The risks of paracervical anesthesia; intoxication and neurological injury of the newborn. Pediatrics, *55*:533, 1975.

22. Hamilton, L. A., and Gottschalk, W.: Paracervical block: advantages and disadvantages. Clin. Obstet. Gynecol., *17*:199, 1974.

23. Harley, J. D., and Celermajer, J. M.: Neonatal methaemoglobinaemia and the "red-brown" screening test. Lancet, *2*:1223, 1970.

24. Hellman, L. M.: Electronics in obstetrics and gynaecology. J. Obstet. Gynaecol. Br. Commonw., *72*:896, 1965.

25. Hollmen, A., Korhonen, M., and Ojala, A.: Bupivacaine in paracervical block—plasma levels and changes in maternal and foetal acid-base balance. Br. J. Anaesth., *41*:603, 1969.

26. ———: Fetal acidosis after paracervical block. Br. J. Anaesth., *41*:1013, 1969.

27. Hollmen, A., Ojala, A., and Korhonen, M.: Paracervical blockade with Marcaine/adrenaline. Acta Anaesthesiol. Scand., *13*:1, 1969.

28. Jagerhorn, M.: Paracervical block in obstetrics. An improved injection method: a clinical and radiological study. Acta Obstet. Gynecol. Scand., *54*:9, 1975.

28a. Joyce, T. H., Aquino, N., and Kuchling, A.: The effect of local anesthetics on gravid human uterine artery strips in vitro. Abstracts of Scientific Papers. P. 539. American Soc. of Anesthesiologists, 1976.

29. Kobak, A. J., and Sadove, M. S.: Combined paracervical and pudendal nerve blocks—a simple form of transvaginal regional anesthesia. Am. J. Obstet. Gynecol., *81*:72, 1961.

30. Kobak, A. J., Sadove, M. S., and Mazeros, W. T.: Anatomic studies of transvaginal regional anesthesia. Obstet. Gynecol., *19*:302, 1962.

31. Le Hew, W. L.: Paracervical block in obstetrics. Am. J. Obstet. Gynecol., *113*:1079, 1972.

32. Levinson, G., and Shnider, S. M.: Placental transfer of local anesthetics—clinical implications. *In* Marx, G. F. (ed.): Parturition and Perinatology, Clinical Anesthesia. Vol. 10, No. 2, p. 173. Philadelphia, F. A. Davis, 1973.

33. McGowan, G. W.: Uterosacral or paracervical block for obstetrical anesthesia. West. J. Surg., *70*:307, 1962.

34. McKenzie, R.: Jet injection of lidocaine for paracervical block. Sixth World Congress of Anesthesiology, Mexico City, 1976. P. 114. Amsterdam, Excerpta Medica, 1976.

35. Morishima, H. O., and Adamsons, K.: Placental clearance of mepivacaine following administration to the guinea pig fetus. Anesthesiology, *28*:343, 1967.

36. Morishima, H. O., *et al.*: Toxicity of lidocaine in the fetal and newborn lamb and its relationship to asphyxia. Am. J. Obstet. Gynecol., *112*:72, 1972.

37. Murphy, P. J., Wright, J. D., and Fitzgerald, T. B.: Assessment of paracervical nerve block anaesthesia during labour. Br. Med. J., *1*:526, 1970.

38. Nyirjesy, S., *et al.*: Hazards of the use of paracervical block anesthesia in obstetrics. Am. J. Obstet. Gynecol., *87*:231, 1963.

39. Page, E. P., Kamm, M. L., and Chappell, C. C.: Usefulness of paracervical block in obstetrics. Am. J. Obstet. Gynecol., *81*:1094, 1961.

40. Paul, R. H., and Freeman, R. K.: Fetal cardiac response to paracervical block anesthesia: Part II. Am. J. Obstet. Gynecol., *113*:592, 1972.

41. Petrie, R. H., *et al.*: Placental transfer of lidocaine following paracervical block. Am. J. Obstet. Gynecol., *120*:791, 1974.

42. Pitkin, R. M., and Goddard, W. B.: Paracervical and uterosacral block in obstetrics—a controlled, double-blind study. Obstet. Gynecol., *21*:737, 1963.

43. Poppers, P. J., and Finster, M.: The use of prilocaine hydrochloride (Citanest) for epidural analgesia in obstetrics. Anesthesiology, *29*:1134, 1968.

44. Rogers, R. E.: Fetal bradycardia associated with paracervical block anesthesia in labor. Am. J. Obstet. Gynecol., *106*:913, 1970.

45. Rosefsky, J. B., and Petersiel, M. E.: Perinatal deaths associated with mepivacaine paracervical-block anesthesia in labor. N. Engl. J. Med., *278*:530, 1968.

46. Rosenfeld, C. R., Barton, M. D., and Meschia, G.: Circulatory effects of epinephrine in the pregnant ewe. Am. J. Obstet. Gynecol., *124*:156, 1976.

47. Rosenfeld, S. S.: Paracervical anesthesia for relief of labor pains. Am. J. Obstet. Gynecol., *50*:527, 1945.

48. Ruoss, C., and Beasley, J. M.: Paracervical block with bupivacaine. [Correspondence] Br. Med. J., *2*:622, 1968.

49. Shnider, S. M., and Gildea, J.: Paracervical block anesthesia in obstetrics. III. Choice of drugs: fetal bradycardia following administration of lidocaine, mepivacaine, and prilocaine. Am. J. Obstet. Gynecol., *116*:320, 1973.

50. Schnider, S. M., *et al.*: High fetal blood levels of mepivacaine and fetal bradycardia. N. Engl. J. Med., *279*:947, 1968.

51. ———: Paracervical block anesthesia in obstetrics. I. Fetal complications and neonatal morbidity. Am. J. Obstet. Gynecol., *107*:619, 1970.

52. Shulman, L.: Comment on paracervical block. *In* Davis, J. E., *et al.*: The combined paracervical-pudendal block anesthesia for labor and delivery. Am. J. Obstet. Gynecol., *89*:360, 1964.

53. Smith, E. B., Henhre, F. W., and Hess, O. W.: Convulsions associated with anesthetic agents during labor and delivery. Anesth. Analg., *43*:476, 1964.

54. Steffenson, J. L., Shnider, S. M., and De Lorimier, A. A.: Transarterial diffusion of mepivacaine. Anesthesiology, *32*:459, 1970.

55. Stern, L., Outerbridge, E. W., and Fawcett, J. S.: Paracervical block in obstetrics. Lancet *2*:322, 1969.

56. Tafeen, C. H., Freedman, H. L., and Harris, H.: Combined continuous paracervical and continuous pudendal nerve block anesthesia in labor. Am. J. Obstet. Gynecol., *100*:55, 1968.

57. Teramo, K.: Studies on foetal acid-base values after paracervical blockade during labour. Acta Obstet. Gynecol. Scand. [Suppl.] *48*(3):80, 1969.

58. ———: Fetal acid-base balance and heart rate during labour with bupivacaine paracervical block anesthesia. J. Obstet. Gynaecol. Br. Commonw., *76*:881, 1969.

59. ———: Effect of paracervical blockade in the fetus. Acta Obstet. Gynecol. Scand. [Suppl.], *16*:1, 1971.

60. Teramo, K., and Widholm, O.: Studies on the effects of anaesthetics on foetus. 1. The effect of paracervical block with mepivacaine upon foetal acid-base values. Acta Obstet. Gynecol. Scand. [Suppl.], *46*(2):1, 1967.

61. Thiery, M., and Vroman, S.: Paracervical block analgesia during labor. Am. J. Obstet. Gynecol., *113*:988, 1972.

62. ———: Fetal bradycardia after paracervical block analgesia in labor. Acta Anaesthesiol. Belg., *24*:288, 1973.

63. Usubiaga, J. E., *et al.*: Passage of procaine hydrochloride and para-aminobenzoic acid across the human placenta. Am. J. Obstet. Gynecol., *100*:918, 1968.

64. Vasicka, A., *et al.*: Fetal bradycardia after paracervical block. Obstet. Gynecol., *38*:500, 1971.

65. White, C. A., and Pitkin, R. M.: Paracervical block anesthesia in obstetrics. Postgrad. Med., *33*:585, 1963.

66. Zourlas, P. A., and Kumar, D.: An objective evaluation of paracervical block on human uterine contractility. Am. J. Obstet. Gynecol., *91*:217, 1965.

17

General Analgesia and Anesthesia

Robert Bryan Roberts, M.D., F.F.A.R.C.S.

INHALATIONAL ANALGESIA

When Queen Victoria imperiously informed her Privy Council "Gentlemen, We are having the baby and We are having the chloroform," she set both sovereign and ecclesiastic stamps of approval on the use of inhalational analgesics in labor. After the birth of Prince Leopold, the Queen announced herself "mightily pleased" with John Snow's ministrations of chloroform on a silk handkerchief with each contraction, thus establishing a vogue in "chloroform a la reine."

While chloroform has long since been relegated to the history books (in most places), inhalational analgesia still provides a highly effective and safe technique for pain relief in childbirth. One of the following agents is usually employed: nitrous oxide, trichloroethylene, methoxyflurane, or, more recently, enflurane or isoflurane.

INHALATIONAL ANALGESIC AGENTS

Nitrous Oxide

For many years, 50 per cent nitrous oxide in air was a standard agent despite the obvious disadvantage of reducing the fraction of inspired oxygen concentration to 0.1. In the United Kingdom, where the midwife with her "gas and air" machine precariously strapped to her bicycle was a familiar figure, the mother had to be certified by a doctor that she was "fit" for the intermittent periods of imposed hypoxia. The old idea that the analgesic effect of nitrous oxide depended primarily on concomitant hypoxia died hard. As late as 1962 workers[6] still drew attention to the decreased arterial oxygen saturation during the use of gas and air. In the early 1960's, special machines such as the Lucy-Baldwin (British Oxygen Company) were constructed to deliver a 50 per cent mixture of nitrous oxide and oxygen. The major advance, however, was the production of premixed nitrous oxide and oxygen in the same cylinder, a mixture called Entonox.[42]

Entonox is a highly stable mixture delivering constant percentages of nitrous oxide and oxygen unless the cylinder is allowed to cool excessively during transportation or storage. The critical temperature (i.e., the temperature above which no amount of increased pressure will produce liquefaction) of nitrous oxide is 36.5° C., that of oxygen is $-118.8°$ C., and that of the mixture is $-7°$ C. If the mixture is allowed to cool below $-7°$ C., partial liquefaction occurs, after which even if the mixture is rewarmed the proportions of gases released are no longer constant. A relatively high concentration of oxygen is initially given off, but with time there is a gradual fall off to below 21 per cent. Agitation of the tank has no beneficial effect.[12] The only effective method of reconstituting the correct mixture after cooling is by leaving the tank *horizontal* for 24 hours at a temperature of above 5° C.[5]

It is unfortunate that the federal bureaucracy has so far barred the use of this valuable agent in the United States; 50/50 nitrous oxide/oxygen can still be used but each anesthesiologist must mix his or her own gases using rotameters or a mixing device.

Trichloroethylene (Trilene)

Trichloroethylene has also been used as an inhalational analgesic in obstetrics. In 1943, Freedman[16] reported its satisfactory use in over 2,000 patients. Its obvious advantages over nitrous oxide were the increased potency and the lack of necessity for accompanying hypoxia. Seward[39] at Oxford showed that a maximum concentration of trichloroethylene in air of 0.5 per cent by volume was sufficient and that 0.33 per cent v/v was adequate after a period of inhaling the 0.5 per cent mixture. From this work developed the Emotril and Tecota machines which in 1954 were approved by the Central Midwives Board for use by midwives in domiciliary practice in Britain.

Although the interaction of trichloroethylene with soda lime producing the toxic products of phosgene and dichloroacetylene has limited its use in the United States (where soda lime is often an integral and irremovable part of the anesthetic machine), the agent is still in considerable use and has one overwhelming advantage—its inexpensiveness.

Methoxyflurane (Penthrane)

Methoxyflurane was introduced into obstetric analgesia in 1962[4,38] and soon proved to be a superior analgesic. An inhaled concentration of 0.35 per cent v/v in air was established as providing significantly better analgesia than a concentration of 0.25 per cent while an inhaled concentration of 0.45 per cent produced

unacceptable drowsiness.[25] Major and her colleagues[24] had already demonstrated a more positive response to methoxyflurane than to trichloroethylene by patients, anesthesiologists, and midwives.

Nephrotoxicity following the use of methoxyflurane in surgical patients was first reported in 1966.[9] Whereas both inorganic fluoride and oxalic acid are products of the biodegradation of methoxyflurane in the body, it is the inorganic fluoride that is almost certainly responsible for the renal failure reported following methoxyflurane administration.[28] The dose of methoxyflurane required to produce this syndrome of vasopressin-resistant polyuria, hypernatremia, serum hyperosmolality, and increased serum urea nitrogen is that resulting in a serum inorganic fluoride level of over 50 μM./l.[8]

Studies on inorganic fluoride levels in obstetric patients following the use of methoxyflurane, either for delivery only or during labor as an intermittent inhalational analgesic in the late first stage and second stage, have reassuringly remained well below the 50 μM./l. level.[32]

Methoxyflurane concentrations of up to 0.5 per cent used during cesarean section produce similarly low levels of inorganic fluoride.[44]

Other Agents

Isoflurane[18] and enflurane[3] have both been used recently as analgesics in obstetrics. Their effectiveness appears to be comparable to 40 to 50 per cent nitrous oxide in oxygen. Unless a high concentration of oxygen were indicated, they appear to have very little advantage over 50/50 nitrous oxide/oxygen. Furthermore, in equi-MAC doses they appear to exert as much myometrial depression as does halothane.[30]

ADVANTAGES OF INHALATIONAL ANALGESICS

1. Profound analgesia and amnesia can be obtained.

2. Laryngeal and cough reflexes are maintained.

3. The fetus is rarely affected.

4. Uterine contractility is not significantly depressed.

5. Expulsive powers are not affected; the parturient can often push better if pain is obtunded.

6. The low concentrations used avoid toxicity.

7. Most low forceps obstetric manipulations can be performed using inhalational analgesics combined with pudendal block.

8. They can be used with increased oxygen concentrations, thus raising the maternal PaO_2

ADMINISTRATION OF INHALATIONAL ANALGESIC AGENTS

During the late second stage when delivery is imminent, it is advantageous for the anesthesiologist to administer the analgesic agent continuously. Between contractions a lower concentration of the agent should be given, increasing the concentration as each contraction starts. In this way there will be less delay in achieving an analgesic concentration in the blood during each contraction.

Adding methoxyflurane or any other potent analgesic to a mixture of nitrous oxide and oxygen is fraught with the danger of producing general anesthesia rather than the desired analgesic planes. This is particularly true if the newer plastic circuits are being used rather than the rubber circuits which absorb larger amounts of methoxyflurane and thus keep the inspired concentration down.

Continued verbal contact should be kept with the patient. Not only will this provide constant reassurance but will also allow for monitoring of the depth of anesthesia.

GENERAL ANESTHESIA

A general anesthetic in the delivery room should be a rare occurrence, totally avoided in unskilled hands and *never* used for obstetrician convenience. The disadvantages of general anesthesia are numerous:

1. The patient is exposed to the danger of pulmonary aspiration.

2. The placenta is no barrier to general anesthetics and the fetus and neonate are thus always exposed to the risk of medullary depression.

3. Pushing ability of the mother is lost.

4. Uterine contractility may be diminished, and increased bleeding may result.

5. The patient is exposed to all the other complications of general anesthesia such as arrhythmias, hypotension, and respiratory inadequacy.

The dangers of general anesthesia are the same whether it is used for forceps delivery or cesarean section, and certain general principles apply to both situations:

1. The airway must be protected at all times.

2. The possibility of *acid* aspiration in particular must be guarded against.

3. Choice of agents and depth of anesthesia must be carefully gauged to cause minimum neonatal depression.

4. Maternal hypotension must be avoided.

Avoidance of vomiting, regurgitation, and aspiration has been thoroughly discussed in Chapter 8. However, some points will bear reemphasizing. Oral antacids very significantly reduce the risk of *acid* aspiration.[35,36] If it has not been stated before, let it be stated now: an obstetric patient who develops acid aspiration pneumonitis following general anesthesia and in whom *no* prior attempt was made to neutralize her gastric contents is the victim of negligence. In over 50 per cent of patients the pH of the gastric contents is below 2.5. Between 25 and 35 per cent of patients also have a gastric volume of at least 25 ml., and some may have a gastric volume of over 500 ml. The time between the patient's last meal and the onset of labor or time of delivery is *not* an indication of gastric contents volume

(Figs. 17-1 and 17-2). The patient most at risk may be the woman who has not eaten for over 24 hours and whose stomach contains only acid gastric juice. Patients for elective cesarean section are as much at risk as those for emergency cesarean section. Antacid, 15 to 30 ml., given regularly at 2 to 3 hour intervals during labor or 1 hour prior to elective cesarean section reduces the number of patients at risk significantly (Table 17-1). The use of glycopyrrolate instead of atropine as premedication may further add to the patient's safety due to its superior inhibition of gastric acid production.[40] Certain H_2 receptor antagonists whose future use is at the moment clouded may in time provide additional valuable prevention. In the United Kingdom, the use of metoclopramide (Maxolon) to increase the rate of gastric emptying has become common.[12] (Metoclopramide is not available in the United States at present.)

Since none of the methods used to reduce the risk of acid aspiration prevent nonacid aspiration, all other measures designed to protect the airway must also be used—prevention of a rise in intragastric

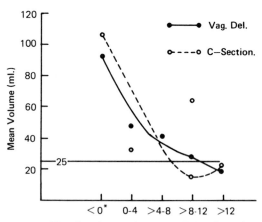

Fig. 17-2.   Mean gastric contents volume at delivery in 146 patients in labor related to the time between last meal and onset of labor. (Roberts, R. B., and Shirley, M. A.: The obstetrician's role in reducing the risk of aspiration pneumonitis. Am. J. Obstet. Gynecol., *124*:611, 1976)

pressure, rapid smooth induction, skillful quick intubation for every obstetric case requiring general anesthesia (as opposed to inhalational analgesia), and recovery of reflexes and, if possible, consciousness prior to extubation.

We can now look at the other prerequisites of general anesthesia, primarily the avoidance of neonatal depression.

Preoxygenation

Preoxygenation provides many benefits. Not only does it allow us not to ventilate the patient until the endotracheal tube is in place, but it provides insurance against maternal and fetal hypoxia during induction and intubation. It may also improve fetal oxygenation though probably not very significantly.

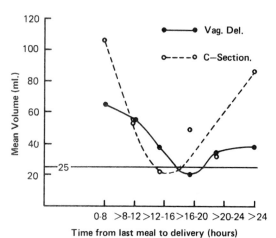

Fig. 17-1.   Mean gastric contents volume at delivery in 146 patients in labor related to the time between last meal and delivery. (Roberts, R. B., and Shirley, M. A.: The obstetrician's role in reducing the risk of aspiration pneumonitis. Am. J. Obstet. Gynecol., *124*:611, 1976)

Induction

Sodium thiopental in a dose of less than 4 mg./kg. of maternal body weight has little if any demonstrable effect on the full-term nonacidotic fetus.[15,22] In the presence of acidosis in the fetus, thiopental can cause neonatal hypotension and ketamine is a

Table 17-1. Number of Patients at Risk to Pulmonary Aspiration Whose Gastric Contents Volume Was More Than 25 ml. and Gastric pH Was Less Than 2.5*

	In Labor			*Elective Cesarean Section*
Antacid†	*Cesarean Section*	*Vaginal Delivery*	*Total*	
Within 4 hr. of delivery	1 (3%) n = 31	1 (2.5%) n = 39	2 (3%) n = 70	0 (0%) n = 31
More than 4 hr. before delivery	4 (36%) n = 11	1 (10%) n = 10	5 (24%) n = 21	—
			18 (24%) n = 76	
No antacid	4 (18%) n = 22	9 (28%) n = 33	13 (24%) n = 55	7 (29%) n = 24

*Roberts, R. B., and Shirley, M. A.: The obstetrician's role in reducing the risk of aspiration pneumonitis. Am. J. Obstet. Gynecol., *124*:611, 1976.

†WinGel, 15 ml.

wiser choice for induction.[27] In the rare case where general anesthesia is absolutely essential despite a premature fetus, intravenous induction agents are best avoided altogether in favor of a nitrous oxide/oxygen induction. There is mounting evidence that thiopental is a broad-based neurobehavioral depressant to the neonate.[20]

Ketamine has recently been used[2] in small doses (0.25–1.0 mg./kg.) as an induction agent and sole anesthetic for vaginal delivery and as an induction agent for cesarean section.[33] There is little doubt that the effect of small doses (less than 1 mg./kg. of maternal body weight) on the fetus is minimal.[20] Despite the assertion that ketamine maintains laryngeal reflexes,[7] aspiration during its use has been reported[34] and is an ever-present danger. Ketamine provides rapid induction and excellent analgesia. In the low doses used in obstetrics, the incidence of postoperative delirium and unpleasant dreams has been low. A major disadvantage is the moderate increase in blood pressure which occurs in a majority of patients and which contraindicates the use of this agent in the preeclamptic patient.

In those areas where its flammability has not proscribed its use, cyclopropane can provide a rapid and smooth induction. Apart from its flammability, however,

there is also the danger of neonatal depression, particularly if narcotics have been used during labor (see also Chap. 3, Placenta and Placental Transfer of Drugs at Term).

Muscle Relaxation

As a rule, the high degree of ionization and high lipophobic characteristics of muscle relaxants prevent their crossing the placenta in any significant concentration. Succinylcholine in therapeutic doses does not cross the placenta.[23] Even the deliberate injection of up to 50 mg. of succinylcholine into the uterine artery at cesarean section produced no relaxant effect on the neonate.[41] Neither curare[17] nor pancuronium[31] appears to cross the placenta and both are safe drugs to use in obstetrics. Maternal blood pressure may be better maintained with pancuronium than with curare.[31]

Gallamine triethiodide (Flaxedil), however, can cross the placenta in appreciable concentrations.[11] Although neonatal weakness has not been reported, it is safer to avoid this agent in obstetrics.

A large dose of succinylcholine should be used to render intubation as easy as possible. Because the fasciculations produced can raise intragastric pressure,[37] leading to regurgitation of gastric contents, a small dose of an antidepolarizing agent such as

3.0 mg. of *d*-tubocurarine should be administered 5 minutes prior to induction. A clear mask, a moderate head-up position, and cricoid pressure are further essential ancillaries to safe intubation. Further doses of succinylcholine either as intermittent boluses or as a continuous infusion may be used to maintain relaxation as required during the obstetric procedure. Alternatively, once evidence of the wearing off of the succinylcholine is seen, relaxation may be continued with *d*-tubocurarine or pancuronium.

Succinylcholine may demonstrate a prolonged action in obstetric patients because the pseudocholinesterase level is normally reduced during pregnancy, hence delaying the normal enzymatic breakdown of the agent. If a continuous infusion of oxytocin has been used, certain patients may demonstrate an altered response to succinylcholine. Neuromuscular depression with the characteristics of a nondepolarizing block, reversible by neostigmine, can occur.[19] Since these problems are rarely encountered, succinylcholine has been widely and safely used in obstetrics (see also Chap. 3).

Maintenance

For many years, 70 per cent nitrous oxide and 30 per cent oxygen has been the standard maintenance regimen, at least until after the baby was delivered, at which time a stronger inhalation agent was introduced or a narcotic agent such as meperidine (50–75 mg.) or fentanyl (0.05–0.1 mg.) was given. Recent evidence, however, suggests that such concentrations of nitrous oxide may have much more of a depressant effect on the neonate, as shown by neurobehavioral testing, than was previously suspected. Marx[26] has shown that 33 per cent nitrous oxide in 66 per cent oxygen may be an optimum concentration. Because this concentration is not sufficient to obtund awareness, a low concentration of an inhalation agent (methoxyflurane, 0.5%, or enflurane, 1%) must be used.

Halothane, 0.5 per cent, may also be used,[29] reportedly without increased uterine blood loss. The latter agent's depressant action on the uterine muscle, however, makes this author particularly wary of its routine use, and this agent is perhaps best reserved for those cases where uterine relaxation is particularly necessary (see Chap. 10, The Oxytocic and Tocolytic Agents).

Awareness in the paralyzed patient during cesarean section has been reported with alarming frequency.[10,43] The temptation to reduce the nitrous oxide concentration (if nitrous oxide/oxygen is being used) for a minute or so before delivery must be resisted. It has practically no effect on fetal oxygenation but may allow the mother to wake up to the most frightening situation in anesthesia—being conscious but totally paralyzed. Wilson and Turner[43] in 1969 studied 150 cases in which thiopental, succinylcholine, and various concentrations of nitrous oxide and oxygen were used. They found that 2 per cent of patients had factual recall, 17.3 per cent had unpleasant recall, some of which were in the form of unpleasant dreams, and 6.6 per cent had pain recall. Recall was much less frequent if at least 75 per cent of nitrous oxide had been used, but recall incidence bore no relation to the induction dose of thiopental which varied from 250 mg. to 500 mg.

The most significant factor in the incidence of recall was the preoperative use of narcotics, only one case of recall out of 32 cases occurring if a narcotic had been given within 6 hours of surgery. In the absence of narcotics, however, there were 25 cases of recall out of 118 cases (21.1%). These studies also suggested that scopolamine may be preferable to atropine as a premedicant because any recall which did occur tended to be more pleasant if the former agent had been used.

Abouleish and Taylor[1] in 1976 studied 68 patients undergoing cesarean section under thiamylal, relaxant, and 67/33 nitrous oxide/oxygen after atropine premedication, and in whom no narcotic had been administered within the previous 6 hours. Immediately following delivery 0.2 mg./kg. of morphine and 0.1 mg./kg. of diazepam were separately administered intravenously to a maximum of 15 mg. and 7.5 mg. respectively. The incidence of unpleasant recall was 3.8 per cent consisting of one patient who reported painless awareness of the abdominal incision and one patient with unpleasant dreams. Two other patients had pleasant dreams. The authors found no correlation between recall and movement, changes in blood pressure, or pupil size.

Other authors[13,14] have failed to detect recall during anesthesia even when a strong auditory stimulus was presented during a period of known light anesthesia as shown by galvanic skin responses. The only recall in the one series[13] was in a patient who opened her eyes during the procedure and winked at the anesthesiologist! These authors suggest that recall does not occur during general anesthesia and that the presence of recall is evidence that the patient was, at least for a period, not anesthetized.

In our zeal to protect the fetus we must remember our responsibility to the mother and be acutely aware of the fact that light anesthesia may occasionally lighten to no anesthesia. This is particularly apt to occur if a small dose of induction agent is followed by a long and difficult intubation. A further small dose of the induction agent is then indicated and justified.

Emergence

As already mentioned, recovery of reflexes and, if at all possible, full consciousness should be achieved prior to extubation because the danger of aspiration is again present. The lack of sedative premedication and the light anesthesia used for cesarean section allow for very rapid recovery. The lack of analgesic medication, however, also means considerable early pain for these patients. In case no narcotic

has been intravenously injected during surgery, intramuscular narcotics for postoperative pain should be given early, preferably on the operating table.

SUMMARY

Inhalational agents are extremely valuable as analgesics in obstetrics. General anesthesia with unconsciousness, however, is a technique which should be reserved for those cases where anesthesia is indicated and regional anesthesia is either contraindicated or refused. Pulmonary aspiration of gastric contents is the most common significant complication, and all precautions must be taken to reduce gastric acidity, prevent regurgitation, and prevent aspiration. Oral antacids, positioning, rapid induction, and mandatory endotracheal intubation are all factors in the prevention of aspiration pneumonia.

The specific agents used for analgesia and anesthesia are less important than the skill and judgment of the administrator. Care must be taken that justifiable concern for neonatal depression does not result in the mother being paralyzed while not adequately anesthetized.

REFERENCES

1. Abouleish, E., and Taylor, F. H.: Effect of Morphine-diazepam on signs of anesthesia, awareness and dreams of patients under N_2O for cesarean section. Anesth. Analg., *55*:702, 1976.
2. Akamatsu, T. J., *et al.*: Experience with the use of ketamine for parturition: 1. Primary anesthetic for vaginal delivery. Anesth. Analg., *53*:284, 1974.
3. Ball, G. F., Marcias-Loza, M. D., and Cohen, H.: Enflurane analgesia in obstetrics. Abstracts of Scientific Papers. The Society for Obstetric Anesthesia and Perinatology, Orlando. 1976.
4. Boisvert, M., and Hudon, F.: Clinical evaluation of methoxyflurane in obstetrical anesthesia: a report on 500 cases. Can. Anaesth. Soc. J., *9*:325, 1962.
5. Bracken, A., Broughton, G. B., and Hill, D. W.: Safety precautions to be observed with cooled premixed gases. Br. Med. J., *3*:115, 1968.
6. Cole, P. V., and Nainby-Luxmore. R. C.: The hazards of gas and air in obstetrics. Anaesthesia, *17*:505, 1962.
7. Corssen, G., and Oget, S.: Dissociative anesthesia

for the severely burned child. Anesth. Analg., 50:95, 1971.

8. Cousins, M. J., and Mazze, R. I.: Methoxyflurane nephrotoxicity: a study of dose-response in man. J.A.M.A., 225:1611, 1973.

9. Crandell, W. B., Papper, S. G., and MacDonald, A: Nephrotoxicity associated with methoxyflurane anesthesia. Anesthesiology, 27:591, 1966.

10. Crawford, J. S.: Awareness during operative obstetrics during general anesthesia. Br. J. Anaesth., 43:179, 1971.

11. Crawford, J. S., and Gardiner, J. E.: Some aspects of obstetrical anaesthesia. Part II. The use of relaxant drugs. Br. J. Anaesth., 28:154, 1956.

12. Crawford, J. S., et al.: Effects of cooling on the safety of premixed gases. Br. Med. J., 2:138, 1967.

13. Dubovsky, S. L., and Trustman, R.: Absence of recall after general anesthesia. Implications for theory and practice. Anesth. Analg., 55:696, 1976.

14. Eisele, V., Weinreich, A., and Bartle, S.: Perioperative awareness and recall. Anesth. Analg., 55:513, 1976.

15. Finster, M., et al.: Plasma thiopental concentrations in the newborn following delivery under thiopental-nitrous oxide anesthesia. Am. J. Obstet. Gynecol., 95:621, 1966.

16. Freedman, A.: Trichloroethylene-air analgesia in childbirth. An investigation with a suitable inhaler. Lancet, 2:696, 1943.

17. Harroun, P., and Fisher, O.W.: The physiological effects of curare, its failure to pass the placental membrane or inhibit uterine contractions. Surg. Gynecol. Obstet., 89:73, 1949.

18. Hicks, J. S., Schnider, S. M., and Cohen, H.: Isoflurane (Forane) analgesia in obstetrics. Annual Meeting of the American Society of Anesthesiologists, 1975. Pp. 99–100. Abstracts of Scientific Papers.

19. Hodges, R. J. H.: Interaction of suxamethonium and oxytocin. Br. Med. J., 1:1416, 1958.

20. Hodgkinson, R., et al.: Neonatal neurobehavioral tests following vaginal delivery under ketamine, thiopental and extradural anesthesia. Anesth. Analg., 56:548, 1977.

21. Howard, F. A., and Sharp, D. S.: Effects of metoclopramide on gastric emptying during labour. Br. Med. J., 1:446, 1973.

22. Kosaka, Y., Takahashi, T., and Mark, L. C.: Intravenous thiobarbiturate anesthesia for cesarean section. Anesthesiology, 31:489, 1969.

23. Kvisselgard, N., and Moya, F.: Investigation of placental thresholds to succinylcholine. Anesthesiology, 22:7, 1961.

24. Major, V., Rosen, M., and Mushin, W. W.: Methoxyflurane as an obstetric analgesic: a comparison with trichloroethylene. Br. Med. J., 2:1554, 1966.

25. ———: Concentration of methoxyflurane for obstetric analgesia by self-administered intermittent inhalation. Br. Med. J., 4:767, 1967.

26. Marx, G. F., and Matteo, C. V.: Effects of different oxygen concentrations during general anesthesia for cesarean section. Can. Anaesth. Soc. J., 18:587, 1971.

27. Marx, G. F., et al.: Neonatal blood pressures. Anaesthesist, 25:318, 1976.

28. Mazze, R. I., Toudell, J. R., and Cousins, M. J.: Methoxyflurane metabolism and renal dysfunction: clinical correlation in man. Anesthesiology, 35:247, 1971.

29. Moir, D. D.: Anaesthesia for cesarean section (an evaluation of a method using low concentrations of halothane and 50% oxygen). Br. J. Anaesth., 42:136, 1970.

30. Munson, E. S., and Embro, W. J.: Enflurane, isoflurane and halothane and isolated human uterine muscle. Anesthesiology, 46:11, 1977.

31. Neeld, J. B., et al.: A clinical comparison of pancuronium and tubocurarine for cesarean section anesthesia. Anesth. Analg., 53:7, 1974.

32. Palahniuk, R. J., and Cumming, M.: Plasma fluoride levels following obstetric use of methoxyflurane. Can. Anaesth. Soc. J., 22:291, 1975.

33. Peltz, B., and Sinclair, D. M.: Induction agents for cesarean section: a comparison of thiopentone and ketamine. Anaesthesia, 28:37, 1973.

34. Penrose, B. H.: Aspiration pneumonitis following ketamine induction. Anesth. Analg., 51:41, 1972.

35. Roberts, R. B., and Shirley, M. A.: Reducing the risk of acid aspiration during cesarean section. Anesth. Analg., 53:859, 1974.

36. ———: The obstetrician's role in reducing the risk of aspiration pneumonitis. With particular reference to the use of oral antacids. Am. J. Obstet. Gynecol., 124:611, 1976.

37. Roe, R. B.: The effect of suxamethonium on intra-gastric pressure. Anaesthesia, 17:179, 1962.

38. Romagnoli, A., and Korman, D.: Methoxyflurane in obstetrical anesthesia and analgesia. Can. Anaesth. Soc. J., 9:414, 1962.

39. Seward, E. H.: Self-administered analgesia during labour with special reference to trichloroethylene. Lancet, 2:781, 1949.

40. Sun, D. C. H.: Comparative study of the effect of glycopyrrolate and propantheline on basal gastric secretion. Ann. N.Y. Acad. Sci., 99(1):153, 1962.

41. Thesleff, S.: The pharmacological properties of succinylcholine iodide. Acta Physiol. Scand., 26:103, 1952.

42. Tunstall, M. E.: Obstetric analgesia. The use of a fixed N_2O and O_2 mixture from one cylinder. Lancet, 2:964, 1961.

43. Wilson, J., and Turner, D. J.: Awareness during cesarean section under general anesthesia. Br. Med. J., 1:281, 1969.

44. Young, S. R., et al.: Methoxyflurane biotransformation and renal function following methoxyflurane administration for vaginal delivery or cesarean section. Anesth. Analg., 55:415, 1976.

18

Psychologic Methods of Analgesia: Prepared Childbirth, Hypnosis, and Acupuncture

Ezzat Abouleish, M.D.

At the present time there is much interest in the psychologic methods of analgesia for childbirth. Many couples, especially young ones, express their desire to go through the process of childbirth without the aid of pain-relieving medication. The reasons are fear of drug action on the baby and their willingness to share the whole process together, especially the delivery. At Magee-Womens Hospital the percentage of deliveries under prepared childbirth increased from 2 per cent in 1970 to 8 per cent in 1976. The techniques of psychologic analgesia are: prepared childbirth, hypnosis, and acupuncture.

PREPARED CHILDBIRTH
DEFINITION

Prepared childbirth is a method which prepares the mother-to-be to control her pains during parturition by psychologic means rather than by drugs.

Prepared childbirth, natural childbirth, Lamaze method of childbirth, Lamaze-Pavlov method for painless childbirth, and the psychoprophylactic method of childbirth are all synonymous. Prepared childbirth aims at reducing the amount of analgesic and anesthetic drugs required during labor and delivery, and at making childbirth an enjoyable event.

PRINCIPLES OF ACTION IN PREPARED CHILDBIRTH

The main principles of action in relieving pain in prepared childbirth are education, training, conditioning, distraction, motivation, suggestion, and expectation. The best results for increasing a person's endurance to pain are obtained by using the multiple approach in which all these principles are utilized.[31f]

Education

The parturient's understanding of pregnancy, labor, delivery, nursing of the baby, and the hospital environment is called *cognitive rehearsal*. This is a known psychological tool for reducing anxiety, thus increasing pain tolerance.[31d,31e] In six to eight sessions she learns about these topics by means of lectures and audiovisual aids such as movies. This course is similar to the "parents teaching classes" provided by large institutions for pregnant women and their husbands, who are all welcome to attend. By the time the mother is ready for labor and delivery, she knows what to expect and what is expected from her.

Fear initiates a vicious circle of skeletal and vascular muscle spasm, hypoxia, and pain. By removing the apprehension of having to face an unknown situation, the foundation for bearable childbirth is established.

Training

Training includes:

Practice in Relaxation. Relaxation decreases the level of anxiety.[31e] In such a mental state, the subject is presumably less fearful of the pain stimuli; therefore, the mind actually decreases its awareness of the painful sensation.[3a]

The gravida is taught how to relax her body as a whole and in particular those muscles associated with labor and delivery, e.g., the abdominal, back and pelvic muscles. Tension in these muscles exaggerates or even initiates pain. At home she practices relaxation 15 minutes per day. She lies on a recliner or on the floor with one pillow under her head and one under her knees. First, she tightens her muscles to be aware of them and then voluntarily relaxes them. She begins with a localized group of muscles, for example, those of one hand, and proceeds to a whole limb, then the whole body. With practice she can relax her muscles without initially tightening them and can simultaneously relax the whole body. When an arm is well relaxed, it is completely limp; and when the whole body is fully relaxed, she feels as if she is "floating in air." These relaxation exercises are very beneficial, not only for pain relief during prepared childbirth, but also for any form of analgesia. For example, during a subarachnoid block, when the patient relaxes her back muscles she can arch her back better, making it easier for the anesthesiologist and for herself. Relaxation, if performed properly, dissipates tension that has built up consciously or subconsciously during the day. If the gravida practices this relaxation shortly before

bedtime, it helps her sleep. During labor, relaxation is a form of distraction since it requires concentration. Also, the relaxed mother is in a hypnoid state in which she is amenable to suggestion. During delivery, the ability to relax the pelvic floor leads to an easy process for both the mother and fetus. The instructor, also the husband, conduct the exercise and check the relaxation. This technique can be used as a conditioned reflex during labor and delivery if practiced prenatally over a period of weeks. For example, when the husband or instructor says "relax" or touches a portion of the body, the woman relaxes because this is the way the exercise has been practiced prenatally.

Muscular Exercises. The aim of muscular exercises is to strengthen the muscles of the back, abdomen, buttocks, and perineum as well as loosen the joints, particularly those of the hips and pelvis. By performing these exercises the gravida develops a sense of well-being and self-control. She has better bearing-down ability during the second stage of labor, less backache during pregnancy and after delivery, better bowel control, and faster healing possibility of the episiotomy. There are many books that describe these exercises. However, it is easier and safer to learn these exercises in groups under the guidance of a qualified person because, if performed incorrectly, exercises can be harmful. Thereafter, these exercises are practiced twice daily for a total of 30 minutes.

Breathing Exercises. The gravida learns how to breathe properly and concentrate on it during childbirth (see below).

Practice in Bearing Down, "Pushing." The exercise of how to push can be learned during pregnancy but no force should be exerted (see below).

Conditioning

By conditioning, an association is developed between breathing and the painless uterine contractions during pregnancy (Braxton-Hicks contractions). When the gravida feels such a contraction, she puts her hand on her abdomen and breathes regularly, quietly, and deeply. By repeating this throughout pregnancy, a conditioned reflex is created. When the first stage of labor starts, this conditioned reflex is used to the mother's advantage to reduce pain. Therefore, when the gravida feels a contraction during labor, she places her hand on her abdomen and breathes again regularly, quietly, and deeply; since a conditioned reflex has been established, the contractions of the first stage of labor will feel mild.

Two types of breathing patterns are usually taught. The first is *deep, slow breathing*. The patient breathes quietly and slowly (10 breaths/min.) while relaxing the abdominal wall. This abdominal relaxation helps in relieving pain and allows the uterus to contract forward and to push the fetus toward the pelvis. The second type is *rapid, shallow breathing* (panting). The rate here is about 60 breaths per minute. This pattern is resorted to when the slow, deep respiration is no longer effective in relieving pain, and in certain situations during the second stage of labor when pushing is not required, e.g., during spinal block or during the delivery of the head to avoid its sudden exit. Breathing exercises have another beneficial effect, namely distraction. As the mother concentrates on breathing she pays less attention to the painful stimuli. Neither type of breathing should be overdone; otherwise the mother develops tetany and the fetus becomes acidotic.[22]

Distraction

Distraction is called by some authors *attention focusing* since *distraction* may imply a passive character.[31e] Distraction can be achieved by either:

1. The Dissociation Strategy. The person concentrates upon the nonpainful character of the nociceptive stimulus. For example, the parturient is instructed to think of labor as muscular contractions of the uterus rather than as labor pains.

2. The Interference Strategy. The person's attention is focused on something else than the nociceptive impulse, thus making awareness of pain a peripheral matter.[15a]

Both strategies are applied with prepared childbirth. The first is enforced into the patient's mind throughout the antenatal course. The second is utilized in many ways. As mentioned above, by concentrating on the breathing pattern, the patient's mind is distracted from the uterine contractions. Also, the patient's husband learns to massage her back and press on certain points on her back and sides. If pressing is applied properly during labor, it can help to relieve pain by "jamming" the pain impulses ascending to the brain. In a sense, it is similar to "pressure acupuncture" in which pain relief is produced by applying manual pressure, instead of inserting needles, at specific points. Massage of the back helps to relax the parturient and distract her mind.

Distraction is more effective early in labor when the pain builds up gradually, is less frequent, and less intense than later during the acceleration phase.[31c]

Motivation

The attention and enthusiasm of the obstetrician, prepared-childbirth instructor, and/or the husband increase the parturient motivation, a process called *Hawthorn effect*.

The motive for attending the childbirth classes varies. Some gravidas who request prepared childbirth are highly motivated and want to accomplish it successfully. However, most of them want to reduce the need for drugs and experience childbirth as a family affair in which both the wife and husband are able to participate.

Suggestion

During the whole course for prepared childbirth it is suggested to the patient that labor and delivery are normal physiologic mechanisms; therefore, the uterine contractions can be tolerated.

Expectation

The use of this tool to increase pain endurance is called *subjective cognitive rehearsal.*[31e] The patient is taught that with the onset of labor, the uterine contractions should feel just like menstrual cramps and cause only variable degrees of discomfort but no pain. This is what the patient will learn to expect and therefore she is not apprehensive, fearful, or tense. Although expectation does not affect the pain sensation, it changes the reaction toward pain.[7]

MECHANISM OF ACTION OF PREPARED CHILDBIRTH

Recently, naturally occurring substances, e.g. enkephalin, endorphin, and SR-13, have been found to have analgesic properties.[7a] They are secreted by neurons in the brain stem especially around the aqueduct and the floor of the fourth ventricle. They inhibit pain pathways, thus called the *endogenous antinoceptive factors.* The determination of the levels of these substances in the parturients who require no analgesics compared to those who need iatrogenic methods of pain relief awaits investigation.

TECHNIQUE[11,12,19,36]

Early in the first stage of labor, when contractions are mild and infrequent, simple distraction is usually sufficient, such as knitting. When the contractions become stronger, the patient relaxes and concentrates on breathing slowly and deeply. If this does not help, she resorts to shallow breathing. The husband helps by giving her moral support, massaging her back, and applying pressure at tender points. The patient is never left alone and is always encouraged that she is doing well and everything is progressing as expected.

When the cervix is fully dilated the patient is asked to push. She is taught that pushing is twice as strong as the uterine contractions, and that without pushing, the second stage is much prolonged. With prepared childbirth, pushing is involuntary; the patient feels marked fullness and weight in the pelvis and an irresistible desire to evacuate that mass by bearing down. It is explained to her that during pushing she has to hold her breath. The contraction of the abdominal and chest muscles against a closed glottis builds pressure within the chest and abdomen and evacuates the abdominal contents, including the fetus. The patient is instructed that she cannot breathe or talk while pushing because if she does, the glottis opens and air escapes. She is asked to take a deep breath and exhale deeply, then take another deep breath, hold it, and push down as forcibly as she can.

During pushing, the contents of the bowel and urinary bladder may escape because of the high pressure built-up inside the abdomen. That is why the parturient is usually given an enema when she first arrives in the labor suite.

To perform pushing efficiently, the patient's hips as well as her knees are widely separated. The head and shoulders are raised, the hands are held either to her legs or to a bar, and she is instructed to push strongly and uninterruptedly for as long as possible. If the contraction is a long one, she takes a deep breath, holds it, and pushes again. Also, to make pushing most effective, the muscles of the perineum are relaxed when bearing down so that minimal resistance is met by the advancing fetus. The patient is asked to relax completely between contractions and to start pushing again with the onset of another contraction.

ANALGESIC AND ANESTHETIC REQUIREMENTS WITH PREPARED CHILDBIRTH

When prepared childbirth was used as a routine method, in 10 to 20 per cent of cases the patients delivered without any anesthetic or analgesic drugs; in 30 to 40 per cent of cases the patients were relaxed and required less analgesics than unprepared parturients; and in 50 per cent of cases pain relief was not altered and patients required another form of analgesia.[4a] These percentages vary with different obstetricians; the attitude and preference of the individual obstetrician affect the ultimate method of pain relief.

However, obstetricians, nurses, physiotherapists, and psychologists who are enthusiastic about prepared childbirth and teach it are to be commended. On the whole, a patient who has attended the course for prepared childbirth, whether she needs anesthesia or not, is a much better patient than the one who has no knowledge of childbirth and hospital environment. The former is usually more relaxed, more cooperative, and has a more positive attitude.

EFFECT ON THE MOTHER

In the following sections, it is relevant not only to discuss the maternal and fetal effects of prepared childbirth, but also to compare them with other conventional anesthetic techniques.

The early proponents of prepared childbirth claimed that the technique has no effect on the maternal physiology. However, if pain is experienced, physiologic changes occur in almost every body system (see Chap. 1). They also stated that with prepared childbirth there is no associated mortality and morbidity compared with anesthesia. However, properly administered vertebral or general anesthesia has no mortality or morbidity; in fact, mortality and morbidity are reduced because of the adequate analgesia and the better conditions for obstetric management.[4a]

To improve the maternal-infant attachment, both have to be able to experience the sensations of touch and eye contact in a reciprocal manner as early as possible after delivery.[16a] Therefore, it is advantageous to have both the mother and baby awake at the time of delivery. It is thus claimed that prepared childbirth adds to the joy of childbirth and increases the parental-infant binding by having the mother conscious during the delivery. However, with epidural or subarachnoid block, better conditions are present because the mother is still awake, yet not distracted by any pain.

Spontaneous delivery, thus avoiding the use of forceps, is considered to be one advantage of prepared childbirth. However, the use of epidural analgesia does not increase the need for forceps delivery.[30] Moreover, it is less traumatic for both the mother and the fetus to perform an episiotomy and resort to low forceps delivery than to allow for a prolonged second stage with the possibility of uncontrolled perineal tears and fetal acidosis.[44]

EFFECT ON THE FETUS

It is claimed that neonates delivered under prepared childbirth are in better condition than those delivered under anesthesia. Proponents of prepared childbirth often refer to the anesthesia literature.[28] A commonly misquoted article is that of Scanlon *et al.* (1974) which gives the results of a study in which infants delivered without anesthesia had better neurobehavior responses than those delivered under epidural analgesia with lidocaine or mepivacaine.[31a] However, when the same authors repeated a similar study using bupivacaine for epidural analgesia, this superiority of prepared childbirth was absent.[31b] Moreover, the acid-base status of babies born under epidural analgesia is better than that of those babies delivered without analgesia.[33,44] Excessive pain can be harmful to the fetus by reducing the uterine blood flow and causing hyperventilation (see p. 15).

EFFECT ON THE COURSE OF LABOR

Prepared childbirth does not interfere with the course of labor; it is claimed to even shorten it. However, if pain is excessive, the regular uterine contractions may change into dysrhythmic ones. In such a case, epidural analgesia will improve the course of labor (see p. 249).

Recently Scott and Rose (1976) compared 129 primiparas who completed prepared childbirth classes with an equal number of matched controls who had not. Although the former group required less analgesics and anesthetics, the course of labor, the maternal complications, and the fetal outcome as assessed by the Apgar scores were not different.[31c]

ROLE OF PREPARED CHILDBIRTH

Prepared childbirth is a useful technique provided its limitations are recognized. The golden rule of "no pain, no anesthesia" also applies here. However, the gravida should be taught to look at anesthesia in childbirth with an open mind; if she is hurting, she should ask for pain relief. The drugs and techniques used today are safe for both the mother and infant. The gravida should be told that there are many factors beyond her control that can make her labor and/or delivery painful, e.g., the size and position of the fetus. She may also need anesthesia for an emergency delivery of the baby. Failure to explain these possibilities before childbirth causes many of these mothers to panic when told of its need and to have postpartum depression when they fail to go throughout labor without requiring analgesia.

Better conditions are obtained by combining prepared childbirth with minimal chemical analgesia, e.g., prepared childbirth for the first stage of labor and spinal or pudendal block for the second stage.

In recent teachings, the role of prepared childbirth as described above is explained to and accepted by the patients. In our institution, the obstetric anesthesia department works hand in hand with the teachers of prepared childbirth. The author considers prepared childbirth and obstetric anesthesia to complement each other. Each patient is a rule by herself; her safety and comfort are the aim of all concerned. During labor and delivery, the options of no medication to full analgesia should be available to every woman. Prepared childbirth is a safer and better technique for both the mother and baby than is "twilight sleep." Therefore, prepared childbirth can play an important role for the control of pain during parturition because of the present shortage in manpower, lack of interest, and limited experience in obstetric anesthesia.

LEBOYER TECHNIQUE[20]

The Leboyer technique of childbirth is a new method which has recently been described by a French obstetrician named Leboyer. Much interest has been directed toward this new technique in which lights are dimmed; voices are subdued; the umbilical cord is left uncut for several minutes; the baby is immediately handed to the mother to hold; the baby is given a bath; and the baby's cry is interpreted as signifying pain and suffering. Some of the features of this technique are good, some doubtful, and some harmful.

First, the good features: placing the baby on the mother's abdomen and giving the baby to the mother to hold, touch, and see is healthy and desirable. As said before, it has been proven that eye-to-eye contact between mother and baby in the first moments after birth strengthens the bond between the two.[16a]

Secondly, the doubtful features: these are the dimming of lights and whispering in the delivery room. There is no proof, by Dr. Leboyer or any other person, that adequate light and the normal tone of the human voice hurt the baby. It is true that hospital personnel should watch every word they utter in the delivery room lest the mother be frightened unintentionally. Certainly flash bulbs in the delivery room and yelling are not allowed. If the situation should require the use of brighter lights for the safety of the mother or resuscitation of the baby, or the ordinary tone of voice for better communication in an emergency situation, one can foresee that the mother and father might panic if they were prepared for childbirth by Dr. Leboyer's method.

The time for cutting the umbilical cord depends on the situation and the preference of the obstetrician at the time of delivery. For example, if the placenta is diseased and the baby is compromised, waiting for several minutes before severing the umbilical cord which is not functioning properly can endanger the baby. It is better under these circumstances to separate the baby and hand him to the anesthesiologist or neonatologist to start his resuscitation.

Thirdly, the harmful features: this is the impression that the baby does not need more than one or two cries at birth and that any further crying means pain or suffering. There is no proof for this assumption. Until a controlled study is performed in which babies delivered according to the Leboyer method are followed for a number of years and compared with babies delivered in the traditional way, Dr. Leboyer cannot assume the superiority of his technique. One should be concerned about the impact of this theory because the mother may suffer psychological trauma if her baby cries more than a few times at birth. She may misinterpret this as a sign that her baby is suffering.

Giving a baby a warm bath immediately after delivery could be harmful if the temperature of the bath is not accurately measured.

Before hospitals start to change their delivery rooms and before the public demands this change, one should wait and see the scientific comparison between Leboyer's technique and the standard techniques which have withstood the test of time.

HYPNOSIS

DEFINITION

Hypnosis is a state of altered consciousness; it is not a state of sleep. When the patient is hypnotized she is awake, her awareness is very restricted, and she is deeply concentrating.

HISTORY

Hypnosis is an ancient medical art which was developed during one of the earliest civilizations in human history, the Egyptian civilization.[43] It was first practiced by priests in the Egyptian "temple sleep" during which curative suggestions were made to patients. These temples rapidly became popular and spread to Greece and countries of the Middle East.

In 1776 Mesmer, an Austrian, published his theory of animal magnetism which states that disease is due to a disturbance in the magnetic balance of special fluids in all animal bodies; health is restored by reestablishing harmony of these fluids.[26] This theory is similar to the Chinese theory of energy and acupuncture.

Mesmerism, the early name of hypnosis, was used to produce anesthesia as early as 1829.[4a] This was called *magnetic anesthesia.* In 1831, magnetic anesthesia was successfully used for pain relief in labor.

In 1843, Braid refuted Mesmer's fluid theory and explained the method in a more scientific way. He gave it the present name, hypnosis. Hypnosis was used successfully for many operations; for example, in 1850 James Esdaile performed thousands of minor and more than 350 major operations on patients under hypnosis. Therefore, acupuncture is not the only nonchemical method of analgesia for surgery or childbirth; hypnosis has been used for more than 100 years.

At about the same time that hypnosis was first used for surgery, in the middle of the nineteenth century, the discovery of chemical anesthesia prevented the widespread acceptance of hypnosis for surgery.

PRINCIPLES OF ACTION OF HYPNOSIS

The mechanism of hypnosis is unknown because it is related to human behavior which is still not fully understood. However, certain factors play important roles in hypnosis, similar to those in other forms of psychologic analgesia. These factors are:

Suggestion and Expectation

The more suggestible a patient is, the better a subject she is for hypnosis. At first, suggestion is from the hypnotist to the patient. Later on, the patient is trained to suggest to herself, a procedure called "autosuggestion" and thus she can induce herself into a trance. This is important when labor starts at home because the patient can thus keep herself comfortable until the hypnotist arrives at the hospital. Also, suggestion can be from other mothers in whom hypnosis has been used successfully. Semantics play an important role in both hypnosis and prepared childbirth by eliminating unhappy words such as pain and cutting; uterine contractions are never mentioned as causing pain; they can cause cramps or discomfort but not pain.

Motivation

There must be good rapport between the hypnotist and the patient. He encourages her, listens to her, and shows interest in her desires and demands. On the other hand, she wants to please him by achieving her assignment. Since she is supposed to have no pain during childbirth, she is going to succeed by not having pain. If she feels pain, she fails and disappoints the hypnotist to whom she looks up and who has spent much time and effort to make her comfortable.

Conditioning

In "glove anesthesia," especially when rehearsed in the delivery room, a conditioned reflex is established before labor (see Technique, below).

Deep Concentration

When the patient is in a trance, her awareness is restricted; except for the voice of the hypnotist, all inputs to the brain, including pain sensations, are blocked. Therefore, sudden noise may distract the patient's concentration and disturb the procedure; a quiet atmosphere is important for hypnosis.

Therefore, the best patient for hypnosis is a suggestible one with average intelligence who is willing to be hypnotized, is able to concentrate, has no fear of hypnosis, and has absolute confidence in the operator.

TECHNIQUE

There are many methods for inducing hypnosis. *The first method is the direct induction* which depends on eye fixation on a certain object with subsequent fatigue and relaxation of muscles. This is the oldest method of hypnosis but is too time-consuming.

The second method is indirect induction. The patient imagines a person completely relaxed, and with the help of the hypnotist, a gradual shift is made from this person to the patient, thus relaxing her.

The third method is the mechanical induction in which visual, auditory, or tactile repetitive stimuli are used to induce hypnosis, such as rhythmic light flashing. Today many electronic devices are used for this purpose.

When hypnosis is used for childbirth, six prenatal sessions should be completed before childbirth. These are usually started at about the fifth month of pregnancy. During the first session the patient is selected after an interview during which certain tests are performed to find out her susceptibility. During the second session, the hypnotist suggests that the patient relax and she is induced into a state of "trance" in which her eyelids feel very heavy, her eyes close, and the entire body completely relaxes.

During the third session, while the patient is in a trance the hypnotist suggests to her that one of her hands feels numb and anesthetized, called "glove anesthesia."

Then, it is suggested to the patient that whatever part of her body she touches with this hand will also be numb and anesthetized. Therefore, the anesthesia is transmitted from her hand to her abdomen, back, and thighs.

During the fourth and fifth sessions, the same procedure is repeated, that is, getting into a state of trance, "glove anesthesia," and transfer of anesthesia.

During the sixth session, the same procedure is repeated in the delivery room.

Since this method is time-consuming, some clinics resort to *group hypnosis*. In the first session the patient is interviewed, and then she attends one of the group sessions. Some members of the group have had successful delivery under hypnosis. She watches and listens to their discussions. This gives her confidence in the technique, the same as in acupuncture anesthesia when the patient is visited by another patient in whom acupuncture was successfully used. In this group, newcomers' questions about hypnosis are mostly answered not by the hypnotist but by those who have experienced hypnosis in previous childbirths.

One obstetrician who is a clinical expert in hypnosis for childbirth stresses that he personally prefers trance state only rather than "glove anesthesia" or transfer of anesthesia.[40a] By simply relaxing the patient and suggesting to her that she is going to be comfortable during labor and delivery, he achieves adequate results. When the patient is in labor, he induces her into a state of trance very quickly, in 30 seconds to 2 minutes, and she stays in such a state until the delivery is accomplished.

SUCCESS RATE OF HYPNOSIS

Studies have been performed on the use of hypnosis as a routine method for analgesia in childbirth. On the whole, 15 per cent of the patients could not be hypnotized. Of those who were hypnotizable, 50 per cent had a comfortable labor and delivery, and 50 per cent failed.[42]

ADVANTAGES OF HYPNOSIS

On the whole, hypnosis is safe for the baby and the mother if no contraindications are present. Studies have shown that babies born under hypnosis or epidural analgesia are in a better condition than those delivered under general anesthesia.[28] Hypnosis has an insignificant effect on the course of labor. Minimal equipment is required and the cooperation of the patient is preserved.

DISADVANTAGES OF HYPNOSIS

Hypnosis cannot be used as a routine method of analgesia in childbirth because it has a limited success rate and is time-consuming. During delivery, the presence of the hypnotist is essential, and this cannot be guaranteed in every case. Hypnosis requires a special hospital atmosphere providing minimal distractions of the patient's concentration, e.g., enthusiastic nursing staff and quiet labor suite and delivery rooms.

CONTRAINDICATIONS FOR THE USE OF HYPNOSIS

The main contraindications are psychosis and hysteria because the patient's condition may worsen after hypnosis.[37]

ROLE OF HYPNOSIS IN CHILDBIRTH

Many patients are attracted to hypnosis because they want an unusual method for childbirth to brag about to their neighbors and friends. Some are curiosity seekers. Some think that during hypnosis they are asleep and someone is going to take care of their pains, such as during general anesthesia. They do not realize that during hypnosis they are awake, conscious, and concentrating deeply, and that much of the success of hypnosis depends on their effort to autosuggest comfort and relaxation. A good hypnotist can select his patients properly, excluding those in whom hypnosis is contraindicated or will be inadequate. Therefore, hypnosis can be effective in alleviating pain and anxiety of childbirth in specially selected cases provided there is an enthusiastic, qualified, and experienced hypnotist as well as interested hospital personnel.[33a]

ACUPUNCTURE

The term acupuncture is derived from the Latin *acus* meaning needle and *punctura* meaning puncture.

PRINCIPLE OF ACUPUNCTURE

Acupuncture is an art and a philosophy; it is not yet a science. It has been practiced in China for 4,000 to 5,000 years for diagnosis and treatment of various diseases as well as for pain relief.[2,23] Acupuncture has been used for anesthesia in surgery only since 1958.[13] According to Chinese theory, each organ has a certain amount of energy. A proportion of this energy is used locally by the organ and the remainder travels in a circular pathway away from and then back to the same organ. These pathways, called "meridians," run longitudinally, more or less parallel, and are located beneath the skin. Along the meridians, the energy reaches the skin surface at certain points called "acupuncture points." When an organ is diseased or a source of pain, the energy produced by that particular organ is said to be disturbed, either too much or too little. The insertion of acupuncture needles at certain points along the corresponding meridian (the acupuncture points) can restore energy to a normal level, thus relieving the pain or curing that particular organ. There is a total of 12 meridians on each side of the body, corre-

sponding to the 12 months, and there are two central meridians, one on the back and one on the front. Therefore, the total number of meridians is 26. Classically, the total number of acupuncture points on the body is 365, corresponding to the days of the year. It is said that energy reaches the body surface at one certain point every day and then moves on to another point on the subsequent day. Recently, it has been shown that the ear pinna is particularly sensitive and has many points corresponding to almost every organ in the body. The number of acupuncture points now exceeds 1,000 and each acupuncture center in China is utilizing its own combination of points, which differs from other centers, to achieve the same result.

MECHANISM OF ACTION OF ACUPUNCTURE

There is a marked similarity between hypnosis, prepared childbirth, and acupuncture. In all of them suggestion, expectation, distraction, motivation, and conditioning play important roles but in different degrees. However, these are not the only explanations for acupuncture. There are many other theories; a popular one is "the gate control theory of pain."[25a] Vibration of the acupuncture needle closes this gate or gates in the central nervous system,[23] thus preventing entry of pain sensation (see Chap. 1). In explaining the mechanism of hypnosis, West (1960) stated that when attention is fixed to a narrow range of stimuli, monotonously presented, there is a gradual but definite decrease in reactivity to other stimuli. The vibration of the acupuncture needle, by providing such a source of stimuli, can act in the same way.

TECHNIQUE
The Acupuncture Points Utilized for Vaginal Delivery

Acupuncture Points for the Uterine Pain (Fig. 18-1A). The points chosen are those usually used to treat dysmenorrhea

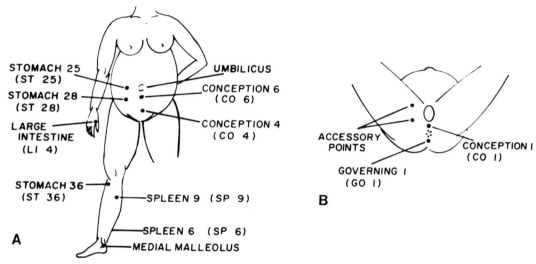

Fig. 18-1. *A.* Acupuncture points for uterine pain. *B.* Acupuncture points for perineal pain. (Abouleish, E., and Depp, R.: Acupuncture in obstetrics. Anesth. Analg., *54*:83, 1975)

and to produce anesthesia for cesarean section.[16,25,31,41]

1. *Stomach 25 (St 25)* is about 5 cm. lateral to the umbilicus.

2. *Stomach 28 (St 28)* is midway between St 25 and the inguinal ligament.

3. *Conception 4 (CO 4)* lies at the junction of the lower and middle thirds of a line joining the umbilicus with the symphysis pubis.

4. *Conception 6 (Co 6)* lies at the junction of the upper and middle thirds of the same line mentioned above.

5. *Large Intestine 4 (LI 4)* lies in the web between the first and second metacarpi, near the radial side of the second metacarpal bone.

6. *Stomach 36 (St 36)* is one finger width below the tibial tuberosity, between the upper ends of tibia and fibula.

7. *Spleen 9 (Sp 9)* is in the tibial fossa, below the medial condyle of the tibia.

8. *Spleen 6 (Sp 6)* is four finger breadths above the medial malleolus, along the posterior ridge of the tibia.

Acupuncture Points for Perineal Pain. The points are:[8]

1. *Governing 1 (Go 1)* is in front of the tip of the coccyx and behind the anus (Fig. 18-1B).

2. *Conception 1 (Co 1)* is in front of the anus and behind the vulva.

3. *Accessory points* are on either side of the vulva.

Equipment Needed for Acupuncture

The equipment used for acupuncture includes needles and a vibrator. The needles used are of different materials, sizes, and shapes according to the country from which they were obtained, the site of insertion, and the purpose of their use (Fig. 18-2). The needles used in the United States are stainless steel, disposable, 32-gauge needles (about 0.25 mm. in diameter). The acupuncture needles are not hollow like a regular needle used for injection but solid like a very fine sewing needle. They are usually supplied in sterile packages containing 12 needles. To augment the effect of acupuncture, the needles are usually vibrated after insertion either manually or by a battery-driven electric machine. The use of a *vibrator* allows for the simultaneous vibration of many needles by one person, either at the same or at different rates and for as long as required. Commonly used vibrators are the Chinese Acupuncture Anesthesia Apparatus, Model 71-1, using 9-volt DC dry bat-

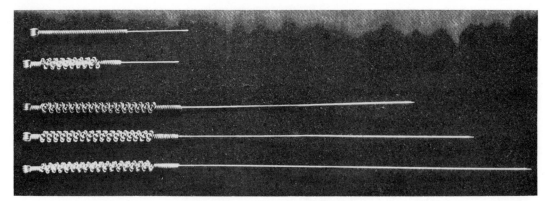

Fig. 18-2.   Acupuncture needles.

teries (Fig. 18-3), and the NeuroAMP Model 102 A, Lock Electro-Acupuncture Devices, San Francisco, California.

Method

The needles are inserted at the selected points to a depth of 1 to 2.5 cm. depending on the site of insertion and the size of the patient. Extra care should be taken during insertion of the needle in the abdomen lest it injures an intra-abdominal organ or the fetus. Sterile technique should be followed. The angle, depth, or site of insertion of the needle should be changed until "Teh-Chi" is obtained. "Teh-Chi" is a peculiar sensation felt by the patient in the form of warmth, numbness or tightness at the site of insertion, sometimes radiating along the corresponding meridian; the operator also feels tightness around the needle. It indicates that the needle is at the right spot. The total number of points used in each patient is usually eight. The electrical output from the acupuncture machine is gradually increased until the patient feels the needle vibrating without associated discomfort. If the output is too great, the unpleasant sensation of the vibration is worse than the labor pain itself. According to the patient's tolerance, the voltage usually varies between 1 and 5 volts, the amperage between 10 and 50 microamps, and the frequency between 1 and 5 cycles per second. The two electrodes from each socket of the machine are attached to needles only on the same side of the patient to avoid conduction of electricity across the body.

SUCCESS RATE OF ACUPUNCTURE

There are few reports on the use of acupuncture for labor and delivery, yet they are conclusive;[1,38] the success rate of acupuncture for childbirth is limited. In one report, electric acupuncture was used in 12 parturients during normal labor. On the average it produced 66 per cent analgesia in 7 patients for 139 minutes.[1] In another report, 19 out of 21 patients had inadequate analgesia following use of either electric or manual acupuncture.[38]

EFFECT ON THE MOTHER

Acupuncture does not cause any change in the mother's vital signs. However, with electric acupuncture there is interference with the recording of the maternal electrocardiogram corresponding to the rate of impulses discharged from the acupuncture machine. Lead I is spared except in cases where hand points are used (Fig. 18-4).

Acupuncture has been well accepted by

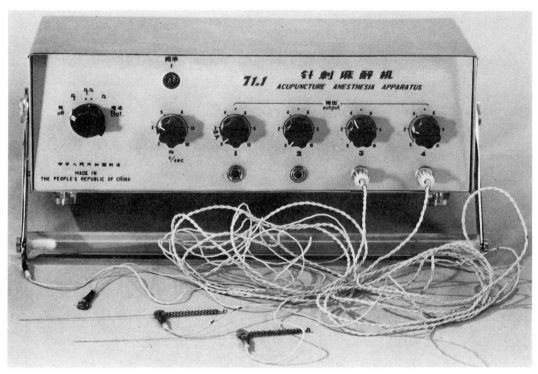

Fig. 18-3.   Chinese acupuncture vibrator.

most of the patients who experienced it, despite the inadequate pain relief.[1,38]

EFFECT ON THE FETUS

Acupuncture has no significant effect on fetal heart rate, baseline variability, or pattern. However, electric acupuncture may cause interference with electronic fetal monitoring (Fig. 18-5). Although the fetal electrocardiogram showed no premature beats or significant changes in the RR interval, the electric impulse from the acupuncture machine was recorded in two out of 10 cases (Fig. 18-6).[1] Acupuncture has no significant effect on the neonatal condition as estimated by Apgar scores and time to sustained breathing.[1,38]

EFFECT ON THE COURSE OF LABOR

There are claims that acupuncture shortens the course of labor.[18] However, by continuously monitoring and recording the uterine contractions, acupuncture was found to have no significant effect on the baseline muscle tonus, force, or frequency.[1]

ACUPUNCTURE FOR CESAREAN SECTION

There are sporadic reports on the use of acupuncture for cesarean section, both in China and elsewhere.[13,15,25,31] To perform acupuncture anesthesia, the points for the relief of uterine pain during labor are utilized. The needles are vibrated for 20 minutes prior to surgery. The abdominal needles are removed while remote needles in the limbs and ear pinna continue to be vibrated until the end of the surgical procedure.

It is doubtful that acupuncture will

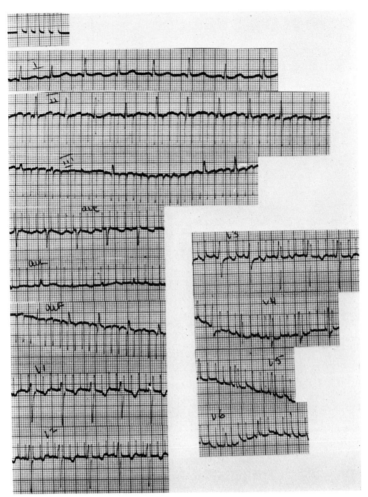

Fig. 18-4. Electric acupuncture interfering with maternal electrocardiogram. The interference signal is apparent in all leads except lead I. (Abouleish, E., and Depp, R.: Acupuncture in obstetrics. Anesth. Analg., *54*:83, 1975)

replace pharmacologic anesthesia for cesarean section.

ACUPUNCTURE FOR INDUCTION OF LABOR

Acupuncture, with or without electrical stimulation, could induce labor in pregnant women.[35] This is not unique only to acupuncture since hypnosis was used for the same purpose.[6] However, the mechanism of induction of labor is still unknown. Various endocrine, psychologic, and nervous factors not only can affect the onset of labor, but also its course.

ADVANTAGES OF ACUPUNCTURE

For childbirth, acupuncture presents favorable theoretical advantages: no drugs are administered; the technique seems simple and inexpensive; maternal vital signs are stable; the patient is alert; aspiration pneumonitis is not a problem; and the fetus is not adversely affected.

DISADVANTAGES OF ACUPUNCTURE

In obstetrics, acupuncture is inferior to regional analgesia such as epidural or spi-

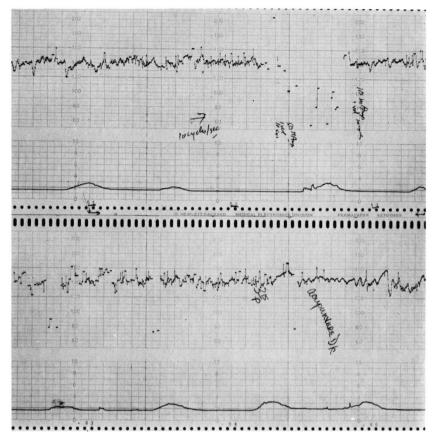

Fig. 18-5. Electric acupuncture interfering with electronic fetal monitoring. Increasing the intensity of the current from 10 microamps to 50 microamps interrupted the fetal heart rate recording which reappeared by reducing the amperage. (Abouleish, E., and Depp, R.: Acupuncture in obstetrics. Anesth. Analg., *54*:83, 1975)

nal block.[1] Acupuncture has the following disadvantages:

1. Acupuncture analgesia is incomplete, unpredictable, and inconsistent.
2. Acupuncture is time-consuming.
3. Acupuncture needles are apt to become dislodged.
4. The patient's movements are restricted.
5. Added wires and machinery are attached to the parturient.
6. Interference with maternal and fetal electronic monitoring occurs.

ROLE OF ACUPUNCTURE AS A METHOD OF ANALGESIA

There has been much interest in acupuncture in many fields of medicine including anesthesiology.[24] The impression that acupuncture is used routinely in China to produce analgesia for all types of surgery is erroneous. It has recently been stated that acupuncture is used in only 20 per cent of surgical patients, while regional analgesia, such as spinal and epidural, makes up the highest percentage of anesthetic techniques.[4] Even in China, despite

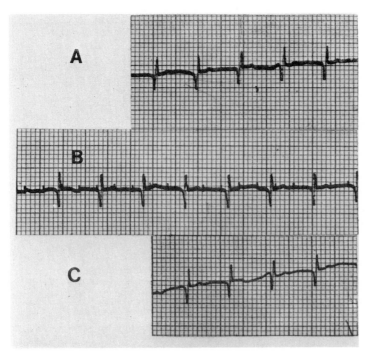

Fig. 18-6. Electric impulse from acupuncture vibrator imposed on fetal electrocardiogram. *A.* Fetal electrocardiogram before acupuncture. *B.* Fetal electrocardiogram during acupuncture showing the electric signal from the vibrator imposed on the ECG. *C.* Fetal electrocardiogram after discontinuing electric acupuncture. (Abouleish, E., and Depp, R.: Acupuncture in obstetrics. Anesth. Analg., *54*:83, 1975)

proper selection of patients, adequate preparation, experience, and cultural background, the success rate of acupuncture in producing analgesia for surgery is limited (60 to 70%).[39] Acupuncture is least effective in the lower part of the body.[26a]

There is no complete relief from pain under acupuncture but there is a state of hypalgesia, depending on the pain threshold of the patient. However, even this state of hypalgesia is doubted. Recent studies in dogs have shown that acupuncture does not affect halothane MAC.[32] In human volunteers, a team of American and Chinese scientists found that acupuncture has no influence on the perception of pain.[9] The experimental design minimized or eliminated factors other than the needles themselves, i.e., medications were not given and the subjects were scientists accustomed to objectivity. Moreover, the autonomic response to pain, as evidenced by measuring the galvanic skin resistance, is not changed by acupuncture. Some scientists consider that the sole effect of acupuncture is to cause the subjects to raise their pain criterion in response to the expectation that acupuncture works.[7,9]

The concept of the importance of accurate localization of the acupuncture is even doubted. Anatomically, there is no difference between the acupuncture points and other parts of the body.[40] The efficacy of acupuncture for the treatment of chronic pain does not depend on whether the needles are inserted at specific points in the traditional meridians or at any arbitrary distant point.[21]

The practicality of acupuncture in obstetrics is questionable.[1,38] The patient may be enthusiastic about the technique, the operator may be a Chinese expert in acupuncture, and still the results are inadequate and unpredictable.[38] Educated childbirth or hypnosis gives the same results as acupuncture with less trouble.

REFERENCES

1. Abouleish, E., and Depp, R.: Acupuncture in obstetrics. Anesth. Analg., *54*:83, 1975.
2. Armstrong, M. E.: Acupuncture. Am. J. Nurs., *72*:1582, 1972.
3. Atlee, H. B.: Natural Childbirth. Springfield, Ill., Charles C Thomas, 1956.
3a. Bobey, M. J., and Davidson, P. O.: Psychological factors affecting pain tolerance. J. Psychosom. Res., *14*:371, 1970.
4. Bonica, J. J.: Anesthesiology in the People's Republic of China. Anesthesiology, *40*:175, 1974.
4a. Bonica, J. J.: Principles and practice of obstetric anesthesia and analgesia. Pp. 763-820. Philadelphia, F. A. Davis, 1967.
5. Braid, J.: Neurypnology. London, J. Churchill, 1843.
6. Carter, J. E.: Hypnotic induction in labor. Am. J. Clin. Hypn., *5*:322, 1963.
7. Clark, W. C., and Yang, J. C.: Acupunctural analgesia: evaluation by signal detection theory. Science, *184*:1096, 1974.
7a. Cohn, M. L., and Cohn, M.: Comparison of pain regulation by enkephalin, and endorphin and SR-13, three naturally occurring compounds. Abstracts of Scientific Papers. P 471. American Society of Anesthesiologists, 1976.
8. Darras, J. C.: Acupuncture in obstetrics and gynecology; presented in The First World Symposium on Acupuncture and Chinese Medicine, San Francisco, California, 1973.
9. Day, R. L., et al.: Evaluation of acupuncture anesthesia: a psychophysical study. Anesthesiology, *43*:507, 1975.
10. DeSoldenhoff. R.: The assessment of relaxation in obstetrics. Practitioner, *176*:410, 1956.
11. Dick-Read, G.: Childbirth Without Fear. Ed. 4. New York, Harper & Row, 1972.
12. ———: The Practice of Natural Childbirth (Abridgement of Childbirth Without Fear, Ed. 4). New York, Harper & Row, 1976.
13. Dimond, E. G.: Acupuncture anesthesia. J.A.M.A., *218*:1558, 1971.
14. Esdaile, J.: Hypnosis in Medicine and Surgery. New York, Julian Press, 1957 (*reissue*). (*Original issue*: Mesmerism in India. Hartford, Silas Andnes & Co., 1850.)
15. Kakizaki, K., et al.: Caesarean section by acupuncture anesthesia. Am. J. Acupuncture, *1*:108, 1973.
15a. Kanfer, F. H., and Seidner, M. L.: Self-control: Factors enhancing tolerance of noxious stimulation. J. Pers. Soc. Psychol., *25*:381, 1973.
16. Kao, F. F.: Acupuncture Therapeutics. Pp. 33, 38, 40, and 73. New Haven, Eastern Press, 1973.
16a. Klaus, M. H., et al.: Maternal attachment: Importance of the first-postpartum days. New Engl. J. Med., *286*:460, 1972.
17. Kline, M., and Guze, H.: Self-hypnosis in childbirth: a clinical evaluation of a patient-conditioning program. J. Clin. Exp. Hypn., *3*:142, 1955.
18. Kubista, E., and Cusera, H.: Acupuncture preparation of primigravidae as a means of shortening labor. Am. J. Acupuncture, *1*:181, 1973.
19. Lamaze, F.: Painless Childbirth. Chicago, Henry Pegnery, 1970.
20. Leboyer, F.: Birth Without Violence. New York, Alfred A. Knopf, 1975.
21. Lee, P. K., et al.: Treatment of chronic pain with acupuncture. J.A.M.A., *232*:1133, 1975.
22. Levinson, G., et al.: Effects of maternal hyperventilation on uterine blood flow and fetal oxygenation and acid-base status. Anesthesiology, *40*:340, 1974.
23. Man, P. L., and Chen, C. H.: Mechanism of acupunctural anesthesia: the two-gate control theory. Dis. Nerv. Syst., *33*:730, 1972.
24. Matsumoto, T., Levy, B., and Ambruso, V.: Clinical evaluation of acupuncture. Am. Surg., pp. 400–405, 1974.
25. Mayrhofer, O.: Personal communication.
25a. Melzack, R., and Wall, P. D.: Pain mechanisms: A new theory. Science, *150*:971, 1965.
26. Mesmer, F. A.: Memoire sur la Decouverte du Magnetisme Animal. Paris, Didot le Jeune, 1779.
26a. McIntyre, J. W. R.: Observations on the practice of anesthesia in the People's Republic of China. Anesth. Analg., *53*:107, 1974.
27. Michael, A. M.: Hypnosis in childbirth. Br. Med. J., *1*:734, 1952.
28. Moya, F., and James, L. S.: Medical hypnosis for obstetrics. J.A.M.A., *174*:2026, 1960.
29. Portnuff, J. C.: The trained obstetrical patient. Am. J. Obstet. Gynecol., *67*:268, 1954.
30. Potter, N., and Macdonald, R. D.: Obstetrical sequences of epidural analgesia in nulliparous patients. Lancet, *1*:1031, 1971.
31. Roccia, L.: Personal experience with acupuncture in general surgery. Am. J. Chin. Med., *1*:329, 1973.
31a. Scanlon, J. W. et al.: Neurobehavioral responses of newborn infants after maternal epidural anesthesia. Anesthesiology, *40*:121, 1974.
31b. Scanlon, J. W., Ostheimer, G. W., Lurie A. O., et al.: Neurobehavioral responses and drug concentrations in newborns after maternal epidural anesthesia with bupivacaine. Anesthesiology, *45*:400, 1976.
31c. Scott, J. R., and Rose, N. B.: Effect of psychoprophylaxis (Lamaze preparation) on labor and delivery in primiparas. New Engl. J. Med., *294*:1205, 1976.
31d. Staub, E., and Kellet, D. S.: Increasing pain tolerance by information about adversive stimuli. J. Pers. Soc. Psychol., *21*:198, 1972.
31e. Stevens, R. J.: Psychological strategies for management of pain in prepared childbirth, I: A review of the research. Birth Family J., *3*:157, 1976.
31f. Stevens, R. J.: Psychological strategies for management of pain in prepared childbirth, II: A study of psychoanalysis. Birth Family J., *4*:4, 1977.
32. Stoelting, R. K., et al.: The influence of acupuncture on halothane MAC in dogs. Anesthesiology, *39*:661, 1973.

33. Thalme, B., Raabe, N., and Belfrage, P.: Lumbar epidural analgesia in labour: II. Effects on glucose, lactate, sodium, chloride, total protein, haematocrit and haemoglobin in maternal, fetal and neonatal blood. Acta Obstet. Gynecol. Scand., *53*:113, 1974.

33a.Tinterow, M. M.: Techniques of hypnosis; Evaluation. *In* Bonica, J. J. (ed.): Principles and practice of obstetric analgesia and anesthesia, Pp. 769-775. Philadelphia, F. A. Davis, 1967.

34. Tom, K. S.: Hypnosis in obstetrics and gynecology. Obstet. Gynecol., *16*:222, 1960.

35. Tsuei, J. J., and Lai, Y.-F.: Induction of labor by acupuncture and electrical stimulation. Obstet. Gynecol., *43*:337, 1974.

36. Vellay, P.: Childbirth Without Pain. New York, E. P. Dutton & Co., 1960.

37. Wahl, C. W.: Contraindications and limitations of hypnosis in obstetric analgesia. Am. J. Obstet. Gynecol., *84*:1869, 1962.

38. Wallis, L., *et al.*: An evaluation of acupuncture analgesia in obstetrics. Anesthesiology, *41*:596, 1974.

39. Wang, J. K.: The practice of acupuncture in China. Anesth. Analg., *53*:111, 1974.

40. Warren, F. Z.: Anatomy of a dermal puncture point. Acupuncture News Digest, *3*(12):4, 1973.

40a.Weber, J.: Personal communication, 1976.

41. Wei-P'ling, W.: Chinese Acupuncture. P. 50. Rustington, Sussex, England, Health Science Press, 1962.

41a.West, L. J.: Psychophysiology of hypnosis, J.A.M.A., *142*:672, 1960.

42. Winkelstein, L. B.: Routine hypnosis for obstetrical delivery. Am. J. Obstet. Gynecol., *76*:152, 1958.

43. Wolberg, L.: Medical Hypnosis: the Principles of Hypnotherapy. vol. 1. New York, Grune & Stratton, 1948.

44. Zador, G., and Nilsson, B. A.: Low dose intermittent epidural anaesthesia in labour. II. Influence on labour and acid-base status. Acta Obstet. Gynecol. Scand. [Suppl.], *34*:17, 1974.

Part Three

The Postpartum Period

19

Neonatal Resuscitation

William Oh, M.D.

Resuscitation of the newborn is an emergency procedure that requires clear understanding of the pathophysiology of fetal and neonatal asphyxia, sound clinical judgment for immediate selection of the correct therapeutic approach, and technical proficiency in resuscitative procedures. The importance of understanding the pathophysiology of asphyxia is obvious, because the selection of treatment modalities is aimed at the resolution of pathologic sequelae of asphyxia. It is also apparent that the understanding of the physiology of the neonate's first breath is an important consideration in clearly comprehending the pathology of asphyxia. Clinical judgment for the specific procedures for resuscitation is dependent on the accurate assessment of the neonate in the first minutes of life. These assessments include not only the physical examination of the infant, but also the history of the pregnancy and intrapartum period that might relate to the fetal status and neonatal condition at birth. In this chapter we will discuss these various aspects in relation to the resuscitation of the newborn infant, particularly in the delivery room setting.

FETAL AND NEONATAL CIRCULATIONS

During fetal life, oxygenated blood from the placenta flows through the umbilical vein into the fetus. A small portion of the umbilical venous blood flow reaches the hepatic circulation, and a majority of it is shunted across the ductus venosus entering the inferior vena cava and the right atrium, and preferentially diverted across the foramen ovale into the left atrium. Additional right to left shunt also occurs through the ductus arteriosus so that a relatively large amount of oxygenated blood is preferentially channeled into the systemic circulation, particularly that supplying the head and the upper portion of the trunk. It has been estimated that pulmonary blood flow only accounts for 12 per cent of the total cardiac output while placental blood flow through the umbilical arteries accounts for 50 per cent of the cardiac output.

When the umbilical cord is clamped at the time of birth, the blood flow across the ductus venosus rapidly declines and this accessory vessel functionally closes during the first 2 to 3 days of life.[15] The onset of respiration is followed by a prompt 15-fold increase in the pulmonary blood flow and a significant fall in pulmonary vascular resistance, along with a gradual decline in the pulmonary arterial pressure during the first few days of life. The increase in pulmonary blood flow and a rise in arterial oxygen saturation will cause a functional constriction of the ductus arteriosus. The closure will eliminate the shunt across the ductus arterious in either direction. Within the first hours after birth, the right atrial pressure also falls, creating a pressure gradient in favor of the left atrium.[3] Therefore within the first six hours after birth, this pressure gradient from the left to the right atrium will result in the closure of the foramen ovale by the approximation of the valve located on the left side of the foramen ovale. When these physiologic events occur and proceed normally, the circulation will be converted from a fetal arrangement (in parallel) to a neonatal (in series) pattern.

Perinatal asphyxia and failure to initiate the first breath would alter the normal transition of the fetal to neonatal circulation. Hypoxia and acidosis will impair the closure of the ductus arteriosus; the failure to initiate proper inflation of the alveoli will result in pulmonary hypoperfusion. These events produce a right to left shunt, compounding the severity of hypoxemia produced by inadequate pulmonary adaptation.

THE NEONATE'S FIRST BREATH

The neonate's first breath is probably one of the most dramatic events in life. The ability of a newly born infant to initiate the first breath and to sustain subsequent respiration will dictate whether the infant will require resuscitative measures or not. Therefore, it is of importance to understand the physical, physiologic and chemical factors involved in the initiation of the first breath. It is well known that the respiratory centers in the neonate, including in those born prematurely, are well developed[7] and are responsive to chemical stimuli.[4,20] It has been shown that a high carbon dioxide tension and a low oxygen tension will initiate hyperventilation in the newborn. At the time of delivery, the fetal Po_2 is generally low and the Pco_2 is high. When the umbilical circulation is interrupted by clamping of the cord or by the diminution of umbilical venous

blood flow, the Po_2 will continue to fall and the Pco_2 will rise. The combined effect of a falling Po_2 and a rising Pco_2 is responsible for the chemical stimulation of the respiratory center to initiate the first breath. There are also other nonchemical stimuli (tactile, thermal, and painful) which could increase the number of efferent impulses from the respiratory centers to the lungs to help induce the onset of the first breath. When the umbilical circulation is interrupted, a rise in systemic blood pressure usually ensues. This rise in blood pressure may start a baroreceptor response generating efferent stimuli from the respiratory center and contributes to the initiation of the first breath. When the lung is inflated, the Hering-Breuer reflex will also participate in maintaining the respiratory functions.

The successful and smooth transition from fetal to neonatal life requires the immediate stabilization of cardiopulmonary function within the first few minutes after birth. The establishment of a normal cardiopulmonary function requires the fulfillment of the following factors immediately after birth: (1) normal responsiveness of the respiratory centers to the various chemical or nonchemical stimuli described above; (2) the initiation of the effector response (respiratory muscles) for the expansion of the thoracic cage with adequate change in transpulmonary pressure for the initiation of the first breath (25–30 cm. H_2O); (3) adequate pulmonary biochemical maturity releasing a sufficient amount of surfactants to maintain alveolar stability during the expiratory phase; and (4) prompt increase of pulmonary blood flow to maintain adequate pulmonary perfusion. If any of these four requirements were unmet, neonatal asphyxia would ensue, requiring immediate resuscitation.

In a full-term infant, the most common cause of inability to establish pulmonary function is fetal asphyxia due to intrapartum fetal distress, and/or heavy maternal premedication or anesthesia which depresses the fetal central nervous system with suppression of the respiratory center's response to the respiratory stimuli. The etiology and pathogenesis of fetal distress and asphyxia are described elsewhere in this book. From the standpoint of management, it is important to recognize the etiology of neonatal asphyxia in order to implement a specific mode of treatment. For instance, in an infant with respiratory depression secondary to heavy maternal premedication with narcotics, the specific treatment will be the utilization of an antinarcotic agent during the process of resuscitation.

PATHOPHYSIOLOGY AND SEQUELAE OF PERINATAL ASPHYXIA

Fetal hypoxemia and acidosis are the hallmarks of fetal asphyxia. Cerebral hypoxemia, secondary to fetal hypoxia and/or decreased fetal cardiac output and cerebral blood flow, may result in cerebral edema and in some instances cerebral hemorrhage. Cerebral edema and/or cerebral hemorrhage are the reasons for the frequent observation of neurologic signs and symptoms in the postasphyxia state.

The presence of fetal acidosis, hypoxia, cerebral edema are the most common reasons for the difficulty in initiating the first breath. The chemical and nonchemical stimuli for the initiation of the first breath would be ineffective because of the profound suppression of the respiratory centers. If the resuscitative measures are not properly performed, the continuum of physiologic and biochemical abnormalities resulting from fetal asphyxia will add to the effects of the neonatal asphyxic episodes. Neonatal asphyxia will further increase the severity of acidosis, hypoxia, and the manifestations of cerebral injury.

It has been shown in experimental sheep models that intrauterine fetal hypoxia may result in the pooling of blood in the fetal vascular compartments resulting in a net placental transfusion of blood from the placenta to the fetus *in utero*.[18] Therefore, hypervolemia with polycythemia and hyperviscosity is not an infrequent finding in infants who have had perinatal asphyxia. There is data showing that infants born with low Apgar scores have a higher blood volume[22] and a lower placental residual blood volume.[19] Hypervolemia and hyperviscosity may exaggerate the signs and symptoms of cardiopulmonary compromise in the newborn infants who have had asphyxia at birth.

In addition, other abnormalities may occur as a result of perinatal asphyxia. These include shock, thermal instability, neonatal hypoglycemia, and neonatal hypocalcemia. Shock is a common finding in infants with severe asphyxia. Thermal instability may be due to several reasons, including central nervous system injury, increased oxygen consumption as a result of asphyxia, and impairment of chemical thermogenesis in the presence of adverse physiologic conditions. Hypoglycemia is a result of increased substrate utilization and impaired glucose production *de novo,* because of hypoxemia and acidosis. The neonatal hypocalcemia is secondary to several factors: (1) relative hypoparathyroidism present in almost all newborn infants in the first day of life;[12a,21] (2) increased endogenous phosphate production in the presence of a stress situation; (3) increased serum phosphate level because of a decrease of phosphate excretion; (4) enhanced production of thyrocalcitonin which has the physiologic effect of driving calcium ions into the intracellular compartment due to asphyxia; and (5) the abrupt change in the distribution of calcium ion in the presence of a changing tissue pH.[18,21] In the presence of acidosis, calcium tends to ionize into the extracellular compartment, therefore creating a falsely high or normal calcium level in the serum; when the acidosis is corrected, the rising pH will result in the ionization of calcium into the intracellular fluid compartment, resulting in an abrupt fall in the serum calcium level.

PREPARATIONS FOR THE RESUSCITATION OF THE NEWBORN

Part of the preparation for an effective resuscitation of the distressed newborn infant is the maintenance of an organized communication system between the obstetrician, anesthesiologist, pediatrician, other primary care physicians, and the nursing personnel. The importance of this communication system is apparent, because the possibility of the birth of a distressed infant is often recognizable from a careful assessment of the history and clinical course of the parturient mother during prepartum and intrapartum periods, and

this possibility should be relayed to the various personnel involved. In this regard, it is important that when a high-risk mother is admitted to the labor room and delivery suite, the perinatal team should be notified. A brief historical and clinical assessment and other pertinent information should be given to those who are responsible for the resuscitation and immediate care of the newborn infant. Several high-risk pregnancy scoring systems are currently available and can be used for the assessment.[12,17] Tables 19-1 and 19-2 are the lists for prenatal and intrapartum high-risk factors designed by Hobel and coworkers. These authors have shown that a statistically valid predicative association has been found between the scores assigned to the prenatal factors and the out-

Table 19-1. High-Risk Prenatal Factors*

Factor	Score†	Factor	Score†
Cardiovascular and renal factors		Epilepsy	5
Moderate to severe toxemia	10	Fetal anomalies	1
Chronic hypertension	10		
Moderate to severe renal disease	10	*Anatomical abnormalities*	
Severe heart disease, Class II–IV	10	Uterine malformation	10
History of eclampsia	5	Incompetent cervix	10
History of pyelitis	5	Abnormal fetal position	10
Class I heart disease	5	Hydramnios	10
Mild toxemia	5	Small pelvis	5
Acute pyelonephritis	5		
History of cystitis	1	*Miscellaneous factors*	
Acute cystitis	1	Abnormal cervical cytology	10
History of toxemia	1	Multiple pregnancy	10
		Sickle cell disease	10
Metabolic factors		Maternal age over 35 years or	
Diabetes (≥Class A-II)	10	under 15 years	5
Previous endocrine ablation	10	Viral disease	5
Thyroid disease	5	Rh sensitization only	5
Prediabetes (A-I)	5	Positive serology	5
Family history of diabetes	1	Severe anemia (<9 g. Hgb)	5
		Excessive use of drugs	5
Previous histories		History of tuberculosis or positive purified	
Previous fetal exchange transfusion for Rh		protein derivative test >10 mm.	5
incompatibility	10	Maternal weight under 100 or over 200	
Previous stillbirth	10	pounds	5
Postterm (>42 weeks)	10	Pulmonary disease	5
Previous premature infant	10	Flu syndrome (severe)	5
Previous neonatal death	10	Vaginal spotting	5
Previous cesarean section	5	Mild anemia (9–10.9 g. Hgb)	1
Habitual abortion	5	Smoking ≥1 pack of cigarets per day	1
Infant weighing more than 10 pounds	10	Alcohol (moderate)	1
Multiparity (>5 fetuses)	5	Emotional problem	1

*Hobel, C. J., *et al.*: Prenatal and intrapartum high risk screening. 1. Prediction of the high risk neonate. Am. J. Obstet. Gynecol., *117*:1, 1973.

†Assignment of numerical score is arbitrarily determined by these authors to reflect degree of risk in relation to neonatal outcome. High score means greater risk.

come of the neonates at birth and during the neonatal period.

When intrapartum monitoring data has revealed abnormal fetal conditions, the perinatal team should be alerted for possible need of resuscitation in the delivery room. The methods of intrapartum monitoring of the fetus are described elsewhere in this book.

In the construction of the perinatal intensive care unit, it is important to incorporate the resuscitation area into the delivery room suite so that the distance between the delivery table and the resuscitation table is minimal. The resuscitation area should be spacious enough to accommodate a radiant warmer, one or two portable equipment pieces such as respiratory or transport incubator, and three or four members of the resuscitating team. The resuscitation room should be well lighted, and an overhead lamp should be available for good illumination of the resuscitation area or table.

The nursing supervisor in the perinatal resuscitation area should make certain that the following equipment is in "ready to go" condition: (1) the radiant warmer should always be on the "on" position; (2) the warm humidified oxygen should be available; (3) the suction apparatus should be in operating condition; (4) the resuscitation tray should be prepacked (Fig. 19-1 shows the contents of the resuscitation tray); (5) the medication tray for resuscitation and the umbilical arterial catheterization tray should be readily available; and (6) other optional equipment that is on call basis should include portable respirator, thoracocentesis tray, and blood pressure apparatus.

RESUSCITATION EQUIPMENT AND MEDICATIONS

Resuscitation Equipment Tray

Figure 19-1 shows equipment for resuscitation. The pediatric-size laryngoscope should have a premature size blade at-

Table 19-2. High-Risk Intrapartum Factors*

Factor	Score†
Maternal factors	
Moderate to severe toxemia	10
Hydramnios or oligohydramnios	10
Amnionitis	10
Uterine rupture	10
Mild toxemia	5
Premature rupture of membrane >12 hours	5
Primary dysfunctional labor	5
Secondary arrest of dilation	5
Demerol >300 mg.	5
MgSO$_4$ >25 g.	5
Labor >20 hours	5
Second stage >2½ hours	5
Clinically small pelvis	5
Medical induction	5
Precipitous labor <3 hours	5
Primary cesarean section	5
Repeat cesarean section	5
Elective induction	1
Prolonged latent phase	1
Uterine tetany	1
Oxytocin augmentation	1
Placental factors	
Placenta previa	10
Abruptio placentae	10
Postterm (>42 weeks)	10
Meconium-stained amniotic fluid (dark)	10
Meconium-stained amniotic fluid (light)	5
Marginal separation	1
Fetal factors	
Abnormal presentation	10
Multiple pregnancy	10
Fetal bradycardia >30 minutes	10
Breech delivery, total extraction	10
Prolapsed cord	10
Fetal weight <2,500 grams	10
Fetal acidosis, pH ≤7.25 (Stage I)	10
Fetal tachycardia >30 minutes	10
Operative forceps or vacuum extraction	5
Breech delivery, spontaneous or assisted	5
General anesthesia	5
Outlet forceps	1
Shoulder dystocia	1

*Hobel, C. J., *et al.*: Prenatal and intrapartum high risk screening. 1. Prediction of the high risk neonate. Am. J. Obstet. Gynecol., *117*:1, 1973.
†See Table 19-1 for the meaning of numerical score.

tachment (10 mm. width). The battery power for the laryngoscope should be checked daily and fresh batteries should be available in the resuscitation area. There have been some discussions recently regarding the propriety of using a straight (portex) or tapered-end (Foregger-Cole)

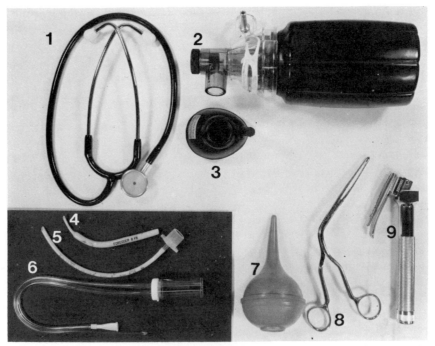

Fig. 19-1. The contents of the resuscitation tray are: 1. Stethoscope. 2. Positive-pressure bag. 3. Face mask. 4. Foregger-Cole tube. 5. Portex tube, 6. DeLee suction tube. 7. Bulb syringe. 8. Magill forceps. 9. Laryngoscope.

endotracheal tube for intubation. The advantage of using a straight tube is ease of intubation and avoidance of irritation of the larynx and vocal cords produced by the tapered portion of the Foregger-Cole tube. However, a distinct disadvantage of the straight tube is that there is a risk of inserting the tube too far, passing beyond the carina and entering the right primary bronchus. For this reason, there is a distinct advantage to using the Foregger-Cole tube, particularly if the operator is familiar with this tube and there is a certainty that the intubation and the need for the placement of the tube are temporary. If a prolonged period of intubation is required, the straight tube is recommended to avoid constant irritation of the larynx by the tapered portion of the Foregger-Cole tube. The aspiration of nasal passages and oropharyngeal cavities is best achieved by the use of the rubber bulb syringe shown in Figure 19-1. The DeLee suction tube

should be used only for aspiration of the stomach contents and the endotracheal tube. The use of the DeLee suction tube for oropharyngeal or nasopharyngeal suction can sometimes irritate the vagal innervation of the posterior pharyngeal area, resulting in a vagal response and bradycardia. If it is necessary to use the DeLee suction tube for the aspiration of the pharyngeal area, one should be extremely gentle in handling the plastic tubes to avoid this complication. The positive-pressure resuscitation bag is an important piece of equipment for resuscitation. The resuscitation bag shown in Figure 19-1 has the disadvantage of being unable to deliver inspired air of more than 40 per cent oxygen concentration. For this reason, there are others who prefer the use of an anesthesia bag which can deliver inspired air with an oxygen concentration as high as 100 per cent. In many centers, the bag shown in Figure 19-1 has been modified to allow delivery of a higher oxygen concentration by attaching an accessory tubing permitting recirculation of the oxygen inflow. The Magill forceps are used by those who prefer nasotracheal rather than orotracheal intubation. In addition to the equipment shown on the tray, appropriate-size tapes, tincture of benzoin, and sutures with needles and scissors should be available for securing the endotracheal tube. An oral airway is also useful in cases where macroglossia and/or micrognathia are the cause of airway obstruction.

Medication Tray

The medication tray should contain the following preparations in appropriate concentrations:

1. Sodium bicarbonate, 0.9 molar solution
2. Epinephrine hydrochloride, 1:10,000 solution
3. Glucose solution, 5 per cent
4. Glucose solution, 10 per cent
5. Calcium gluconate solution, 10 per cent
6. Neonatal naloxone, 0.02 mg./ml. of solution
7. Albumin or Plasmanate solution
8. Normal saline and sterile water as diluent.

Adequate amounts of each preparation should be available and the medication tray should be kept simple and well marked (Fig. 19-2) so that personnel can quickly locate the appropriate medication desired.

TECHNIQUE OF INTUBATION

The use of a laryngoscope for the direct visualization of the glottis is the best method of endotracheal intubation in a distressed newborn. With practice and experience, the intubation can be accomplished promptly with minimal complications. The infants should be placed in the supine position and the head placed very close to the edge of the resuscitation table. A roll of diapers can be placed under the back of the neck to provide a hyperextended position. With the right hand holding the biparietal portion to keep the head of the infant steady, the laryngoscope is held in the operator's left hand and the blade is placed in the right corner of the infant's mouth, depressing the tongue while advancing the blade for approximately 2 cm. As the blade is introduced, it is swung into the midline; and as it reaches the junction of the epiglottis and the base of the tongue, the blade is tipped slightly to lift the epiglottis anteriorly to expose the glottis. The glottis is a vertical black hole bordered posteriorly by the arytenoid cartilages which usually appear pink. When the glottis is identified, a quick visual inspection should be done to identify the patency of the airway. If mucus or meconium is present, a quick suction should be performed to clear the airway. The endotracheal tube is then introduced into the glottis with the right hand until the tapered portion of the Foregger-Cole tube rests immediately above the opening of the glottis. If a portex tube is used, the intended length of the tube to be inserted beyond the glottis should be predetermined according to the approximate size of the infant.[16]

Following the placement of the endotracheal tube, a mouth-to-tube resuscitation can be performed by blowing brief puffs of air into the tube to produce rise of the neonate's chest wall. One may enrich the inspired air with oxygen by allowing an oxygen source to flow into the operator's mouth. Very often the infant may take a good gasp and begin to breathe on his own following a brief period of mouth-to-tube resuscitation. If this does not occur, a more prolonged resuscitation effort can be done by attaching the endotracheal tube to a positive-pressure bag for further resuscitation. Following the placement of the tube and during the resuscitation, it is important to determine that the tube is indeed in the trachea and not in the esophagus by

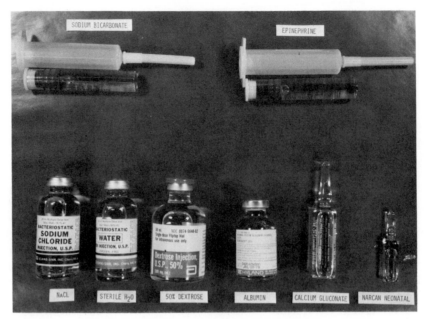

Fig. 19.2   Typical contents of a medication tray for the neonatal resuscitation area.

observing the movement of the chest wall and by auscultating the upper part of the chest for the presence of breath sounds during the ventilation.

PROCEDURE FOR RESUSCITATION

The assessment of the neonatal condition during the first 60 seconds of life is the most important step in the choice of resuscitation procedure for an asphyxiated infant. Dr. Virginia Apgar designed an objective scoring system bearing her name for this purpose.[2] This scoring system (Table 19-3) is useful not only in the assessment of the neonatal condition in the first minute of life, but also in the assessment of the infant at 3, 5, or 10 minutes of life as a reflection of the effectiveness of resuscitation procedure. Based on the initial Apgar score, one could systematically select the appropriate step in the management of the asphyxiated infant. A schematic approach to resuscitation is shown in Figure 19-3.

If the Apgar score is 0, meaning there is no heart tone or respiratory effort and the infant is extremely limp, hypotonic and cyanotic, the presence of fetal heart tone a few minutes prior to delivery of the mature nondeformed fetus would probably indicate immediate cardiopulmonary resuscitation. If the fetal heart tone has not been heard for a long time before the delivery of the fetus, or if the fetus is extremely immature or has obvious major malformations, it is probably inappropriate to apply heroic measures for resuscitation. The specific details for cardiorespiratory resuscitation can be described as follows:

The infant should be intubated immediately and the upper airway should be maintained patent. One person should use an anesthesia bag to deliver positive-pressure ventilation while a second person applies closed cardiac massage. The appropriate method of cardiac massage is to apply two fingers on the chest, at the second and third interspace just to the left of

Table 19-3. The Apgar Scoring System*

Sign	> Points <		
	0	*1*	*2*
Heart rate	Absent	Less than 100/min.	More than 100/min.
Respiration	Absent	Slow, irregular	Good, crying
Muscle tone	Limp	Some flexion of extremities	Active movement
Reflex irritability (response to catheter in nose)	Absent	Grimace	Cough and sneeze
Color	Blue, pale	Body pink, extremities blue	Completely pink

*Apgar, V.: A proposal for a new method of evaluation of the newborn infant. Anesth. Analg., *52*:379, 1958.

the sternum, and the force of the fingers should be directed backward and slightly upward. The cardiac massage should synchronize with the positive-pressure ventilation at a ratio of 3 to 1, i.e., for every three strokes of cardiac massage, one breath is applied. This will maintain a normal ratio of 120 beats per minute heart rate and 40 breaths per minute respiration. One should bear in mind that the purpose of cardiopulmonary resuscitation is to drive adequate amounts of blood from the ventricles to the aorta as well as to the pulmonary artery. For every amount of blood that is delivered to the pulmonary artery and returned to the left atrium, the ventilation will hopefully raise the PaO_2 level. When the PaO_2 is raised to a level of adequate oxygen saturation, oxygenation of the myocardium will initiate myocardial activity. When the heart rate is initiated (even at a low rate), administration of intracardiac epinephrine (1:10,000 dilution) may produce an adequate inotropic effect

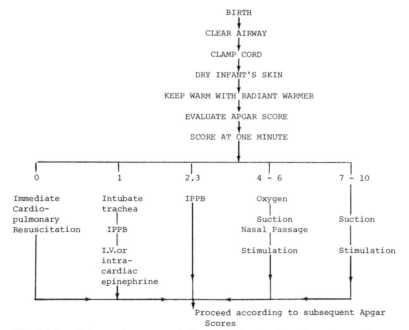

Fig. 19-3.   Schematic approach for resuscitation based on the 1-minute Apgar score result.

to raise the heart rate to normal range and establish an adequate cardiac output. As soon as the heart rate is normalized, cardiac resuscitation should be terminated and pulmonary resuscitation alone should be maintained.

If the Apgar score is 1, that is if a heart rate of less than 100 beats per minute is the only item responsible for the Apgar score, immediate intubation is necessary followed by intracardiac epinephrine administration if bradycardia persists in spite of appropriate ventilation. If the heart rate completely stops, cardiopulmonary resuscitation, as described above, should be instituted.

If the Apgar score is 2 or 3, intermittent positive-pressure breathing with the use of a positive-pressure bag is often enough to initiate the first breath by the Hering-Breuer reflex with an improvement of the respiratory status of the infant. If the Apgar score continues to deteriorate in spite of positive-pressure ventilation, intubation should be done and resuscitative measures applied according to the Apgar score, as described previously.

If the Apgar score is between 4 and 6, provision of a high oxygen concentration in the inspired air is often sufficient to increase the ventilatory function of the infant.

If the Apgar score is greater than 7, active resuscitation is probably not necessary. Attempts should be made to maintain the patency of the airway, and in most cases all that is necessary is to apply external stimulation, such as gentle flicking of the toes.

In all circumstances, the following items should be part of the resuscitation procedure:

1. Clamping of the umbilical cord can be done immediately if there is a need for it. For instance, in the presence of a nuchal cord, the umbilical cord can be clamped immediately when the infant is delivered. In the absence of emergency indications, a 30-second interval between the delivery of the fetal buttocks and clamping of the cord

is advisable since this duration of intact umbilical circulation will provide an extra 10-15 ml./kg. of blood transfusion to the infant. Excessive placental transfusion, such as milking of the cord, should be avoided particularly in the presence of asphyxia, a condition which might have increased the fetal blood volume *in utero*.

2. Immediately following the clamping of the cord, the infant's body should be dried quickly with a sterile towel and the infant should be placed in the radiant warmer (Fig. 19-4) for temperature control.

3. To maintain patency of the upper airway, nasopharyngeal suction should be done with the use of the rubber bulb syringe.

DRUG THERAPY DURING RESUSCITATION

During the process of resuscitation, ventilation should always be the primary concern since the establishment of pulmonary function is the most important priority for resuscitation. However, there are instances in which drugs may be necessary to overcome specific underlying factors or complications of neonatal asphyxia. These medications should always be used with appropriate indications based on objective evidence and should not replace ventilation as the primary priority. The drugs that are often used during the resuscitation process include the following:

Sodium Bicarbonate

It is known that during perinatal asphyxia due to fetal distress, metabolic acidosis is an important biochemical complication, and its prompt identification and correction may improve the outcome of the infants during the neonatal course.[1,11] As the respiratory acidosis is being treated with appropriate ventilation, metabolic acidosis can be corrected with intravascular infusion of sodium bicarbonate. Ideally, the dosage of sodium bicarbonate should

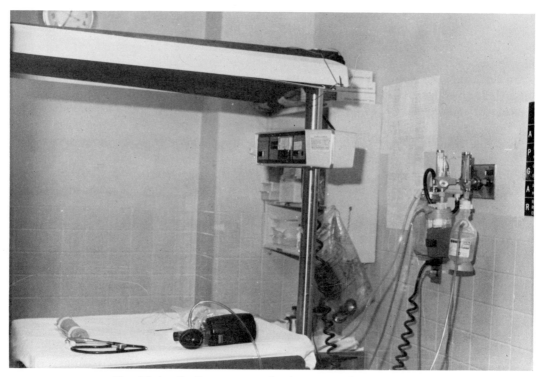

Fig. 19-4.   Radiant warmer in the neonatal resuscitation area.

be calculated on the basis of acid-base deficit determined by analysis of arterial blood. For this purpose, fetal scalp blood samples or cord arterial blood obtained at birth may be used to determine the acid-base status. The formula for the calculation of base deficit is as follows: dose of sodium bicarbonate (mEq.) = base deficit (mEq./l.) × 0.4 × body weight (kg.). The sodium bicarbonate can be infused through an umbilical artery catheter or an umbilical venous catheter placed in the inferior vena cava. The sodium bicarbonate can be best administered in the form of a half-strength solution (1 part 0.9 M sodium bicarbonate and 1 part sterile water) and at a rate no faster than 1 mEq. for every 2-minute period. Giving the sodium bicarbonate through a needle or a short catheter inserted into the umbilical vein is not an appropriate method since the blood flow through the umbilical vein usually ceases following the clamping of

the umbilical cord. Furthermore, with the reduction of flow through the ductus venosus, there is a high probability that the sodium bicarbonate may enter the portal sinus which may cause hepatic necrosis.[10] Therefore, injection of $NaHCO_3$ is preferable through a catheter introduced in the umbilical artery than in the umbilical vein. In the absence of blood gas determination and in cases of severe asphyxia, one may administer 2 mEq./kg./dose of sodium bicarbonate in the manner described above, provided the infant is being ventilated properly.

Epinephrine Hydrochloride

Epinephrine hydrochloride is a useful drug for the treatment of infants with asphyxia associated with cardiac arrest. The dosage of epinephrine hydrochloride is 0.01 mg./kg. administered intracardiacly at a dilution of 1:10,000. It should be accompanied with closed cardiac massage in order to circulate it through the coronary circulation and help achieve its direct effect on the myocardium. In infants with profound bradycardia, the epinephrine may be given intravenously. Arterial administration of this drug is not recommended.

Volume Expanders (Blood, Plasma, Plasmanate, Albumin Solution, or Normal Saline Solution)

Hypotension due to hypovolemia is a common complication of perinatal asphyxia. The hypotension is particularly profound in infants of low birth weight. If asphyxia is associated with pallor, tachycardia, feeble or weak pulse, and hypotension, administration of volume expanders is an important mode of treatment during resuscitation. The specific choice for the volume expander will depend on the etiology of shock and the availability of the material. In cases where hemorrhage is the obvious cause of hypotension, whole blood is the drug of choice. Nevertheless, in an emergency situation when blood is unavailable, plasma or any of the volume expanders will suffice as a temporary measure and blood can be transfused as an elective procedure to correct the anemia. In infants of low birth weight, it has been shown that a large number of infants with asphyxia are hypovolemic[5] and volume expanders are useful as part of the resuscitative procedures. However, it is important that prior to administration of the volume expander, hypotension should be documented by measurement of blood pressure. It has been shown recently that random administration of volume expander (albumin solution) in infants of low birth weight with hypoalbuminemia did not reduce neonatal morbidity and mortality.[6]

Blood pressure can be measured in several ways; the most accurate method is the use of a transducer-recorder system in measuring the blood pressure by means of an umbilical artery catheter. In the absence of this system, a spinal puncture monometer may be used and connected to an arterial catheter. The displacement of a water column in mm. H_2O divided by 13.6 (mercury density) will provide the mean blood pressure in mm. Hg. The normal values and the two-standard deviation of the mean of arterial mean blood pressure in neonates of various gestational age during the first 12 hours of life has been measured[13] and should be used as a criterion for the diagnosis of hypotension. This arterial blood pressure chart (Fig. 19-5) should be made readily available in the perinatal resuscitation area for quick reference. If an arterial catheter is not available, an alternative methods of determining blood pressure utilizing ultrasonic waves, e.g., Doppler is also valid although not as accurate. The flush method of blood pressure measurement is the least desirable since the accuracy is poor, particularly if the blood pressure is in the hypotensive range.

Glucose Infusion

As indicated previously, hypoglycemia during the first 6 to 12 hours of life is a common complication in infants with asphyxia. Therefore it is of importance to provide a glucose infusion soon after the resuscitation procedure to prevent or ameliorate this metabolic complication. A hypertonic glucose solution as a bolus infusion can be used as long as one is not dealing with an infant of a diabetic mother. In the latter case, a bolus infusion of hypertonic glucose may result in rebound hypoglycemia. In most instances, the best approach is to provide a continuous infusion of 10 per cent glucose through a peripheral venous or umbilical arterial catheter, whichever route is feasible, giving a dose of 6 to 7 mg./kg./min. of glucose. The blood glucose should be monitored during the first 12 hours of life, e.g., by the use of a semiquantitative method of blood glucose determination (Dextrostix).

Neonatal Naloxone (Narcan)

Naloxone is a narcotic antagonist and is very useful if the infant is depressed as a result of administration of narcotics such as morphine or meperidine to the mother during labor. It is important to establish the diagnosis prior to the administration of this antagonist. The diagnosis can be established by the history of administration of a narcotic agent to the mother prior to the delivery of the infant, the clinical manifestations of an infant who has irregular respiration, lack of meconium staining and pallor, and the presence of neurologic signs such as hypotonia, lethargy, and depression. Administration of this antagonist often produces a prompt improvement of the infant's condition. Other narcotic antagonists include nalorphine (Nalline) and levallorphan (Lorfan), but these agents are less desirable since they have a respiratory-depressant effect if they are given to infants whose respiratory depression is not due to narcotic agents.

Other Agents Useful in Resuscitation of the Newborn

Other agents that may be useful in the resuscitation procedures include atropine, isoproterenol, and calcium gluconate, but these agents are of secondary importance.

POST-RESUSCITATION PROCEDURES

When normal cardiopulmonary functions are established following effective resuscitation, the presence of hypotension, hypothermia, respiratory distress, seizure, and other clinical abnormalities should be promptly recognized and the etiology of the symptoms determined. In addition, the physician should perform a thorough evaluation of the neonate to detect the presence of congenital abnormalities. Below is a list of congenital abnormalities that may result in neonatal asphyxia at the time of birth. These conditions should be considered particularly if the asphyxia is persistent and the resuscitation is difficult.

Following the evaluation, it is advisable to gently insert a nasogastric tube for the aspiration of gastric contents. The procedure of gastric aspiration may have some diagnostic values in that: (1) If a gastric tube cannot be introduced, esophageal atresia should be suspected. (2) In the presence of large amounts of gastric aspi-

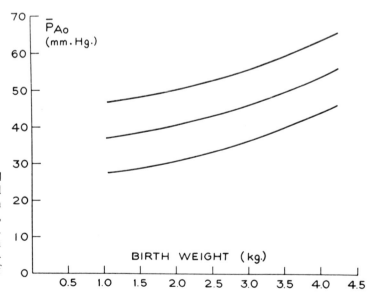

Fig. 19-5. Mean arterial blood pressure and standard deviation in relation to birth weight. (Kitterman, J. A., Phibbs, R. H., and Tooley, W. H.: Aortic blood pressure in normal newborn infants during the first twelve hours of life. Pediatrics, *44*:959, 1969)

Congenital Abnormalities That May Result in Neonatal Asphyxia

1. Diaphragmatic hernia
2. Potter's syndrome
3. Congenital hypoplastic lungs
4. Polycystic kidneys
5. Bilateral posterior choanal atresia
6. Congenital pulmonary lymphangiectasia
7. Congenital laryngeal stenosis

---

rate (in excess of 30 ml.) the possibility of a congenital obstructive lesion of the gastrointestinal tract should be considered. (3) In the presence of prolonged rupture of the membranes, the gastric aspirate may be a useful biologic fluid for bacteriological analysis and staining for the presence of polymorphonuclear cells as well as bacteria. (4) If the infant has respiratory distress, the analysis of gastric aspirate for surface-active material can be useful in making the differential diagnosis of respiratory distress. It has been shown that in the presence of a negative foam-stability test (indicating absence of surface-active material in the gastric aspirate) the infant's respiratory distress is most likely due to hyaline membrane disease.[8,9]

Umbilical artery catheterization is indicated if the infant develops persistent respiratory distress following resuscitation and requires a high concentration of oxygen to maintain a pink color. The catheterization should be done under sterile conditions, after the infant's status is stable, and preferably under the radiant warmer to maintain the infant's body temperature.

MECONIUM ASPIRATION

In the presence of meconium-stained amniotic fluid, it is advisable to clear the infant's upper airway as thoroughly as possible prior to delivery of the thorax. In cases of severely asphyxiated infants in whom laryngoscopy and intubation are necessary, aspiration of the trachea should be done to clear the meconium from the upper airway. If the meconium is extremely tenacious in consistency, it may be useful to instill 0.5 to 1.0 ml. of normal saline into the trachea, quickly followed by aspiration of the instilled solution. As a rule, inspection of the larynx should be performed in every case of suspected meconium aspiration. The exception is if the neonate has started crying, has a good Apgar score, and the meconium is thin. The harmful effects of laryngoscopy, e.g., neonatal bradycardia, laryngospasm, and trauma, outweigh the expected beneficial effects. By then the suction of meconium is rather difficult to achieve since it has reached inaccessible parts of the neonate's lungs.

COMPLICATIONS OF RESUSCITATION

Following active resuscitative measures such as intubation and positive-pressure bagging, a number of possible complications should be looked for. These include: (1) pneumomediastinum pulmonary interstitial emphysema or pneumothorax; (2) trauma to the pharynx, the vocal cords, or larynx as a result of attempted laryngoscopy and intubation; and (3) although uncommon, the possibility of esophageal perforation from faulty intubation may also occur.

REFERENCES

1. Adamsons, K.: Treatment of acidosis with alkali and glucose during asphyxia in foetal rhesus monkeys. J. Physiol., *169*:679, 1963.
2. Apgar, V.: A proposal for a new method of evaluation of the newborn infant. Anesth. Analg., 52:379, 1958.
3. Arcilla, R. A., *et al.*: Portal and atrial pressures in the newborn. A comparative study between infants born with early and late cord clamping. Acta Paediatr. Scand., 55:615, 1966.
4. Avery, M. E., Chernick, V., and Young, M.: Fetal respiratory movement in response to rapid changes of CO_2 in the carotid artery. J. Appl. Physiol., 20:225, 1965.
5. Ballard, B. R., *et al.*: Observations on hypovolemia in the newborn. Clin. Res., 20:278, 1972.

6. Bland, R. D., Clarke, T. L., and Harden, L. B.: Rapid infusion of sodium bicarbonate and albumin into high risk premature infants soon after birth: a controlled, prospective trial. Am. J. Obstet. Gynecol., *124*:263, 1976.

7. Boyd, J. D.: The development of the human carotid body. Contrib. Embryol. Carnegio Inst., *26*:1, 1937.

8. Cowett, R. M., and Oh, W.: Gastric aspirate foam stability test as an aid in the diagnosis of respiratory distress syndrome. Pediatr. Digest, *18*:13, 1976.

9. Cowett, R. M., *et al.*: Foam stability test on gastric aspirate and the diagnosis of respiratory distress syndrome (RDS). N. Engl. J. Med., *293*:413, 1975.

10. Erkan, V., Blankenship, W., and Stahlman, M. T.: The complication of chronic umbilical vessel catheterization. Pediatr. Res., *2*:317, 1968.

11. Hobel, C. J., *et al.*: Early vs. late correction of neonatal acidosis in low birth weight infant. J. Pediatr., *81*:1178, 1972.

12. ———: Prenatal and intrapartum high risk screening. 1. Prediction of the high risk neonate. Am. J. Obstet. Gynecol., *117*:1, 1973.

12a. Hohenauer, L., and Oh, W.: Calcium and phosphorous homeostasis in the first day of life. Biol. Neonate, *15*:49, 1970.

13. Kitterman, J. A., Phibbs, R. H., and Tooley, W. H.: Aortic blood pressure in normal infants during the first twelve hours of life. Pediatrics, *44*:959, 1969.

14. Leake, R., Williams, P., and Oh, W.: Validity of neonatal blood pressure obtained by the manometric method. Pediatrics, *52*:293, 1973.

15. Lind, J., Stern, L., and Wegelius, C.: Human Foetal and Neonatal Circulation. Springfield, Ill., Charles C Thomas, 1964.

16. Lowe, A., and Thibeault, D. W.: A new and safe method to control the depth of endotracheal intubation in the neonates. Pediatrics, *54*:506, 1974.

17. Nesbitt, R. E. L., Jr., and Aubrey, R. H.: High risk obstetrics II value of a semi-objective grading system in identifying the vulnerable group. Am. J. Obstet. Gynecol., *103*:972, 1969.

18. Oh, W., *et al.*: Placenta to lamb fetus transfusion in utero during acute hypoxia. Am. J. Obstet. Gynecol., *122*:316, 1975.

19. Philip, A. G. S., Yee, A. B., and Rosy, M.: Placental transfusion as an intrauterine phenomenon in deliveries complicated by foetal distress. Br. Med. J., *2*:11, 1969.

20. Purves, M. J.: The effects of hypoxia in the newborn lamb before and after denovation of the carotid chemoreceptor. J. Physiol., *185*:60, 1966.

21. Tsang, R. C., and Oh, W.: Neonatal hypocalcemia in low birth weight infants. Pediatrics, *45*:773, 1970.

22. Yao, A., *et al.*: Placental transfusion in the premature infant with observation on clinical course and outcome. Acta Paediatr. Scand., *58*:561, 1969.

20

The Neonatal Intensive Care Unit

William Oh, M.D.

During the past decade, the concept of regionalization of perinatal care facilities has effectively crystallized with the specific goal of reducing perinatal morbidity and mortality. The concept of regionalization is based on the principle that within a well-defined population base and/or geographic delineation, a network of health care facilities relating to obstetrics and neonatal medicine can be organized to allow each facility in the network the capability of delivering an appropriate level of care. The rationale for this concept is based on statistical data from the various centers in the United States and Canada, showing a significant reduction in perinatal mortality when a neonatal intensive care unit was established in a maternity hospital and/or when high-risk neonates were referred to a neonatal intensive care unit for diagnosis and management.[6,15] More recently, the American College of Obstetrics and Gynecology, the American Academy of Pediatrics, and the American Academy of General Practice have taken an official position by endorsing the concept of perinatal care regionalization, and a document to be used as a guideline for this regionalization has been published.[12] The document proposes that within the region, three levels of perinatal facilities can be established:

1. *Level I Facilities.* These are hospitals with the capabilities for handling uncomplicated pregnancies. The critical factors for these facilities are the capabilities for detecting high-risk pregnancies during the prenatal period for prompt referral to the level III hospitals. Studies have shown that a significant number of high-risk neonates were the products of uneventful pregnancies and were not detected or suspected during the prenatal screening.[1,3,8] Therefore, another important factor in the level I facility is the availability of facilities and personnel for emergency care of mothers and high-risk newborn infants when needed.

2. *Level II Facilities.* These are hospitals with larger obstetric services and are usually situated in the urban and suburban areas. They provide the full range of obstetric and neonatal care for uncomplicated pregnancies and for the majority of complicated obstetric and neonatal illnesses. The volume of deliveries in these hospitals may not be large enough to justify the establishment of a perinatal and neonatal intensive care unit. Therefore, the more seriously ill newborn will need to be referred to a level III hospital.

3. *Level III Facilities or Tertiary Care Center.* The region served by the level III facility should have at least 10,000 live births per year, including those delivered in the tertiary care center. The level III facility provides service for uncomplicated as well as complicated pregnancies, but the major charge to this institution is the establishment of: (1) a well-equipped perinatal and

neonatal intensive care unit; (2) leadership in the educational process for the perinatal health care personnel within the region; and (3) an active research program relating to perinatal medicine.

It should be pointed out that the implementation of this regionalization concept and plan is sometimes hampered by logistic difficulties arising from political, religious, social, and other factors, and that in some instances flexibilities and modifications may have to be made to fit into local conditions and circumstances. In following the plan for regionalization of perinatal care, the establishment of a neonatal intensive care unit in the tertiary care center is an important step. In this chapter, the details in the establishment of this unit will be described.

PHYSICAL FACILITIES OF THE NEONATAL INTENSIVE CARE UNIT

Location

Within a well-defined region, there should be an appropriate number of level III or tertiary care facilities depending on the geographic and population needs. Figure 20-1 shows the schematic arrangement of the various components of a tertiary care center. Within this level III or tertiary care center, the labor and delivery rooms should be constructed as an integrated unit (perinatal intensive care unit) for the care of normal as well as high-risk mothers and fetuses. The neonatal intensive care unit should be adjacent to the perinatal intensive care unit and the resuscitation area. The distance between the maximal care area of the neonatal intensive care unit and the resuscitation area should be as short as possible. To facilitate the visitation of the critically ill neonates by their mothers, the postpartum care area for these mothers should also be as close to the neonatal intensive care unit as possible. The mothers of critically ill infants should be in private rooms within the postpartum area to allow for privacy during the grieving process. In recent years, the issue of mother-infant in-

teraction after birth as it pertains to distressed infants has been explored and the data seem to favor the need for immediate, close, and frequent contact between the mother (and father) and the infant.[4]

Bed Requirements

In planning the establishment of a neonatal intensive care unit, certain guidelines can be used to determine the number of beds required for a specific region. The most useful base of reference in determining the bed requirement is the number of live births within the region. However, it is apparent that a precise formula cannot be used to calculate this requirement, since this formula may vary according to the level of risk of the population involved, the pattern of referrals to the neonatal intensive care unit from other institutions, census fluctuation, and several other related factors. Nevertheless, guidelines can be used for initial planning, and the precise need can be adjusted as the planner or organizer gains experience during the actual operation of the unit.

In the initial planning stage, the following guidelines can be used to estimate the number of beds required for the neonatal intensive care unit. It has been estimated that approximately 10 per cent of the total live births in a level III hospital may require admission to the neonatal intensive care unit.[15] The experience at Women and Infants Hospital of Rhode Island confirms this estimate; in 1975, some 500 infants (out of 5,000 live births at the hospital) were admitted to the neonatal intensive care unit. The patient days generated from the 500 admissions totalled 8,500 per year.[9] The bed requirement for the infant born in this obstetric service is therefore 22 (8,500 divided by 365). For the extramural admissions (admissions from the other community hospitals) the referral rate is generally smaller (2% of total live births) but the number of patient days generated from this population is longer, since only the sicker infants are referred to this neonatal intensive care unit. In a region

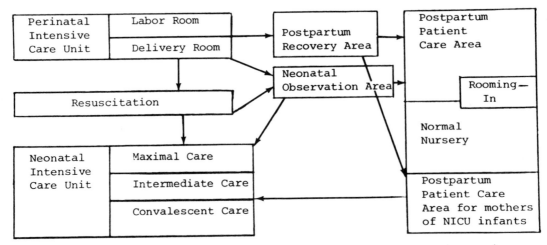

Fig. 20-1. Schematic representation of the layout for the patient care area in a tertiary care center.

with 10,000 live births per year, approximately 200 infants will be transferred to the neonatal intensive care unit. In our experience, this number of referrals would generate approximately 6,000 patient days per year, requiring an additional 16 beds to accommodate these admissions. The total bed requirement is therefore 38 for a region having 15,000 live births (10,000 in the various community hospitals and 5,000 in the level III hospital). This figure is lower than the formula proposed by Swyer who gave an estimate of 5.7 beds per 1,000 live births. The discrepancy is partly accounted for by the active retransfer of convalescing infants to the referring hospitals in the region served by Women and Infants Hospital of Rhode Island, and more importantly, it also reflects the variations resulting from local circumstances in each region. Allowance for the day-to-day fluctuation of bed occupancy should also be considered in estimating the bed requirements.

Designation of Patient Care Areas and Space Requirement

The neonatal intensive care unit should be separated into three different patient care areas (Fig. 20-1) for maximal, inter-

mediate, and convalescent care. The maximal care area is designed for infants who have the most serious illness, requiring assisted ventilation and close monitoring of vital signs including blood pressure. The space requirement for this area is at least 50 and ideally 100 square feet per patient. The intermediate care area is designed for infants who are recovering from the most serious conditions, but who still require close monitoring. The space requirement is between 40 to 60 square feet per patient. The convalescent care area is designed for infants who are not acutely ill and are generally the premature infants who are recovering from their illness and are detained in the hospital until they gain sufficient weight. The space requirement for this area is 25 to 30 square feet per infant. The main rationale for this progressive patient care concept is to allow the aggregation of patients categorized by the degree of severity of their illness for the appropriate distribution of space, personnel, and equipment.

Individual Life-Support Modules

In the maximal and intermediate care areas, the construction of individual life-support systems for patient care is extremely useful. Figure 20-2 shows a typical life-support module designed for the care of one infant requiring maximal or intermediate care. This module has 2 oxygen outlets, 1 air outlet, and 1 suction device outlet. It also has 12 duplex electrical outlets with appropriate grounding.

The counter top for each module should be constructed with two different height levels, one to allow the placement of the monitoring equipment in an easily visible level, and the other to be used as a writing space for the nursing as well as medical personnel at the bedside. In our experience, the module system is very effective in maintaining organization and efficiency in the delivery of care to acutely ill infants.

Environmental Requirements

The major considerations for the control of environment in the neonatal intensive care unit are to provide comfortable working conditions for the personnel, optimal setting for temperature control for the seriously ill infants, and maintenance of an atmosphere for the prevention of nosocomial spread of infection.

The lighting of the intensive care unit should provide adequate illumination to allow close observation of the infants without creating an artificial lighting that may hamper the interpretation of an infant's color in cases such as cyanosis and jaundice. In most instances, a fluorescent daylight lamp is satisfactory and the illumination should be approximately 100-foot candle at the infant's level.

The airflow pattern within the intensive care unit is also an important feature in the construction of the unit. The input of air should be near the ceiling while the outflow of air should be near the floor. The reason for this is to minimize the contamination of environmental air in the unit as a result of airflow from the floor toward the ceiling (the floor area is the dirtiest portion

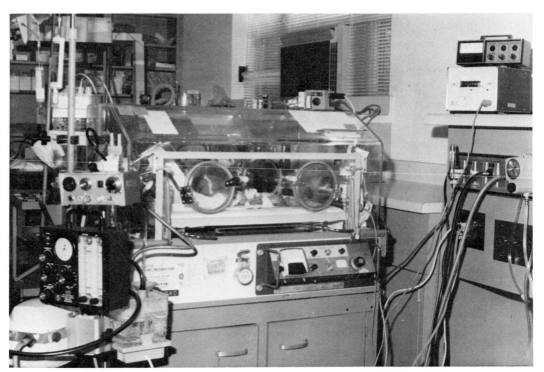

Fig. 20-2.   Individual life-support module in the neonatal intensive care unit.

of the room). A minimum of 12 air changes per hour should be maintained within the neonatal intensive care unit to assure the freshness of the environment. The temperature in the intensive care unit should be thermostatically controlled at 80 to 85°F. The relative humidity should be maintained at approximately 50 per cent. It is apparent that an air conditioning system is necessary to maintain four-season temperature and humidity control.

The acoustical factor is another consideration in the construction of the neonatal intensive care unit. The use of various electronic monitors and respirators can generate a significant amount of noise within the nursery.[16] To protect the nursery personnel from damage to hearing, the noise level in the unit should be maintained below 75 decibels. This can be accomplished by providing an acoustic ceiling structure and lowering the intensity of the alarm noise level in the monitoring equipment.

Supporting Areas

The following supporting areas should be incorporated into the neonatal intensive care unit: (1) various office areas for the neonatologists, director or supervisor of nursing services, social worker, public health nurse, respiratory therapist, and unit manager; (2) sleeping quarters for the house officers near the intensive care unit; (3) a nurse's lounge with lockers for the nursing staff; (4) a conference room for teaching as well as for parent interviews; and (5) an adequate area for storage.

Equipment

The equipment listed below should be available in the neonatal intensive care unit:

1. *Radiant Warmer.* Each intensive care unit should have a radiant warmer in the admitting area. The advantage of a radiant warmer is the easy accessibility to the infant for procedures and the adequacy of temperature control. In some nurseries,

the radiant warmer is also used for the long-term care of the ill infants. Higher insensible water loss has been documented in infants treated with a radiant warmer;[17] therefore, close monitoring of intake and output for fluid balance is essential.

2. *Incubator.* The conventional type of incubator is most commonly used in the neonatal intensive care unit (Fig. 20-2). One can adequately maintain the body temperature of seriously ill infants with the use of this form of incubator. An additional advantage is that the infant is enclosed in an isolated environment and the risk of infection is lower. However, the conventional incubator has the disadvantage of allowing less efficient accessibility to the infant inside and the possibility of thermal instability if one has to open the incubator for procedures at frequent intervals.

3. *Cardiorespiratory Monitors.* There are various forms of cardiorespiratory monitors on the market. Most of them are satisfactory for the monitoring of cardiac and respiratory rates in infants. One major consideration in the selection of a specific type of monitor is the availability of servicing and maintenance for these instruments. One frequent complication in the use of these monitors is the skin irritation and subsequent secondary lesions in the infants of very low birth weight secondary to frequent changes of adhesives for the application of the sensors.

4. *Intravenous Infusion Pump.* This is a useful piece of equipment for the delivery of parenteral fluid to small or sick infants. The infusion pump should have a wide flexibility and versatility as well as accuracy in the amount of fluid that can be delivered.

5. *Phototherapy Unit.* This is a very frequently used piece of equipment for the treatment of jaundice in the neonate. There are portable models available. However, a ceiling track can be used to store the phototherapy lamp and the advantage to this is that the lamp can be moved in a

horizontal or vertical direction for versatility and space-saving purposes (Fig. 20-3).

6. *Respirator.* There are several forms of respirators to deliver positive-pressure or negative-pressure ventilation. The positive pressure respirators cause chest expansion by applying positive pressure to the airway. The negative-pressure respirators produce chest expansion by applying negative pressure to the thoracic wall which it surrounds. The positive-pressure respirators (volume-constant or pressure-constant varieties) are more popular than the negative-pressure respirators. However, it has been shown that the negative-pressure respirator offers the advantage of having a lower complication rate in reference to pneumothorax and bronchopulmonary dysplasia.[7,10] In its current state of development, the negative-pressure respirator has some technical flaws that make its usage more difficult than the positive-pressure respirator. It should be pointed out that the effectiveness of a ventilatory program in an intensive care unit is dependent not so much on the type of respirators used but rather on the team of personnel who manages the respirator program.

7. *Blood Pressure Apparatus.* Each neonatal intensive care unit should have different forms of equipment that could measure blood pressure of critically ill infants. A standard sphygmomanometer can be used to measure blood pressure by the flush method; a Doppler method for measuring blood pressure has also been used. In infants with an umbilical arterial catheter in place, a transducer-recorder system for measuring the blood pressure is probably the most desirable means of obtaining this data (see also Chap. 19).

8. *Oxygen Monitor and Controller.* This is an important piece of equipment for ap-

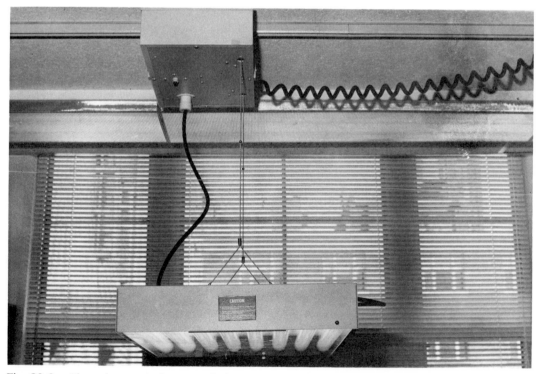

Fig. 20-3.   Photolherapy unit suspended on a ceiling track. The unit can be adjusted horizontally and vertically for greater flexibility.

propriate control of oxygen therapy. The oxygen monitor can analyze the oxygen concentration in the inspired air, and in most devices, an alarm system has been incorporated. The oxygen controller has the capacity to adjust the oxygen and compressed air inflow into the incubator or oxygen hood in order to maintain the oxygen concentration at a preset level. An alarm system is also available in this model.

Other equipment that should be available in the neonatal intensive care unit includes a metric system scale, a portable suction apparatus, and a portable electronic thermometer. The latter is most useful in monitoring the body temperature of an infant during the admission procedure.

PERSONNEL REQUIREMENTS IN THE NEONATAL INTENSIVE CARE UNIT

Medical Staff

The neonatal intensive care unit should be directed by a full-time board-eligible or board-certified neonatologist. Depending on the size of the unit, the neonatologist should have one or more assistant neonatologists on his or her staff. In most instances, the primary discipline of these neonatologists is pediatrics; however, this does not preclude the well-trained or qualified anesthesiologist, surgeon, or obstetrician from supervising the day-to-day function of this unit.

The availability of the pediatric house staff to the unit is an essential requirement. In recent years the increasing demand on house staff for patient care is beginning to create a proportionately larger rotation of house staff through neonatology in relation to the overall pediatric residency training program. As this trend continues, it may become necessary to develop a core of extended-role nurses who will complement the pediatric house staff for the patient care in these units.

A fellowship training program is also an important integral part of the perinatal tertiary care center. The director of the center has the responsibility of providing these trainees with experience in patient care, teaching, research, as well as administrative skills. The fellows should have equal exposure to patient care and research and, in most centers, the fellow is effectively utilized as a junior member of the faculty for the entire training program.

In addition to the core neonatal staff, the neonatal intensive care unit should have the services of the various pediatric disciplines that will provide the subspecialty services. This includes surgery, cardiology, endocrinology-metabolism, infectious diseases, allergy-immunology, genetics, neurology, neurosurgery, and hematology.

Nursing Staff

The quality of a neonatal intensive care unit is heavily dependent on its nursing staff. The nursing staff should be under the direction of a director or supervisor.

The adequate staffing of nurses is an important factor in the quality of the nursing care in the unit. The formula for the staffing is based on the progressive patient care concept and can be arranged as follows: for the maximal care area, a nurse-patient ratio of 1 to 1 or 1 to 2 is needed. For the intermediate care area, a nurse-patient ratio of 1 to 2 to 1 to 4 is adequate, while in the convalescent care area a nurse-patient ratio of 1 to 4 to 1 to 6 will suffice. It is important that this nurse-patient ratio is maintained throughout the three nursing shifts during a 24-hour period and on a 7 days per week basis. The adequacy of nursing staff is a common problem among the neonatal intensive care units. There are several ways of maintaining an adequate nursing staff but the most important factors include: (1) providing optimal pay scale and fringe benefits for the nurses; (2) creating an *esprit de corps* in the intensive care unit to maintain high morale; and (3) instituting an ongoing in-service program to maintain the quality as well as the interest of the nursing staff for patient care.

The smooth operation of the neonatal intensive care unit also requires the presence of several paramedical personnel who are especially trained and exclusively assigned to the neonatal area. This paramedical personnel should include the respiratory therapist, social workers, public health nurses, physical therapists, and pharmacists.

In a large-size neonatal intensive care unit, the availability of a unit manager to assist the unit director in his administrative functions is also essential.

SUPPORTING SERVICES

Laboratory Medicine

Ideally, a member of the pathology staff within the institution should be given the responsibility of coordinating the service, teaching, and research components of perinatal pathology.

The laboratory facilities should have the capability of determining the various biochemical analyses by micromethods requiring small samples of blood. The most common biochemical determinations required for patient care in the neonatal intensive care unit include: bilirubin, complete blood count, glucose, calcium, electrolytes, blood urea nitrogen, and blood gases. The latter is the most commonly employed laboratory test and the analysis should preferably be done within the neonatal intensive care unit for efficiency and prompt reporting of the results to the clinicians. The laboratory services should also provide microbiology and blood-banking supports for the unit.

Radiological Services

A full-time pediatric radiologist familiar with neonatal radiology should be assigned to the neonatal intensive care unit. A portable roentgenographic machine should also be available and placed within the intensive care unit for its exclusive use. A 24-hour radiological consultation service should be available for cases where the radiological interpretations require the radiologist's expertise. The radiology service should also provide facilities for cardiac catheterization and other special procedures for diagnostic purposes.

Follow-Up Clinic

Each tertiary care center should have a follow-up clinic for the high-risk infants. In recent years, the neurological and developmental outcomes of graduates from the intensive care unit have improved significantly and this improvement has been attributed to the intensive care provided to these infants.[11] The maintenance of a follow-up clinic provides continuity of care to these infants and it also provides a yardstick for the performance of the intensive care unit. The follow-up clinic should be directed by a pediatrician who has experience in primary health care as well as neonatal medicine. The other members of the follow-up team should include a pediatric neurologist, a psychologist, a public health nurse, and a social worker. A close liaison should be maintained between the follow-up clinic and the team at the neonatal intensive care unit as well as the primary care physicians in the community. The director of the neonatal intensive care unit should have the overall responsibility of the follow-up clinic.

STATISTICAL COLLECTION AND ANALYSIS

The tertiary care center should maintain a program for the ongoing collection of data on admissions, deaths, transfers from the regions, and retransfers of infants to the community hospital. A periodic assessment and analysis of the data should be done to evaluate the performance of the tertiary care center as the leader in perinatal care within the region. If the volume of patients within the region is sufficiently large, it may be justified and necessary to utilize a computerized system for the storage and analysis of the statistics. The results of the statistical analysis should be shared with the various parties involved in perinatal care in the region. One could also utilize these data as the subject for discussion in the periodic educational activities between the various perinatal care facilities.

EDUCATIONAL COMPONENTS

The educational program at the tertiary care center should consist of three components: (1) a teaching program for the medical students of the affiliated university, and a postgraduate program for the house staff and fellows. This component is the cornerstone of the entire educational program since the quality of the tertiary care center and the quality of the other components of the teaching program are heavily dependent on the quality of the medical student, house staff, as well as the neonatology fellow within the intensive care unit. The neonatal teaching program should be integrated with the other subspecialities within the framework of the department of pediatrics, the department of obstetrics and gynecology, the department of anesthesiology, the department of pathology, the department of radiology, and other related disciplines. (2) An in-service program should also be organized for the nursing personnel as well as other allied health professionals, such as respiratory therapists, physical therapists, and ambulance drivers. The in-service teaching program should be under the leadership of the directors of the various allied health professional groups in conjunction with the director of the neonatal intensive care unit. (3) A teaching program for the community physicians, nurses, and other allied health professionals should also be organized to specifically achieve three goals: the first goal is to promulgate the most modern advances in the care of the well and sick neonates; the second goal is to as-

sure that the facilities and procedures for care of the infants in the nurseries of the level I and II hospitals are optimal. The latter can be achieved by an organized outreach teaching program by which the faculty members from the tertiary care center will visit the community hospitals for on-site teaching and demonstrations. And the third goal is to strengthen the relationship between the staff of the level I and II hospitals and the tertiary care center, and to encourage the former to refer cases to and seek advice from the latter center.

INFANT TRANSPORT SYSTEM

Ideally, mothers with high-risk pregnancies should be delivered at the tertiary care center. However, a certain number of high-risk infants are not predictable during the prenatal period. Therefore, there are a number of distressed infants who require transfer to the neonatal intensive care unit. The transport of these infants should be the responsibility of the tertiary care center and a system of infant transport should be organized. [13]

The ideal vehicle for transfer of high-risk infants depends on the geographic distance between the hospitals in the region served by the tertiary care center and the center itself. If the distance is within 1 to 2 hours' driving time, a well-equipped ambulance should suffice. Otherwise, a fixed-wing transport system may be considered for transport for greater distances. [14] In most instances, a transport incubator (as shown in Fig. 20-4) equipped to maintain the body temperature of the infant during transport is used. Other additional requirements include the provisions to allow the use of high concentrations of oxygen during transport, the ability to infuse intravenous fluid, and the capability of monitoring the cardiorespiratory signs and the oxygen concentration of the inspired air during transport. The personnel from the neonatal intensive care unit should be responsible for the transport since they are

Fig. 20-4. Infant transport incubator.

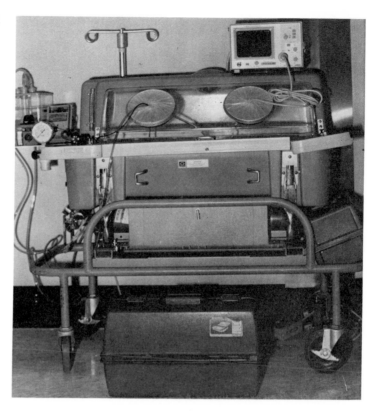

well trained and are most familiar with the care of a seriously ill neonate. Depending on the circumstances, a fellow, a member of the house staff, a nurse, or a respiratory therapist, or all of the above, may be required to accompany the infant. A well-organized infant transport system can effectively reduce the additional risk of morbidity and mortality during this particular procedure.

Retransfer of an Infant to the Community Hospital

To minimize the overcrowding in the neonatal intensive care unit, it is a good policy to make arrangements for the transfer of the convalescent infants from the neonatal intensive care unit to the community hospital from which the infants came. To do this, it must be assured that the nursery in the community hospital is capable of handling the category of infants who are being retransferred. In general, infants who do not require oxygen, intravenous nutrition, or other more sophisticated modes of therapy are considered candidates for retransfer. It is also important to make sure that these infants are free of infectious disease to protect the community hospital nurseries from nosocomial infections. The retransfer of infants to the community hospital is also an effective means of building the collaboration between the community hospital and the tertiary care centers. A recent study by Leake and coworkers [5] has shown that the risk of the retransfer practice to the infants is negligible and should be encouraged by all the parties concerned.

REFERENCES

1. Butler, N. R., and Alberman, E. D.: Perinatal Problems: The Second Report of the 1958 British Perinatal Mortality Survey. P. 44. Edinburgh and London, E. & S. Livingstone, 1969.
2. Butler, N. R., and Bonham, D. G.: Perinatal Mor-

tality: The First Report of the 1958 British Mortality Survey. [Under the auspices of the National Birthday Trust Fund] Edinburgh and London, E. & S. Livingstone, 1963.

3. Hobel, C. J., *et al.*: Prenatal and intrapartum high risk screening. 1. Prediction of the high risk neonate. Am. J. Obstet. Gynecol., *117*:1, 1973.

4. Klaus, M. H., and Kennel, J. H.: Mothers separated from their newborn infants. Pediatr. Clin. North Am., *17*:1015, 1970.

5. Leake, R. D. Loew, A. D., and Oh, W.: Retransfer of convalescent infants to the community intermediate care nursery. Clin. Pediatr. *in press*.

6. Meyer, B. P., *et al.*: Statewide reduction of neonatal mortality through effective regionalization of newborn intensive care. (Abst.) Pediatr. Res., *404*:1973.

7. Monin, P. J. P., *et al.*: Assisted ventilation in the neonate—comparison between positive and negative respirators. Pediatr. Res., *10*:464, 1976.

8. Nesbitt, R. E. L., Jr., and Aubrey, R. H.: High risk obstetrics. II Value of a semi-objective grading system in identifying the vulnerable group. Am. J. Obset. Gynecol., *103*:972, 1969.

9. Oh, W. : Unpublished data.

10. Outerbridge, E. W. Roloff, D. W., and Stern, L.: Continuous negative pressure in the management of severe respiratory distress syndrome. J. Pediatr., *81*:384, 1972.

11. Rawlings, G., *et al*: Changing prognosis for infants of very low birth weight. Lancet, *1*:516, 1971.

12. Ryan, G. M.: Toward improving the outcome of pregnancy. Recommendations for the regional development of perinatal health services. Obstet. Gynecol., *46*:375, 1975.

13. Segal, S. (ed.): Manual for the transport of high risk newborn infants. Can. Pediatr. Soc., 1972.

14. Shepard, K. S.: Air transportation of high risk infants utilizing a flying intensive care nursery. J. Pediatr., *77*:148, 1970.

15. Swyer, P. R.: The regional organization of special care for the neonate. Pediatr. Clin. North Am., *17*:761, 1970.

16. Vidyasager, D., Joseph, M. E., and Hamilton, L. R.: Noise level in the neonatal intensive care unit. J. Pediatr., *88*:115, 1976.

17. Williams, P. R., and Oh, W.: The effects of radiant warmer on insensible water loss in newborn infants. Am. J. Dis. Child., *128*:511, 1974.

21

Postpartum Tubal Ligation

Ray McKenzie, M.D., F.F.A.R.C.S.

Due to changing attitudes of both patients and physicians, the incidence of tubal ligation is increasing, and over half the sterilization procedures are performed in the immediate postpartum period.[42] The majority of sterilizations performed in the United States at present are done on a voluntary basis, the procedure being requested by the patient and her husband due to medical indications, multiparity, or socioeconomic reasons.[64] There are multiple reasons why tubal ligation is one of the most frequent operations performed today. These reasons include the cost of child care and education, standards of upbringing, the convenience for both parents, awareness of world overpopulation, protection for females at risk from further pregnancy, and the inadequacies of the contraceptive devices, including the dangers of birth control pills.

The estimated world population in 1971 was 3.7 billion. Continuation of the world population growth rate predicts a doubling of the human population in 35 years. The rate of doubling can be seen from the following figures published in 1975:

8,000 B.C. to 1 A.D.	60,000 years to double
1 A.D. to 1750 A.D.	13,000 years to double
1750 A.D. to 1800 A.D.	163 years to double
1850 A.D. to 1900 A.D.	129 years to double
1900 A.D. to 1950 A.D.	82 years to double
1950 A.D. to 1985 A.D.	35 years to double

For the world as a whole, the death rate is now less than half the birth rate.[27]

In 1964 Campbell estimated that in the United States about 200,000 pregnancy-preventing operations were performed annually in females between the ages of 18 and 39 years, with over half the operations being solely for sterilization purposes.[12] The incidence of sterilization in the postpartum period was 3.2 per cent of live births according to Starr and Kosasky[62] and 1.7 per cent according to Moore and Russell.[51] Medical indications for sterilization included multiparity, multiple cesarean sections, heart disease, hypertension, diabetes, psychiatric illnesses, and a miscellaneous group including treated carcinoma of the cervix. Some sterilizations were done because of potential future fetal defects and others were done for socioeconomic reasons. A decade ago it was standard procedure to perform postpartum tubal ligation if the female was 45 years of age or older and after her fourth child, 35 to 40 years of age and after her fifth child, and at any age after the sixth child.[64] These criteria were all conservative and are now obsolete. Today, criteria for performing postpartum tubal ligation are based on the will of the wife and husband to give their consent. In 1971, Little indicated that there were an estimated 265,000 female sterilizations performed in the United States.[42] Paterson in 1969 quoted that 2 to 3 per cent of obstetric patients in Australia undergo sterilization during the puerperium.[54] In the 1975 United Kingdom survey of anesthetic services to obstetrics in the Birmingham region, Crawford and Opit calculated that 100 anesthetics for postpartum sterilization per year would result from every 3 thousand live births per year, a percentage of 0.33.[17] Comparing this with the ratio of delivery to sterilization of 5 to 1 in Florida in 1973, it is obvious that there is more demand for postpartum sterilization in the United States.[42] Thus, the obstetric anesthesiologist is frequently made aware that the anesthesia designed for delivery may be followed by a second procedure, that of tubal ligation. Foresight develops, enabling him to plan ahead, thereby reducing the patient's stress, hospital stay, and overall medical bills.

TIMING OF POSTPARTUM TUBAL LIGATION

The optimum time for postpartum tubal ligation depends in part on the type of delivery.

Tubal Ligation Accompanying Cesarean Section

Provided informed consent has been obtained and the delivery results in an apparently normal infant, tubal ligation at the section is the most convenient time for the patient, obstetrician, and anesthesiologist. Many obstetric units follow the dictum, "once a section, always a section," which enables the obstetrician to perform tubal ligation at delivery when requested, thus avoiding another procedure.

Puerperal Sterilization

The optimum time for sterilization is 24 to 36 hours postdelivery. It is claimed that a 6-hour wait after delivery reduces the likelihood of bleeding and permits rest for the mother following her labor.[64] There is a relative contraindication to postpartum

tubal ligation more than 48 hours after labor, since bacteria are present in the uterus. Other relative contraindications include a predisposition to infection, prolonged rupture of membranes, intrapartum fever, and manual removal of the placenta.[64]

Interval Sterilization

Patients with cardiac disease, marked hypertension, severe renal disease, or acute toxemia are commonly advised to undergo interval tubal ligation when their medical conditions have stabilized. In this group of patients, interval sterilization is performed when complete involution of the uterus has taken place, i.e., 6 months after delivery.

Radiation Sterilization

Radiation sterilization is infrequently performed and is reserved for women over 40 years of age who are very bad surgical risks.

Immediate Postdelivery Bilateral Tubal Ligation

In a large obstetric hospital with 24-hour anesthesiologist coverage, postpartum tubal ligation is conveniently regarded as a semi-emergency operation, which can be scheduled during daylight hours. In smaller institutions when anesthesiologist availability is limited, difficulties can arise. Thirty members of the Society of Obstetricians, Anesthesiologists and Pediatricians surveyed did not regard the operation as an acute emergency procedure as far as infection was concerned.[59] They recommended expediency in scheduling, citing bed space, hospital stay, and cost of hospitalization as the main reasons.

In answer to the question "should postpartum tubal ligation be done immediately following delivery?" 22 out of 30 answers were affirmative, provided a properly functioning continuous epidural was in place. Six out of the 30 members surveyed recommended immediate postdelivery tubal ligation with the proviso that general endotracheal anesthesia be used. The risk of aspiration pneumonitis should preclude induction of general anesthesia for tubal ligation following delivery by conduction techniques. It is salutary to report that 4 out of 30 anesthesiologists encountered aspiration of stomach contents in patients with general anesthesia in the immediate postpartum period.[59]

In subsequent correspondence with the surveyed members it became clear that the decision to perform immediate postdelivery bilateral tubal ligation must be tempered by the condition of the delivered infant. Neonatal or infant death can change the parental attitudes. One patient was reported to have implored her obstetrician to "untie her tubes" following her infant's death.[60] Conversely, interval tubal ligation has resulted in an unwanted pregnancy, conception having occurred during the waiting period.[61] The consensus of opinion suggests a delay of 8 to 24 hours to be optimum.

EFFECT OF MATERNAL FACTORS ON MATERNAL AND INFANT SURVIVAL

Public health figures relating maternal and infant morbidity and mortality to maternal age, parity, and birth interval have been published. In summary, the risk of maternal death is increased when the mother is less than 20 years of age. Between the ages of 20 and 24, there is a minimal maternal death rate which increases 4 to 5 times when the pregnancy occurs in the maternal age group of over 40. Maternal mortality increases with parity beyond the third child regardless of maternal age. Interestingly enough, prematurity, infant death, and congenital defects approximately parallel maternal mortality, i.e., increases when the mother is under 20 or over 40 years of age. The infant risk increases when birth intervals are less than 12 months, since there is an increased rate of prematurity. The lower

fetal mortality occurs when there is a 3- to 4-year gap between pregnancies.[47a] Although a woman's age, parity and the length of the birth interval affect maternal and fetal survival, other factors including economic circumstances, cultural practices, genetic makeup, health and nutritional status, environment and medical care, all play their role. Nevertheless, the maternal factors of age and parity can support the decision for planned postpartum tubal ligation.

MORTALITY RATE FOR POSTPARTUM TUBAL LIGATION

The mortality rate for sterilization ranges between 0.3 per cent for all sterilization procedures including hysterectomy, to 0.012 per cent for interim laparoscopic procedures, i.e., 12 patients in every 100,000 will die.[42] All those involved in the sterilization procedure should do everything possible to reduce these catastrophes since a young woman's life is on the line. In Wylie's survey of anesthesia-related deaths in 1974, over 50 per cent of the deaths occurred in patients who were healthy preoperatively.[67]

EFFECTS OF PARTURITION ON THE MOTHER

Abrupt important maternal physiologic changes occur after parturition. Bonica states that cardiac output is increased in the immediate postpartum period due to continuing tetanic contractions of the mother's empty uterus, the removal of obstruction to venous return, the need for diuresis, and pain or apprehension.[8] Left ventricular work is increased and remains so until after the fourth postpartum day. Stroke volume remains 25 per cent above normal. Although the blood pressure remains constant, the peripheral resistance falls from 1053 dynes per second/cm.^{3} to 945 dynes per second/cm.^{3}; the central venous pressure remains elevated for several days. The pulmonary or central blood volume immediately postpartum is increased by almost 400 ml. The hemoglobin increase during delivery is attributed to fluid shifts into the interstitial fluid and increased fluid loss from perspiration. This rise in hemoglobin can be maintained during the postpartum period, dependent on the amount of blood loss at delivery, fluid load, and renal function. The white cell count increases to 15,000 during delivery and is associated with a fall in circulating eosinophils, the degree depending on the stress response of the parturient. Platelets and fibrinogen increase, reducing the likelihood of late postpartum bleeding. Blood sugar decreases unless restored by intravenous glucose. Renal tract changes during pregnancy and delivery include compression of the ureters, ureteral dilatation, hydroureter, and hydronephrosis. The elongated urethra may be compressed and bruised, and the bladder is frequently enlarged and hypotonic, making urinary retention commonplace. The mucosa is edematous and hyperemic. A postpartum diuresis continues for 4 to 5 days. Proteins are usually absent from the urine after 48 hours. Acetonuria often seen postdelivery disappears in 3 days. Hormonal changes are believed to be responsible for the increase in $PaCO_2$ following delivery; however, $PaCO_2$ does not reach normal levels for 10 to 14 days. A moderate respiratory alkalosis is present at the time of postpartum tubal ligation, with $PaCO_2$ values averaging 34 mm. of Hg. The basal metabolic rate of oxygen consumption returns to normal within the first two weeks. A weight loss of 5 to 7 pounds occurs.[9]

The puerperium is associated with strong emotional reactions which occur most frequently during the 24- to 48-hour postpartum phase and affect over 60 per cent of parturients. This emotional adjustment is self-limiting and disappears when the mother goes home. Apprehension and tension can cause many complaints (e.g., backache, headache, fatigue), all of which may be confused with the aftermath of anesthesia. For discussion of other maternal changes during the puerperium, see Chapter 2, Changes in Maternal Physiology During Pregnancy, Parturition, and the Puerperium.

GENERAL ANESTHESIA FOR POSTPARTUM TUBAL LIGATION

Most patients prefer general anesthesia for postpartum tubal ligation. Since the postpartum patient can be regarded as being in the prime of life, meticulous attention must be given to the preoperative preparation, intraoperative care, and postoperative recovery. Maternal anesthesia should be designed so that the infant's care is disturbed as little as possible. Unfortunately, a significant mortality rate still exists when physical status 1 patients (American Society of Anesthesiologists' classification) are given a general anesthetic.[67]

Preoperative Preparation

The patient's chart must be thoroughly checked. Pertinent medical history and clinical examination determine the presence of significant medical conditions. Review of antepartum care provides the anesthesiologist with information on complications during pregnancy, since recorded blood pressure, edema, proteinuria, glycosuria, and weight gain are all documented. All complications must be noted, but particular attention should be paid to those patients who have had a recent intercurrent illness. Fluid balance should be reviewed with care. Preeclamptics during pregnancy may convulse in the postpartum period. Their treatment must be thoroughly reviewed. Magnesium sulfate acts as a competitive neuromuscular blocking agent as well as a central nervous system depressant. If a patient was preeclamptic or had significant hemorrhage during vaginal delivery, it is preferable to postpone tubal ligation.

Preoperative anesthesia questionnaire forms completed by the patient help the anesthesiologist define pertinent potential problems.[61] Diabetics require blood sugar estimation. Insulin sensitivity is markedly increased in the immediate postpartum period, and when insulin requirements during labor are continued into the first postpartum day, hypoglycemia occurs. The cardiac patient has proven myocardial reserve if she has no complication during her pregnancy and delivery. Clinical assessment and examination will confirm the presence or absence of preexisting disease and reveal significant intercurrent postpartum debilities.

Essential laboratory studies include postpartum hemoglobin and hematocrit since blood loss at delivery is difficult to determine with accuracy. Blood typing and screening are essential predelivery tests available in the patient's record. A preoperative chest x-ray is necessary to confirm clinical findings provided the results of a recent chest x-ray are not available. Any questions pertaining to anesthesia should be discussed frankly with the patient and informed consent must be obtained.

Light premedication is required since many postpartum patients are fatigued from hard work during their intrapartum period and lack of sleep. When a narcotic is chosen, an antiemetic sedative should be given. There is a paucity of information on gastric emptying and gastric acidity in this period. Recently Blouw and coworkers,[7] compared gastric emptying in 21 postpartum patients with 11 nonpregnant females and found no significant differences in gastric volume and pH. They concluded that gastric emptying occurs during the 8 hours immediately following delivery and that the postpartum patient is at no greater risk than the prepared elective surgical patient. Antacids have been recommended by Hester and Heath for all prepared patients scheduled for general anesthesia.[28]

In the operating room a functioning intravenous drip, chest stethoscope, and electrocardiogram monitor along with routine monitoring of vital signs meet minimal standards for the induction of anesthesia. We believe it is mandatory to have these aids in every case scheduled for general anesthesia.

General Anesthesia Technique

Intravenous induction can be achieved with a short-acting barbiturate, diazepam or ketamine.[22]

Nitrous oxide-oxygen anesthesia base is standard. The supplement chosen depends on the patient's history. Halothane is considered to be the most potent uterine muscle relaxant.[58] However, blood loss during therapeutic abortion is equally high with enflurane or methoxyflurane.[46] Although methoxyflurane is an accepted inhalational agent for delivery, Galloon has shown that, provided administration of this drug is long enough, it will cause uterine relaxation.[24] The concentrations recommended by Lowe are followed when methoxyflurane is used.[43] Methoxyflurane is avoided in patients with renal problems. The high biodegradability (30 to 50% metabolized)[30] increases the amount of fluoride in the mother's milk. Halothane anesthesia[57] (20% metabolized) results in a prolonged bromide level[33] which is also passed with the milk to breast-fed infants. Enflurane (2.4% metabolized)[13] is contraindicated in the epileptic patients, and there have been no studies concerning the effect of enflurane on previously toxemic patients. It seems prudent to avoid enflurane for this group since we are not sure that enflurane is harmless to the kidney, although current literature implies safety in the majority of patients.[15] Overall, the best selection of volatile anesthetic agents from a metabolic point of view is enflurane. Gold[25] prefers to examine the amounts recoverable rather than assuming the percentage metabolized. Thus, 83 per cent enflurane, 37 percent halothane, and 19 per cent methoxyflurane are exhaled.[25]

No one has been able to trace 100 per cent of the dose of any inhalational agent administered.

The author does not recommend intubation for the routine case given an inhalational anesthetic. There is no doubt that laryngoscopy adds to the list of minor complications in the postoperative period. Some anesthesiologists prefer to intubate all patients to protect the lungs from possible aspiration. Bersen and Adriani in 1954 assessed a 7 per cent silent regurgitation rate in their nonintubated surgical patients.[6] Until further evidence is produced, there are no strict guidelines for intubation.

There is no contraindication to narcotic anesthesia. Fentanyl with nitrous oxide-oxygen is our combination of choice, since the operation rarely lasts more than 45 minutes. This time period equates with the duration of the action of fentanyl. However, the minimal alveolar concentration equivalent of fentanyl estimated from Fraioli's work on the MAC equivalent of morphine is 14 cc. or 0.7 mg.[23] Should this dose be administered, postoperative ventilatory assistance would be necessary. We recommend intubation when fentanyl anesthesia is used, so that 2 to 3 cc. or 0.10 mg. to 0.15 mg. becomes adequate.

Relaxant agents are seldom necessary. Succinylcholine drip or gallamine triethiodide can be given so that the duration of action does not exceed the time of surgery. Both drugs are highly ionized, and minimal quantities reach the mother's milk. Neither drug relaxes the smooth muscle of the uterus.

Recommended Treatment of Patients in the Recovery Room

Postpartum patients are best placed on their side in the Sims position, thereby providing drainage from the larynx to the lower corner of the mouth. Laryngeal reflexes may be obtunded from anesthesia or relaxant drugs, making the patient vulnerable to respiratory obstruction or inhalation of vomitus. In this position, the tongue falls away from the airway, and any secretions or vomitus will drain from the dependent lower corner of the mouth. Also, many postpartum tubal ligation patients have painful episiotomies and they are more comfortable when lying on their side. Care must be taken to avoid pressure on the perineal nerve as it crosses the fibula. The upper part of the dependent arm should lie close to the chest wall, since dislocation of the shoulder has been reported when turning patients on their side. Oxygen 6 to 10 liters per minute is given by face mask or nasal catheters and analgesic drugs for pain are dispensed as required. Fluid balance must be maintained until the patient can take oral fluids. Recovery room visits by anesthesia personnel with notation must be made.

SPINAL ANESTHESIA FOR POSTPARTUM TUBAL LIGATION

In many institutions, spinal anesthesia is used for delivery. There is no contraindication to repeating a subarachnoid puncture to provide analgesia for postpartum tubal ligation. A block level up to T10 provides adequate conditions for surgery since the abdominal incision for tubal ligation is made in the area of the T11 nerve supply and the fallopian tubes lie just beneath the peritoneum. There is minimal stimulation to the unblocked vagus, phrenic and sympathetic nerves (see Chap. 15, Subarachnoid Block). Postpartum tubal ligation should not be viewed as a major abdominal procedure since there is no necessity to insert abdominal packs or examine the abdominal contents. It causes no harm to induce a higher block up to and including T5. The dose of spinal anesthetic agent is increased when compared with the dose used for delivery. Following years of obstetric anesthesia practice, Phillips recommended 50 mg. of 5 per cent lidocaine for a 150-cm. (5-feet) female to obtain a T6 block for cesarean section increasing the dose to 80 mg. of 5 per cent lidocaine for the 165-cm. (5 feet 6 inch) female.[56] Also, Assali and Prystowski quote dose reduction of one third the standard dose for the pregnant female at term.[4] In our experience with postpartum patients at least 75 mg. of 5 per cent lidocaine (Xylocaine) is necessary to obtain a T10 level in the average patient, with a dose range of 60 to 90 mg. depending on her height. Tetracaine 6 to 9 mg. with 10-per cent glucose achieves similar safe block heights. Judicious use of the head-down tilt within the first 5 minutes can cause a rise in the block level of two to four segments. After 5 minutes the block level with lidocaine is fixed. With tetracaine this can take a few minutes longer.

Clinical and patient impression implies that lidocaine has a delayed onset in the postpartum female compared with her intrapartum state. It is not uncommon to wait for 5 minutes for the full development of the block. Tetracaine may take 10 minutes for practical effectiveness. (For technique, needle size, and complications see Chap. 15, Subarachnoid Block.)

EPIDURAL ANESTHESIA FOR POSTPARTUM TUBAL LIGATION

The ideal time for postpartum tubal ligation is within 48 hours following delivery.[64] Epidural catheters have been kept in place without recorded infection for many days in the treatment of debilitating chronic pain. To avoid repeating an epidural block for tubal ligation, the catheter inserted at the time of delivery can be left in place and used again for providing analgesia during the tubal ligation. Pain relief may be provided in the postoperative period without narcotics by injecting suitable refill doses.[26] Catheter placement,[50,55] catheter leakage,[1] and infection[16,20] are fully discussed in Chapter 14, Epidural Analgesia.

Reinduction of Epidural Anesthesia

Before attempting reinduction of epidural anesthesia resuscitation equipment to treat complications including con-

vulsions or respiratory or cardiac arrest must be on hand. The intravenous line must be running freely. Gentle aspiration must be performed in an attempt to determine if the epidural catheter tip has entered a blood vessel or the subarachnoid space.

Injecting the Test Dose of Local Anesthetic

A test dose of 2 to 4 ml. of the local anesthetic should be injected with the patient either in the horizontal or slightly head-down position. The specific gravity of the local anesthetic for epidural anesthesia can be less than the cerebrospinal fluid, and when the patient is in a head-up position, a hypobaric-type spinal could result.[48] Pulse and blood pressure should be checked at minute intervals. Five minutes after the test dose a selected dose of the local anesthetic can be injected. Since the operative procedure is short, 3 per cent chloroprocaine, 1.5 to 2 per cent lidocaine, or 1.5 to 2 per cent mepivacaine can be used. The use of bupivacaine, 0.5 to 0.75 per cent, for surgery reduces postoperative discomfort.

Obtaining the Block Height Necessary

A minimal practical sensory block height at T10 is necessary and T8 is preferable. It is unwise to induce a block above T5. Surgery can begin after checking the extent of the block with pinprick. It is prudent to allow 20 to 30 minutes for the block to reach maximum effectiveness. With spinal anesthesia the postpartum patient requires an increase of almost 50 per cent in dose to obtain the same height of block as when she is pregnant.[4] With epidural in the nonpregnant female, 1.5 to 1.8 ml. per segment equates with 1 to 1.2 ml. per segment in the pregnant state for an age range of 20 to 40 years.[10]

Need for Sedation or Anesthesia

The anesthesiologist must be prepared to provide sedation for any patient discomfort. Remember that usually no conduction technique blocks either the vagus or phrenic nerves. Air under the diaphragm may cause shoulder tip pain. A gentle surgeon reduces noxious pressure sensations. Diazepam, 2.5 to 10 mg. intravenously usually suffices. Ketamine is the only intravenous anesthetic agent able to completely abolish pain.[45] Failure of conduction anesthesia either from root sparing or inadequate block may require the induction of general anesthesia.

Postoperative Care

Postoperative pain relief may be provided by top-up doses of local anesthetic agents. Bupivacaine, 0.125 to 0.25 per cent, is satisfactory for this purpose.

Removal of the Epidural Catheter

Since the epidural catheter has been in place for many hours, it is usually removed after the first dose of pain relief is given. A thorough inspection of the catheter is essential to be sure it is complete with nothing sheared off or broken and left in the epidural space. Most manufactured catheters are radiopaque, so subsequent x-rays of the back may show any catheter fragments left in the epidural space. Litigation could be initiated years after the event. The patient's records should always be completed with the statement, "Catheter removed, checked and found to be complete." For a full discussion of epidural technique and problems associated with the epidural catheter, see Chapter 14, Epidural Analgesia.

TUBAL LIGATION IN THE PUERPERIUM BY LAPAROSCOPY

As early as 1970, Keith in the United States and Steptoe in England recommended puerperal laparoscopic sterilization.[34,63] Clark and coworkers compared the results of laparoscopy and abdominal tubal ligation in the immediate postdelivery period and concluded that both procedures were safe, practical, and acceptable methods of tubal sterilization.[14] The claimed advantages of laparoscopy included the reduction in hospital stay and low mortality. Paterson in Australia added that greater mobility of the patient was an important factor in reducing thromboembolic complications.[54] McKenzie suggested that the laparoscopic procedure had the advantages of low infection rate and minimal adhesion formation.[44]

The disadvantages of laparoscopy tubal ligation include difficulty in visualization of the tubes if done before the fifth postpartum day.[53] Cruikshank and coworkers reported on a small series of 26 patients successfully sterilized from 2 to 48 hours postpartum which resulted in 3-day hospital stays.[18] Keith in a larger series recommended the second or third postpartum day for the procedure.[36] Other disadvantages of performing laparoscopy during the puerperium include pelvic bleeding, difficulty in safe leverage to change the bulky uterine position, fixing the vulsellum to the vascular cervix, increasing likelihood of infection, and the breaking down of partly healed perineal wounds due to increased intra-abdominal pressure. The volume of gas necessary for displacement of abdominal viscera increased by 50 per cent since vascular absorption is increased and the abdominal wall is lax.[53]

Whitney recommends the use of synthetic oxytocin to facilitate the movement of the uterus and reduce its size.[66] Although enthusiasts stress the virtues of laparoscopy for postpartum tubal ligation, the majority of obstetricians favor a conservative rather than an optimistic approach to increasing the use of this technique. After all, the fallopian tubes in the postpartum patient are readily accessible through a small abdominal incision since they lie immediately beneath the peritoneum, an inch or so below the umbilicus.

Carbon Dioxide or Nitrous Oxide for Inducing Pneumoperitoneum

Carbon dioxide was formerly the popular gas used for peritoneal insufflation because of its absorption in the body, reducing the duration of so called afterpains, and, since carbon dioxide is a fire extinguisher and does not support combustion, fulguration could be used for the tubal section without fear of extensive burns. Disadvantages in its use soon became apparent. Measurements made by Alexander, Noe, and Brown[3] verified the increase in $PaCO_2$ of approximately 10 torr. McKenzie[44] suggested that carbon dioxide is a soluble gas, absorbed at a rapid rate, and is physiologically active. Acidosis and catecholamine stimulation from a rising $PaCO_2$ could be responsible for the incidence of cardiac changes including hypertension, hypotension, arrhythmias, and even cardiac arrest.[29] Although hyperventilation will reduce the increased carbon dioxide blood levels, Alexander and Brown suggested that since there was no increase when nitrous oxide was used as the insufflating gas, increased $PaCO_2$ resulted from peritoneal absorption.[2] Lay and Taylor[40] used nitrous oxide, a gas which supports combustion, for inducing pneumoperitoneum and concluded that nitrous oxide was safer (no acidosis or catecholamine release), easier to administer, more readily available, and less expensive than carbon dioxide. In our experience, the anesthesia is less fraught with problems of sweating, hypotension, hypertension, and cardiac arrhythmias when nitrous oxide is used. Our statistics show that carbon dioxide-induced pneumoperitoneum and halothane cause more arrhythmias (some ventricular in origin) than do nitrous oxide-induced pneumoperitoneum and halothane.

At first we believed that unexplained deaths in patients undergoing laparoscopy were due to gaseous emboli. We monitored many of our patients with ultrasound detectors without recording any disturbance. If carbon dioxide emboli occur, then nitrous oxide should increase the embolic incidence. Nitrous oxide is relatively insoluble and is slowly absorbed whereas carbon dioxide is relatively soluble and rapidly absorbed. Thus a carbon dioxide

bubble traveling in a vein would tend to reduce in size while a nitrous oxide bubble would not. The lack of detection of gas embolus regardless of the nature of the insufflating gas leads us to believe that gas embolus does not occur during laparoscopy unless the Verres needle is placed in one of the veins and gas is directly injected. In cases of sudden collapse at the time of insufflation, gas embolus cannot be ruled out.

Carbon dioxide combines with water and can cause acid irritation of the peritoneum. Most cases of shoulder pain occur during the first 24 hours postlaparoscopy and are caused by gas irritating the peritoneal surface of the diaphragm. Although nitrous oxide absorption is slower than carbon dioxide absorption, there is no difference in the incidence of shoulder tip pain when the two groups are compared. The surgeon should pay strict attention to compress the abdomen and release as much gas as possible prior to the removal of the laparoscope. This is the most important step in reducing the incidence of afterpains. A recent study by Brown and coworkers[11] led to the conclusion that nitrous oxide produced less discomfort than carbon dioxide in awake patients having laparoscopy with local anesthesia and mild sedation.

Nitrous oxide can be used in the same apparatus designed for carbon dioxide insufflation, since both gases have a molecular weight of 44.

We have been most satisfied with nitrous oxide-induced pneumoperitoneum because of the benign anesthesia course. PaO_2 is maintained at approximately 200 torr by using a 50:50 nitrous oxide-oxygen base for the inhalational anesthetic.

Ventilation During Pneumoperitoneum

Pneumoperitoneum increases intraabdominal pressure to 20 torr in the average case. This pressure tends to push the diaphragm upward and causes an increase in pleural pressure. The lungs are compressed. Increased ventilation pressure must compensate for the decreased chest compliance[29] when general anesthesia is used. Brown and coworkers[11] have shown the ability of the awake patient to compensate not only for the restriction of ventilation, but also in the ability to breathe fast enough to clear carbon dioxide from carbon dioxide-induced pneumoperitoneum. Oxygen saturation and pH were maintained within normal physiologic range, but there was concern over the bradycardia caused by stimulation of the vagus at the time of intra-abdominal manipulation. Positive-pressure ventilation tends to reduce venous return and cardiac output can be affected adversely. Ventilating pressures must be kept to the lowest pressures required to maintain a minute volume of 8 to 10 liters. Increased $PaCO_2$ levels can result from hypoventilation, compression of the lungs by the diaphragm, or from the absorption of carbon dioxide from the peritoneum.[3] Acidosis caused by carbon dioxide can be prevented by adequate ventilation. In view of these data we believe that it is unwise to schedule patients with compromised pulmonary function for laparoscopy.

Cardiovascular Changes With Pneumoperitoneum

The central venous pressure tends to rise when pneumoperitoneum is induced. Venous blood flow is at first maintained by extra venous intra-abdominal pressure squeezing the contents of the abdominal veins into the thoracic veins. The inferior vena cava is compressed and blood flow in it is reduced. The pressure on the abdominal part of the inferior vena cava is 15 to 20 torr, while the normal intraluminal value is 6 to 10 cm. of water.

Venous blood returning to the heart from the legs must pass primarily through the vertebral system of veins. Femoral venous pressure increases above that of the inferior vena cava, reestablishing blood flow. During these physiologic changes the heart may be starved of blood. Indeed,

narrowing of pulse pressure often occurs.[2] The stage is set for cardiac arrest. Anesthesiologists must be aware that ventilating pressure must return to zero between ventilations with an adequate respiratory pause to allow for maximum pulmonary blood flow during this critical readjustment period. Since pleural pressure is increased by the ascent of the diaphragm caused by pneumoperitoneum, the right atrial pressure cannot be used as an index of venous return. Right atrial pressure reflects a composite of pleural and intra-abdominal pressures, as well as venous pressure.[31]

In 1972 Kelman and his associates[37] reported on the physiologic changes occurring with a progressive increase in intra-abdominal pressure. They studied 21 patients in the horizontal position and 18 patients in a 25 degree head-down tilt position. All were premedicated and anesthetized with the $PaCO_2$ kept at 25 torr. The central venous pressure increased from 4.6 to 10.2 cm. of water; intrathoracic pressure increased from 1.8 to 3.2 cm. of water; and femoral venous pressure paralleled the increase in intra-abdominal pressure up to 40 cm. of water. With intra-abdominal pressures of greater than 40 cm. of water, the central venous pressure and cardiac output began to fall. These data suggest that limitation of intra-abdominal pressure to 30 cm. of water is desirable and that the head-down position makes little difference.

A most comprehensive article was produced by Ivankovich and coworkers.[31] These workers used both carbon dioxide- and nitrous oxide-induced pneumoperitoneum in 15 mongrel dogs, subjecting them to progressive increases in intra-abdominal pressure up to 40 mm. Hg. Cardiac output and inferior vena caval flow were increased immediately following insufflation. Both flows fell precipitously as inflation pressure increased, with a 60 per cent fall in cardiac output at 40 mm. Hg intra-abdominal pressure. Physiologic compensation was evident from the increased peripheral resistance which was elevated by approximately 200 per cent. No cardiostimulatory effect of carbon dioxide was found in this study in spite of significant rises in $PaCO_2$, and it was concluded that the absorption of carbon dioxide was insufficient to stimulate the heart in the presence of decreased venous return and increased peripheral resistance. Ivankovich stressed that intra-abdominal pressures of more than 20 mm. Hg were dangerous and should be avoided at all times. One of the most practical observations of this study was that all cardiovascular parameters returned to normal within 1 minute of release of intra-abdominal pressure.

In 1972, Marshall and coworkers[47] reported a consistent fall in cardiac output and a rise in mean arterial pressure, central venous pressure, and heart rate with nitrous oxide-induced pneumoperitoneum in humans. Carbon dioxide-induced pneumoperitoneum caused no fall in cardiac output. In contrast to Ivankovich in his study using dogs, Marshall attributed the difference to increased sympathetic activity caused by carbon dioxide absorbed from the intra-abdominal surface in a sufficient amount to initiate a catecholamine response. Species difference could explain the differing results.

Using dye dilution techniques in humans with carbon dioxide-induced pneumoperitoneum, Motew and coworkers[52] found that cardiac output was unchanged at 20 mm. Hg intra-abdominal pressure, and recorded an insignificant decrease at 30 mm. Hg. Motew recommended limitation of insufflating pressure to 20 mm. Hg. These findings conflict with Kelman's results since he demonstrated an increase in cardiac output at intra-abdominal pressures up to 30 cm. of water with a sharp fall above 40 cm. of water (approximately 30 mm. Hg).

In 1976 Lenz and associates[41] examined stroke volume and cardiac output using impedance cardiography during laparoscopy. Impedance cardiography is a technique based on the observation that when an alternating current is passed through the thorax, a change in electrical impedance results with each cardiac cycle. A constant sinusoidal current of 4 milliamperes at 100 kilohertz is passed from a circular diaphragmatic electrode to a similar electrode around the neck. The changes in thoracic impedance to this constant current are measured from two electrodes encircling the thorax and neck between the outer current electrodes. The resulting impedance change with each cardiac cycle is correlated with the point on the trace corresponding to the second heart sound derived from a synchronous phonocardiogram. The stroke volume can be calculated from the formula of Kubicek.[39] Twenty-four patients were examined. Stroke volume began to fall and continued falling throughout the whole procedure. Although the average fall was 23 per cent, the stroke volume in one patient fell by 51 per cent. The cardiac output fell by an average of 17 per cent, while the maximum fall recorded was 45 per cent. It was interesting to note that the usual intraoperative cardiovascular monitoring of blood pressure and pulse rate, and the clinical assessment of the circulation gave no indication of any fall in cardiac output in any of the patients including the one in which the cardiac output fell by 45 per cent.

In summary all anesthesiologists and laparoscopists should understand the pathophysiology of pneumoperitoneum.

1. Use nitrous oxide which is less physiologically active than carbon dioxide.

2. Ventilate all anesthetized patients adequately.

3. Never exceed 4 liters of insufflating gas.

4. Do not exceed 20 mm. Hg intra-abdominal pressure.

5. Realize that as soon as intra-abdominal pressure is released, all car-

diovascular and respiratory parameters rapidly return to normal.

Anesthesia for Laparoscopy

All types of anesthesia have been used. Dey recommends sedation with intramuscular meperidine (Demerol) followed by diazepam (Valium) in combination with local infiltration using 20 cc. of 1 per cent prilocaine hydrochloride.[21] Cruikshank recommends 15 mg. of alphaprodine (Nisentil) intravenously followed by 15 mg. of diazepam and has used 500 mg. of lidocaine by intraperitoneal instillation in postpartum women.[18] Blood lidocaine levels reached 5.30 μg./ml., a figure below the toxic dose of 9 to 10 μg./ml. reported by Merrifield[49] and Bromage.[10] In cats, diazepam increases the convulsive dose of intravenous lidocaine as reported by de Jong.[19] In monkeys, intravenous diazepam prophylaxis increases the convulsive dose of lidocaine by 27 per cent.[5] Some individuals are more susceptible than others, and we have noted dizziness and tremors around the mouth during interval laparoscopic sterilization with lidocaine. It must be noted that 1,000 mg. of lidocaine given to nonpregnant females for interval laparoscopic sterilization results in lower central venous blood levels.[18] This underlines the increased absorption rate in the puerperal patient caused by increased pelvic vascularity.

Spinal anesthesia has been used for laparoscopy without reported complications apart from headache. Theoretically, the loss of vascular tone below the block could result in a disastrous sudden drop in venous return when pneumoperitoneum is produced.[31] A similar criticism could apply to the selection of epidural analgesia for laparoscopy. However, Clark and coworkers.[14] in 1974 recommended laparoscopy utilizing the conduction anesthesia induced for delivery. They eliminated the second anesthetic in 29 patients and stated that this method of anesthesia for postpartum tubal ligation is safe, practical, and acceptable.

Keith, in the 1972 series of 172 patients, used general anesthesia for laparoscopy.[35] He listed hypotension (a drop of greater than 30 mm. Hg secondary to gaseous insufflation) as the commonest anesthetic complication, affecting 40 per cent of patients. One patient's operation was cancelled when her blood pressure became unrecordable. Arrhythmias, tachycardia, difficult intubation, and sore throat were the next most frequent anesthesic complications. Our unpublished studies indicate an increased likelihood of arrhythmias when carbon dioxide is used as the insufflating agent. There is an increased incidence of arrhythmias when halothane is used, and some of these are ventricular in origin. Innovar and fentanyl have a low arrhythmic rate, and only supraventricular arrhythmias have been reported with their use. Enflurane holds an intermediate position. Nitrous oxide used for inducing pneumoperitoneum reduces the rate of arrhythmias with all agents. Compared with carbon dioxide, nitrous oxide is physiologically benign. Our choice of anesthetic agent is therefore fentanyl with a preference for the addition of droperidol in small doses to reduce the nausea and vomiting reported to occur frequently when fentanyl is used alone.[48] Our recommendations discussed elsewhere,[65] include chest stethoscope, electrocardiograph monitor, preoxygenation for 3 to 5 minutes and d-tubocurarine 3 mg. or gallamine triethiodide 20 mg. given 3 minutes before induction of anesthesia. Thiamylal sodium 250 to 400 mg. followed by succinylcholine 100 mg. is injected and intubation performed without ventilation. If difficulty is encountered and the patient needs ventilation before intubation, a gastric tube is passed after successful intubation to deflate the stomach. Anesthesia is maintained with nitrous oxide 3 liters per minute and oxygen 2 liters per minute.

Innovar, fentanyl or enflurane supplement the anesthesia according to the patient's needs.

FUTURE DEVELOPMENTS

The prevailing socioeconomic conditions are expected to continue, and therefore, a steady patient demand for bilateral tubal ligation may be expected.

It is time to reconsider the staffing patterns so that a 24-hour service of all personnel—obstetrician, anesthesiologist, nurses, technicians and auxiliary staff—is available in sufficient numbers to perform this service. Communication by the obstetrician to the anesthesiologist will enable those physicians to decide ahead of time the most suitable method of anesthesia for delivery and bilateral tubal ligation. The consensus of opinion of anesthesiologists is that a continuous epidural allows both flexibility and safety for the mother. Proper conduction anesthesia protects the parturient from inhalation of gastric contents. It is difficult to fully justify the use of spinal analgesia for both procedures since T10 is a sufficient block height for delivery, and to maintain this level for 1 to 2 hours requires a higher level of block for the delivery. There is no contraindication to repeat the block, should the level be deemed inadequate before the start of the bilateral tubal ligation. However, little is known about the control of block height at the second injection. We have used sedation with 50:50 nitrous oxide-oxygen along with Innovar, fentanyl or methoxyflurane 0.1 to 0.2 per cent to supplement a receding block.

Any attempt to anesthetize the patient for immediate postdelivery bilateral tubal ligation requires endotracheal intubation with all the precautions to prevent aspiration. No prudent anesthesiologist likes to face this situation when safer methods of anesthesia can be available or a wait of 8 to 48 hours would remove this risk. Immediate postpartum bilateral tubal ligation by the laparoscopic method under general anesthesia presents even more dangers than abdominal bilateral tubal ligation, since intra-abdominal pressure is increased, the vena caval blood flow pattern is changed, and ventilatory problems exist from the elevated diaphragm. The increasing enthusiasm for interval bilateral tubal ligation performed with local infiltration of the abdominal wall and application of local anesthesia for both fallopian tubes has few physiological problems. The risk of aspiration is avoided, the patient is able to initiate vasoconstriction of the blood vessels of the lower limb during laparoscopy (which increases 200% in animal studies), and maintain normal physiological control of respiration. It is difficult to justify immediate laparoscopic postpartum bilateral tubal ligation unless performed under local infiltration anesthesia.

In summary, the obstetrician, anesthesiologist, and hospital administrators agree that the ideal time to perform tubal ligation is immediately following delivery, provided that the neonate is normal and consent forms are presigned. The cost savings to the patient, third parties and hospitals are considerable. In larger centers, where continuous epidurals are a common practice, immediate postpartum bilateral tubal ligation is expected to increase by the use of the abominal approach.

REFERENCES

1. Abouleish, E.: Preventing and detecting leakage in epidural catheters. Anesth. Analg., *53*:474, 1974.
2. Alexander, G. D., and Brown, E. M.: Physiologic alterations during pelvic laparoscopy. Am. J. Obstet. Gynecol., *105*:1078, 1969.
3. Alexander, G. D., Noe, F. E., and Brown, E. M.: Anesthesia for pelvic laparoscopy. Anesth. Analg., *48*:14, 1969.
4. Assali, N. S., and Prystowsky, H.: Studies on autonomic blockade; comparison between effects of tetraethylammonium chloride (TEAC) and high selective spinal anesthesia on the blood pressure of normal and toxemic pregnancy. J. Clin. Invest., *29*:1354, 1950.

5. Ausinsch, B., Malagodi, M. H., and Munson, E. S.: Diazepam in the prophylaxis of lignocaine seizures. Br. J. Anaesth., *48*:309, 1976.

6. Berson, W., and Adriani, J.: "Silent" regurgitation and aspiration during anesthesia. Anesthesiology, *15*:644, 1954.

7. Blouw, R., *et al.*: Gastric volume and pH in postpartum patients. Anesthesiology, *45*:456, 1976.

8. Bonica, J. J.: Principles and Practice of Obstetric Analgesia and Anesthesia. Vol. 1, pp. 80–81. Philadelphia, F. A. Davis, 1967.

9. ———: Principles and Practice of Obstetric Analgesia and Anesthesia. Vol. 2, p. 924. Philadelphia, F. A. Davis, 1967.

10. Bromage, P. R., and Robson, J. G.: Concentrations of lignocaine in the blood after intravenous intramuscular epidural and endotracheal administration. Anaesthesia, *16*:461, 1961.

11. Brown, D. R., *et al.*: Ventilatory and blood gas changes during laparoscopy with local anesthesia. Am. J. Obstet. Gynecol., *124*:741, 1970.

12. Campbell, A. A.: The incidence of operations that prevent conception. Am. J. Obstet. Gynecol., *89*:694, 1964.

13. Chase, R. E., *et al.*: The biotransformation of Ethrane in man. Anesthesiology, *35*:262, 1971.

14. Clark, D. H., Jr., Schneider, G. T., and McManus, S.: Tubal sterilization: comparison of outpatient laparoscopy and postpartum ligation. J. Reprod. Med., *13*:69, 1974.

15. Cousins, M. J., *et al.*: Metabolism and renal effects of enflurane in man. Anesthesiology, *44*:44, 1976.

16. Crawford, J. S.: Particulate matter in the extradural space. Br. J. Anaesth., *47*:807, 1975.

17. Crawford, J. S., and Opit, L. J.: A Survey of the Anaesthetic Services to Obstetrics in the Birmingham Region. Birmingham, England, J. W. Tuckey & Sons, 1975.

18. Cruikshank, D. P., Laube, D. W., and De Backer, L. J.: Intraperitoneal lidocaine anesthesia for postpartum tubal ligation. Obstet. Gynecol., *42*:127, 1973.

18a. Day, L. H.: Population dynamics. In Romney, S. L. (ed.): Gynecology and Obstetrics: The Health Care of Women. Chap. 3, p. 23. New York, McGraw-Hill, 1975.

19. de Jong, R. H., and Heavner, J. E.: Diazepam prevents local anesthetic seizures. Anesthesiology, *34*:523, 1971.

20. Desmond, J.: The use of micropore filters in continuous epidural anaesthesia. Can. Anaesth. Soc. J., *19*:97, 1972.

21. Dey, A., and Makay, G.: Postpartum tubal ligation and local anaesthesia. [Letter] Br. Med. J., *3*:252, 1974.

22. Figallo, E. M., *et al.*: Ketamine as a sole anesthetic agent in laparoscopic sterilization: reappraisal of the effects of the premedication and the incidence of its adverse emergency reactions. A double-blind study of 135 cases. Br. J. Anaesth., *in press.*

23. Fraioli, R. L., Sheffer, L. A., and Steffenson, J. L.: The MAC equivalent of morphine. American Society of Anesthesiologists Annual Meeting, 1973. P. 253. Abstracts of Scientific Papers, 1973.

24. Galloon, S.: Ketamine and the pregnant uterus. Can. Anaesth. Soc. J., *20*:141, 1973.

25. Gold, M. I.: A symposium on Ethrane and Forane. Anesth. Rev., *2*:23, 1975.

26. Griffiths, D. P. G., Diamond, A. W., and Cameron, J. D.: Postoperative extradural analgesia following thoracic surgery: a feasibility study. Br. J. Anaesth., *47*:48, 1975.

27. Romney, S. L. (ed.) Gynecology and Obstetrics: The Health Care of Women. Pp. 23, 549. New York, McGraw-Hill, 1975.

28. Hester, J. B., and Heath, M. L.: Pulmonary acid aspiration syndrome: should prophylaxis be routine? Br. J. Anaesth., *47*:630, 1975.

29. Hodgson, C., McClelland, R. M. A., and Newton, J. R.: Some effects of the peritoneal insufflation of carbon dioxide at laparoscopy. Anaesthesia, *25*:382, 1970.

30. Holaday, D. A., Rudofsky, S., and Treuhaft, P. S.: The metabolic degradation of methoxyflurane in man. Anesthesiology, *33*:579, 1970.

31. Ivankovich, A. D., *et al.*: Cardiovascular effects of intraperitoneal insufflation with carbon dioxide and nitrous oxide in the dog. Anesthesiology, *42*:281, 1975.

32. Jamil, A. K.: Information on patients due for anaesthesia. [Correspondence] Anaesthesia, *30*:826, 1975.

33. Johnstone, R. E., *et al.*: Increased serum bromide concentration after halothane anesthesia in man. Anesthesiology, *42*:598, 1975.

34. Keith, L., Webster, A., and Lash, A.: A comparison between puerperal and nonpuerperal laparoscopic sterilization. Int. Surg., *56*:325, 1971.

35. Keith, L., *et al.*: Laparoscopy for puerperal sterilization. Obstet. Gynecol., *39*:616, 1972.

36. ———: Puerperal tubal sterilization using laparoscopic technique: a preliminary reqort. J. Reprod. Med., *6*:69, 1974.

37. Kelman, G. R., *et al.*: Cardiac output and arterial blood-gas tension during laparoscopy. Br. J. Anaesth., *44*:1155, 1972.

38. Kim, Y. I., Mazza, N. M., and Marx, G. F.: Massive spinal block with hemicranial palsy after a test dose for extradural analgesia. Anesthesiology, *43*:370, 1975.

39. Kubicek, W. G., *et al.*: Impedance cardiography as a non-invasive means to monitor cardiac function. J. Assoc. Adv. Med. Instrum., *4*:79, 1970.

40. Lay, C. L., and Taylor, D. L.: Prevention of deaths from cardiac arrest or cardiac arrhythmias during laparoscopy. Ob-Gyn Collected Letters, International Correspondence Society of Obstetricians and Gynecologists, Series XII, 1971.

41. Lenz, R. J., Thomas, T. A., and Wilkins, D. G.: Cardiovascular changes during laparoscopy. Studies of stroke volume and cardiac output using impedance cardiography. Anaesthesia, *31*:4, 1976.

42. Little, W. A.: Current aspects of sterilization: the

selection and application of various surgical methods of sterilization. Am. J. Obstet. Gynecol., *123*:12, 1975.

43. Lowe, H. J., and Hagler, K.: Clinical and laboratory evaluation of an expired anesthetic gas monitor (Narko-Test). Anesthesiology, *34*:378, 1971.

44. McKenzie, R.: Laparoscopy. N.Z. Med. J., *74*:87, 1971.

45. McKenzie, R., and Tantisira, B.: Culdoscopy: a new use for ketamine. Anesth. Analg., *52*:351, 1973.

46. McKenzie, R., and Wemyss-Gorman, P.: Unpublished data.

47. Marshall, R. L., *et al.*: Circulatory effects of peritoneal insufflation with nitrous oxide. Br. J. Anaesth., *44*:1183, 1972.

47a. Meeker, C. I.: Birth control and sterilization. In Romney, S. L., (ed.): Gynecology and Obstetrics: The Health Care of Women. Chap. 29, p. 549. New York, McGraw-Hill, 1975.

48. Mercer, J. P., *et al.*: An outpatient program for laparoscopic sterilization. Obstet. Gynecol., *41*:681, 1973.

49. Merrifield, A. J., and Carter, J. J.: Intravenous regional analgesia: lignocaine blood levels. Anaesthesia, *20*:287, 1965.

50. Moore, D. C.: Bupivacaine vs. etidocaine anesthesia for vaginal delivery. Audiodigest, Vol. 17, No. 8, April 21, 1975.

51. Moore, J. G., and Russell, K. P.: Maternal medical indications for female sterilization. Clin. Obstet. Gynecol., *7*:54, 1964.

52. Motew, M., *et al.*: Cardiovascular effects and acid-base and blood gas changes during laparoscopy. Am. J. Obstet. Gynecol., *115*:1002, 1973.

53. Neely, M. R., and Elkady, A. A.: Modified technique to puerperal laparoscopic sterilization. J. Obstet. Gynaecol. Br. Commonw., *79*:1025, 1972.

54. Paterson, P. J., and Grimwade, J. C.: Laparoscopic sterilization during the puerperium. Med. J. Aust., *2*:312, 1972.

55. Pathy, G. V., and Rosen, M.: Prolonged block with recovery after extradural analgesia for labour. Br. J. Anaesth., *47*:520, 1975.

56. Phillips, O. C.: Regional vs. general in C-section. Annual Refresher Course Lectures. P. 203-A. American Society of Anesthesiologists, 1976.

57. Rehder, K., *et al.*: Halothane. Biotransformation in man: a quantitative study. Anesthesiology, *28*:711, 1967.

58. Shnider, S. M.: Halothane and uterine hemorrhage. Anesthesiology, *32*:99, 1970.

59. S.O.A.P. Newsletter, July 1, 1973.

60. S.O.A.P. Newsletter, September 1, 1973.

61. S.O.A.P. Newsletter, December 1, 1973.

62. Starr, S. H., and Kosasky, H. J.: Puerperal sterilization. Am. J. Obstet. Gynecol., *88*:944, 1964.

63. Steptoe, P.: Laparoscopic tubal sterilization—a British viewpoint. I.P.P.F. Medical Bulletin, *5*:4, 1971.

64. Te Linde, R. W., and Mattingly, R. F.: Operative Gynecology. Ed. 4. Philadelphia, J. B. Lippincott, 1970.

65. Wadhwa, R., McKenzie, R., and Wadhwa, S. R.: Anesthesia for laparoscopy. Pa. Med., *76*:69, 1971.

66. Whitney, P. F.: Laparoscopic sterilization in the puerperium. J. Obstet. Gynaecol. Br. Commonw., *79*:166, 1972.

67. Wylie, W. D.: "There, but for the grace of God. . . ." Ann. R. Coll. Surg. Engl., *56*:171, 1975.

Index

Page numbers in *italics* indicate figures; "t" indicates tabular matter.

427